ECMO

Extracorporeal Cardiopulmonary Support in Critical Care

3rd Edition

Krisa Van Meurs, M. D.
Kevin P. Lally, M. D.
Giles Peek, M. D.
Joseph B. Zwischenberger, M. D.

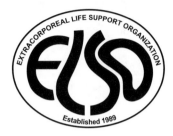

Senior Editor: Krisa Van Meurs
Editors: Kevin P. Lally, Giles Peek, Joseph B. Zwischenberger
Senior Manuscript Editor: Mary Nelson
Manuscript Editors: Frances Rucks, Annalise Farmer, Betty Littleton, Arlene Sheehan, Peter Farmer, Andrew
    Farmer
Layout: Peter Rycus
Production: Jesse Suber

©2005 Extracorporeal Life Support Organization, Ann Arbor, Michigan

Previous editions 1996, 2000

Printed in the United States of America

ISBN 0-9656756-2-9

Cover photography (from top):
"Adult Patient, End of a Veno-venous ECLS Run. The neck cannula withdrawing blood from the right atrium, the tracheostoma, and
    the naso-gastric tube are easily seen. The patient is fully awake and able to communicate. Submitted by Bjorn Frenckner,
    MD, Astrid Lindgren Children's Hospital, Karolinska Institutet, Stockholm, Sweden
"ECMO Family Reunion, WFUBMC, June 2000" Douglas R Hansell, ECMO Coordinator, Wake Forest University Baptist Medical
    Center, Winston-Salem, NC
"Long-distance ECMO Transport of Critically Ill Neonate Inside USAF Aircraft" Cody Henderson, MD, Major, USAF, MC, Wilford
    Hall USAF Medical Center, Lackland AFB, TX
"Waiting...Child on ECMO Support" Steve Barbour, MD, Pediatric Infectious Diseases, Phoenix Children's Hospital, Phoenix, AZ
"ECMO Pump" WFUBMC, January, 2000" Wake Forest University, School of Medicine, Creative Communications, Winston-Salem,
    NC
Cover design: Mary E. Nelson, Stanford University School of Medicine, Division of Neonatology & Developmental Medicine,
    Stanford, CA

Dedication

The editors and authors wish to dedicate this edition of the "Red Book" to Robert H. Bartlett, M.D. Such a simple tribute is true to Dr. Bartlett's humble style; however, those who know Bob realize he exudes much more than an encyclopedic knowledge of medicine and biotechnology. Rather, he embraces a philosophy of innovation, honesty, introspection, and critical analysis that has cut across all disciplines of critical care for the past four decades. We salute the man who evolved from a pioneer in the day of gooseneck lamps in back treatment rooms to a proponent of prospective, randomized multi-center trials and outcomes analysis. For the thousands of physicians he has impacted, the tens of thousands of patients who are alive today due to ECMO, and the millions who have benefited from his critical care teachings, Bob Bartlett is **the** critical care physician.

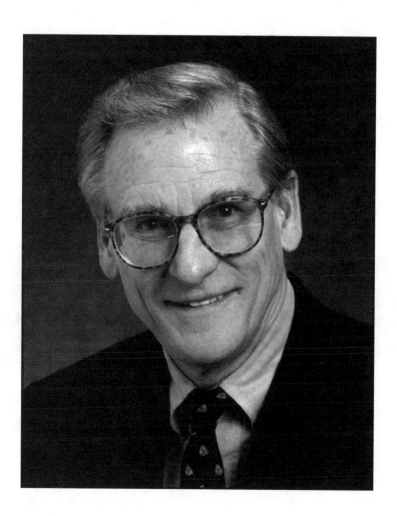

List of Contributors

Scott K. Alpard, M.M.S.
Surgical Research Fellow
Department of Surgery
University of Texas Medical Branch - Galveston
Galveston, Texas

Gail M. Annich, M.D., M.S.
Assistant Professor of Pediatrics
Division of Pediatric Critical Care
University of Michigan
CS Mott Children's Hospital
Ann Arbor, Michigan

Denis Azzopardi, M.D.
Senior Lecturer in Paediatrics and Neonatal Medicine
Division of Paediatrics Obstetrics and Gynaecology
Hammersmith Campus
Imperial College
London, United Kingdom

Robert H. Bartlett, M.D.
Professor of Surgery
Department of Surgery
University of Michigan Medical School
Ann Arbor, Michigan

Thomas D. Black, B.S.
Medical Student
School of Medicine
University of Texas Medical Branch - Galveston
Galveston, Texas

Desmond Bohn, M.B., F.R.C.P.C.
Chief, Department of Critical Care Medicine
Professor of Anesthesia and Pediatrics
The Hospital for Sick Children, Toronto
Toronto, Canada

Jeanne E. Braby, R.N., M.S.N., C.C.R.N.
Cardiopulmonary Support Clinician
Pediatric Intensive Care Unit
Children's Hospital of Wisconsin
Milwaukee, Wisconsin

Judith Brown, N.N.P.
Child Development Program
Department of Psychiatry and Behavioral Medicine
Children's National Medical Center
Washington, D.C.

Dorothy Bulas, M.D.
Professor of Pediatrics and Radiology
The George Washington University School of Medicine
Children's National Medical Center
Washington, D.C.

Timothy E. Bunchman, M.D.
Professor
Director Pediatric Nephrology and Transplantation
DeVos Children's Hospital
Grand Rapids, Michigan

Andrew I.M. Campbell, M.D., F.R.C.S.
Assistant Professor, Faculty of Medicine
Department of Surgery
University of British Columbia
Pediatric Cardiovascular and Thoracic Surgeon
BC Children's Hospital
Vancouver, Canada

Robin Chapman, R.N.
University of Michigan
Ann Arbor, Michigan

Dai Chung, M.D.
Associate Professor of Surgery
Department of Surgery- Division of Pediatric Surgery
University of Texas Medical Branch- Galveston
Galveston, Texas

Steven A. Conrad, M.D., Ph.D.
Professor of Medicine, Emergency Medicine, and
Pediatrics
Director, ECLS Program
Louisiana State University Health Sciences Center
Shreveport, Louisiana

Chris Cordle, Ph.D.
Clinical Psychologist
Department of Psychology
University of Leicester
Leicester, United Kingdom

Charles S. Cox Jr., M.D.
The Children's Fund Distinguished Associate Professor of Surgery and Pediatrics
The University of Texas-Houston Medical School
Houston, Texas

Heidi J. Dalton, M.D.
Professor of Pediatrics
George Washington University
Medical Director, Pediatric Intensive Care Unit
Director, Pediatric ECMO Program
Children's National Medical Center
Washington, D.C.

Susan E. Day, M.D.
Associate Professor of Pediatrics (Critical Care)
Medical College of Wisconsin
Medical Director, ECMO Program
Children's Hospital of Wisconsin
Milwaukee, Wisconsin

Brittany B. DeBerry, M.D.
Chief Resident in General Surgery
Department of Surgery
University of Texas Medical Branch - Galveston
Galveston, Texas

Robert J. DiGeronimo, M.D.
Lieutenant Colonel, U.S.A.F., M.C.
Division of Neonatology
Wilford Hall U.S.A.F. Medical Center
Lackland A.F.B., Texas

Brian W. Duncan, M.D.
Surgical Director, Pediatric Cardiac Transplant and
Heart Failure
Pediatric and Congenital Heart Surgery
The Cleveland Clinic Foundation
Cleveland, Ohio

Francine Dykes, M.D.
Associate Professor of Pediatrics
Emory University School of Medicine
Medical Director, Neonatal Intensive Care Unit and
Neonatal ECMO
Children's Healthcare of Atlanta at Egleston
Atlanta, Georgia

Patricia A. English, M.S., R.R.T.
ECLS Program Coordinator
Respiratory Care Department
Massachusetts General Hospital
Boston, Massachusetts

Kathryn N. Farrow, M.D.
Assistant Professor of Pediatrics
Division of Neonatology
Northwestern University
Children's Memorial Hospital
Chicago, Illinois

Richard K. Firmin, M.B.B.S., F.R.C.S.
Consultant Cardiothoracic Surgeon
ECMO Director
Glenfield Hospital
University of Leicester
Leicester, United Kingdom

James D. Fortenberry, M.D., F.C.C.M., F.A.A.P.
Clinical Associate Professor of Pediatrics
Emory University School of Medicine
Division Director, Critical Care and Pediatric ECMO
Children's Healthcare of Atlanta at Egleston
Atlanta, Georgia

Björn Frenckner, M.D., Ph.D.
Professor of Pediatric Surgery
Astrid Lindgren Children's Hospital
Karolinska Institutet
Stockholm, Sweden

Penny Glass, Ph.D.
Associate Professor of Pediatrics
The George Washington University School of Medicine
and Health Sciences
Child Development Program
Department of Psychiatry and Behavioral Medicine
Children's National Medical Center
Washington, D.C.

Edward B. Goldman, J.D.
Associate Vice-President and Deputy General Counsel
University of Michigan
University of Michigan Health System
Ann Arbor, Michigan

Peter H. Grubb, M.D.
Lieutenant Colonel, U.S.A.F., M.C.
Division of Neonatology
Wilford Hall U.S.A.F. Medical Center
Lackland A.F.B., Texas

Barbara M. Haney, R.N.C., M.S.N., C.P.N.P.
Clinical Nurse Specialist, ECMO Coordinator
Neonatal-Perinatal Medicine
Children's Mercy Hospitals and Clinics
Kansas City, Missouri

Douglas R. Hansell, B.S., R.R.T.
Director, Pulmonary Services
Monroe Carell Jr. Children's Hospital at Vanderbilt
University
Nashville, Tennessee

Samantha Harris, M.Sc.
ECMO Co-ordinator
Heartlink ECMO Centre
Glenfield Hospital
Leicester, United Kingdom

Chris Harvey, M.B.B.S., F.R.C.S.
Senior ECMO Fellow
Glenfield Hospital
Leicester, United Kingdom

Cody L. Henderson, M.D.
Major, U.S.A.F., M.C.
Division of Neonatology
Wilford Hall U.S.A.F. Medical Center
Lackland A.F.B., Texas

Michael H. Hines M.D., F.A.C.S.
Associate Professor of Cardiothoracic Surgery and
Pediatrics
Wake Forest University School of Medicine
Director of ECMO and Perfusion Services
Brenner Children's Hospital and WFU/Baptist
Medical Center
Winston-Salem, North Carolina

Susan R. Hintz, M.D.
Assistant Professor of Pediatrics
Division of Neonatology and Developmental Medicine
Stanford University School of Medicine
Lucile Packard Children's Hospital
Palo Alto, California

Ronald B. Hirschl, M.D., M.S.
Professor of Surgery
Section of Pediatric Surgery
University of Michigan
Mott Children's Hospital
Ann Arbor, Michigan

Tom Jaksic, M.D., Ph.D.
Pediatric Surgeon
Associate Professor of Surgery
Harvard Medical School
Children's Hospital Boston
Boston, Massachusetts

Rajiv Jalan, M.B.B.S., M.D., F.R.C.P., F.R.C.P.E., Ph.D.
Senior Lecturer in Hepatology
Institute of Hepatology
University College London Medical School
Universtity College London Hospitals
London, United Kingdom

Nikki Jones, M.B.Ch.B., A.F.R.C.S.(Ed)
Specialist Registrar
Department of Cardiothoracic Surgery
Western Infirmary
Glasgow, United Kingdom

Amir M. Khan, M.D.
Assistant Professor of Pediatrics
Division of Neonatology
The University of Texas-Houston Medical School
Houston, Texas

Tracy K. Koogler, M.D.
Assistant Professor of Anesthesia and Pediatrics
Section of Pediatric Critical Care
The University of Chicago Pritzker School of Medicine
Chicago, Illinois

Robert L. Kormos, M.D.
Professor of Surgery, Division of Cardiothoracic Surgery
Co-Director Heart Transplantation
Director Artificial Heart Program
Medical Director McGowan Institute for Regenerative Medicine
University of Pittsburgh Medical Center
Pittsburgh, Pennsylvania

Kevin P. Lally, M.D.
Professor of Surgery and Pediatrics
Division of Pediatric Surgery
The University of Texas-Houston Medical School
Houston, Texas

John Lantos, M.D.
Professor of Pediatrics
Chief, General Pediatrics
The University of Chicago Pritzker School of Medicine
Chicago, Illinois

James E. Lynch, B.S., R.R.T.
ECMO Coordinator
Department of Critical Care Nursing
University of Texas Medical Branch - Galveston
Galveston, Texas

David Machin, B.Sc., A.C.P.
Senior Perfusionist
Glenfield Hospital
Leicester, United Kingdom

Judiann Miskulin, M.D.
Assistant Professor
Department of Surgery
Indiana University Medical Center
Indianapolis, Indiana

Inger Mossberg, C.R.N.A., I.C.C.R.N., B.Sc.
ECMO Specialist
ECMO Department
Karolinska University Hospital
Stockholm, Sweden

Palle Palmér, M.D.
Department of ECMO
Astrid Lindgren Children's Hospital
Karolinska Institutet
Stockholm, Sweden

Giles J. Peek, M.D., F.R.C.S., C.Th.
Consultant in Cardiothoracic Surgery and ECMO
Glenfield Hospital
Leicester, United Kingdom

Robert Pettignano, M.D., F.A.A.P., F.C.C.M., M.B.A.
Associate Professor of Pediatrics
Emory University School of Medicine
Pediatric Critical Care
Hughes Spalding Children's Hospital
Atlanta, Georgia

Thomas Pranikoff, M.D.
Associate Professor of Surgery and Pediatrics
Brenner Children's Hospital
Wake Forest University School of Medicine
Winston-Salem, North Carolina

Ravi S. Radhakrishnan, M.D.
Surgical Research Rellow
Department of Surgery
The University of Texas-Houston Medical School
Houston, Texas

Robert T. Remenapp, R.N., B.S.N.
Clinical Nurse III
ECMO Program
University of Michigan Hospitals
Ann Arbor, Michigan

Stephen J. Roth, M.D., M.P.H.
Assistant Professor of Pediatrics
Division of Pediatric Cardiology
Department of Pediatrics
Stanford University School of Medicine
Lucile Packard Children's Hospital
Palo Alto, California

Peter T. Rycus, M.P.H.
ELSO Registry Manager
Extracorporeal Life Support Organization
University of Michigan
Ann Arbor, Michigan

Babak Sarani, M.D.
Fellow in Trauma and Critical Care Surgery
Department of Critical Care Medicine
University of Pittsburgh Medical Center
Pittsburgh, Pennsylvania

Matthew C. Scanlon, M.D.
Assistant Professor of Pediatrics
Division of Critical Care
Medical College of Wisconsin
Patient Safety Officer
Children's Hospital of Wisconsin
Milwaukee, Wisconsin

Arlene M. Sheehan, R.N., N.N.P., M.S.
ECMO Coordinator
Lucile Packard Children's Hospital
Palo Alto, California

Billie Lou Short, M.D.
Professor of Pediatrics
Division of Neonatology
The George Washington University School of Medicine
Children's National Medical Center
Washington, D.C.

Thomas L. Spray, M.D.
Alice Langdon Warner Endowed Chair in Pediatric
Cardiothoracic Surgery
Chief, Division of Cardiothoracic Surgery
Children's Hospital of Philadelphia
Philadelphia, Pennsylvania

Robin H. Steinhorn, M.D.
Professor of Pediatrics
Division of Neonatology
Northwestern University
Children's Memorial Hospital
Chicago, Illinois

Jeffrey B. Sussmane, M.D., F.C.C.M.
Assistant Clinical Professor of Pediatrics
Division of Critical Care Medicine
Miami Children's Hospital
Miami, Florida

Dick Tibboel, M.D., Ph.D.
Professor of Experimental Pediatric Surgery
Director of Pediatric Surgical Intensive Care
Erasmus Medical Center, Sophia Children's Hospital
Rotterdam, Netherlands

Ravindranath Tirouvopaiti, M.B.B.S., F.R.C.S.
CESAR Trial Fellow
Department of Surgery
Glenfield Hospital
University of Leicester
Leicester, United Kingdom

Susan P. Tourner, M.D.
Clinical Fellow
Division of Pediatric Critical Care Medicine
Department of Pediatrics
Stanford University School of Medicine
Lucile Packard Children's Hospital
Palo Alto, California

Krisa P. Van Meurs, M.D.
Professor of Pediatrics
Division of Neonatology and Developmental Medicine
Stanford University School of Medicine
Lucile Packard Children's Hospital
Palo Alto, California

Anke WinklerPrins, B.A., R.N., B.S.N.
Interim Nurse Manager and Education Coordinator
ECMO Program
University of Michigan Hospitals
Ann Arbor, Michigan

Birgit Wittenstein, Dr. Med.
Fellow in Paediatric Intensive Care
Great Ormond Street Hospital
London, United Kingdom

Joseph B. Zwischenberger, M.D.
Professor of Surgery, Medicine, and Radiology
Leroy Hillyer Endowed Chair in Surgery
Director of General Thoracic Surgery and ECMO
Program
University of Texas Medical Branch
Galveston, Texas

Preface to the 3rd Edition

The third edition of the ECMO Redbook entitled *ECMO: Extracorporeal Cardiopulmonary Support in Critical Care* follows the previous editions published by ELSO in 1996 and 2000. Again, the goal has been to provide an exhaustive treatise on extracorporeal life support for use as a reference for ECMO practitioners worldwide. The last 5 years have produced significant changes in extracorporeal life support, and thus we have added 10 new chapters to this volume on topics including neuroprotection with hypothermia, plasmapheresis, safety issues, nursing care, management of pain and sedation, and new applications of ECLS. The majority of the remaining chapters have been substantially updated and revised.

We wish to thank the many authors who contributed their time to this endeavor. Additionally, the invaluable assistance from the following individuals has been essential in the editorial preparation of the textbook: Mary E. Nelson, Frances Rucks, Annalise Farmer, Arlene Sheehan, Peter Farmer, James Lynch, Betty Littleton, Andrew Farmer, Jesse Suber, and Peter Rycus. It was a pleasure to work with each of them.

As with the previous editions, in the spirit of academic collaboration, any of the figures tables, or text, not previously bound by copyright, may be reproduced in scientific publications without further permission.

Krisa Van Meurs, M.D.
Kevin Lally, M.D.
Giles Peek, M.D.
Joseph Zwischenberger, M.D.

Stanford, California
August 2005

Table of Contents

1

Extracorporeal Life Support: An Overview

Joseph B. Zwischenberger, M.D. and Robert H. Bartlett, M.D.

Introduction

Various terms are used to describe mechanical life support. Extracorporeal life support (ECLS) is a general term used to describe prolonged but temporary (<30 days) support of heart or lung function using mechanical devices. When the heart/lung machine is used in the OR in venoarterial mode to provide total support of heart and lung function to facilitate cardiac surgery, the technique is called cardiopulmonary bypass (CPB). When used with extrathoracic cannulation for respiratory and/or cardiac support, the technique has been called extracorporeal membrane oxygenation (ECMO), extracorporeal lung assist (ECLA), and extracorporeal CO_2 removal ($ECCO_2R$). When used with extrathoracic cannulation for emergency cardiac support, the technique has been called cardiopulmonary support (CPS) or extracorporeal cardiopulmonary resuscitation (ECPR). Blood pumps alone can be used as left ventricular assist devices (LVAD), right ventricular assist devices (RVAD), or biventricular assist devices (BiVAD). Although all of these applications are discussed in this book, the abbreviations ECLS and ECMO will be used interchangeably to mean treatment of cardiac or pulmonary failure by prolonged extracorporeal circulation with mechanical devices. Generally, all of these device applications include vascular access catheters, connecting tubing, a servo-regulating blood pump, a gas exchange device (usually incorrectly called an oxygenator), a heat exchanger, and various measuring and monitoring devices. Systemic anticoagulation (most commonly using heparin) is required to reduce the blood-surface interaction between the coagulation mechanisms and the foreign surface of the circuit; therefore, the balance between thrombosis and bleeding is always a major concern.

ECLS can be used for mechanical assistance during cardiac or pulmonary failure occurring in newborn infants, older children, or adults. Depending on the application, ECLS can be used in a venoarterial (VA) mode, venovenous (VV) mode, or arterial-venous (AV) mode. In general, ECLS is indicated for acute, severe reversible cardiac or respiratory failure when the risk of dying from the primary disease despite optimal conventional treatment is high (50-100%). Since ECLS is used only in patients who are otherwise likely to die, the results focus on survival. Long-term quality-of-life studies show favorable results for the majority of survivors. The current reported survival rate for neonatal respiratory failure is 77%, for pediatric respiratory failure 56%, for adult respiratory failure 53%, for pediatric cardiac failure 43%, and for adult cardiac failure 32%.

The Extracorporeal Life Support Organization (ELSO) was founded in 1989 as a volunteer study group comprised of clinical centers using ECLS. There are currently 109 member centers from 17 countries. The most important activity of ELSO is to maintain a large central database for all active centers including their submitted cases (>30,000 to date), devices and complications, and patient outcomes. ELSO coordinates prospective studies; publishes guidelines for ECLS referral and practice; facilitates teaching, standardization, and communication; and serves as the professional voice for ECLS technology. In 1993, members of ELSO published a textbook on extracorporeal life support edited by Arensman and Cornish, entitled "Extracorporeal Life Support". In 1996 and 2001, ELSO published a comprehensive text, entitled "ECMO: Extracorporeal Cardiopulmonary Support in Critical Care", known as the "Red Book". Here is the third edition of the "Red Book".

This edition is focused on the application of ECLS. Sections include a detailed review of ECLS physiology and pathology; the devices and logistics required; legal, ethical, economic, and regulatory issues; and related clinical and laboratory research. The details of ECLS management, indications, and results are presented for cardiac and respiratory support in neonates, pediatric, and adult populations. This book is prepared and published by ELSO, and the authors were selected from the ELSO membership. The invited chapters were edited; however, the opinions and style expressed in each chapter were retained.

History

John Gibbon's development of the CPB machine marks the beginning of cardiopulmonary support.[1] The history of perfusion is riddled with challenges and esteemed by accomplishments. Few have chronicled the history as well as Dr. Walton Lillehei, M.D, Ph.D., in the first ECLS textbook, edited by Arensman and Cornish.[2]

From crude-cross circulatory support, in which a child's parent is used as a biological heart-lung machine, to the use of heterologous biological oxygenators such as explanted dog or monkey lungs, and finally to the modern development of membrane oxygenators and centrifugal pumps, Dr. Lillehei recalls first-hand 60 years of progress.

As cardiopulmonary support progressed, so did the emerging field of critical care. The positive pressure ventilator allowed physicians to study and treat severe respiratory failure. The ventilator was soon modified for application in neonates, contributing to the decline in mortality associated with newborn respiratory failure. Unfortunately, positive pressure ventilation also inflicted unintended changes in cardiopulmonary physiology. In patients that did survive, morbidity in the form of bronchopulmonary dysplasia became common. Many physicians sought a balance that allowed the ventilator to be used as a life-saving treatment without causing long-standing pulmonary damage.

A major step in moving CPB from the OR to the bedside was the development of a long-term gas exchange device or "oxygenator". Gas exchange devices that did not separate the gas from the blood caused hemolysis when used for more than a few hours at a time. Pioneering work by Kolff, Kolobow, and others demonstrated the long-term benefits of a spiral coil-type silicone membrane.[3] Reports of the first patients supported by bedside CPB began to appear in the literature in 1972.[4]

Early trials of ECMO were marked by both success and failure. In one of the earliest randomized trials of ECMO sponsored by the NIH, ECMO was compared to conventional treatment in adults with ARDS.[5] This trial found no difference in survival and was terminated before even one third of the planned enrollment was accrued. There were numerous problems with the trial, including the lack of prior ECMO experience by some of the centers involved, uncontrolled bleeding, and the predominance of influenza pneumonia in enrolled patients. Clearly, patient selection and technology needed improvement, but the trial halted the use of ECMO to treat adult respiratory failure for decades.

In 1976, Bartlett et al. reported the successful use of CPB on an abandoned newborn nicknamed "Esperanza" (Spanish for *Hope*) by the nursing staff.[6] With this case, a new era of bedside CPB called ECMO was born. Neonates with diagnoses such as meconium aspiration syndrome (MAS), persistent pulmonary hypertension of the newborn (PPHN), and congenital diaphragmatic hernia (CDH) presented the opportunity to treat severe respiratory failure in a population with little hope of survival using conventional therapies. Their disease was often reversible with just a few days of ECMO support. In 1982, Bartlett published the initial ECMO experience with 45 newborns.[7] In this series of patients, ECMO was only utilized after maximal conventional therapy had failed and the infants were considered moribund by the attending neonatologist. With >50% survival in patients considered to have a 90% mortality, the interest in ECMO for newborn respiratory failure was high. Yet even with these early promising results, the lack of a randomized trial caused many physicians to continue to doubt its safety and efficacy.

Clinical trials addressing a seemingly lifesaving technique troubled many investigators. In an attempt to satisfy those calling for a randomized trial, Bartlett et al. used a strategy of "play the winner", comparing ECMO to conventional treatment.[8] With this strategy, the more successful treatment was favored in the randomization scheme. After the death of one infant in the conventional treatment arm, 12 consecutive patients were successfully treated with ECMO. Amid much controversy, O'Rourke and colleagues conducted a prospective, randomized trial in neonates with severe respiratory failure using a conventional 50/50 randomization strategy, comparing ECMO to conventional ventilator management. The trial

was stopped by the data safety monitoring board because of the clear superiority of ECMO in this patient population.[9] Another group of patients with high mortality and morbidity were infants with low cardiac output following a complex congenital heart repair. The first reported use of ECMO for cardiac support was by Baffes et al. in 1970; however, by the 1990s, ECMO became the technique of choice for this population.[10]

With the success of ECMO in the neonatal population, its use expanded rapidly throughout the late 1980s and early 1990s. Subsequently, the role of ECMO for adult respiratory failure in adults was once again revisited. Reports initially appeared as small case series. In 1997, for example, Kolla et al. reported 54% survival in 100 adult patients treated at the University at Michigan utilizing a ventilator management algorithm that included ECMO.[11]

As interest in ECMO grew, a voluntary alliance formed among active centers to pool data, compare information, and exchange ideas. A steering committee and bylaws formalized ELSO in 1989. Since the formation of ELSO and the ELSO Registry database, many publications addressing the safety and efficacy of ECMO have been published in the medical literature. Using data from the ELSO Registry, Stolar et al. showed a survival rate of 83% in 3500 newborns with respiratory failure with a predicted mortality of 80%.[12] Zwischenberger et al. reported 46% survival in 553 cases following cardiac surgery.[13] In 1991, an NIH conference on the diffusion of ECMO technology was held. A clear consensus was reached that the use of ECMO should continue. With over 30,000 patients currently in the database, ELSO continues to accumulate valuable information for comparing center-specific results with the international experience. Some recent trends include a rise in the number of cardiac patients treated with ECLS, the use of ECLS for resuscitation of acute cardiorespiratory failure, and decreased utilization for neonatal respiratory failure.

ECLS patients represent a constantly shifting population. Rarely today are newborns placed on ECMO for simple respiratory failure. Patients receive an array of therapeutic efforts prior to ECMO such as high-frequency oscillatory ventilation (HFOV), inhaled nitric oxide (iNO), prone positioning, and surfactant. As our understanding of the pathophysiology of severe cardiac and respiratory failure improves, patients are more likely to benefit from disease-specific therapies. In the future, ECLS is likely to continue as a rescue tool for patients of all ages who fail such therapies.

References

1. Gibbon JH, Jr. Application of a mechanical heart and lung apparatus to cardiac surgery. *Minn Med* 1954; 37:171-185.
2. Lillehei CW. *History of the development of extracorporeal circulation.* 1st ed. Boston: Blackwell Scientific Publications; 1993.
3. Kolff WJ, Effler DB, Groves LK, Peereboom G, Moraca PP. Disposable membrane oxygenator (heart-lung machine) and its use in experimental surgery. *Cleve Clin Q* 1956; 23:69-97.
4. Kolobow T, Spragg RG, Pierce JE, Zapol WM. Extended term (to 16 days) partial extracorporeal blood gas exchange with the spiral membrane lung in unanesthetized lambs. *Trans Am Soc Artif Intern Organs* 1971; 17:350-354.
5. Hill JD, O'Brien TG, Murray JJ, et al. Prolonged extracorporeal oxygenation for acute post-traumatic respiratory failure (shock-lung syndrome). Use of the Bramson membrane lung. *N Engl J Med* 1972; 286:629-634.
6. Zapol WM, Snider MT, Hill JD, et al. Extracorporeal membrane oxygenation in severe acute respiratory failure. A randomized prospective study. *JAMA* 1979; 242:2193-2196.
7. Bartlett RH. Esperanza. Presidential address. *Trans Am Soc Artif Intern Organs* 1985; 31:723-726.
8. Bartlett RH, Andrews AF, Toomasian JM, Haiduc NJ, Gazzaniga AB. Extracorporeal membrane oxygenation for newborn respiratory failure: forty-five cases. *Surgery* 1982; 92:425-433.
9. O'Rourke PP, Crone RK, Vacanti JP, et al. Extracorporeal membrane oxygenation and conventional medical therapy in neonates with persistent pulmonary hypertension of the newborn: a prospective randomized study. *Pediatrics* 1989; 84:957-963.
10. Baffes TG, Fridman JL, Bicoff JP, Whitehill JL. Extracorporeal circulation for support of palliative cardiac surgery in infants. *Ann Thorac Surg* 1970; 10:354-363.
11. Kolla S, Awad SS, Rich PB, Schreiner RJ, Hirschl RB, Bartlett RH. Extracorporeal life support for 100 adult patients with severe respiratory failure. *Ann Surg* 1997; 226:544-564; discussion 65-66.
12. Stolar CJ, Snedecor SM, Bartlett RH. Extracorporeal membrane oxygenation and neonatal respiratory failure: experience from the extracorporeal life support organization. *J Pediatr Surg* 1991; 26:563-571.
13. Zwischenberger JB, Cox CS, Jr. ECMO in the management of cardiac failure. *Asaio J* 1992; 38:751-753.

2

Physiology of ECLS

Robert H. Bartlett, M.D.

Introduction

Management of extracorporeal life support (ECLS) is the ultimate in the application of physiology to the care of critically ill patients. The medical team must be experts in all aspects of critical care. A thorough understanding of respiratory, hemodynamic, renal, and coagulation pathophysiology is a prerequisite for the management of these patients and is discussed in the other chapters of this book. This chapter provides a review of physiologic and pathophysiologic principles required specifically for the management of ECLS. The principles are applied similarly to all patient groups (newborn infants, children, or adults). Therefore, selected examples from each patient group are used. Likewise, the principles apply to venoarterial (VA) and venovenous (VV) bypass, and also to respiratory or cardiac support, and examples are drawn from each of these modes of support. Although our use of these principles has resulted in improved technology and improved management over the last three decades, the physiologic principles remain the same as those presented in previous publications.[1,2]

ECLS is performed by draining venous blood, removing CO_2 and adding O_2 through an artificial lung, and returning the blood to the circulation via a vein (VV) or artery (VA). When used in the VA mode, most of the venous blood

is diverted from the central circulation, hence the term cardiopulmonary bypass (CPB).

Modes of vascular access and perfusion

In VA, the functions of both heart and lungs are replaced by artificial organs, either totally or partially. During partial VA bypass, perfusate blood mixes in the aorta with left ventricular blood which has traversed the lungs. Hence, the content of oxygen and CO_2 in the patient's arterial blood represents a combination of blood from these two sources, and the total systemic blood flow is the sum of the extracorporeal flow plus the amount of blood passing through the heart and lungs.

In VV, the perfusate blood is returned to the venous circulation and mixes with venous blood coming from the systemic organs, raising the oxygen content and lowering CO_2 content in the right atrial blood. Some of this mixed blood is returned to the extracorporeal circuit, termed "recirculation," and some of it passes into the right ventricle, the lungs, and into the systemic circulation. Since the volume of blood removed is exactly equal to the volume of blood re-infused, there is no net effect on central venous pressure, right or left ventricle filling, or hemodynamics. The content of oxygen and CO_2 in the patient's arterial blood represents that of right ventricle blood modified by any pulmonary function that might exist. The systemic blood flow is the native cardiac output and is unrelated to the extracorporeal flow.

Arteriovenous (AV) extracorporeal circulation is commonly used for hemodialysis or hemofiltration, but not for cardiac or pulmonary support. The AV route can be used for gas exchange provided the arterial blood is desaturated, and the cardiovascular system can tolerate the AV fistula with a large enough flow to achieve adequate gas exchange. This is, after all, the mechanism of gas exchange in the placenta and fetus. Because of the blood flow requirements for gas exchange support, the AV route is not a reasonable approach to total extracorporeal respiratory support, except when the patient can tolerate a large AV shunt and an increase in cardiac output. However, AV flow through a membrane lung can provide CO_2 removal, decreasing the need for mechanical ventilation.[3]

Comparison of CPB and VA ECLS

The physiology and pathophysiology of total VA bypass for cardiac surgery has been well documented.[4] While the principles of gas exchange and blood flow are the same, there are several important differences between the conduct of ECLS and OR bypass. Some of the important differences are summarized in Table 1. Because the sole purpose of CPB in the OR is to permit heart surgery, total VA bypass is always used, with airtight occlusion of the venous drainage catheters and arterial access, usually directly into the aorta. Because there is total stagnation of blood in the pulmonary circulation, some chambers of the heart, and parts of the extracorporeal circuit, total anticoagulation is required and is achieved by administrating a large dose of heparin. This anticoagulation, and uncontrolled blood flow into the operative field from the coronary sinus, bronchial veins, and thebesian veins, results in continuous bleeding which is managed by aspiration and filtration of the shed blood with return to the venous reservoir (referred to as coronary suction or autotransfusion). To minimize bleeding into the field, and to minimize risks associated with high blood flow, it is common practice to manage systemic perfusion at abnormally low levels of blood flow (2-2.4 $l/m^2/min$) and abnormally low

Table 1. Comparison of CPB for cardiac surgery and VA ECLS in the ICU.

	OR CPB	ICU ECLS / ECMO
Venous reservoir	Yes	No
Heparin (ACT)	↑ Dose (>600)	Titrated (120-180)
Autotransfusion	Yes	No
Hypothermia	Yes	No
Hemolysis	Yes	No
Anemia	Yes	No
Arterial filter	Yes	No
Venous drainage	Right atrium	Right atrium
Pump control	Perfusionist/Reservoir	Perfusionist/Servo-control
Gas exchange	Membrane lung	Membrane lung
Heat exchanger	Yes	Yes
Monitors	SvO_2, pressure	SvO_2, pressure

hematocrit (typically 20%). This combination of low blood flow and low hematocrit leads to very low systemic oxygen delivery, which could result in oxygen debt and metabolic acidosis except that total body hypothermia is usually implemented, maintaining the ratio of delivery to consumption in the normal range of 5:1. A very efficient heat exchanger and a large water bath are required for CPB for heart surgery.

There is a risk of inadvertently aspirating large amounts of air into the venous catheters, and it is necessary to rapidly raise or lower the entire blood volume at times during cardiac operations. Therefore, a large venous reservoir is included in the venous drainage line, both to trap aspirated air and to allow frequent variations in intracorporeal vs. extracorporeal blood volume. Because the blood is anticoagulated, it does not clot. It is common practice during cardiac surgery to arrest the heart to permit a still operating field, and it is common practice to clamp the aorta above the coronary ostia but below the perfusion catheter to minimize coronary blood flow for the purpose of allowing operations directly on the coronary vessels and to minimize coronary sinus flow during operations on the right side of the heart. Because the myocardium is without blood flow during aortic cross clamping, various techniques must be employed to minimize ischemic damage to the myocardium. This has resulted in an entire field of research related to myocardial perfusion and protection during VA bypass for cardiac surgery. The cornerstone of all these techniques is direct myocardial hypothermia achieved by a combination of topical cooling and cold coronary perfusate. Because the aorta is cross clamped during most of the cardiac operation, bronchial and thebesian blood flow will cause gradual filling and eventual overdistention of the left atrium and left ventricle. Left unchecked, this overdistention damages the endocardium and myocardium so that some system of left-sided venting of this blood is a necessary component of CPB for cardiac surgery.

In contrast, ECLS uses partial rather than total CPB. This is achieved by extrathoracic cannulation conducted at normothermia, normal blood flow, and normal hematocrit, emphasizing normal systemic oxygen delivery to match metabolic needs. Heparinization is titrated to very low levels, and bleeding should be an infrequent complication. The design of the extracorporeal circuit eliminates venous reservoirs, coronary suction apparatus, and large heat exchangers. Left-sided venting is not possible under most circumstances, so normal left ventricular contractility must be maintained. In VV bypass, the entire circulation is dependent on normal myocardial function.

Aside from these differences in perfusion technology, the entire approach to management of extracorporeal circulation is quite different when comparing CPB to ECLS. CPB is conducted in the OR with the sole intention of operating upon the heart. There is an appropriate sense of urgency to minimize the time on bypass. Complications including myocardial damage, renal failure, liver failure, hemolysis, and abnormal bleeding increase proportionately with the amount of time on bypass. Unlimited amounts of bleeding in the operating field are tolerated and managed by autotransfusion, with the realization that the effect of heparin will be reversed by protamine at the end of the procedure. An interval of 1-2 hours for rewarming or and attempts to come off bypass would be considered unacceptably long. Sometimes huge doses of catecholamines are given to assist a poorly functioning heart to come off bypass. If the patient cannot be weaned off bypass within a few hours, the only alternative is a chronic mechanical support system. Since the patient is anesthetized and paralyzed, it is impossible to directly evaluate neurologic function.

In contrast, ECLS is managed in the ICU by a team expecting days or weeks of continuous care. The patient is maintained awake or is awakened at regular intervals to evaluate neurologic function. Feeding, ventilation, antibiotic management, and renal function are important aspects of ECLS care. The use of inotropic drugs and high ventilator settings is minimal, and weaning from bypass may proceed over a period of hours or days. The patient commonly lacks heart, lung, or renal function for days, and futility is conceded only after many days of vital organ failure.

Oxygen kinetics and tissue respiration

Normal values for oxygen consumption and delivery in adults are shown in Figure 1. Oxygen consumption (VO_2) is controlled by tissue metabolism, and hence is decreased by rest, paralysis, and hypothermia, and is increased during muscular activity, infection, hyperthermia, and increased levels of catecholamine and thyroid hormones. The metabolic rate is defined as the VO_2. VO_2 x 5 cal/l = estimated energy expenditure. The VO_2 in normal resting humans is 5-8 cc/kg/min in newborn infants, 4-6 cc/kg/min in children, and 3-5 cc/kg/min in adults. Although VO_2 may increase up to 10-fold with

exercise, VO_2 increases by only 50-60% during sepsis or with catecholamine use. The amount of oxygen absorbed across the lung in the process of pulmonary gas exchange is exactly equal to the amount of oxygen consumed by peripheral tissues during metabolism (the Fick principle) regardless of the status of pulmonary function. Hence, VO_2 can be measured at the airway or calculated as the product of arterial venous oxygen content difference times cardiac output (The Fick equation).

Systemic oxygen delivery

Systemic oxygen delivery (DO_2) is the amount of oxygen delivered to peripheral tissues each minute or the product of arterial oxygen content times cardiac output. DO_2 is controlled by cardiac output, hemoglobin concentration, hemoglobin saturation, and dissolved oxygen, in that order. The normal value for DO_2 is 4-5 x VO_2 regardless of patient size. Since the oxygen content of normal arterial blood is the same for all ages and sizes of patients (20 cc O_2/dl), variations in oxygen delivery for patients of different size and metabolic activity are caused by variations in cardiac output. The oxygen content is rarely measured directly for clinical applications, and it is standard practice to describe blood oxygenation in terms of PaO_2 (partial pressure of oxygen in arterial blood) or hemoglobin saturation. However, oxygen content is the most important measurement in the physiologic management of critically ill patients. The relationship of PaO_2, saturation, and oxygen content is described in Figure 2. Typical values for venous and arterial blood at different levels of hemoglobin are identified. Note that there is more oxygen in normal blood with a PaO_2 of 40 mm Hg than in anemic blood with a PaO_2 of 100 mm Hg. A unique aspect of cardiorespiratory homeostasis is the tendency to maintain systemic oxygen delivery at the normal level. In anemia, cardiac output will increase until DO_2 is normalized. In hypoxia, the cardiac output increases, and in chronic hypoxia, RBC mass increases under the influence of eryth-

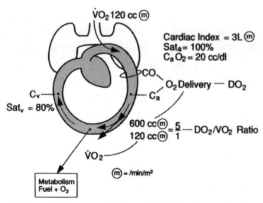

Figure 1. Oxygen delivery (DO_2) is the product of cardiac output (CO) times arterial oxygen content (Ca). Oxygen consumption (VO_2) is the amount of oxygen consumed across the lungs, which is identical to the amount of oxygen consumed in systemic metabolism. Normally the oxygen delivery is 4-5 times the amount of oxygen consumption. The venous blood saturation measures the ratio between DO_2 and VO_2.

ropoietin until systemic oxygen delivery is again normalized. These compensatory mechanisms should be recognized and assisted in the critically ill patient. For example, the best treatment for a ventilated patient who is hypoxic, anemic, tachycardic, hypotensive, and hypermetabolic is usually red blood cell (RBC) transfusion (rather than using inotropic drugs or increasing FiO_2).

The normal relationship between DO_2 and VO_2 is shown in Figure 3. The normal ratio is 5:1, and when VO_2 changes secondary to variations in metabolism, DO_2 readjusts by increasing or decreasing cardiac output to maintain the normal ratio. If systemic oxygen delivery is moderately decreased (e.g., by decreasing cardiac output), there is no change in oxygen consumption; hence, the amount of oxygen extracted from each deciliter of arterial blood is greater. There could be a situation in which the rate of tissue metabolism exceeded the rate of oxygen delivery, which would result in anaerobic metabolism, limitation of VO_2 based on decreased oxygen supply, and oxygen "debt." In theory, this would occur whenever the ratio of delivery to consumption is less than 1:1.

In practice, this situation occurs when the ratio is less than 2:1. The difference is explained by the fact that some of the systemic oxygen delivery goes to tissue that uses little oxygen (e.g., skin, fat, and tendons). Between this critical point at a DO_2/VO_2 ratio of 2:1 and the normal ratio of 5:1, decreased delivery is compensated for by increased extraction, maintaining normal hemodynamic and respiratory stability. Since mixed venous blood oxyhemoglobin saturation reflects this ratio exactly, it is the most important indicator for managing critically ill patients. If the arterial blood is fully saturated, the venous saturation decreases proportionate to the amount of oxygen extracted from arterial blood. Thus, if the oxygen extraction ratio is 20%, the venous saturation will be 80%; if the oxygen extraction ratio is 33%, the venous saturation will be 67%, and so on. These levels of venous saturation and corresponding DO_2/VO_2 ratios are identified in Figure 4.

CO_2 production

The amount of CO_2 produced during systemic metabolism per minute (VCO_2) is approximately equal to the amount of oxygen consumed. The ratio of CO_2 production to oxygen consumption is known as the respiratory quotient; depending

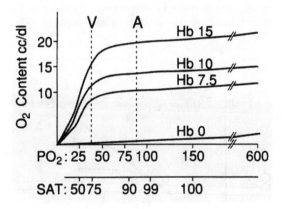

Figure 2. The amount of oxygen in blood can be expressed as oxygen content, PO_2, or saturation of hemoglobin. In this figure all 3 measurements are applied to blood, ranging from normal hemoglobin (15 gm/dl) to anemia hemoglobin (7.5 gm/dl) to plasma hemoglobin (0). The typical values for normal arterial (A) and venous (V) blood are shown. Notice that PO_2 and saturation are normal in anemic blood even though oxygen content is severely decreased.

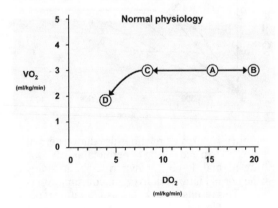

Figure 3. The normal relationship between VO_2 and DO_2. A is the normal 5:1 DO_2/VO_2 relationship: if DO_2 increases (A→B) or decreases (A→C), VO_2 is unchanged. If DO_2 is less than twice VO_2, VO_2 decreases (C→D).

on the energy substrate, it varies from 0.7 for fat to 0.8 for protein to 1.0 for carbohydrate. Under normal conditions, the rate and depth of breathing are controlled to maintain the $PaCO_2$ (the partial pressure of CO_2 in arterial blood) at 40 mm Hg. Even a slight increase in metabolically produced CO_2 will result in a proportionate increase in alveolar ventilation, sufficient to increase the amount of CO_2 excretion so that $PaCO_2$ remains at 40 mm Hg. Unlike systemic oxygen delivery, CO_2 excretion is not affected by hemoglobin concentration or blood flow but is very sensitive to changes in ventilation. For this reason, and because CO_2 excretion is more efficient than oxygenation in the lung, CO_2 removal can be maintained at normal levels even during severe lung dysfunction.

Gas exchange on ECLS

Oxygen delivery

During ECLS, oxygen delivery is controlled by the combination of blood oxygenation in the membrane lung, flow through the extracorporeal circuit, oxygen uptake through the native lung, and cardiac output through the native heart.

Blood oxygenation in the membrane lung is a function of membrane geometry, the thickness of the blood film, the membrane material and thickness, FiO_2, the residence time of RBCs in the gas exchange area, the hemoglobin concentration, and the inlet saturation (the latter two defining the oxygen uptake capacity of each deciliter of blood). All of these factors are included in a single descriptor of membrane lung function called rated flow.[5] Rated flow is the amount of normal venous blood that can be raised from 75%-95% oxyhemoglobin saturation in a given time period. This concept is illustrated in Figure 5. In this example, typical data for the 0.8 m^2 and 1.5 m^2 membrane lungs are shown. The structure of the 0.8 membrane lung is such that the rated flow is 1000 cc/min, corresponding to an actual oxygen transfer of 50 cc/min. This information is used to plan which membrane lung to use for ECLS and to evaluate membrane lung performance during perfusion.

As long as the extracorporeal blood flow is less than the rated flow of the membrane lung, the blood leaving the lung will be fully saturated and the amount of systemic oxygen delivery via the extracorporeal circuit will be controlled by blood flow and the oxygen uptake capacity. The

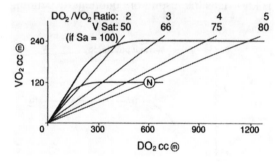

Figure 4. DO_2/VO_2 relationships during normal metabolism and during hypermetabolism. During normal, hypo-, or hypermetabolic states, the normal ratio of delivery to consumption is 5:1. This results in 80% venous saturation if the arterial blood is 100% saturated. The isobar for the 5:1 ratio is demonstrated in this diagram, as well as the isobar for 4:1, 3:1, and 2:1 ratios. Corresponding levels of venous saturation are shown. A state of decreasing oxygen consumption occurs when the ratio is less than 2:1.

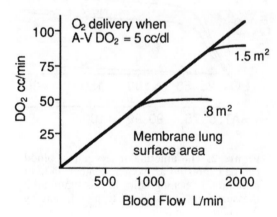

Figure 5. The amount of oxygen delivery for any membrane lung is fixed by the geometry of the device. In this example, oxygen delivery for 2 different membrane lungs is demonstrated. In this example, it is assumed that the AVO_2 difference is 5 cc/dl.

amount of oxygen that can be taken up in each deciliter equals hemoglobin gm/dl x unsaturated fraction x 1.36 cc/g. When the outlet blood is 100% saturated, the uptake capacity is the same as the $AVDO_2$ (arterio-venous difference in oxygen content). If the hemoglobin concentration is low or the venous blood saturation is high, the amount of oxygen that can be taken up in the membrane lung is decreased. It is possible to compensate for decreased oxygen-binding capacity by increasing blood flow. Conversely, we can achieve oxygen delivery at low blood flow by increasing oxygen-binding capacity. This is detailed in Figure 6, where oxygen delivery for VA and VV bypass in a typical newborn infant is demonstrated. The oxygen requirement for this infant is 20 cc/min. All of the oxygen requirements can be supplied by VA bypass at a flow of 400 cc/min or by VV bypass at a flow of 660 cc/min.

The resulting systemic PaO_2 and systemic oxygen delivery are a function of oxygen delivery through the extracorporeal circuit and through the native heart and lung. In planning the size of the circuit and extracorporeal flow rate, it is assumed that there will be no gas exchange across the native lung. With this assumption, in VV bypass, PaO_2

and saturation will be identical to the values in the mixed venous (right ventricle or pulmonary artery) blood. Because of the nature of VV bypass, this saturation will never be higher than 95%, and typically will be closer to 80% with a PaO_2 of approximately 40 mm Hg. Consequently, it is common for a patient on VV ECLS to be cyanotic and hypoxic. Systemic oxygen delivery is perfectly adequate as long as there is a compensatory increase in cardiac output. Improvement in native lung function results in increasing arterial oxygenation, and the amount of native lung function during VV bypass can be identified as the difference between venous and arterial saturation.

In VA bypass, the interpretation of arterial blood gases is more complicated. The perfusate blood is typically 100% saturated with a PO_2 (partial pressure of oxygen) of 500 mm Hg. When the lung is not functioning, the left ventricular

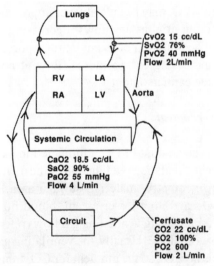

Figure 7. A diagrammatic representation of VA bypass in which half of the venous return goes through the extracorporeal circuit, and half goes through the right ventricle, into the pulmonary circulation, and into the left ventricle. In this example, the lungs have no oxygen exchange; therefore, the amount of oxygen in pulmonary arterial blood, pulmonary venous blood, and aortic root blood is the same. This desaturated blood mixes with completely saturated perfusate blood in the aortic arch, resulting in arterial saturation of 90% in the systemic circulation.

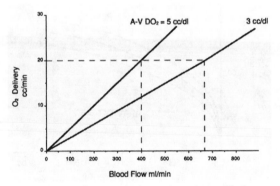

Figure 6. When a membrane lung is used below its maximal rated flow, the amount of oxygen delivery is inversely related to the saturation in venous blood. In this example, the blood flow required to achieve 20 cc/min oxygen delivery is shown for 2 different venous saturation conditions. $AVDO_2$ 5 cc/dl is typical for VA perfusion. $AVDO_2$ 3 cc/dl is typical for VV perfusion.

ejected blood is identical to right atrial blood, typically with a saturation of 75% and a PO_2 of 35 mm Hg. An example is shown in Figure 7; if the hemoglobin is 15 g/dl, the perfusate oxygen content is 22 cc/dl and the right atrial and left ventricular oxygen contents are both 15 cc/dl. The resulting arterial blood gases reflect the relative amounts of perfusate and native lung flow. Therefore, if 50% of the venous return is routed through the extracorporeal circuit, the oxygen content of systemic arterial blood will be 18.5 cc/dl, corresponding to a saturation of 90% and a PaO_2 of 55 mm Hg. The systemic oxygen content is determined by the following formula: Systemic O_2 content = Perfusate O_2 content x (ECC Flow / Total Flow) + LV Blood O_2 content x (Lung Flow / Total Flow), where ECC is extracorporeal circuit flow and LV is left ventricle.

Thus, during VA bypass, an increase in systemic PaO_2 may be indicative of improving lung function at constant flows, decreasing native cardiac output at constant extracorporeal flow, or increasing extracorporeal flow at constant native cardiac output.

CO_2 removal

The amount of CO_2 eliminated in extracorporeal circulation is a function of the membrane lung geometry, material, surface area, blood PCO_2, and, to a lesser extent, blood flow and membrane lung ventilating gas flow (referred to as sweep flow). Usually, the ventilating gas contains no CO_2, so the gradient for CO_2 transfer is the difference between the blood PCO_2 and zero (when the gas flow rate is high). As the PCO_2 drops during the passage of blood through the membrane lung, the gradient decreases, so CO_2 excretion is less at the blood outlet end of the device than at the inlet end. Consequently, the amount of CO_2 transfer is relatively independent of blood flow and only moderately dependent on inlet PCO_2, with the major determinant of CO_2 elimination being total surface area and

the flow rate of the sweep gas (Figure 8). CO_2 removal for a typical membrane lung at different levels of PCO_2 is shown over a range of blood flows. Notice that the capacity for CO_2 removal is considerably greater than the capacity for oxygen uptake at the rated flow (Figure 3). For any silicone rubber or microporous membrane oxygenator, CO_2 clearance will always be more efficient than oxygenation when the oxygenator is well ventilated and functioning properly.

The extracorporeal circuit is generally designed to supply total oxygen requirements. For this reason, the membrane lung is capable of removing an excess of CO_2. Increasing sweep flow and the total surface area of the membrane lung in the extracorporeal circuit can selectively increase CO_2 transfer, but not oxygen delivery.

Following the rationale for oxygen delivery and assuming that there is no gas exchange across the native lung, the arterial PCO_2 will be the same as venous PCO_2 in VV bypass, and it will be a function of mixing perfusate and cardiac output blood in VA bypass. However, because of the efficiency of extracorporeal CO_2 removal, the systemic PCO_2 can effectively be set at any level by matching the membrane lung surface

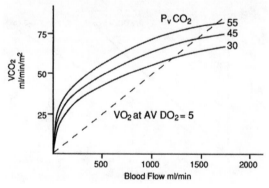

Figure 8. CO_2 clearance is better than oxygen uptake at any blood flow below the maximal rated flow for an oxygenator. In this example, the oxygen uptake at $AVDO_2$ 5 cc/dl is shown in the dotted line. The rated flow for this oxygenator is 50 cc/O_2/dl. CO_2 clearance exceeds oxygen uptake at all blood flows. The higher the pCO_2 of the venous blood, the greater CO_2 transfer.

area and gas flow with the systemic production of CO_2. In practice, the system is over-designed for CO_2 removal, and if bypass is run to supply total oxygen requirements, CO_2 removal will be excessive, resulting in significant respiratory alkalosis. This situation may be controlled by adding CO_2 to the sweep gas, thus decreasing the gradient, or by decreasing the sweep flow rate; both decrease total CO_2 transfer.

If the native lung can supply oxygen absorption and the intent of extracorporeal circulation is primarily CO_2 removal, this can be accomplished with VV access and relatively low blood flow. This is referred to as extracorporeal CO_2 removal, or $ECCO_2R$.[6]

ECLS equipment

Tubing and catheters

Blood flow through the extracorporeal circuit is limited by the size of the venous drainage catheter. Resistance to blood flow varies directly with the length of the catheter and inversely with the fourth power of the radius of the catheter. Consequently, the shortest and largest internal diameter catheter that can be placed in the right atrium will allow the highest rate of extracorporeal blood flow. The superior vena cava allows

the most direct access to the right atrium, and the right internal jugular vein usually has a large diameter. A catheter placed in the right internal jugular vein will usually permit venous drainage equivalent to the normal resting cardiac output for patients of all ages and sizes. Blood drains through the venous tubing to a pump which directs the blood through the membrane lung and back into the patient. There is significant resistance to flow through the membrane lung and across the reinfusion catheter, so the pressure on the arterial side of the circuit increases with increasing blood flow. In practice, the pump is set to deliver the desired flow and the post-pump pressure is continuously monitored. Pressures as high as 300 mm Hg are considered safe, although the higher the pressure, the higher the likelihood of blood leaks or circuit disruption. A standard system for describing pressure/flow characteristics of catheters and tubing, referred to as the M number, has been described by Montoya et al.[7,8] (Figures 9 and 10).

Pumps

Some measures must be taken to assure that the pump does not apply excessive suction to the venous catheter, as negative pressure >200 mm Hg will cause cavitation (bubble formation)

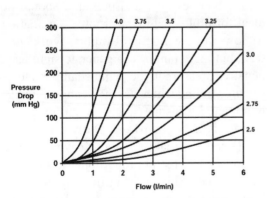

Figure 9. Pressure drop in cannulas with various M numbers as a function of blood flow. The M number is a dimensionless number that describes pressure flow characteristics of vascular access catheters. In this figure, catheters for pediatric and adult perfusion are shown.

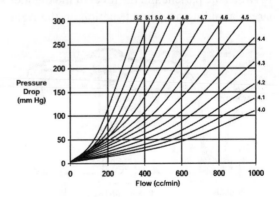

Figure 10. Pressure drop in cannulas with various M numbers as a function of blood flow. This figure shows the M number for catheters commonly used for ECLS.

which causes hemolysis; the right atrium and vena cava may become sucked into the catheter, causing endothelial damage; and negative pressure anywhere in the system always increases the risk of air entrainment and embolism. In cardiac surgery, these problems are avoided by including a large blood reservoir into which the venous line drains and air bubbles float to the top. A large reservoir is unacceptable for ECLS because of the risk of thrombosis in the stagnant blood and because the extracorporeal circuit must be maintained at a constant volume. The occlusive roller pumps which are usually used for extracorporeal support could potentially generate direct suction on the venous catheter. In practice, this problem is avoided by the inclusion of a small collapsible bladder positioned at the lowest point of the venous line. The bladder, or a transducer directly in the venous line, is attached to an electrical switch that slows or stops the roller pump whenever the pump suction results in negative pressure, and then restarts the pump instantly when the filling pressure exceeds the pump suction (i.e., the venous drainage flow exceeds the pump flow) (Figure 11).

The above system has two important advantages. Whenever the bladder collapses or the transducer senses negative pressure, and the pump stops, the suction effect of the siphon between the patient and the level of the bladder stops, avoiding any direct suction on the right

atrium. Secondly, because the pump motor is slowed or turned off whenever the bladder is collapsed, the pump cannot generate negative pressure in the blood between the pump and the bladder, which would cause cavitation and hemolysis. Thus, this bladder and electrical switching mechanism provides servo-regulation and some measure of safety for prolonged perfusion with a roller pump. The pump is adjusted to provide the desired level of gas exchange or cardiac support. As long as the venous drainage is adequate, the bladder remains distended and the desired flow is delivered. If venous drainage is impeded for any reason (hypovolemia, pneumothorax, kinking of the venous catheter), the pump stops and an alarm sounds. Flow resumes as soon as venous drainage is reestablished. Early in the course of extracorporeal circulation, flow is increased to the point at which the bladder collapses, thus identifying the flow limitation of venous drainage for the system. This flow rate is usually considerably greater than the flow actually required for extracorporeal support. However, if maximal flow through the system is inadequate after optimizing volume status and increasing the distance between patient and pump, another venous catheter must be added to augment the flow.

Centrifugal pumps, in which a spinning rotor generates flow and pressure, should be ideal for prolonged extracorporeal circulation. At low flow, centrifugal pumps work very well, but these pumps can generate significant negative pressure in the pump chamber and associated tubing whenever the venous drainage is impaired, causing cavitation and extensive hemolysis in the pump head. The risk of generating damaging negative pressure, cavitation, and hemolysis is directly proportional to the rotor pump speed.[9] Although centrifugal pumps have been used for prolonged support, the potential for hemolysis is significant. This problem can be avoided by incorporating a small bladder in the venous drainage line as described above, or by including a servo-regulation system in which

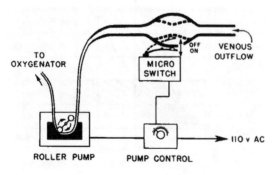

Figure 11. Diagrammatic representation of the "bladder box" system for servo-regulation of the inlet pressure for a roller pump.

pump speed is decreased when excessive negative pressure is generated.[10] When centrifugal pumps are used for cardiac surgery, it is not necessary to include venous line bladders or negative pressure sensors because the pump attaches directly to the venous reservoir and servo-regulation is provided by level sensing or by the pump operator. For this reason, the pump manufacturers have not provided mechanisms for servo-regulation during prolonged use; venous controllers or venous pressure sensors must be incorporated to permit centrifugal pumps to be used for ECLS.

A pumping system with all the advantages of the servo-regulated roller pump but without the extra bladder and hardware is the passively-filling propulsion pump, which is a combination roller pump and peristaltic pump. In the past, this type of pump was devised and marketed by the Rhone-Poulenc Company of France[11] and was used extensively for cardiac surgery in that country. A modification of this type of pump with several important improvements is currently marketed by Baxter-Bentley Laboratories (Irvine, CA) in the U.S.[12] This unique pump uses a flaccid but distensible pump chamber tube which is stretched over rollers without a raceway to push against. The pumping chamber fills passively, allowing the generation of flow and pressure. However, if the venous drainage is inadequate, the pumping chamber simply collapses without generating negative pressure. As the pumping chamber becomes more round during free filling and high flow, the amount of pressure generated reaches a plateau which can be adjusted by the operator. For example, if the pressure plateau is set at 400 mm Hg, flow decreases above this pressure and arterial line rupture cannot occur. Because of the passive filling of the pump chamber, air cannot be entrained or pumped, and the risk of air embolism is minimal. The entire pumping chamber can be incorporated into a solid enclosure that permits controlled inflow suction if desired. Because of the many advantages of this type of pumping

system, it is likely that the propulsion pump will become the safest pump for ECLS and cardiac surgery.

It can be seen that both building and monitoring the ECLS circuit requires knowledge of the pressure, flow, and resistance characteristics of each of the blood conduit components. Although these relationships can be calculated for straight tubes of known diameters, most access catheters have irregular diameters and side holes which require individual characterization. As previously mentioned, the M number provides a standard system for describing pressure/flow relationships in blood access devices.[7,8] If the M number for a specific catheter is known, the pressure and flow over the full range of use can be determined from a nomogram (Figures 9-10).

Non-pulsatile flow

The effect of VA bypass on systemic perfusion is reflected in the pulse contour and pulse pressure. The extracorporeal pump creates a flow that is essentially non-pulsatile. Consequently, as more blood is routed through the extracorporeal circuit, the systemic arterial pulse contour becomes flatter, then intermittent, then stops altogether when total bypass is reached. At total bypass, the left ventricle gradually distends with bronchial and thebesian flow and ejects

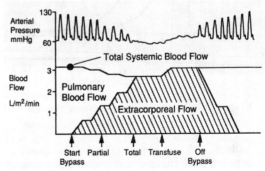

Figure 12. As extracorporeal flow increases, systemic pulse pressure decreases. In this example, total CPB is associated with a flat systemic pulse contour.

when it is full, leading to an occasional pulsatile beat (Figure 12). In practice, it is unusual to reach total bypass for any sustained period with extrathoracic cannulation as long as there is cardiac function. Typically, VA ECLS is run at about 80% of normal resting cardiac output, which allows 20% or more of the blood to pass through the lungs and left heart, resulting in a diminished but discernible pulse contour. As long as total blood flow is adequate, the presence of a pulse contour is not physiologically important.[13-15] The discussion concerning pulsatile and non-pulsatile flow has been the subject of much research over the last three decades. The results of some of these studies are summarized in Figure 13. As long as total blood flow to the patient or research animal is on the high to normal side (typically >100 cc/kg/min), there is no difference between pulsatile and non-pulsatile perfusion. Similarly, if total blood flow is very low (<40 cc/kg/min), inadequate oxygen delivery, shock, anaerobic metabolism, and acidosis occur regardless of the type of

perfusion. At low but less than adequate blood flow, the effects of hypoperfusion and acidosis are somewhat ameliorated by pulsatile flow. The reason for this is the fact that non-pulsatile flow results in greater stimulation of the aortic and carotid sinus pressor sensors, resulting in greater release of endogenous catecholamines with deleterious effects on the microcirculation. During ECLS, all of the management effort is placed on maintaining normal or excessive systemic oxygen delivery; therefore, non-pulsatile perfusion does not have any deleterious effects. In fact, non-pulsatile perfusion can be maintained for months as long as total blood flow is adequate.[16,17] The kidney is the organ most sensitive to non-pulsatile flow, and the moderate anti-diuresis which occurs from non-pulsatile flow stimulating the juxtaglomerular apparatus can usually be overcome with small doses of diuretics.

Left ventricle function

As mentioned earlier, draining blood from the left atrium and left ventricle is an essential part of CBP in the OR. As long as the left ventricle is ejecting blood adequately, left-sided venting is not an issue during VA ECLS. If ECLS is being used for cardiac support, or if the preceding period of hypoxemia has resulted in myocardial stun with severe malfunction, the left side of the circulation can be become overdistended, resulting in cardiac damage and pulmonary edema. When this occurs, or ideally before this occurs, left sided decompression must be instituted. This is rarely a significant problem in VA ECLS in neonates, probably because the left-sided circulation decompresses through the patent ductus arteriosus. Periods of non-pulsatile flow in the neonate on VA bypass may exist for 12-24 hours without obvious, severe, left-sided myocardial injury from overdistension. Conversely, even a few minutes of left-sided over-distention will result in myocardial damage and obvious pulmonary edema in

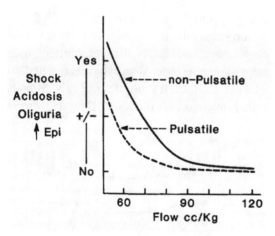

Figure 13. Diagrammatic representation of the incidence of acidosis, oliguria, and increased catechol secretion related to pulsatile/non-pulsatile flow. There is no significant difference between pulsatile and non-pulsatile flow so long as the total systemic blood flow is normal. At moderately decreased flow, pulsatility affords some protection against the systemic signs of shock.

older children and adults. For this reason, it is important to maintain left ventricular function and ejection during partial VA bypass. If myocardial failure does not allow ejection against the pressure generated by VA bypass, arterial resistance should be decreased by vasodilation, or left-sided venting should be promptly initiated. The left side can be vented by thoracotomy and direct cannulation of the left atrium, or by transseptal atriotomy, creating a small atrial septal defect in the catheterization laboratory. Another approach used in the laboratory by Kolobow is catheterization of the pulmonary artery by a small catheter to allow retrograde decompression into the right atrium.[18]

VV and VA access

VV bypass has no effect on hemodynamics. Blood is drained from and returned to the venous circulation at the same rate because the extracorporeal circuit is non-compliant. This is true whether VV bypass is achieved with 2 separate catheters or with a single double lumen catheter. An interesting variation of VV bypass proposed by Kolobow et al.[19] and used by Durandy et al.[20] is the tidal flow system. In tidal flow VV extracorporeal circulation, a single venous catheter in the right atrium is used. Venous blood is drained for approximately 1 second, a valve changes the access, and oxygenator blood is re-infused through the same catheter over a shorter time, typically 0.5 seconds. This system results in significant fluctuations in right atrial pressure, but this does not interfere with right ventricular or left-sided hemodynamics. Recent studies by Kolla et al.[21] show that tidal flow can be used for total support, even in large animals.

The physiology of hemodynamics and gas exchange during VA bypass is shown in Figure 14. In this example, before ECLS, VO_2 is significantly elevated because of endogenous and exogenous catecholamines and the systemic effects of hypoxia; arterial saturation is 85%, and venous saturation is 50%. As soon as VA bypass is instituted, both arterial and venous saturations increase to normal levels. When exogenous catecholamine infusions and ventilator settings are decreased, VO_2 falls to normal metabolic levels. The adequacy of flow is monitored by normal mixed venous blood saturation in the extracorporeal circulation, and flow can be decreased to maintain venous saturation at ~75%. During an episode of seizure activity, oxygen consumption increases. With no change in systemic blood flow, venous saturation decreases (i.e., oxygen extraction increases) during this period of increased muscle activity. Bleeding is characterized by a decrease in venous return, necessitating a decrease in total systemic blood flow. This results in impaired oxygenation, manifested by a fall in venous saturation. Blood is transfused until adequate extracorporeal flow can be maintained. In the example in Figure 14, an excess transfusion volume was given. At stable VA extracorporeal flow, this extra blood volume results in increased transpulmonary blood flow, resulting in systemic hypoxemia, which ultimately is reflected as venous hypoxemia as well. This change in delivery can be compensated by an increase in extracorporeal flow, although this combination of increasing flow, then blood volume, then flow, then blood volume is the classic example of a physiologic vicious circle known as tail-chasing. In the example in Figure 14, a drop in arterial then venous saturation following oxygenator failure would be expected. Weaning from extracorporeal circulation is illustrated as progressively decreasing flow while maintaining normal arterial and venous saturation during constant oxygen consumption.

The physiology of hemodynamics and gas exchange during VV bypass is diagrammed in Figure 15. In this example, the pre-ECLS status is the same as in the previous examples. Institution of VV bypass results in improvement of both venous and arterial saturation, which become equivalent at ~85% saturation.

This level of systemic oxygen delivery allows ventilator settings and catecholamine infusions to be decreased, resulting in a return-to-normal systemic oxygen consumption. Increased muscular activity with seizure activity results in increased VO_2, reflected as a decrease in both arterial and venous saturation. Bleeding results in impaired venous return and a decrease in both arterial and venous saturation as the right atrial blood becomes desaturated. Transfusion does not return these factors to normal, but transfusion of excess volume does not significantly impair oxygenation as it did during VA circulation. Oxygenator failure is accompanied by a decrease in both arterial and venous saturation, and weaning from VV ECLS follows the same pattern as VA bypass.

Some of the major differences between VA and VV access are shown in Table 2. One of the important differences is that arterial perfusion pressure and therefore systemic vascular resistance are maintained at fairly high levels during VA circulation. Moreover, if the carotid artery is used, the jet of the arterial infusate may concentrate directly on the aortic arch or even on the cusps of the aortic valve. This combination of events may lead to difficulty in left ventricular emptying and decreased coronary artery blood flow because the left ventricular myocardium does not sufficiently relax to allow coronary perfusion. Cornish and others have studied these phenomena in detail.[22,23] They have shown that myocardial damage can result simply from prolonged VA bypass. These problems can be avoided with the use of VV bypass, assuming that myocardial function is adequate to sustain systemic perfusion. When VV and VA access

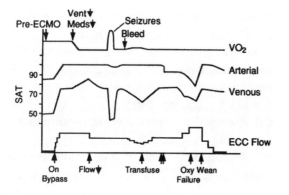

Figure 14. Typical events during VA bypass cause changes in oxygen consumption and in arterial and venous saturation, depending on the extracorporeal flow. In this example, oxygen consumption (VO_2) decreases with the onset of ECLS because there is less metabolic stress and less exogenous catecholamine infusion. During VA bypass, arterial saturation is maintained over 95% and flow is adjusted to maintain arterial and venous saturation. Increased oxygen consumption associated with seizures causes a decrease in venous saturation but minimal change in arterial saturation. Bleeding causes a decrease in venous return associated with lower oxygen delivery, manifested primarily by a decrease in venous saturation. Transfusion allows return of flow to normal. Over-transfusion at a constant extracorporeal flow results in increased patient lung blood flow. When the lungs are not functioning, arterial saturation decreases (Figure 7). When the native lungs have recovered, it is possible to wean extracorporeal flow while maintaining adequate arterial and venous saturation.

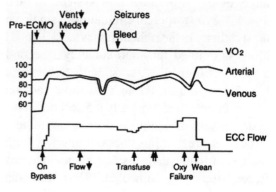

Figure 15. The same events described in Figure 14 are shown here during VV bypass. Unlike VA bypass, the arterial and venous saturation levels are nearly the same during VV bypass. Changes related to increased oxygen consumption, bleeding, and transfusion reflect arterial and venous saturation in the same fashion. When the native lung recovers, arterial saturation improves and extracorporeal flow is weaned down.

have been compared in neonatal ECLS, the survival rate is consistently better with patients treated with VV access. This is somewhat misleading because patients that begin ECLS with severe cardiac failure receive VA access to provide cardiac support. When large groups of patients from the ELSO Registry were compared, and when the difference in pre-bypass cardiac status was considered, no difference in survival was found between VV and VA ECLS.[24]

Coagulation control

Whenever blood contacts a prosthetic surface, the physiologic mechanism of thrombosis begins. Blood proteins adhere instantly to the prosthetic surface, creating a molecular protein layer which forms the blood-surface interface for the rest of the period of exposure. The proteins in this layer affect subsequent events. Some proteins such as albumin pacify or passivate the surface, minimizing subsequent adherence or activation of fibrinogen, Factor 12, complement, and platelets. The thrombogenicity of prosthetic surfaces is related to the amount of fibrinogen which adheres during blood exposure. Platelets adhere to fibrinogen on an artificial surface and are stimulated to release platelet granule material, attracting other platelets and stimulating the formation of fibrin. If no anticoagulant is present in the blood and the flow is slow or absent, a platelet fibrin mesh grows in seconds, trapping RBCs and white blood cells (WBCs) in the process and leading to a blood clot. If there is no anticoagulant in the blood but the flow is very fast, there is

Table 2. Differences between VA and VV ECLS.

	VA	VV
Hemodynamics		
Systemic perfusion	Circuit flow and cardiac output	Cardiac output only
Arterial BP	Pulse contour damped	Pulse contour full
CVP	Not very helpful	Accurate guide to volume status
PA pressure	Decreased in proportion to ECC flow	Not affected by flow
Effect of R-L shunt	Mixed venous into perfusate blood	None
Effect of L-R (PDA) shunt	Pulmonary hyperperfusion may require increased flow	No effect on ECC flow, usual PDA physiology
Selective R arm, brain perfusion	Occurs	Does not occur
Gas exchange		
Typical blood flow for full gas exchange	80-100 cc/kg/min	100-120 cc/kg/min
Arterial oxygenation	Sat. controlled by ECC flow	80-95% sat. common at max flow
CO_2 removal	Depends on sweep gas and membrane lung size	Same as VA
Oxygenator	0.4 or 0.6	0.6 or 0.8
Decrease initial vent settings	Rapidly	Slowly

insufficient time for the growth of a clot before the aggregated platelets are washed away, so significant clotting does not occur.

When fibrin formation is inhibited by heparin, the growth of the clot is impeded even in areas of slow flow, so aggregates of platelets and WBCs grow in stagnant zones without the fibrin glue which leads to solid thrombosis. When the platelet-WBC aggregate extends into the stream of rapidly flowing blood, it grows, and then waves in the stream, and eventually breaks off. This platelet-WBC aggregate embolizes into the patient and disaggregates in the first capillary bed; the effete platelets recirculate until they are removed by the reticuloendothelial system.[25] Platelet transfusion is usually required to maintain the platelet count >80,000/mm^3 during ECLS.

Although ECLS can be conducted for long periods without systemic anticoagulation so long as high flow is maintained with no stagnant areas,[26] the clinical practice is to give systemic heparin continuously in a dose to maintain the whole blood activated clotting time (ACT) at ~200 seconds, or ~1.5 x normal. Generally this requires 30-60 units/kg/hr of heparin. Heparin is bound to platelets and is excreted in the urine, so higher heparin doses are required during diuresis and platelet transfusion, while lower heparin doses are required for renal failure and thrombocytopenia. Obviously, the heparin effect, rather than the exact heparin concentration, is the important parameter. The heparin effect must be measured in whole blood, such as whole blood ACT, rather than in plasma, such as partial thromboplastin time (PTT) or thrombin time. The use of heparin-bonded circuits and other non-thrombogenic coatings may change the practice of anticoagulation in ECLS in the future. Coagulation and anticoagulation in ECLS is discussed in detail in Chapter 3.

Physiologic principles in ECLS management

Based on an understanding of the physiology of ECLS and of the pathophysiology of the patient's primary disease, it is obvious that the goal of ECLS is to maintain systemic oxygen delivery and CO_2 removal in the proper proportion to systemic metabolism. This is achieved at low ventilator settings or inotropic drug dosages which could not be tolerated otherwise. This process should eliminate any further ventilator-induced lung injury and improve systemic perfusion, allowing time for the native lung or heart to recover from the acute illness.

Planning and priming the circuit

Although total support may never be necessary, the circuit must be configured with the option of total support being available. The tubing, connectors, and pump must be capable of adequate blood flow, typically 100 cc/kg/min for newborn infants, 75 cc/kg/min for children, and 50 cc/kg/min for adults (Table 3). If VV access is used for respiratory support, these estimates of blood flow should be increased by 20%, since higher blood flow will be required for adequate oxygenation because of recirculation. The venous access catheter should be large enough to deliver this amount of blood flow with the assistance of 100 cm of siphon, and the arterial or reinfusion catheter should be large enough to permit this level of blood flow at line pressures <300 mm Hg proximal to the membrane lung. The membrane lung must have a rated flow higher than the maximal anticipated blood flow. At present, the spiral coil membrane lung designed by Kolobow and manufactured by the Avecor Corporation (Minneapolis, MN) is the one primarily used for ECLS in the U.S. Other types of membrane lungs have been used successfully for ECLS. Specifically, membrane lungs made from microporous materials are more efficient than the solid silicone rubber membrane lung, easier to prime, easier to manufacture, and have lower bedside pressure drop. The disadvantage to microporous membrane lungs is that plasma leakage can occur through the micropores in an unpredictable fashion. Various types of membrane lungs and their function are discussed in Chapter 6.

Once the circuit components have been selected and assembled in sterile fashion, the system is ready for priming. First, the system is filled with CO_2 gas to displace any nitrogen which would form bubbles. Then, a saline clear prime is used to displace the CO_2. The system is de-bubbled during circulation through a priming reservoir. A small amount of albumin is then added to decrease subsequent fibrinogen adsorption during initial blood exposure. In newborn infants, this clear prime is usually displaced with one adult unit of packed RBCs to maintain the hematocrit in normal range during the initiation of ECLS. The blood is recirculated through the priming reservoir until the temperature is 37°C and the electrolytes and blood gases are near normal. At this time, the circuit is ready for connection to the patient. In older children and adults (and in some neonatal emergencies), ECLS is initiated with a clear crystalloid and albumin prime. Once this solution is evenly mixed with the patient's blood,

significant dilution of platelets, proteins, and RBCs invariably occurs. RBC transfusion is necessary to return the hematocrit to normal levels. The resultant intracorporeal and extracorporeal blood volume sustained with packed RBCs, platelet concentrate, and colloid solution excretes the fluids by diuresis. Initiating bypass with clear prime is normally recommended for children and adults. It is important to ensure that the ionized calcium in the prime is in normal range;[27] otherwise, acute, severe myocardial depression and even cardiac arrest can follow the initiation of ECLS.

Cannulation

While the circuit is being primed, vascular access cannulas are placed. For the reasons outlined above, the right internal jugular vein is primarily used for venous access. The largest internal diameter, shortest catheter that can be placed into the jugular vein usually permits the desired blood flow. A smaller catheter is preferable if the M number is less than that dictated by the desired flow rate. If VA circulation is to be used, the advantage of the right common carotid artery is that it provides flow directly into the aortic root. Both the jugular vein and

Table 3. Typical flow and gas exchange requirements for pediatric patients with the Avecor oxygenator.

Patient size (kg)	Medtronic membrane lung surface area size	Rated flow* (l/min)	Gas exchange† (cc/min)
	0.4	0.5	30
3-10	0.8	1	60
	1.5	2	120
10-30	2.5	3	180
	3.5	4	240
30+	4.5	5	300

*Rated flow = maximal flow of 75% saturated venous blood which can be fully oxygenated.
† O_2 and CO_2 exchange at $AvDO_2$ vol % and RQ 1.0. Potential CO_2 exchange is higher.

common carotid artery can be ligated distally. Both arterial and venous collateral circulations are adequate in almost all patients. Femoral vein access can provide total venous drainage if the catheter is large and long enough. Femoral artery access can be used for cardiac support, but will result in aortic root hypoxemia in cases of respiratory failure.

If VV access is used for respiratory support, perfusate blood can be returned directly to the jugular vein catheter using the tidal flow system or a double lumen catheter. Alternatively, the perfusate can be returned to any large systemic vein. Usually, the femoral vein is catheterized for 2-vein VV access. In 2-vein cannulation, recirculation is minimized when drainage is from the inferior vena cava and reinfusion is into the right atrium.[28]

Monitoring

ECLS requires several monitors in addition to patient vital signs, blood gases, and ventilator settings. Blood flow is monitored continuously, usually by the rpm on the roller pump. Although routinely used, this method of measuring flow can be grossly incorrect if the rollers are not occlusive or if the tubing is not round. Pressure should be monitored on the arterial side of the circuit, preferably before and after the membrane lung. An increasing pressure gradient across the membrane lung suggests thrombosis. The expected post-oxygenator pressure should be predicted for any given flow based on the M number of the return catheter. If the pressures are higher than expected, the arterial line or catheter is kinked or occluded. The most important parameter is continuous monitoring of mixed venous saturation. This is measured by placing an Oximetrix fiberoptic catheter (Hospira, Inc., Lake Forest, IL) through a Touhy Borst adapter into the venous line. Since venous drainage blood represents a mixture of blood from the superior vena cava, the inferior vena cava, and the coronary sinus, the mixed venous

saturation (SvO_2) is an accurate representation of the DO_2/VO_2 ratio during VA bypass. With VA access, as long as the SvO_2 is in the range of 75% and all aspects of perfusion are going well, it is not necessary to measure systemic or circuit blood gases more frequently than every 12 hours. If the system includes a transcutaneous oximeter and an online PCO_2 monitor, sampling of the blood for gas analysis is rarely necessary. During VV bypass, the mixed venous saturation is higher because of recirculation. With VV bypass, the ideal is to maintain the venous saturation as high as possible, usually ~85-90%. If cardiac output is normal, this level of saturation is sufficient to maintain normal systemic oxygen delivery. When SvO_2 is combined with transcutaneous oximetry in a patient on VV bypass, the adequacy of extracorporeal support and the amount of lung function can be assessed simultaneously. Measurement of end tidal CO_2 at the airway is another helpful monitor of native lung function. During the initial days of an ECLS run, end tidal CO_2 may be ≤5 mm Hg. As functioning lung units resume ventilation or as pulmonary blood flow to ventilated units increases, end tidal CO_2 will increase. When end tidal CO_2 is near normal (>35 mm Hg), a trial of weaning off ECMO should be considered.

Measuring whole blood ACT hourly monitors the status of anticoagulation. Platelet count is measured every 8-12 hours. Details of monitoring and management are shown in Figure 16.

Patient management on ECLS

The blood flow is set at a level that will provide total oxygen and CO_2 exchange, and mechanical ventilation is reduced to minimal or lung rest settings. Patient arterial blood gases are checked and continuous monitors are calibrated. Thereafter, venous saturation is maintained at the desired level by increasing or decreasing extracorporeal blood flow. $PaCO_2$ is maintained at ~40 mm Hg by adjusting the flow rate and composition of sweep gas. Systemic blood pressure is maintained at the desired level by adjusting blood volume. Hemoglobin is maintained between 14-15 g/dl. Platelet count is maintained at >75,000/mm³ and ACT is maintained at ~200 seconds. A major decrease in venous saturation with no change in the other settings is usually caused by an increase in metabolic rate, which may be transient (e.g., during crying or seizures) or sustained. A sustained increase in metabolic rate can be matched by an increase in circuit blood flow or can be treated with sedation, paralysis, and/or hypothermia. A major increase in venous saturation with no change in other settings is usually caused by a decrease in metabolic rate or the onset of native lung function. Hypovolemia, catheter kinking or malposition, pneumothorax, or pericardial tamponade may cause a sudden decrease in venous drainage. A gradual decrease in systemic oxygenation or an increase in $PaCO_2$ may be a sign of deteriorating membrane lung function. Membrane lung function is assessed by measuring oxygen and CO_2 transfer and comparing the results to the

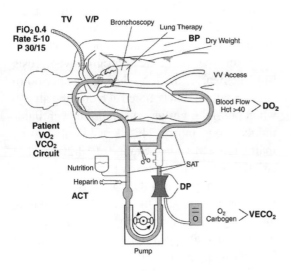

Figure 16. Typical VV ECLS is shown in this diagram. Extracorporeal flow is adjusted to maintain a desired level of systemic arterial and venous saturation.

expected transfer at that level of blood flow and CO_2 gradient. If the membrane lung is deteriorating, a new lung should be inserted, although this is an infrequent occurrence.

The native lung during ECLS

When ECLS is used solely for cardiac support, the lung usually remains in normal condition throughout the time on bypass, including its radiographic appearance and physiologic function. Since cardiac support always involves VA bypass, this normal native lung function is masked by a very extensive ventilation perfusion mismatch in which low normal levels of ventilation are excessive compared to the amount of blood actually flowing through the pulmonary capillaries. This gives the impression of large dead space ventilation which is reflected in low end tidal CO_2. If this mismatch is treated by decreasing mechanical ventilation to very low levels of pressure, then alveolar collapse may eventually occur. For this reason it is best to maintain the end expiratory pressure at 10-15 cm H_2O throughout VA ECLS for cardiac support, carefully limiting inspiratory plateau airway pressure to ≤30 cm H_2O. This will result in a small tidal volume which can be maintained at a low ventilatory rate. Even with these settings, excess CO_2 elimination may occur, and it is often necessary to incorporate CO_2 into the sweep gas during VA bypass when lung function is normal. The fact that lung appearance and function remain normal during VA bypass for cardiac support is ample evidence that there is little or no direct effect of ECLS on lung capillary permeability or lung function.

Usually, however, there is some degree of lung abnormality and respiratory failure ranging from mild cardiogenic pulmonary edema (when ECLS is used for cardiac support) to total and severe lung dysfunction (when ECLS is used for respiratory support). In this situation, as soon as the pre-existing high airway pressure is decreased, small airways and alveoli held open by excessive distending pressures often collapse, leading to the radiographic picture of consolidation and congestion referred to as white out, and the physiologic picture of little or no gas exchange through the native lung. This is true on both VV and VA modes of support. This period of no native lung function makes the patient entirely dependent on the extracorporeal circuit. If ECLS is discontinued, even for 1-2 minutes, profound hypoxemia and cardiac arrest can result. For this reason, back-up ventilator settings are posted to be used in the event that ECLS is interrupted. Typically, these settings are 100% oxygen, peak airway pressure (PIP) of 40 cm H_2O, peak and expiratory pressure (PEEP) 10 cm H_2O, rate 20-30 beats/min. However, if the lung is totally consolidated, no amount of air delivered into the airway will recruit lung volume sufficiently to sustain life, so great attention is devoted to avoiding this possible complication. To minimize total lung consolidation, mean airway pressure (MAP) is maintained in the range of 10-20 cm H_2O. This approach, originally proposed for neonates by Keszler,[29] minimizes the risk of total consolidation, improves the safety factor during the first days of ECLS, and appears to shorten the course of ECLS in newborn infants. Although initial concerns related to high MAP limited the application of this technique, it is now apparent that lung injury from airway pressure results from peak pressures >30 cm H_2O, and chronic distention at mean pressures of 10-20 cm H_2O is not damaging to normal or injured alveoli. ECLS is used primarily to sustain life during this period of severe lung dysfunction. In neonates, the lung function is usually limited by pulmonary vasoconstriction, which generally resolves in a few days for almost all patients. In children and adults, however, parenchymal lung disease often leads to total lung dysfunction for a period of days or weeks. Recovery is related to the amount of lung destruction and the resultant pulmonary fibrosis during the acute fibroproliferative phase of lung injury.[30]

Various methods have been proposed to minimize lung damage and fibrosis based on laboratory experiments, but currently there is no method to prevent progressive lung destruction aside from avoiding high ventilator settings. Almost all these patients are successfully managed with VV access. Therefore, when the lung has not functioned, the mixed venous saturation and the arterial saturation are identical and minimal end tidal CO_2 is detected. When pulmonary gas exchange is directly measured via the airway, the amount of oxygen and CO_2 exchanged via the native lung may range from 0-50% of total patient VO_2 and VCO_2. As lung function begins to return, an increase in arterial saturation is seen between venous and arterial blood, some aeration is evident on chest radiograph, and CO_2 appears in the ventilating gas. When direct measurements are made, it is common to see 20-40% of total gas exchange occurring through the native lung 3-7 days after the initiation of ECLS. When native lung gas exchange is <20% of the total patient gas exchange by day 7, the prognosis for lung recovery is poor. Nonetheless, cases have been seen in which lung gas exchange function was minimal for periods of up to four weeks and the patient ultimately recovered. Current research is aimed at identifying patients with poor lung function who will ultimately recover or die of progressive fibrosis. Management of the lung during this period of severe malfunction is aimed at recruiting alveoli when possible, but avoiding further ventilator-induced long injury. This is accomplished by maintaining MAP in the range of 10-20 cm H_2O, strictly limiting peak airway pressure to <40 cm H_2O, and maintaining FiO_2 <50%. Conventional methods of managing the severely injured lung including prone positioning, postural drainage, maintenance at dry weight, full nutrition, and bronchoscopy as needed.

Pulmonary vascular resistance is an important indicator of the prognosis for lung recovery.[31] Even though hypoxic vasoconstriction is at its maximum in the totally consolidated lung, pulmonary vascular resistance is only slightly elevated. Of course, this is only significant during VV bypass, because the full cardiac output is passing through the pulmonary circulation as well as the systemic circulation. For this reason, even if cardiac output is not directly measured, a comparison of the mean systemic artery pressure to the mean pulmonary artery pressure affords a direct comparison of the relationship between systemic and pulmonary vascular resistance. Normally, the systemic vascular resistance is 25 mm $Hg/l/m^2$ and the normal pulmonary vascular resistance is 3 mm $Hg/l/m^2$ corresponding to a mean pulmonary artery pressure 20 mm Hg, wedge pressure of 10 mm Hg, and cardiac index of 3 $l/m^2/min$. During total lung consolidation the pulmonary artery pressure may rise from 3-6 Wood units (with mean pulmonary artery pressure $\leq$30) and may be sustained at this level for several days. If progressive lung destruction and fibrosis occurs, this fibrosis eventually obliterates the pulmonary capillary bed and pulmonary vascular resistance rises to systemic levels. Right ventricular failure occurs and it is virtually impossible to resuscitate the heart, even on full VV bypass. For all these reasons, the ratio between pulmonary and systemic mean blood pressure during ECLS has become a valuable indicator of the likelihood of lung recovery.

During prolonged, uncomplicated ECLS, function of other vital organs is maintained. Specifically, kidney, liver, host defenses, brain, and gut functions remain normal as long as the primary disease does not affect physiology of these organs.

Weaning and decannulation

Indicators of lung recovery include increasing PaO_2 or decreasing $PaCO_2$ without changing ventilator or ECLS settings, increased VO_2 or VCO_2 measured via the airway, increasing lung compliance, and a clearing chest radiograph. Indicators of cardiac recovery include increasing

SvO_2 with no change in VO_2 or other parameters, increasing pulse contour, and improving contractility detected by echocardiography.

When native lung or cardiac function improves, extracorporeal flow is gradually decreased, allowing the native lung to carry more of the load. When 70-80% of the gas exchange is occurring via the native lung (i.e., the extracorporeal flow rate is 20-30% of the initial flow rate), the patient should be trialed off bypass at moderate ventilator settings. In VA bypass, the tubing leading to the patient is clamped, permitting continuing circulation through a bridge. If gas exchange and perfusion are adequate, the catheters can be removed, usually after another period of low flow bypass, to be sure that lung function will be maintained. In VV bypass, a trial off bypass is attempted by capping off gas flow to the membrane lung but continuing extracorporeal flow. With this arrangement, the venous saturation monitor becomes a useful guide to the adequacy of systemic oxygen delivery during the trial.

Using these simple physiologic principles of management, extracorporeal circulation can be maintained in the absence of pulmonary function for 1-6 weeks.

Summary

ECMO represents gas exchange physiology in its purest form. It requires the operators of this technology to be skilled in all aspects of critical care and have a firm grasp of the physiologic principles of the cardio-respiratory system. A thorough understanding of the principles presented in this chapter provides the foundation of knowledge necessary for all who participate in the care for patients on ECLS.

References

1. Bartlett RH and Cilley RE. Physiology of Extracorporeal Life Support. In: Arensman RM, Cornish JD, eds. *Extracorporeal Life Support*. Boston: Blackwell Scientific Publications, 1993:89-104.
2. Bartlett RH. Extracorporeal Life Support for Cardiopulmonary Failure. *Curr Probl Surg*. 1990; 27:621-705.
3. Zwischenberger JB, Alpard SK, Conrad SA, Johnigan RH, Bidani A. Arteriovenous carbon dioxide removal: development and impact on ventilator management and survival during severe respiratory failure. *Perfusion* 1999; 14:299-310.
4. Bartlett RH and Delius RE. Physiology and Pathophysiology of Extracorporeal Circulation. In: Kay PH, ed. *3rd Edition of Techniques in Extracorporeal Circulation*, London: Butterworths, 1992:8-32.
5. Galletti PM, Richardson PD, Snider MT. A standardized method for defining the overall gas transfer performance of artificial lungs. *Trans Am Soc Artif Intern Organs* 1972; 18:359-368,374.
6. Pesenti A, Gattinoni L, Kolobow T, Damia G. Extracorporeal circulation in adult respiratory failure. *Trans Am Soc Artif Intern Organs* 1988; 34:43-47.
7. Montoya JP, Merz SI, Bartlett RH. A standardized system for describing flow/pressure relationships in vascular access devices. *Trans Am Soc Artif Intern Organs* 1991; 37:4-8.
8. Delius RE, Montoya JP, Merz SI, et al. A new method for describing the performance of cardiac surgery cannulas. *Ann Thorac Surg* 1992; 53:278-281.
9. Tamari Y, Lee-Sensiba K, Leonard EF, Parnell V, Tortolani AJ. The effects of pressure and flow on hemolysis caused by Bio-Medicus centrifugal pumps and roller pumps. Guidelines for choosing a blood pump. *J Thor Cardiovasc Surg* 1993; 106:997-1007.
10. Pedersen TH, Videm V, Svenning JL, et al. Extracorporeal membrane oxygenation using a centrifugal pump and a servo regulator to prevent negative inlet pressure. *Ann Thorac Surg* 1997; 63:1333-1339.
11. Butruille Y, Chevallet J, Granger A, et al. Rhone-Poulenc oxygenator and associated pumping system. In: Zapol WM, Qvist J, eds. *Artificial Lungs for Acute Respiratory Failure*. New York: Academic Press, 1976: 223.
12. Montoya JP, Merz SI, Bartlett RH. Laboratory experience with a novel non-occlusive, pressure-regulated, peristaltic blood pump. *ASAIO J* 1992; 38:M406-411.
13. Rudy LW, Heyman MA, Edmunds LH Jr. Distribution of systemic blood flow during cardiopulmonary bypass. *J Appl Physiol* 1973; 34:194-200.
14. Boucher JK, Rudy LW, Edmunds LH Jr. Organ blood flow during pulsatile cardiopulmonary bypass. *J Appl Physiol* 1974; 36:86-90.
15. Tominaga R, Smith WA, Massiello A, Harasaki H, Golding LA. Chronic nonpulsatile blood flow. I. Cerebral autoregulation in chronic nonpulsatile biventricular bypass: carotid blood flow response to hypercapnia. *J Thor Cardiovasc Surg* 1994; 108:907-912.
16. Bernstein EF, Cosentino LC, Reich S, et al: A compact low hemolysis non-thrombogenic system for non-throacotomy prolonged left ventricular bypass. *Trans Am Soc Artif Intern Organs* 1974; 20B:643-652.
17. Golding LR, Murakami G, Harasaki H, et al. Chronic non-pulsatile blood flow. *Trans Am Soc Artif Intern Organs* 1982; 28:81-85.
18. Kolobow T, Rossi F, Borellim M, Foti G. Long term closed chest partial and total cardiopulmonary bypass by peripheral cannulation for severe right and/or left ventricular failure including ventricular fibrilla-

tion. The use of a percutaneous spring in the pulmonary artery position to decompress the left heart. *ASAIO Trans* 1988; 34:485-489.

19. Kolobow T, Borell M, Spatola R, Tsumo K, Prato P. Single catheter venovenous membrane lung bypass in the treatment of experimental ARDS. *ASAIO Trans* 1988; 34:35-38.

20. Durandy Y, Chevalier JY, Lecompte Y. Single-cannula venovenous bypass for respiratory membrane lung support. *J Thorac Cardiovasc Surg* 1990; 99:404-409.

21. Kolla S, Crotti S, Lee A, Gargulinski et al. Total respiratory support with tidal flow extracorporeal circulation in adult sheep. *ASAIO J* 1997; 43:M811-M816.

22. Cornish JD, Heiss KF, Clark RH, Strieper MJ, Boecler B, Kesser K. Efficacy of venovenous extracorporeal membrane oxygenation for neonates with respiratory and circulatory compromise. *J Pediatr* 1993; 122:105-109.

23. Holley DG, Short BL, Karr SS, Martin GR. Mechanisms of change in cardiac performance in infants undergoing extracorporeal membrane oxygenation. *Crit Care Med* 1994; 22:1865-1870.

24. Gauger PG, Hirschl RB, Delosh TN, Dechert RE, Tracy T, Bartlett RH: A matched pairs analysis of venoarterial and venovenous ECLS in neonatal respiratory failure. *ASAIO J* 1995; 41:M573-M579.

25. Hicks RE, Dutton RC, Ries CA, Price DC, Edmunds LH Jr. Production and fate of platelet aggregate emboli during venovenous perfusion. *Surg Forum* 1973; 24:250-252.

26. Whittlesey GC, Kundu SY, Salley SO, Nowlen TT, Klein MD. Is heparin necessary for extracorporeal circulation? *ASAIO Trans* 1988; 34:823-826.

27. Meliones JN, Moler FW, Custer JR, et al. Hemodynamic instability after the initiation of extracorporeal membrane oxygenation: role of ionized calcium. *Crit Care Med* 1991; 19:1247-1251.

28. Rich PB, Awad SS, Crotti S, Hirschl RB, Bartlett RH, Schreiner RJ. A prospective comparison of atrio-femoral and femoro-atrial flow in adult venovenous extracorporeal life support. *J Thorac Cardiovasc Surg* 1998; 116:628-32.

29. Keszler M, Subramanian KN, Smith YA, et al. Pulmonary management during extracorporeal membrane oxygenation. *Crit Care Med* 1989; 17:495-500.

30. Pratt PC, Vollmer RT, Shelburne JD, Crapo JD: Pulmonary morphology in a multihospital collaborative extracorporeal membrane oxygenation project. I. Light microscopy. *Am J Pathol* 1979; 95:191-214.

31. Ichiba S, Dechert R, Bartlett RH. Pulmonary/systemic arterial pressure correlates with outcome in severe respiratory failure. (In preparation.)

3

Coagulation, Anticoagulation, and the Interaction of Blood and Artificial Surfaces

Gail M. Annich, M.S., M.D. and Judiann Miskulin, M.D.

Introduction

The first successful clinical application of extracorporeal perfusion occurred on May 6, 1953, in Philadelphia when Dr. John Gibbon closed an atrial septal defect in Cecelia Bovalak using a heart-lung machine that he and his wife developed.[1] Early operations using extracorporeal perfusion were associated with high morbidity and mortality, in large part because of the consequences of blood contact with the wound and biomaterials in the perfusion circuit. To minimize the side effects of cardiopulmonary bypass (CPB), perfusion times were made as short as possible, but open-heart surgery still caused unique bleeding, fluid, and systemic complications that could not be avoided. CPB was itself an acute "inflammatory multi-systemic disease" and therefore was not considered to be a technology appropriate for long-term circulatory or respiratory support. In 1968, with the development of the Bramson lung (one of the first membrane oxygenators), J.D. Hill and his colleagues used prolonged extracorporeal perfusion to support and save the life of a young cyclist who had developed acute respiratory insufficiency after trauma.[2] This was the beginning of ECLS as we know it. However, to this day, the ability to completely control the interaction between blood and the biomaterials of the extracorporeal circuitry

remains challenging and a barrier to its wider use for highly complex conditions.

During open-heart surgery, the entire blood mass is exposed to the biomaterials of the perfusion circuitry and also to the non-endothelial cells in the wound. Under normal circumstances, blood proteins and cells only interface at the endothelium, which simultaneously maintains the integrity of the vascular system and the normal flow of blood. Endothelial cells maintain this delicate balance in blood, between thrombosis and anticoagulation (hemostasis), by producing both anticoagulants and procoagulants. However, when circulating blood comes into contact with non-endothelial surfaces, be that artificial (CPB circuit) or biological (surgical wound), coagulation is initiated, and if this exposure is ongoing, all of the blood components involved in the body's defense reaction are activated. This intense and explosive reaction of the blood elements results in a massive whole-body inflammatory response.[3]

Although likened to CPB, ECLS differs significantly from open-heart surgery or ventricular assist devices (VADs). The two main differences are the duration of extracorporeal support and the amount of blood exposed to non-endothelial surfaces per unit of time. CPB for cardiac surgery continuously exposes the entire circulating blood volume to the wound and a significant area of the artificial biomaterial circuitry for a few hours or less. Large doses of heparin are required to prevent clotting, and essentially all elements in the blood are activated during this time. VADs expose circulating blood to a relatively small area of the artificial surface. Initially, the amount of blood exposed to the wound varies; however, once the device is placed, the wound blood is not circulated and the non-endothelial surface area of exposure is small. ECLS systems expose part of the blood volume to a large surface area of artificial biomaterial circuitry, but little to no wound blood is circulated. Therefore, some heparin is necessary to prevent clotting within the extracorporeal circuit, but less than that required in CPB because the stimulus to blood component activation is less.

The basic mechanisms of blood protein and cellular activation during different applications of extracorporeal perfusion are identical, but the intensity of these reactions will vary depending upon the duration of the stimuli, the type of anticoagulants, patient variability, and type of artificial circuitry. Activation refers to conversion of blood zymogens to active enzymes, expression of blood cellular receptors, initiation of cell signaling, and release of vasoactive and cytotoxic substances. With long-term applications, a new equilibrium must be reached between activated blood elements and the body's ability to remove and control these substances. The patient's ability to neutralize cell signaling, vasoactive, and cytotoxic substances; to replace consumed cells and proteins; to repair damage; and to restore homeostasis is influenced by age, comorbidities, organ reserves, and other factors.

Much of the present knowledge about ECLS physiology comes from studies of short-term CPB and open-heart surgery. The collective experience with ECLS is ever increasing and expanding and is now beginning to contribute to this knowledge. Although current technology does not allow much control of the blood non-endothelial surface, the understanding of the pathogenesis and chemical dynamics at this interface is increasing and new methods, surfaces, and drugs are actively under investigation. Thus, ECLS is a treatment modality which has the potential to extend the lives of patients who would otherwise succumb from severe but potentially reversible diseases or injuries. This chapter reviews current knowledge about the interactions between blood and the artificial surfaces of ECLS support devices, current anticoagulation management on ECLS, and future systemic anticoagulation and surface technologies.

Pathophysiology of the blood-surface interaction

During ECLS, blood is circulated via a mechanical pump and is independent of physiological controls. This system is in parallel with the native heart. The native heart is responsive to physiologic controls but is only partially utilized, either because of disease or lack of inflow. Mechanisms that normally maintain physiologic homeostasis are disrupted. Intravascular pressures fluctuate outside normal ranges, fluid shifts occur with the extracellular compartment, and capillary permeability increases. ECLS decreases systemic vascular resistance, but this varies between patients. Fluid accumulates in the interstitial space with surprisingly little intracellular accumulation.[4,5] With alterations in temperature, acid-base balance, blood and extracellular fluid volume, and changes in vasomotor tone caused by circulation of vasoactive substances, many physiologic reflexes are modified or negated.[5,6] Pulse pressure will often be attenuated or even obliterated, although its absence causes little harm according to long-term studies of pulseless circulation.[7] At a core temperature of 37°C, pulse pressure does not alter the distribution of blood flow during extracorporeal circulation;[8] however, regardless of pulsatility, blood flow to the stomach, intestines, and adrenal glands is increased during ECLS.[9]

Contact with synthetic, non-endothelial cell surfaces, shear stresses, turbulence, cavitation, and osmotic forces directly injures blood.[10] Surface charge is important in the repulsion or attraction of various charged blood components. The presence or absence of specific chemical groups, the surface tension, wettability of the polymer, and the presence of fillers and plasticizers all contribute to the reaction.[11] Whether the morphology of the surface is smooth, pitted, or rough at both the macroscopic and microscopic level is also important. The rheological pattern of blood flow across the polymer (with laminar flow being uncommon), the presence or absence of stagnation flow points and vortical flow patterns, or a blood-air interface will also contribute to the reaction and the fate of the surface.[11] In addition to these flow dynamics, the effect of shear rate on platelets and other components of coagulation is also critically important. The higher the shear rate, the more platelet deposition and less fibrin deposition, while at lower shear rates the reverse occurs. With respect to shear rates and its effect on the coagulation cascade, factor Xa generation by tissue factor (TF): VIIa is augmented with increases in shear rate.

Plasma proteins and lipoproteins are progressively denatured during ECLS.[12] Protein denaturation increases plasma viscosity, produces macromolecules, decreases protein solubility, and increases protein reactive side groups. Plasma IgG, IgA, IgM, and albumin decrease more than expected from hemodilution.[13] Red blood cells (RBCs) develop reversible echinocytic changes, but some are also hemolyzed by shear forces and activation complement.[14,15] Roller pumps cause more hemolysis than centrifugal pumps[16] although with improved technology this is less of an issue. Platelets and white blood cells (WBCs) are also injured during perfusion, but the consequences of activation of these cells far outweigh the effects of direct injury. These whole-body responses are important to know, as they result from the molecular and cellular activation of blood and its components.

Initial events

As soon as surface contact is made, plasma proteins are instantly adsorbed (<1 second) from heparinized blood onto all non-endothelial cell surfaces to form a monolayer of bound proteins.[17-19] For a specific protein, the amount adsorbed depends upon its concentration in plasma and, as mentioned above, the intrinsic surface activity of the biomedical surface. The specificities of each biomaterial surface for each plasma protein produce an infinite number of adsorbed proteins that are unique for each biomaterial and each patient-specific combination of plasma proteins. The physical and chemical composition of the polymer determines which proteins are most likely to adhere to that surface, which will not necessarily be the proteins of greatest concentration within the plasma. In addition, as every extracorporeal circuit is made up of a variety of different biomaterials, when assessing adsorbed proteins on the various surfaces, the chemical, physical, and morphological properties of each polymer surface must be considered.[11,20]

Adsorbed proteins compete for space on the biomaterial surface, are tightly packed, irreversibly bound, and immobile. The density of adsorbed proteins is 2-3 times greater than the density of proteins calculated within the plasma. Fibrinogen is one of the main proteins adsorbed by most artificial surfaces; it adheres more selectively to hydrophobic rather than hydrophilic materials. These surfaces are constantly changing their protein layer with each pass of blood volume across them (Figure 1). Added to this complexity is the fact that as proteins adhere to the surface, they can undergo specific conformational changes[21,22] that may expose receptor amino acid groups that are recognized by specific blood cells or plasma proteins such as factor XII, complement protein 3, or platelets.[20] For a given adsorbed protein, these uncontrolled conformational changes may vary between biomaterial surfaces and, in turn, vary the reactivity of the adsorbed protein with cells and blood proteins. In contrast, endothelial cells selectively bind specific proteins using specialized receptors in response to cellular signals regulating anticoagulants and procoagulants.

The relative concentrations and topography of these adsorbed proteins affect the thrombogenicity of the surface. Biomaterials vary in thromboresistance, but all eventually stimulate clot formation. The reactivity of surface proteins of the adsorbed layer[23] suggests that the thrombogenic stimulus of biomaterial surfaces varies with time. Little is known about the flux of surface-adsorbed proteins over time in extracorporeal perfusion systems.

Activation of blood elements

ECLS activates at least 6 plasma protein systems and 5 blood cell types as blood passes through the extracorporeal circuit. Much of the morbidity associated with ECLS results from the formation of circulating microemboli, activated enzymes, cell signaling, and the production of vasoactive and cytotoxic substances by these activated plasma protein systems and cells (Table 1). It is, therefore, worthwhile to understand the basics

of these systems in order to understand how to manage the ECLS patient.

Coagulation cascade

Activation of the coagulation cascade occurs immediately with exposure of the blood to non-endothelial cells via surgery and cannulation wounds and as the blood makes contact with the artificial circuit. To break it down, a series of systems and pathways become activated which are both procoagulant and anticoagulant with the end result of an increased propensity for thrombus formation. These pathways can be categorized into 4 basic groups: contact system, extrinsic pathway, intrinsic pathway, and common pathway. There is great complexity and overlap in their functions, but for simplicity this section will focus on the general aspects which influence ECLS (Figure 2).

Contact system

Four proteins – factor XII, prekallikrein (PK), high-molecular-weight-kininogen (HMWK), and C1-inhibitor (C1-INH) – have been shown to play major roles for the activation and inhibition of the surface-mediated

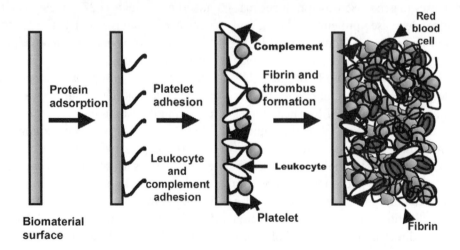

Figure 1. Simplistic representation of the blood-surface interaction during ECLS. This shows the components relevant to thrombosis and even though complement and leukocytes are considered to be involved with inflammation, they are also very relevant participants in thrombosis formation.

Table 1. Cellular and plasma protein systems altered/activated by CPB, open-heart surgery, and ECLS.

Vasoactive substances	• Epinephrine, norepinephrine, dopamine • Vasopressin, bradykinin • Angiotensin II, renin
Cytotoxic substances	• Gamma interferon, TNF α • Interleukin 1-β, 6, 8, 10, 13
Cellular signaling/binding	• Complement 3a, 4a, 5a, leukotriene LTB4 • Histamine, serotonin • Ca^{2+}, K^+, Mg^{2+} • Monocyte chemotactic protein-1, endothelin-1 • Prostacyclin, nitric oxide, PGE_2 • Platelet activating factor, thromboxane A_2 • P-selectin, platelet microparticles
Hormonal	• Corticosteroids, aldosterone • Thyroxine, triiodothyronine • Glucagon • Atrial naturetic factor

In all likelihood plasma concentrations of many of these substances probably return to or toward normal as ECLS continues over days to weeks.

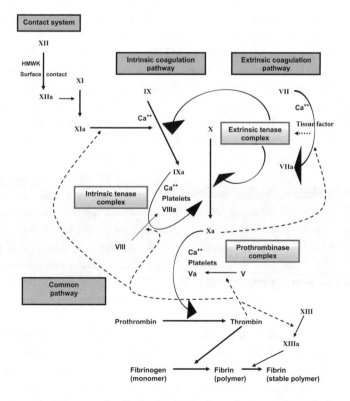

Figure 2. The coagulation cascade. Both the intrinsic pathway and extrinsic pathway lead to the formation of the prothrombinase complex, the common pathway which catalyzes the conversion of prothrombin to thrombin, and fibrinogen to fibrin. The principal pathway stimulated during ECLS is thought to be the intrinsic pathway.

pathway, the "contact system."[24] The role of this system in the initiation of the intrinsic pathway is unclear, as only the deficiency of factor XI causes hemorrhagic abnormalities whereas deficiencies in the contact proteins (factor XII, HMWK, and PK) have not.[11,25-27] It is likely that this system primarily initiates the inflammatory response, complement activation, fibrinolysis, angiogenesis and kinin formation.[24,28,29] The involvement of factor XII in the activation of factor XI is by the binding of factor XII to negatively-charged surfaces which are limited in vivo. The heavy chain of factor XII binds to the surface causing a local increase in the enzyme concentration, autoactivation (XIIa formation), and resultant action on its substrates PK and factor XI to form kallikrein and XIa.[24,30] Factor XIa activates the intrinsic pathway and the formation of the intrinsic tenase complex factor IXa-factor VIIIa. It is noteworthy that factor XI can also be activated by thrombin once the coagulation cascade has been activated.

Factor XIIa also cleaves PK. The cleavage of PK forms kallikrein, and this creates a feedback loop whereby further cleavage of factor XII is accelerated.[31] Kallikrein is also a strong agonist for neutrophil activation. Both HMWK and C1-INH bind to the light chain of kallikrein.[24,32-34] When C1-INH binds to kallikrein, its enzymatic activity is rapidly inactivated, whereas when HMWK binds to kallikrein, it protects kallikrein from the inhibitory effects of C1-INH and other plasma protease inhibitors.[24] The cleavage of HMWK by kallikrein forms bradykinin and activated HMWK, which binds to the surface with 10-fold greater affinity than its cofactor, enhances PK and fibrinolysis activity, and inhibits angiogenesis.[24] It is clear that the activation of factor XI by factor XIIa is a minor event in the initiation of the contact system, and it is well known that deficiencies in factor XII have not been associated with abnormal bleeding. This suggests a more integrally-related coagulation cascade with the extrinsic and intrinsic pathways interacting with one another, rather than independently initiating thrombin formation.

Intrinsic coagulation pathway

The intrinsic system could be defined as coagulation which is initiated by components contained entirely within the vascular system.[24] It has a primary role in the propagation phase of the cascade. Classically, the initiation of the intrinsic pathway has been described as the activation of factor IX by factor XIa in the presence of Ca^{2+}, providing a pathway for fibrin formation which is independent of factor VII. Factor IXa can also be activated by factor VIIa, and this activation requires Ca^{2+} as well as TF embedded within a lipid bilayer (cell membrane). Once factor IX is activated in the presence of calcium, phospholipids, and activated factor VIII (VIIIa), it produces the intrinsic tenase complex (Figure 2).[35,36] The intrinsic tenase complex binds with factor X and activates it (factor Xa). It is a significant contributor to thrombin generation and a primary factor in the cascade's propagation phase.

Once factor X is activated, it slowly cleaves prothrombin to produce thrombin; however, this reaction becomes 300,000 times faster when Xa is anchored by factor Va in the presence of Ca^{2+} onto a phospholipid surface provided by platelets, monocytes, or endothelial cells.[37,38] This complex is called the prothrombinase complex and initiates the activation of the common pathway. Factor V is activated by either factor Xa or thrombin (Figure 2).

Extrinsic system

The principal activation of the coagulation system in vivo is the extrinsic pathway, which involves both blood and vascular elements. In the absence of a major wound, however, the extrinsic coagulation pathway is a lesser stimulus to clotting during ECLS. The most critical component to the activation is TF, an intrinsic membrane protein that functions as a cofactor to factor VIII in the intrinsic system and to factor V in the common pathway. TF is synthesized by macrophages and endothelial cells; this synthesis is induced by cytokines such as interleukin-1 (IL-1), endotoxins, and tumor necrosis factor (TNF).[24,39-41] It is expressed on vascular sub-endothelium and many other cells such as stimulated monocytes and endothelial cells.[42-44]

The major plasma component to the extrinsic system is factor VII, one of the vitamin K-dependent prozymogens (the others being factors IX, X, prothrombin, and protein C). The importance of vitamin K-dependent factors is that they have the ability, once activated, to remain membrane-bound and to also facilitate other reactions in the presence of appropriate cofactors.[24] As a wound is created, TF is expressed and rapidly binds to and converts factor VII to factor VIIa, creating the TF/FVIIa complex or extrinsic tenase complex. This complex, which then forms upon either activated monocytes or perturbed endothelial cells, has 2 main substrates it acts upon, factor IX and factor X,[24] and it then initiates the activation of the common pathway.

As stated above, this pathway plays a minimal role in thrombus formation during ECLS unless a major wound is present; however, it must be noted that as ECLS continues over time, monocytes increase their expression of TF and, thus, the formation of the extrinsic tenase complex, which is responsible for the onset of coagulation.

Common pathway

As the extrinsic tenase complex cleaves either factor IX or X, these serine proteases remain membrane- or phospholipid-bound. The cofactor necessary for factor IXa to catalyze the conversion of factor X to factor Xa is factor VIII, while the cofactor for the factor Xa conversion of prothrombin to thrombin is factor V. Factor VIII exists in plasma, primarily as a noncovalent complex with von Willebrand factor (VWF). Factor V is supplied by activated platelets and is either excreted from the α-granules or fuses with the platelet membrane to bind factor Xa to the platelet, forming the prothrombinase complex and thereby activating the common coagulation pathway by the cleavage of prothrombin (Figure 2).

The cleavage of prothrombin produces α-thrombin and a useful maker of the reaction, protein fragment F1.2. Thrombin is a powerful enzyme known for its procoagulant functions by the cleavage of fibrinogen and activation of platelets, but it must be noted that its formation also leads to anticoagulant activity by the activation of protein C, the stimulation of endothelial cells to produce prostacyclin, and tissue plasminogen activator (t-PA) which initiates fibrinolysis.[11,45,46] In addition, it is also involved in cellular proliferation and inflammation. Within the common pathway, however, thrombin's specific role is to cleave fibrinopeptides, activate factor XIII, potentiate the effects of factor VIII and V, and activate protein C and factor XI.

As aforementioned, thrombin cleaves fibrinogen (i.e., fibrinopeptides). The formation of fibrin strands or monomers is the second phase of hemostasis (the first being platelet aggregation). Fibrinogen is present in high concentrations within plasma and platelet granules and interacts with many different proteins. During ECLS, fibrinogen is one of the more preferentially bound proteins, especially to hydrophobic surfaces.[11] Thrombin binds to the central domain of fibrinogen, cleaving it into fibrinopeptides A and B and producing monomers and polymers of fibrin. These fibrin monomers and polymers interact side-to-side and laterally to form a fibrin mesh which is then crosslinked by factor XIIIa to form a stable hemostatic plug. Add to this the potentiation of factors VIII and V, which produces more tenase and prothrombinase complexes, and the result is a burst in thrombin activity and fibrin formation. For ECLS, this means clot or thrombus formation.

Physiologic inhibitors of coagulation

In order to control the coagulation cascade, plasma contains several protease inhibitors to modulate and inhibit serine proteases. Some of the commonly known are α_1-protease inhibitor, α_2-macroglobulin, heparin cofactor II, and antithrombin III (AT III). AT III is the most important of these as it neutralizes both factor Xa and thrombin by forming a complex with the enzymes and blocking their active sites.[11] AT III also inhibits factor IXa, XIa, and XIIa. Under the conditions of ECLS, this inhibition by complex formation continues but is physiologically too slow to prevent thrombosis unless other agents innate to the endothelium catalyze AT III activity (see anticoagulation section).

Other important inhibitors of coagulation are tissue factor protease inhibitor (TFPI), thrombomodulin, protein C, and protein S. TF-VIIa is not inhibited efficiently by AT III, and therefore has its own inhibitor, TFPI, which has its largest pool present on the luminal surface of the vascular endothelium. However, it is also present in the plasma, 10% in the platelets, and is released by activated monocytes. It has 2 binding sites: one for factor Xa and one for the TF-VIIa complex. However, this inhibition cannot prevent thrombosis when TF-VIIa complexes are being formed at a high rate, such as during ECLS.

The endothelium itself participates in thrombosis regulation via thrombomodulin. Thrombin binds to thrombomodulin on endothelial cells, and the formation of this complex activates protein C, a vitamin K-dependent protein that inactivates factor Va and VIIIa. In order for protein C to function, its cofactor, protein S, another vitamin K-dependent protein, must be present. Once again, this system of thrombosis regulation is inadequate to prevent thrombus formation within the ECLS circuitry.

Fibrinolysis

Fibrinolysis resembles the coagulation cascade with involvement of zymogen-to-enzyme conversions and feedback loops for potentiation and inhibition. Plasminogen is one of the main zymogens in plasma responsible for fibrinolysis, and thrombin is one of the main activators of this system. Thrombin activates protein C, and this activation results in the destruction of Va and VIIIa, thereby reducing the production of tenase and prothrombinase complexes. Thrombin also stimulates endothelial cells to produce t-PA. T-PA binds avidly to fibrin and cleaves plasminogen to plasmin, resulting in the cleavage of fibrin by plasmin. The protein fragment produced from fibrin cleavage is a D-dimer, a useful marker of fibrinolysis. F1.2, D-dimer, and fibrinopeptide A (produced by the conversion of fibrinogen to fibrin) increase during extracorporeal perfusion, indicating ongoing thrombin production, fibrin formation, and lysis,[46,47] which represent a consumptive coagulopathy.

As with all other pathways of the coagulation system, fibrinolysis is regulated by a feedback loop controlled by the native protease inhibitors: α_2-antiplasmin, α_2-macroglobulin, and plasminogen activator inhibitor-1. Plasminogen activator inhibitor-1, produced by endothelial cells, directly inhibits t-PA and urokinase, but little is produced during CPB and open-heart surgery. α_2-antiplasmin rapidly inhibits unbound plasmin and prevents the enzyme from circulating, but inhibits plasmin bound to fibrin poorly. α_2-macroglobulin is a slow inhibitor of plasmin.

In addition to fibrinolysis, plasmin is both an inhibitor and stimulator of platelets, depending upon concentration and temperature.[48] At high concentrations of plasmin, under normothermic conditions, platelets undergo conformational changes which result in the centralization of granules and internalization of GPIb receptors, but not the GPIIb/IIIa receptors.

Complement

The complement system is also activated during ECLS and is generally treated as part of the inflammatory response induced by ECLS. Like the coagulation system, it is comprised of 2 separate pathways that lead to a common pathway. Although both the coagulation cascade and complement cascade are discussed as separate entities, each interacts significantly to modulate the other's activity.[11,49,50] Table 2 summarizes the various interactions between complement and coagulation factors.

Both the alternative and classical complement pathways are activated during ECLS, and produce the gateway protease, C3b.[51,52] The classical pathway is activated by various stimuli, many of which are known to be present or increased during ECLS (e.g., immune complexes, C-reactive protein, and endotoxins). One of these triggers binds the C1 complex, activating the C1s. This leads to C2 and C4 activation and ultimately to the formation of C3 convertase, which cleaves C3 into C3a and C3b.[53] C3b is the active enzyme which cleaves C5 to both C5a and C5b. C5a is a major agonist for neutrophils[54,55] and monocytes, while C5b initiates the formation of the terminal complement complex (TCC) by sequentially binding C6, C7, C8, and several molecules of C9.[56] TCC is capable of producing holes in cellular membranes, causing lysis and cell death. It also accelerates thrombin formation via its action on the prothrombinase complex.[57]

The alternative pathway does not require antibody or immune complexes for activation. It is activated by foreign surfaces, whether they be microbial organisms or elements, particles, or biomaterial surfaces. Complement activation via the alternative pathway occurs spontaneously at a low rate, but as hydrolyzed C3 is formed, factor B becomes activated and then initiates the cleavage of C3 to form C3a and C3b. During ECLS or CPB, with a biomaterial surface to bind C3b covalently to its hydroxyl or amine groups, factor B and D binding occurs, and the alternative C3 convertase (C3bBb) is formed, creating a positive amplification loop. Properdin stabilizes the C3 convertase, and the clustering of C3b on the surface allows the formation of C5 convertase (C5b), with the assembly of TCC to follow as in the classical pathway.[11]

Biomaterial surfaces can be described as either activating (having hydroxyl or amino groups present) or non-activating (negatively charged with carboxyl or sulfate groups, or bound heparin)[11,58] surfaces and complement activation during ECLS or CPB is likely dependent upon the binding of either factor H (cofactor for Factor I which inhibits C4b and C3b) or Factor B to the biomaterial. This is, however, not the entire explanation for complement activation, since even alleged non-activating surfaces such as polyacrylonitrile can activate

Table 2. Interactions between complement and coagulation elements.

Protein	Type of Interaction
Thrombin	Proteolysis of C3, C5, C6, and factor B
Factor XIIa	Proteolysis of C1r, C1s, and C3
Kallikrein	Proteolysis of C1, C5, and factor B
Antithrombin III	Protect RBCs from lysis by mC5b-9
Bb	Proteolysis of prothrombin
C3bBb	Proteolysis of prothrombin
C1 inhibitor	Inactivates FXIIa and kallikrein
S protein (vitronectin)	Stabilizes plasminogen activator inhibitor 1
C4b-binding protein	Binds to vitamin K-dependent protein S

Adapted from Gorbet MB, Sefton MV. Biomaterial-associated thrombosis: roles of coagulation factors, complement, platelets, and leukocytes. *Biomaterials* 2004; 25:5681-5703.

complement.[11] In addition to the chemical make up of the circuitry, membrane oxygenators are less activating than bubble oxygenators when used during ECLS or CPB.[59,60]

The intensity of complement activation varies with the biomaterials used in the perfusion circuit.[61] The heparin-protamine complex activates complement via the classical pathway.[62] C3a, C4a, and C5a produced by complement activation are anaphylatoxins which increase capillary permeability, produce vasodilatation, constrict bronchiolar smooth muscle, and stimulate release of histamine from mast cells.[6] C3a decreases cardiac contractility.[63] Complement is activated at the beginning of extracorporeal perfusion[64] and ECLS.[65] During open-heart surgery, anaphylatoxins increase progressively,[66] but the concentrations of anaphylatoxins following the initiation of ECLS have not been described.

Platelets

Platelets are the mainstay for hemostasis and preservation of vascular wall integrity. They are discoid-shaped, anuclear cellular fragments approximately 3-4 µm in size and are derived from megakaryocytes in the bone marrow. Minimal stimulation is necessary to activate platelets, and there are a wide range of agonists which cause platelet activation and adhesion through a multitude of pathways and receptors.[11] Platelets respond to minimal stimulation and become activated when they encounter a thrombogenic stimulus such as injured endothelium, subendothelium, or artificial surfaces. There are at least 5 physiologic responses that occur at the time of platelet activation:

1) Platelet release into the microenvironment (platelet factor 4, thrombospondin, ß-thromboglobulin, ADP, and serotonin) encouraging platelet chemotaxis and activation

2) P-selectin release and expression on the platelet membrane after α granule secretion; it mediates adhesion to neutrophils, monocytes, and lymphocytes

3) Initiation of the eicosanoid pathway resulting in the liberation of arachidonic acid, and the synthesis and release of prostaglandins and thromboxane B_2; all contribute to further platelet activation

4) Platelet shape change which promotes platelet-to-platelet contact and adhesion, as well as tenase and prothrombinase complex formation upon them

5) Formation of platelet microparticles (PMPs), rich in factor Va, platelet factor 3, and phosphatidyl serine, a phospholipid-like procoagulant; the role of PMPs is unclear, but in vitro they are shown to adhere to fibrinogen and fibrin enhancing further platelet aggregation[11,67]

Among the various platelet receptors for adhesion, GPIb and GPIIb/IIIa have the highest density on platelets and are important in the platelet surface interaction which occurs during ECLS. GPIb mediates the platelet interaction with VWF. It will not bind to plasma VWF unless ristocetin is present; however, it will bind to surface adsorbed or immobilized VWF. The adherence of platelets via GPIb to adsorbed VWF is dependent upon shear stress, which is necessary to provide the conformational change in VWF which allows binding to occur.[11]

GPIIb/IIIa (CD41/CD61) is the dominant platelet receptor, with 40-80,000 receptors present on resting platelets and another 20-40,000 present inside the platelets within the α granules and the membranes of the open canalicular system. It is an integrin receptor. Resting platelets with inactive GPIIb/IIIa have a low affinity for binding to adsorbed fibrinogen. Once the platelet is activated, and conformational shape change of the platelet occurs, the high-affinity binding site of GPIIb/IIIa is exposed and binding of soluble fibrinogen occurs, which in turn leads to platelet aggregation and platelet-leukocyte aggregates by the crosslinking of 2 GPIIb/IIIa receptors or by the crosslinking of GPIIb/IIIa with Mac-1 on the leukocyte The crosslink is made by fibrinogen.

Platelet activation and adhesion, as described above, is known to occur during both CPB and ECLS, as well as with vascular access catheters and grafts. Both adherent platelets and platelet microparticles are procoagulant in nature, and therefore provide continual, ongoing stimulus for the above-described physiologic platelet responses. The number of platelets that adhere to a surface is proportional to the amount of surface-adsorbed fibrinogen,[22] but this density can vary with the chemical and physical composition of the surface. For example, rough surfaces accumulate more platelets than smooth surfaces,[68] and fewer platelets adhere to polyurethane than to silicone rubber.[17] It is known that during ECLS platelet adhesion and aggregate formation reduce the circulating platelet count;[11] however, it should be noted that high consumption and formation of microemboli, rather than occlusive thrombi, can occur even in the event of minimal adhesion to the circuitry surface. As ECLS continues, adherent platelets detach, leaving fragments of platelet membrane behind; these will also detach and circulate. The circulating platelet pool during ECLS consists of decreased numbers of morphologically normal platelets, increased numbers of platelets at various stages of activation (e.g., pseudopod formation, degranulation, and membrane receptor loss), and new larger platelets released from the bone marrow. Bleeding times increase in the presence of structurally normal-appearing platelets[69-71] and as ECLS continues beyond 24 hours, platelet consumption continues.

Endothelial cells

Endothelial cells maintain the fluidity of blood and the integrity of the vascular system. They cover an estimated area of about ~1,000 m^2

in adults. Endothelial cells are activated during CPB by a variety of agonists such as thrombin, C5a[72], IL-1, and TNF.[46,73] Endothelial cells produce prostacyclin, heparin sulfate, t-PA, and TF pathway inhibitor, which regulates the extrinsic coagulation pathway. Thrombomodulin and protease nexin 1, both produced by endothelial cells, remove thrombin. Endothelial cells produce protein S, which is a necessary cofactor for normal Protein C function; protein C is a natural anticoagulant. Endothelial cells also produce vasoactive substances and cytokines such as nitric oxide (NO), prostacyclin, endothelin-1[6,74], IL-1, IL-6,[75] and platelet activating factor (PAF), as well as inactive substances such as histamine, norepinephrine, and bradykinin.[74] Prostacyclin concentrations increase rapidly at the start of CPB and then begin to decrease.[76] During open-heart surgery, endothelin-1 peaks several hours after CPB ends.[77]

Activation of endothelial cells during CPB stimulates expression of protein and cellular receptors, including TF and both P and E selectins. TF is procoagulant; P and E-selectins mediate rolling adhesion of neutrophils and monocytes to facilitate arrest and, eventually, transmigration of these cells to the extravascular space. VCAM-1 and ICAM-1 are endothelial cell integrins that serve as ligands for Mac-1 (CD11b/CD18) and α4β1 receptors on neutrophils and monocytes. Experimentally, ICAM-1 is up-regulated during CPB and in myocardial ischemia-reperfusion sequences; the roles of ICAM-1 and VCAM-1 are not clearly defined.

Leukocytes

Circulating leukocytes are comprised of neutrophils, monocytes, lymphocytes, basophils, and eosinophils. Neutrophils, monocytes, and lymphocytes are the main groups of cells involved in the inflammatory responses during ECLS. Contact with artificial surfaces activates both neutrophils and monocytes. Some of the indicators of this activation are L-selectin shedding and CD11b upregulation, which have been widely demonstrated in hemodialysis[11,78-80] and CPB,[11,81-86] as well as degranulation with the release of elastase and lactoferrin,[11] and the presence of cytokines such as IL-1 and TNFα, as seen in ECLS.[11]

ECLS-induced leukocyte activation also causes an increase in adhesion and a barrier to the leukocytes as the foreign material cannot be engulfed; therefore, an array of potent oxygen metabolites and proteolytic enzymes are released. The material characteristics of the artificial surfaces modulate the adsorption of proteins to the surface and therefore moderate the level of activation, depending upon which proteins are adsorbed. The presence of platelets on the surface may also mediate leukocyte adhesion via the interaction between P-selectin, GPIIb/IIIa, and CD11b.[11,87,88]

The mechanisms by which material-induced leukocyte activation and adhesion occurs during ECLS is unclear. What is known as pertains to neutrophils, monocytes, and lymphocytes follows.

Neutrophils

Neutrophils are the most abundant WBCs, representing 40-60% of the leukocyte population. Because of dilution, neutrophil counts decrease immediately after ECLS initiation and recover slowly thereafter. The principal agonists for activating neutrophils during ECLS are kallikrein and C5a.[59,84,126] Other agonists include factor XIIa, heparin, leukotriene B4, IL1-ß, IL-8, and TNFα. Many of the latter group are also released by activated neutrophils, enhancing the activation process. During ECLS, neutrophils release neutral proteases such as elastase, lysosomal enzymes, myeloperoxidase, hydrogen peroxide, hydroxyl radicals, hypochlorous acid, hypobromous acid, acid hydrolases, and collagenases. The released inflammatory mediators have various properties which include chemoattraction for leukocytes, promotion of adherence

to endothelial cells, further platelet activation, and ongoing mediation of the systemic inflammatory response to ECLS.[11,55,89,90]

During CPB and ECLS, neutrophils also express Mac-1 (CD11b/CD18) receptors, which bind neutrophils to endothelial cells and collagen.[91,92] It also binds factor X and fibrinogen and thus facilitates thrombin formation.[93] During CPB, activated neutrophils express both CD11c/CD18, which binds to fibrinogen and a complement fragment,[94] and L-selectin, a receptor for P-selectin that is expressed by endothelial cells, platelets, and α4ß1 receptors.

Both CPB and ECLS cause accumulation of activated neutrophils in pulmonary perivascular and interstitial tissue. This accumulation is associated with increased capillary permeability, interstitial edema, and large alveolar-arterial oxygen differences during and after perfusion.[90,95]

Monocytes

During open-heart surgery, monocytes are activated to express TF in both the wound and extracorporeal circuit,[96,97] but activation in the circuit is delayed for several hours.[37,38] Blood that is in contact with the surgical field contains higher concentrations of activated proteins from the extrinsic coagulation pathway and from monocytes expressing TF than from simultaneous samples taken from the extracorporeal circuit during CPB.[96] If the amount of field blood added to the perfusate is small, as in ECLS, the increase in the percentage of circulating monocytes expressing TF is low.[97] Agonists for activating monocytes during open-heart surgery include C5a, immune complexes, endotoxin, IL-6, γ-interferon, IL-1ß, TNFα, and monocyte chemotactic protein-1 (MCP-1). Except for C5a, immune complexes, and endotoxin, the other agonists are also produced by activated monocytes. The activated monocytes are found to express Mac-1, L-selectin, and MCP-1;[94,96,98,99] to form aggregates with platelets;[100] and to produce MCP-1, IL-1ß, IL-6, γ-interferon, and TNFα.[101-103] There is evidence that both CPB and open-heart surgery stimulate the production of these cytokines, but peak concentrations occur hours after CPB ends.[103-106]

Lymphocytes

Extracorporeal perfusion decreases the total number of lymphocytes and specific subsets of lymphocytes, particularly B lymphocytes, natural killer cells, helper T-cells, and T-suppressor lymphocytes.[107,108] It increases IL-1 synthesis and production of PGE_2, which act to inhibit certain T-cell lymphocytic functions and to inhibit macrophage antigens.[109] Lymphocyte responses to IL-2 and γ-interferon are attenuated, and CD4+ and IL-2 receptor expression is similarly downregulated. These changes are independent of blood transfusions[108] and indicate depression of the immune response. Corresponding changes in complement and immunoglobulins may also increase the risk of infection for ECLS patients. Lymphocyte counts usually recover within 5 days of weaning from ECLS; slower recovery is associated with a poor prognosis.[110] There are little data for ECLS; however, Kawahito et al. report that IL-6 and IL-10 are elevated in patients prior to beginning ECLS and decrease during ECLS.[106]

Anticoagulation

With all that is known about blood-surface interactions with artificial materials, heparin remains the primary anticoagulant for ECLS; however, it is far from ideal. It has the advantage of being swiftly reversed by protamine or platelet factor 4[111] and is widely available for parenteral use. Heparin accelerates the action of AT III approximately 1,000-fold, but does not prevent thrombin formation; it inhibits thrombin after it is formed. Heparin inhibits coagulation at the end of the coagulation cascade instead of the beginning; therefore, many powerful serine

proteases are already formed by the time heparin binds to AT III. Furthermore, the heparin-AT III complex only inhibits soluble thrombin and does not inhibit thrombin already bound to fibrin.[112] Heparin-catalyzed AT III weakly inhibits factor Xa and factor IXa, but these reactions are relatively slow compared to the inhibition of thrombin. Therefore, thrombin forms continuously and is circulated during ECLS when heparin, low molecular weight heparin (LMWH), or a heparinoid is used for anticoagulation.[113,114]

Standard (unfractionated) heparin has undesirable side effects. The drug activates several blood elements and may produce sometimes devastating allergic reaction in some patients. Heparin increases the sensitivity of platelets to various agonists.[115,116] Heparin is an agonist for factor XII,[117] complement, neutrophils, and monocytes.[118-120] Heparin-induced thrombocytopenia (HIT) occurs in 2-6% of patients (usually adults) who receive the drug; heparin-induced thrombocytopenia and thrombosis rarely occur, but causes catastrophic complications when they do.[121,122] Heparin is not an ideal anticoagulant for ECLS, but current alternatives also have drawbacks, and the vast experience with the use of heparin on ECLS continues to make it the first choice.

Several compounds are available or are in development as alternatives to standard heparin, but reported experience with alternatives in patients on ECLS is minimal.[123-125] LMWHs catalyze ATIII and are better Xa inhibitors than standard heparin,[49] but are weaker blockers of thrombin[126] and poorly reversed by protamine.[127,128] There is evidence that LMWH produces less microvascular bleeding than standard heparin. The plasma half-life is 2-4 times that of standard heparin.[126] Because of poor reversal by protamine, LMWH is contraindicated for open-heart surgery.[127] LMWH may cause HIT, but the incidence is less than with standard heparin.[121] Heparinoids contain dermatan sulfate alone or are mixed with chondrin sulfate and heparin sulfate, the natural heparin produced by endothelial cells. By itself, dermatan sulfate catalyzes heparin cofactor II, which is a direct thrombin inhibitor.[129] Heparinoids do not cause HIT and have been successfully used as an alternative for heparin during cardiac surgery.[130] The primary drawback preventing the approval for use of heparinoids in the U.S. is their long half-life and the fact that their anticoagulant effects cannot be reversed with protamine.

Many compounds have been investigated for anticoagulation efficacy. A large number of reversible and irreversible direct thrombin inhibitors are known[131] and a few have been used clinically during ECLS in patients with heparin allergy. Argatroban is a potent, reversible, direct inhibitor of both bound (fibrin) and unbound thrombin. It is an alternative anticoagulant for those patients with HIT or heparin allergy who require ECLS.[132] It has a short half-life (15-120 hours) and is excreted primarily through the feces. The drawbacks are that time to anticoagulation and steady state is anywhere from one-half to 3 hours, and monitoring is done using activated partial thromboplastin times (aPTT) and anti-IIa activity, with the goal anti IIa level around 1.0.[133] Another direct thrombin inhibitor is recombinant hirudin. It was initially identified as the anticoagulant which allows leeches to attach and remove blood from their host. It binds irreversibly to both bound and unbound thrombin.[123,124] It has a half-life of ~1.3 hours with normal renal function, but this can increase substantially into days with renal insufficiency. Again, as with argatroban, monitoring is done using aPTTs and anti-IIa activity.

Factor Xa is the gateway enzyme for the common coagulation pathway, as previously described. Edmunds et al. screened several potent factor Xa inhibitors in an in vitro model of ECLS.[125] The inhibitors tested included recombinant antistasin (Merck & Co, Whitehouse Station, NJ; Ki for FXa=0.3 nM), recombinant tick anticoagulant peptide (Merck; Ki for FXa=0.5 nM), ecotin (Genentech, South San Francisco, CA; Ki for FXa=54 pM), and boroarginine (DUP 714, E.I. du Pont de Nemours and Company, Wilmington, DE). Their studies all showed that these compounds failed to suppress thrombin formation or activity for any substantial benefit above that provided by standard or LMWH.

Spanier et al. have reported the successful use of a factor IXa inhibitor during thoracotomy and 90 minutes of CPB in a baboon animal model.[134] This inhibitor compound selectively inhibits the intrinsic coagulation pathway and not the extrinsic coagulation pathway, therefore allowing clotting for wound bleeding without thrombus formation within the extracorporeal circuit. This inhibitor may be suitable for ECLS, since the major stimulus for thrombin formation is from the blood-artificial surface interaction rather than a surgical wound.

During ECLS, the anticoagulant effect of heparin on whole blood is best monitored by the activated clotting time (ACT), as opposed to measurements of the effect of heparin on plasma (as measured by aPTT or thrombin time). ACT is a crude monitor of heparin anticoagulation, but the most practical, bedside method available.[135,136] Heparin preparations vary in anticoagulant effectiveness, and patients vary in their sensitivity to and metabolism of heparin.[137] After an initial bolus for cannulation (usually 100 units/kg body weight), a continuous infusion is started to maintain ACT between 180-200 seconds. This typically requires an infusion rate of 25-100 units/kg/hr; the ACT is measured every hour. Higher rates of heparin are required during periods of high urinary output and during platelet transfusions, since the heparin binds to platelets; lesser rates are needed during renal failure and thrombocytopenia. It is not recommended that heparin be withheld even if the upper ACT limit has been exceeded while on the lowest minimal heparin dose. Other causes of ACT elevation may need to be considered at this point (e.g., infection). Patients who receive heparin for a prolonged period (i.e., days) or are poorly nourished may become resistant due to AT III deficiency. Low AT III is treated with fresh frozen plasma transfusions. Additional heparin will be ineffective unless there is enough AT III available to catalyze. Lower levels of anticoagulation may reduce the potential for bleeding but increase the risk for thrombosis in the extracorporeal circuit. The clinician must keep in mind that during ECLS, thrombin is constantly generated and the fibrinolytic system is strongly activated; consequently, each patient on ECLS has some degree of consumptive coagulopathy and must be maintained within a narrow equilibrium between bleeding and thrombosis.[114,138] It must also be cautioned that as older ACT monitoring equipment is replaced by new equipment, ACT measures on the new device must be calibrated within a clinically acceptable range of variation to the device standard used previously.[139]

Consequences of blood activation during ECLS

Bleeding

Bleeding is defined as failure of blood to clot outside of blood vessels, and thrombosis the clotting of blood within vessels. Bleeding and thrombosis are pathologic poles of a spectrum of differing ratios of anticoagulants to procoagulants. Optimum ratios, which allow blood to clot and intravascular blood to flow, are near the center. This sensitive balance between procoagulants and anticoagulants must be well understood by those who manage patients on ECLS. CPB and ECLS produce consumptive coagulopathies that continue as long as blood circulates over non-endothelial cell surfaces. Only the quantities and ratios of anticoagulants and procoagulants vary in the tug-of-war between clotting and bleeding. Interventions to reduce non-surgical bleeding necessarily increase the likelihood that more thrombin will be generated and more fibrin formed. Similarly, therapy that

suppresses coagulation increases the possibility of bleeding.

Deficiency of soluble coagulation factors is a rare cause of bleeding after open-heart surgery, but is not rare in neonatal ECLS.[140] A Boston study discovered that 13 of 19 patients had severe reductions in 2 or more soluble coagulation proteins prior to beginning ECLS and that replacement therapy added to the priming volume did not correct the deficiency in 10 of these patients. Intracranial hemorrhage (ICH) in neonates during ECLS continues to be a major complication of the procedure and is a primary cause of permanent morbidity. Some ECLS centers give additional fresh frozen plasma (FFP) to the priming volume and periodic doses during ECLS.

Non-surgical bleeding complications associated with open-heart surgery are primarily related to heparin, platelets and their function, and fibrinolysis. Fibrinolysis has already been discussed. Heparin-related bleeding is caused by too much heparin or HIT. Heparin overdose is avoided by frequent measurement of ACT and periodic measurement of aPTT. HIT in ECLS patients is a complex and serious problem, particularly if associated with persistent bleeding, which is more common in adults than newborns.[141,142] Platelets are activated during ECLS, and circulating platelets are dysfunctional and are steadily consumed. The resultant bleeding requires platelet transfusion, but blood testing for HIT may be necessary if platelet counts remain low and bleeding continues. High titers of heparin-induced antibodies may cause heparin-induced thrombocytopenia and thrombosis (HITT) with devastating and often fatal complications.[143] If the patient is not bleeding, thrombocytopenia >100,000/μl is not treated. If the patient has HIT, heparin must be stopped and an alternative anticoagulant such as argatroban or recombinant hirudin must be considered. If platelet transfusions are given to patients with HIT but the heparin not removed, bleeding will not be controlled and intravascular (arterial, venous, or both) coagulation may occur.

Emboli and thrombi

Patients on ECLS are spared a variety of emboli that are aspirated from the wound and removed by filtration or washing during open-heart surgery. These emboli include fibrin, free fat, denatured lipoproteins, chylomicrons, platelet and leukocyte aggregates, red cell debris, and spallated biomaterial from roller pumps.[144] The major sources of emboli during ECLS are air, fibrin, platelet aggregates, emboli from blood and blood product transfusions, and the microemboli present in them.

Air emboli may originate from areas of low or sub-atmospheric pressure within the ECLS circuit. Both roller and centrifugal pumps produce negative pressure when venous inflow is obstructed.[145] Pinholes in tubing, cracked connectors, incompletely closed stopcocks, and poorly tied catheter ligatures may allow air to be entrained into the venous drainage circuit upstream of the pump. Membrane tears and excessive pressure in the gas phase of microporous membrane oxygenators are additional sources of air. Air emboli are less soluble in blood than oxygen emboli because of the very low solubility coefficient of nitrogen. On the other hand, CO_2 diffuses rapidly in blood. Massive air embolism usually results from errors in the operation of the perfusion system and can be catastrophic.

Donor blood, even after filtration, contains microemboli of platelets, leukocytes, lysed RBCs, fibrin, and lipid precipitates. Standard blood filters contain 170 μm sized pores and fail to remove most of the particulate emboli from citrated blood.[146] Smaller pore sizes impair blood flow and are not used. Because ACTs are usually maintained between 180-200 seconds, filters are not used in the outflow line during ECLS. At the concentrations of heparin used during ECLS, thrombin forms in areas of cavitation, turbulence, stagnant flow, connector seams, and before and after constrictions in the flow path.[147,148] Under certain conditions of flow, platelets and other non-red cells marginate.[1487] Thrombosis within the circuit is most likely during periods of low pump flow and when the heparin concentration is reduced.

Small arterial emboli lodge in arterioles and precapillaries. They cause death of only a few cells in any one location, and are therefore difficult to detect. During open-heart surgery, microemboli can be observed by retinal examination and sometimes by careful histology.[149,150] Venovenous (VV) ECLS uses the native lung as a filter and thus prevents most of the systemic cellular injury due to particulate and gaseous emboli.[151]

Organ dysfunction

Circulation of vasoactive, cell-signaling, and cytotoxic substances generated by the interaction between blood elements and the non-endothelial surfaces of the perfusion circuit produce an inflammatory response that increases interstitial fluid and causes temporary dysfunction of every organ. These consequences of blood activation from the contact with biomaterials mediate the morbidity of CPB and open-heart surgery. The effects of the duration of elevated concentrations of vasoactive and cytotoxic substances in the circulation during ECLS are largely unexplored, but neonates appear to tolerate ECLS with minimal evidence of a prolonged inflammatory response and minimal need for the transfusion of blood products.[143] Overall results are better in neonates.[152] Patients on ECLS clearly achieve some sort of equilibrium between organ injury and repair as perfusion continues, but survival requires considerable organ functional reserve which may not be present in older patients.[153] Corry et al. have shown that activated complement disappears within a few hours after placing a left VAD, but that IL-6 and IL-8 remain elevated for 1-2 weeks before returning to baseline values.[154] The much larger non-endothelial cell surface area exposed to blood during ECLS is likely to prolong the circulation of various inflammatory mediators.

Other chapters in this book detail the dysfunction of specific organs that may be due to persistence of an inflammatory response or to accumulated microemboli during ECLS. Until more data are available, measures of organ dysfunction related to ECLS will be difficult to separate from organ responses to associated injury or disease.

Strategies to control the blood-surface interface

The endothelial cells maintain the fluidity of blood by producing anticoagulants and removing procoagulants from the blood stream. Circulation of blood through an extracorporeal circuit produces a strong thrombotic stimulus primarily by the activation of the intrinsic coagulation pathway, the activation of platelets, and by stimulating monocytes to produce TF.[93] TF is also expressed by endothelial cells when stimulated by thrombin.[155] Blood is not exposed to a wound, however, so the stimulus to thrombin formation is less than that which occurs during open-heart surgery. This advantage is offset by reducing heparin concentrations and accepting lower ACT in an effort to reduce ongoing, slow bleeding. This practice establishes a consumptive coagulopathy, but the stimuli for thrombin and fibrin formation differ from those during open-heart surgery and, therefore, offer different opportunities for control of the equilibrium between fibrin formation and ongoing fibrinolysis.

Since the properties of the endothelial cell are not likely to be duplicated by a man-made biomaterial, a combination of selective inhibitors of blood reactions and surface modifications offers an attractive strategy for reducing thrombin and fibrin formation and reducing the heparin requirements for ECLS. The factor IXa inhibitor developed by Spanier et al. is especially suited for ECLS since the inhibitor specifically blocks the intrinsic coagulation pathway and does not prevent generation of thrombin from TF expression.[134] So far, this agent has not been used in any large studies either for CPB nor for ECLS, but further investigation of its use in left VADs may help identify its utility.

Suppression of fibrinolysis during ECLS for the purpose of reducing bleeding in infants was investigated by a multi-institutional study using epsilon-amino caproic acid (EACA).[156] Seventeen percent of patients had grade 3 or higher ICH and 7% had thrombotic complications (placebo group). The authors concluded that the antifibrinolyic was safe but not necessarily effective for reducing hemorrhagic complications. Others have reported a case of intravascular thrombosis when EACA was used during ECLS.[157]

Nafamostat mesilate is a broad-spectrum protease inhibitor that suppresses activation of contact proteins during in vitro extracorporeal recirculation.[158] Mellgren et al. evaluated nafamostat mesilate for inhibition of platelets during 24-hour recirculation of fresh, heparinized, human blood.[159] The authors found that the drug attenuated platelet activation and thrombin formation and, therefore, may be helpful during ECLS. Nafamostat mesilate has now been used in 2 small case series for controlling hemorrhagic complications in neonates. It was not used alone, but rather in conjunction with heparin. Once added, it allowed for a decrease in the heparin infusion with no increase in thrombosis within the extracorporeal circuit and a decrease in the bleeding of the patients. In an open-heart surgery study, the drug reduced circulating thrombin-antithrombin complexes and D-dimers with a significant reduction in postoperative blood loss.[160] Another commonly used protease inhibitor used for bleeding complications during ECLS for pediatric cardiothoracic surgery is aprotinin. It, like nafamostat mesilate, is a proteolytic enzyme inhibitor that can help reduce fibrinolysis and also perform as an anticoagulant, thereby decreasing the amount of heparin needed for ECLS. It is important to note, however, that dosing adjustments in the pediatric population must be carefully calculated to prevent any thromboembolic complications while on ECLS.

NO added to the sweep gas of the oxygenator reduces platelet adhesion and activation during in vitro and in vivo extracorporeal circulation.[161-164] In the presence of NO, platelets become reversibly anesthetized, and, therefore, do not become activated during contact with the extracorporeal circuit. The half-life of NO is extremely short in plasma, as hemoglobin very quickly eliminates it (<1 second). This allows for rapid reversal of its inhibitory effects on platelets and allows them to quickly function at the sites where hemostasis is necessary. NO and the creation of NO releasing polymers have been successfully demonstrated in a rabbit model of VV ECLS. MAHMA NO is a diazeniumdiolated compound (Z-1-[N-methyl-N-[6-(N-methylammoniohexyl)amino]]diazen-1-ium-1,2-diolate) that can be incorporated into a polymer matrix of an artificial surface and when exposed to water vapor releases NO at the surface of that polymer. Without systemic heparinization, MAHMA NO-doped circuits showed significantly decreased platelet consumption (Figure 3) when compared to both the heparinized and non-heparinized control groups.[165] On scanning electron microscopic examination of the circuits (Figure 4), Group C, the non-heparinized NO-releasing circuits, was the only group in which platelets retained their spherical, non-activated shape. In contrast, both of the heparinized groups, although demonstrating no fibrin adherence, showed at least partially activated, amorphous-shaped platelets, most likely secondary to heparin and its effect on platelets. Group A demonstrates what happens to blood when it interacts with artificial surfaces in the absence of interventions to attenuate these responses. Newer diazeniumdiolates are currently being developed and explored to identify those which will perform well clinically.[166,167]

Radomski et al. demonstrated a reduction in platelet aggregation when critically ill neonates received NO prior to going on ECLS. Once on ECLS, the thrombocytopenia and platelet activation was no different than in the control patients; however, the release of matrix metal-

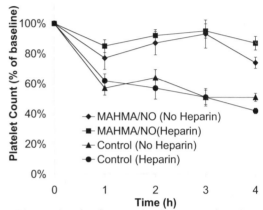

Figure 3. The first study demonstrating the efficacy of NO-releasing polymers. Both MAHMA/NO without systemic heparinization and MAHMA/NO with systemic heparinization groups were compared to heparinized and non-heparinized control groups over a 4-hour period in a rabbit model of extracorporeal circulation.

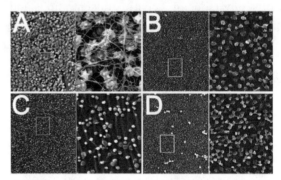

Figure 4. Scanning electron microscopic examination of ECC circuits both NO-doped and controls. The micrographs are representative of the entire circuit and the right side of each is a 5-fold magnification of the area selected on the left. The groups are represented as follows: Group (A) non-heparinized controls; Group (B) heparinized controls; Group (C) non-heparinized NO-releasing circuit; and Group (D) heparinized NO-releasing circuit.

loproteinase-2 (MMP-2), a nonthromboxane, non-adenosine diphosphate (ADP) pathway of platelet activation which is usually very high in ECLS patients not on NO, was significantly reduced.[168] This may be an important step to understanding how to control the platelet response presently seen in ECLS.

Prior to the development of NO-releasing polymers, surface-modifying additives (SMAs) had been the main focus of blood-surface interface control. SMAs are low concentrations of chemicals added to mobile bulk biomaterials during fabrication to reduce interfacial energy. These additives spontaneously migrate to the solid surface and dominate surface molecules. One commercially available SMA uses a triblock-copolymer containing polar and non-polar polymer chains of polycaprolactone-polydimethylsiloxane-polycaprolactone (Cobe Cardiovascular Inc., Arvada, CO).[169] Other formulations with different intrinsic surface activities remain under investigation.[170,171] In a clinical investigation of patients with first-time myocardial revascularization, the available SMA product significantly reduced platelet activation, adhesion, and release; reduced thrombin generations; and reduced t-PA production. No differences in post-operative blood loss were noted.[172]

Heparin-coated extracorporeal circuits are commercially available and have been extensively used and studied in patients during open-heart surgery. The Carmeda process (Medtronic Inc., Minneapolis, MN) covalently bonds partially-degraded heparin to aminated biomaterial surfaces by reduction with sodium cyanoborohydride.[173] Duraflo II heparin-coated circuits (Baxter International, Deerfield, IL) ionically bind heparin to the surface and use a proprietary process to retard leaching.[174] During clinical cardiac surgery, no consistent or significant differences between the 2 methods of heparin bonding are apparent.

In 1996, Edmunds et al. reviewed and cited the voluminous literature reporting experience with heparin-bonded perfusion circuits during open-heart surgery.[175] They found no reports of beneficial experience in ECLS patients. Neither ionic- nor covalent-bound heparin-coated perfusion circuits convincingly reduced the rate of thrombin formation, although the coatings did bind AT III onto the surface.[176] When these circuits were used for life support without systemic heparin, the incidence of visible thrombus within the ventricle or pump head was 27% .[177] Clotting also occurred in other circumstances when heparin coated circuits were used with reduced systemic heparin or no heparin. In addition the literature did not establish any reduction in postoperative bleeding or transfusion requirements when heparin coated perfusion circuits were used during open-heart surgery.[175]

A preponderance of studies indicate that generation of the terminal complement complex is reduced during open-heart surgery when heparin coated circuits are used with or without reduced concentrations of systemic heparin.[175,178] The evidence that other markers of complement activation are attenuated by heparin coating is less persuasive.[175,179] Despite many clinical studies, there is no convincing evidence that consistent and meaningful changes in platelet or granulocyte activation or cytokine production are produced by heparin coating.[175] Lastly, clinical benefits of heparin-coated extracorporeal circuits cannot be shown when standard doses of systemic heparin are used, even when associated with a reduction in the concentration of the terminal complement complex.[179,180] However, when the systemic dose of heparin is reduced, clinical studies are about equally divided with respect to clinical benefit.[175] Since thrombin cannot be measured in vivo in real time and since the anti-thrombotic and anti-inflammatory benefits of heparin-coated circuits have not been equivocally demonstrated in patients undergoing open-heart surgery, there is limited rationale for the use of these circuits during ECLS.

In 1969, Zucker and Vroman observed that adsorbed fibrinogen is necessary for platelet adhesion to glass slides, but that platelets do not adhere to fibrinogen-coated slides if contact with platelets is delayed for 3 minutes.[181] In the same year, Salzman observed that platelets do not adhere to albumin-coated surfaces,[182] but Adrian et al. recently demonstrated this protection is transient.[183] Addonizio et al. used prostacyclin, which has a half-life in plasma of 2-3 minutes, to briefly inhibit platelets during simulated extracorporeal circulation of fresh heparinized human blood. During hour 2 of recirculation, platelets were no longer inhibited but did not react or adhere to surfaces of the extracorporeal circuit.[184] Shigeta et al. used a disintegrin, bitistatin, to initially inhibit platelets during ECLS for 24 hours in sheep and demonstrated that after recovery from inhibition during the first hour, platelets did not begin to react with the circuit until hour 12.[185] Salzman used the phrase "surface passivation" to describe the development of non-reactivity of platelets to surfaces previously exposed to blood.[182] This phenomenon is probably due to conformational changes in surface-adsorbed fibrinogen and suggests that surface-adsorbed proteins are not totally immobile over time. The ability to predict and control the topography of adsorbed plasma proteins on inert biomaterial surfaces greatly diminishes the chances of developing nonthrombogenic biomaterials and serves as a reminder that the endothelial cell uses multiple metabolic processes to simultaneously maintain the fluidity of blood and the integrity of the vascular system.

Summary

During that last 50 years, we have learned to pump and ventilate blood outside of the body, but at present we have not yet conquered the activation of extracorporeally circulated blood constituents. We are closer, but not yet there. This limitation severely restricts the use of ECLS in patients, particularly those who have consumptive coagulopathies and bleeding dyscrasias prior to the initiation of ECLS. Control of the blood-surface interface promises huge benefits to critical care medicine by allowing ECLS to give time for organ recovery. The tools to master the blood-surface interface are at hand, and the goal is well worth it.

References

1. Gibbon JH Jr. Application of a mechanical heart and lung apparatus in cardiac surgery. *Minn Med* 1954; 37:171-185.

2. Hill JD, O'Brien TG, Murray JJ, et al. Prolonged extracorporeal oxygenation for acute post-traumatic respiratory failure (shock lung syndrome). Use of the Bramson membrane lung. *N Engl J Med* 1972; 286:629-634.

3. Blackstone EH, Kirklin JW, Stewart RW, Chenoweth DE. The damaging effects of cardiopulmonary bypass. In: Wu KK, Roxy EC, eds. *Prostaglandins in clinical medicine: Cardiovascular and Thrombotic Disorders*. Chicago, IL: Yearbook Medical Publishers Inc.; 1982: 355.

4. Menninger FJ 3rd, Rosenkranz ER, Utley JR, Dembitsky WP, Hargen AR, Peters RM. Interstitial hydrostatic pressure in patients undergoing CABG and valve replacement. *J Thorac Cardiovasc Surg* 1980; 79:181-187.

5. Smith EE, Faftel DC, Blackstone EH, Kirklin JW. Microvascular permeability after cardiopulmonary bypass. An experimental study. *J Thorac Cardiovasc Surg* 1987; 94:225-233.

6. Downing SW, Edmunds LH Jr. Release of vasoactive substances during cardiopulmonary bypass. *Ann Thorac Surg* 1992; 54:1236-1243.

7. Golding LR, Jacob G, Groves LK, Gill CC, Nose Y, Loop FD. Clinical results of mechanical support of the failing left ventricle. *J Thorac Cardiovasc Surg* 1982; 83:597-601.

8. Boucher JK, Rudy LW Jr, Edmunds LH Jr. Organ blood flow during pulsatile cardio-

pulmonary bypass. *J Appl Physiol* 1974; 36:86-90.

9. Rudy LW Jr, Heymann MA, Edmunds LH Jr. Distribution of systemic blood flow during cardiopulmonary bypass. *J Appl Physiol* 1973; 34:194-200.

10. Leverett LB, Hellums JD, Alfrey CP, Lynch EC. Red blood cell damage by shear stress. *Biophys J* 1972; 12:257-273.

11. Gorbet MB, Sefton MV. Biomaterial-associated thrombosis: roles of coagulation factors, complement, platelets and leukocytes. *Biomaterials* 2004: 25:5681-5703.

12. Lee WH Jr, Hairston P. Structural effects on blood proteins at the gas-blood interface. *Fed Proc* 1971; 30:1615-1622.

13. Clark RE, Beauchamp RA, Magrath RA, Brooks JD, Ferguson TB, Weldon CS. Comparison of bubble and membrane oxygenators in short and long perfusions. *J Thorac Cardiovasc Surg* 1979; 78:655-666.

14. Woodman RC, Harker LA. Bleeding complications associated with cardiopulmonary bypass. *Blood* 1990; 76:1680-1697.

15. Salama A, Hugo F, Heinrich D, et al. Deposition of terminal C5b-9 complement complexes on erythrocytes and leukocytes during cardiopulmonary bypass. *N Eng J Med* 1988; 318:408-414.

16. Kawahito K, Nose Y. Hemolysis in different centrifugal pumps. *Artif Org* 1997; 21:323-326.

17. Uniyal S, Brash JL. Patterns of adsorption of proteins from human plasma onto foreign surfaces. *Thromb Haemost* 1982; 47:285-290.

18. Ziats NP, Pankowsky DA, Tierney BP, et al. Adsorption of Hageman factor (factor XII) and other human plasma proteins to biomedical polymers. *J Lab Clin Med* 1990; 116:687-696.

19. Horbett TA. Principles underlying the role of adsorbed plasma proteins in blood interactions with foreign materials. *Cardiovasc Pathol* 1993; 2:137S-148.

20. Horbett TA. Proteins: structure, properties, and adsorption to surfaces. In: Ratner BD, Hoffman AS, Schoen FJ, Lemons JE, eds. *Biomaterials Science. An Introduction to Materials in Medicine.* San Diego CA: Academic Press; 1996:133-141.

21. Brash JL, Scott CF, Hove P, et al. Mechanism of transient adsorption of fibrinogen from plasma to solid surfaces: role of the contact and fibrinolytic systems. *Blood* 1988; 71:932-939.

22. Lindon JN, McManamaa G, Kushner L, Merrill EW, Salzman EW. Does the conformation of adsorbed fibrinogen dictate platelet interactions with artificial surfaces? *Blood* 1986; 68:355-362.

23. Ratner BD. Characterization of biomaterial surfaces. *Cardiovasc Pathol* 1993; 73:1249-1253.

24. Colman RW, Clowes AW, George JN, Hirsh J, Marder VJ. Overview of Hemostasis. In: Colman, RW, Hirsh J, Marder VJ, Clowes AW, George JN, eds. *Hemostasis and Thrombosis; Basic Principles and Clinical Practice.* 4th ed. Philadelphia, PA: Lippincott Williams & Wilkins; 2001: 3-16.

25. Colman RW, Jameson B, Lin Y, Johnson D, Mousa SA. Domain 5 of high molecular weight kininogen (kininostatin) downregulates endothelial cell proliferation and migration and inhibits angiogenesis. *Blood* 2000; 45:543-550.

26. Colman RW. Biologic activities of the contact factors in vivo--potentiation of hypotension, inflammation, and fibrinolysis, and inhibition of cell adhesion, angiogenesis, and thrombosis. *Thromb Haemost* 1999; 1568-1577.

27. Mandle R Jr, Colman RW, Kaplan AP. Identification of prekallikrein and high-molecular-weight kininogen as a complex in human plasma. *Proc Natl Acad Sci USA* 1976; 73:4179-4183.

28. Colman RW. Surface-mediated defense reactions. The plasma contact activation system. *J Clin Invest* 1984; 73:1249-1253.

29. Colman RW. Contact activation pathway: Inflammatory, fibrinolytic, anticoagulant, antiadhesive, and antiangiogenic activities. In: Colman, RW, Hirsh J, Marder VJ, Clowes AW, George JN, eds. *Hemostasis and Thrombosis; Basic Principles and Clinical Practice. 4th ed.* Philadelphia, PA: Lippincott Williams & Wilkins; 2001: 103-121.

30. Gigli I, Mason JW, Colman RW, Austen KF. Interaction of plasma kallikrein with the C1 inhibitor. *J Immunol* 1970; 104:574-581.

31. Schapira M, Scott CF, James A, et al. Protection of human plasma kallikrein from inactivation by C1 inhibitor and other protease inhibitors. The role of high molecular weight kininogen. *Biochemistry* 1981; 20:2738-2743.

32. Schapira M, Scott CF, James A, et al. High molecular weight kininogen or its light chain protects human plasma kallikrein from inactivation by plasma protease inhibitors. *Biochemistry* 1982; 21:567-572.

33. Bauer KA, Kass BL, ten Cate H, Hawiger JJ, Rosenberg RD. Factor IX is activated in vivo by the tissue factor mechanism. *Blood* 1990; 76:731-736.

34. Limentani SA, Furie BC, Furie B. The biochemistry of Factor IX. In: Colman, RW, Hirsh J, Marder VJ, Salzman EW, eds. *Hemostasis and Thrombosis; Basic Principles and Clinical Practice. 3rd ed.* Philadelphia, PA: Lippincott Williams & Wilkins; 1994: 94-108.

35. Tracy PB, Rohrbach MS, Mann KG. Functional prothrombinase complex assembly on isolated monocytes and lymphocytes. *J Biol Chem* 1983; 258:7264 7267.

36. Tracy PB, Eide LL, Mann KG. Human prothrombinase complex assembly and function on isolated peripheral blood cell populations. *J Biol Chem* 1985; 260:2119-2124.

37. Scandura JM, Walsh PN. Factor X bound to the surface of activated human platelets is preferentially activated by platelet-bound factor IXa. *Biochemistry* 1996; 35:8903-8913.

38. Edwards RL, Rickles FR. Macrophage procoagulants. *Prog Hemost Thromb* 1984; 7:183-209.

39. Colucci M, Balconi G, Lorenzet R, et al. Cultured human endothelial cells generate tissue factor in response to endotoxin. *J Clin Invest* 1983; 71:1893-1896.

40. Bevilacqua MP, Pober JS, Majeau GR, Ctran RS, Gimbrone MA Jr. Interleukin 1 (IL-1) induces biosynthesis and cell surface expression of procoagulant activity in human vascular endothelial cells. *J Exp Med* 1984; 160:618-623.

41. Edgington TS, Mackman N, Brand K, Ruf W. The structural biology of expression and function of tissue factor. *Thromb Haemost* 1991; 66:67-79.

42. Drake TA, Ruf W, Morrissey JH, Edington TS. Functional tissue factor is entirely cell surface expressed on lipopolysaccharide-stimulated human blood monocytes and a constitutively tissue factor-producin neoplastic cell line. *J Cell Biol* 1989; 109:389-395.

43. Grabowski EF, Rodriquez M, Nemerson Y, McDonnell SL. Flow limits Factor Xa production by monolayers of fibroblasts and endothelial cells. *Blood* 1990; 76(Suppl):422a.

44. Coughlin SR, Vu TK, Hung DT, Wheaton VI. Characterization of a functional thrombin receptor. Issues and opportunities. *J Clin Invest* 1992; 89:351-355.

45. Francis CW, Marder VJ. Physiologic regulation and pathologic disorders of fibrinolysis. In: Colman, RW, Hirsh J, Marder VJ, Salzman EW, eds. *Hemostasis and Thrombosis; Basic Principles and Clinical Practice. 3rd ed.* Philadelphia,PA: Lippincott Williams & Wilkins; 1994:1076-1103.

46. Niewiarowski S, Senyi AF, Gilles P. Plasmin-induced platelet aggregation and platelet release reaction. *J Clin Invest* 1973; 52:1647-1659.

47. Urlesberger B, Zobel G, Zenz W, Kuttnig-Haim M, et al. Activation of the clotting system during extracorporeal membrane oxygenation in term newborn infants. *J Pediatr* 1996; 129:264-268.

48. Lu H, Soria C, Cramer EM, et al. Temperature dependence of plasmin-induced activation or inhibition of human platelets. *Blood* 1991; 77:996-1005.

49. Nurmohamed MT, Cate H, Cate JW. Low molecular weight heparin(oid)s. Clinical investigations and practical recommendations. *Drugs* 1997; 53:736-751.

50. Lu H, Du-Bruit C, Soria J, et al. Postoperative hemostasis and fibrinolysis in patients undergoing cardiopulmonary bypass with or without aprotinin therapy. *Thromb Haemost* 1994; 72:438-443.

51. Sims PJ. Plasma Proteins: Complement. In: Hoffman R, Benz EJ Jr, Shattil SF, Furie B, Cohen HJ, eds. *Hematology*. New York, NY: Churchill Livingstone; 1991: 1582-1591.

52. Chenoweth DE, Cooper SW, Hugli TE, et al. Complement activation during cardiopulmonary bypass: evidence for generation of C3a and C5a anaphylatoxins. *N Engl J Med* 1981; 304:497-503.

53. Wachtfogel YT, Harpel PC, Edmunds LH Jr, Colman RW. Formation of C1s-C1-inhibitor, kallikrein-C1-inhibitor and plasmin-alpha 2-plasmin-inhibitor complexes during cardiopulmonary bypass. *Blood* 1989; 73:468-471.

54. Berger M. Complement mediated phagocytosis. In: Volanakis JE, Frank MM, eds. *The Human Complement System in Health and Disease*. New York, NY: Marcel Dekker Inc.; 1998: 285-308.

55. Chenoweth DE, Hugli TE. Demonstration of specific C5a receptor on intact human polymorphonuclear leukocytes. *Proc Natl Acad Sci USA* 1978; 75:3943-3947.

56. Volanakis JE. Overview of the complement system. In: Volanakis JE, Frank MM, eds. *The Human Complement System in Health and Disease*. New York, NY: Marcel Dekker Inc.; 1998: 9-32.

57. Wiedmer T, Esmon CT, Sims PJ. Complement proteins C5b-9 stimulate procoagulant activity through the platelet prothrombinase. *Blood* 1986; 68:875-880.

58. Kazatchkine MD, Carreno MP. Activation of the complement system at the interface between blood and artificial surfaces. *Biomaterials* 1988; 9:30-35.

59. Cavarocchi NC, Pluth JR, Schaff HV, et al. Complement activation during cardiopulmonary bypass. Comparison of bubble and membrane oxygenators. *J Thorac Cardiovasc Surg* 1986; 91:252-258.

60. Jansen NJ, Van Oeveren W, van den Brock L, et al. Inhibition by dexamethasone of the reperfusion phenomena in cardiopulmonary bypass. *J Thorac Cardiovasc Surg* 1991; 102:515-525.

61. Videm V, Scennivig JL, Fosse E, et al. Reduced complement activation with heparin-coated oxygenator and tubings in cornary bypass operations. *J Thorac Cardiovasc Surg* 1992; 103:806-813.

62. Kirklin JK, Westaby S, Blackstone EH, Kirklin JW, Chenoweth DE, Pacifico AD. Complement and the damaging effects of cardiopulmonary bypass. *J Thorac Cardiovasc Surg* 1983; 86:845-857.

63. Downing SW, Edmunds LH Jr. Release of vasoactive substances during cardiopulmonary bypass. *Ann Thorac Surg* 1992; 54:1236-1243.

64. Del Balzo UH, Levi R, Polley MJ. Cardiac dysfunction caused by purified human C3a anaphylatoxin. *Proc Nat Acad Sci USA* 1985; 82:886-890.

65. Valhonrat H, Swinford RD, Ingelfinger JR, et al. Rapid activation of the alternative

pathway of complement by extracorporeal membrane oxygenation. *ASAIO J* 1999; 45:113-114.

66. Tamiya T, Yamasaki M, Maeo Y, Yamashiro T, Ogoshi S, Fujimoto S. Complement activation in cardiopulmonary bypass, with special reference to anaphylatoxin production in membrane and bubble oxygenators. *Ann Thorac Surg* 1988; 46:47-57.

67. Marcus AJ. Platelet activation. In: Fuster V, Ross R, Topol EJ, eds. Atherosclerosis and cornary artery disease. Philadelphia, PA: Lippincott-Raven Publishers; 1996: 607-637.

68. Laufer N, Merin G, Grover NB, Pessachowicz B, Borman JB. The influence of cardiopulmonary bypass on the size of human platelets. *J Thorac Cardiovas Surg* 1975; 70:727-731.

69. Edmunds LH Jr, Ellison N, Colman RW, et al. Platelet function during open cardiac operation; comparison of the membrane and bubble oxygenators. *J Thorac Cardiovasc Surg* 1982; 83:805-812.

70. Kestin AS, Valeri CR, Khuri SF, et al. The platelet function defect of cardiopulmonary bypass. *Blood* 1993; 82:107-117.

71. Anderson HL III, Cilley RE, Zwischenberger JB, et al. Thrombocytopenia in neonates after extracorporeal membrane oxygenation. *ASAIO Trans* 1986; 32:534-537.

72. Saadi S, Platt JL. Endothelial cell responses to complement activation. In: Volanakis JE, Frank MM, eds. The Human Complement System in Health and Disease. New York, NY: Marcel Dekker Inc.; 1998: 335-353.

73. Wenger RK, Lukasiewicz H, Mikuta BS, Niewiarowski S, Edmunds LH Jr. Loss of platelet fibrinogen receptors during clinical cardiopulmonary bypass. *J Thorac Cardiovasc Surg* 1989; 97:235-239.

74. Vane JR, Anggard EE, Botting RM. Regulatory functions of the vascular endothelium. *N Eng J Med* 1990; 323:27-36.

75. Jaffe EA. Endothelial Cell Structure and Function. In: Hoffman R, Benz EJ Jr, Shattil SJ, et al., eds. *Hematology, Basic Principles and Practice.* New York, NY: Churchill Livingstone; 1991: 1198-1213.

76. Faymonville ME, Deby-Dupont G, Larbuisson R, et al. Prostaglandin E2, prostacyclin, and thromboxane changes during nonpulsatile cardiopulmonary bypass in humans. *J Thorac Cardiovasc Surg* 1986; 91:858-866.

77. Hashimoto K, Horikoshi H, Miyamoto H, et al. Mechanisms of organ failure following cardiopulmonary bypass; the role of elastase and vasoactive mediators. *J Thorac Cardiovasc Surg* 1992; 104:666.

78. Rousseau Y, Carreno MP, Poignet JL, Kaztchkine MD, Haeffner-Cavaillon N. Dissociation between complement activation, integrin expression and neutropenia during hemodialysis. *Biomaterials* 1999; 20:1959-1967.

79. Cristol JP, Canaud B, Rabesandratana H, Gaillard I, Serre A, Mion C. Enhancement of reactive oxygen species production and cell surface markers expression due to hemodialysis. *Nephrol Dial Transplant* 1994; 9:389-394.

80. Von Appen K, Goolsby C, Mehl P, Goewert R, Ivanovich P. Leukocyte adhesion molecule as biocompatibility markers for hemodialysis membranes. *ASAIO J* 1994; 40:M609-615.

81. Videm V, Mollnes TE, Fosse E. Heparin-coated cardiopulmonary bypass equipment. I. Biocompatibility markers and development of complications in high-risk population. *J Thorac Cardiovasc Surg* 1999; 117:794-802.

82. Fitch JC, Rollins S, Matis L, et al. Pharmacology and biological efficacy of a recombinant, humanized, single-chain antibody C5 complement inhibitor in patients undergoing coronary artery bypass graft surgery with cardiopulmonary bypass. *Circulation* 1999; 100:2499-2506.

83. Rinder C, Fitch J. Amplification of the inflammatory response: adhesion molecules associated with platelet/white cell responses. *J Cardiovasc Pharmacol* 1996; 27(Suppl 1):S6-12.

84. El Habbal MH, Carter H, Smith L, Elliot MJ, Strobel S. Neutrophil activation in paediatric extracorporeal circuits: effect of circulation and temperature variation. *Cardiovasc Res* 1995;29:102-107.

85. Gillinov AM, Bator JM, Zehr KH, et al. Neutrophil adhesion molecule expression during cardiopulmonary bypass with bubble and membrane oxygenators. *Ann Thorac Surg* 1993; 56:847-853.

86. Cameron D. Initiation of white cell activation during cardiopulmonary bypass: cytokines and receptors. *J Cardiovasc Pharmacol* 1996; 27(Suppl 1):S1-5.

87. Eriksson C, Nygren H. Polymorphonuclear leukocytes in coagulating whole blood recognize hydrophilic and hydrophobic titanium surfaces by different adhesion receptors and show different patterns of receptor expression. *J Lab Clin Med* 2001; 137:296-302.

88. Gemmell CH. Flow cytometric evaluation of material-induced platelet and complement activation. *J Biomater Sci Polym Ed* 2000; 11:1197-1210.

89. Wachtfogel YT, Kucich U, Greenplate J, et al. Human Neutrophil degranulation during extracorporeal circulation. *Blood* 1987; 69:324-330.

90. Craddock PR, Fehr J, Brigham KL, Kronenberg RS, Jacob HS. Complement and leukocyte-mediated pulmonary dusfunction in hemodialysis. *N Engl J Med* 1977; 296:769-774.

91. Gluszko P, Rucinski B, Musial J, Wenger RK, et al. Fibrinogen receptors in platelet adhesion to surfaces of extracorporeal circuit. *Am J Physiol* 1987; 252:H615-621.

92. Fortenberry JD, Bhardwaj V, Niemer P, Cornish JD, Wright JA, Bland L. Neutro-phil and cytokine activation with neonatal extracorporeal membrane oxygenation. *J Pediatr* 1996; 128:670-678.

93. Kappelmayer J, Bernabei A, Gikakis N, Edmunds LH Jr, Colman RW. Upregulation of Mac-1 surface expression on neutrophils during simulated extracorporeal circulation. *J Lab Clin Med* 1993; 121:118-126.

94. Asimakopoulos G, Taylor KM. Effects of cardiopulmonary bypass on leukocyte and endothelial adhesion molecules. *Ann Thorac Surg* 1998; 66:2135-2144.

95. Ratliff NB, Young WG Jr, Hackel D, Mikat E, Wilson JW. Pulmonary injury secondary to extracorporeal circulation. An ultrastructural study. *J Thorac Cardiovasc Surg* 1973; 65:425-432.

96. Chung JH, Gikakis N, Rao AK, Drake TA, Colman RW, Edmunds LH Jr. Pericardial blood activates the extrinsic coagulation pathway during clinical cardiopulmonary bypass. *Circulation* 1996; 93:2014-2018.

97. Barstad RM, Ovrum E, Ringdal MA, et al. Induction of monocyte tissue factor procoagulant activity during coronary artery bypass surgery is reduced with heparin-coated extracorporeal circuit. *Br J Haematol* 1996; 94:517-525.

98. Ernofsson M, Thelin S, Siegbahn A. Monocyte tissue factor expression, cell activation, and thrombin formation during cardiopulmonary bypass: a clinical study. *J Thorac Cardiovasc Surg* 1997; 113:576-584.

99. Ernoffson M, Siegbahn A. Platelet-derived growth factor-BB and monocyte chemotactic protein-1 induce human peripheral blood monocytes to express tissue factor. *Thromb Res* 1996; 83:307-320.

100. Rinder CS, Bonnert J, Rinder HM, Mitchell J, Ault K, Hillman R. Platelet activation and aggregation during cardiopulmonary bypass. *Anesthesiology* 1991; 74:388-393.

101. Insel PA. Analgesic-antipyretic and anti-inglammatory agents and drugs employed

in the treatment of gout. In: Hardman JG, Limbird LE, eds. *Goodman and Gilman's the Pharmacological Basis of Theraputics.* New York, NY: McGraw-Hill Inc.; 1996: 618-619.

102. Fingerle-Rowson G, Auers J, Kreuzer E, et al. Down-regulation of surface monocyte lipopolysaccharide-receptor CD14 in patients on cardiopulmonary bypass undergoing aorta-coronary bypass operation. *J Thorac Cardiovasc Surg* 1998; 115:1172-1178.

103. Haeffner-Cavaillon N, Roussellier N, Ponzio O, et al. Induction of interleukin-1 production in patients undergoing cardiopulmonary bypass. *J Thorac Cardiovac Surg* 1989; 98:1100-1106.

104. Steinberg JB, Kapelanski DP, Olson JD, Weiler JM. Cytokine and complement levels in patients undergoing cardiopulmonary bypass. *J Thorac Cardiovasc Surg* 1993; 106:1008-1016.

105. Frering B, Philip I, Dehoux M, Rolland C, Langlois JM, Desmonts JM. Circulating cytokines in patients undergoing normothermic cardiopulmonary bypass. *J Thorac Cardiovasc Surg* 1994; 108:636-641.

106. Kawahito K, Kawakami M, Fujiwara T, Adachi H, Ino T. Interleukin-8 and monocyte chemotactic activating factor responses to cardiopulmonary bypass. *J Thorac Cardiovasc Surg* 1995; 110:99-102.

107. Roth JA, Golub SH, Cukingnan RA, Brazier J, Morton DL. Cell mediated immunity is depressed following cardiopulmonary bypass. *Ann Thorac Surg* 1981; 31:350-356.

108. DePalma L, Yu M, McIntosh CL, Swain JA, Davey RJ. Changes in lymphocyte subpopulations as a result of cardiopulmonary bypass. The effect of blood transfusion. *J Thorac Cardiovasc Surg* 1991; 101:240-244.

109. Markewitz A, Faist E, Lang S, Endres S, Fuchs D, Reichart B. Successful restoration of cell-mediated immune response after cardiopulmonary bypass by immunomodulation. *J Thorac Cardiovasc Surg* 1993; 105:15-24.

110. Kawahito K, Kobayashi E, Misawa Y, et al. Recovery from lymphocytopenia and prognosis after adult extracorporeal membrane oxygenation. *Arch Surg* 1998; 133:216-217.

111. Bernabei A, Gikakis N, Maione TE, et al. Reversal of heparin anticoagulation by recombinant platelet factor 4 and protamine sulfate in baboons during cardiopulmonary bypass. *J Thorac Cardiovasc Surg* 1995; 109:765-771.

112. Weitz JI, Hudoba M, Massel K, Maraganore J, Hirsh J. Clot-bound thrombin is protected from inhibition by heparin-antithrombin III but is susceptible to inactivation by antithrombin III-independent inhibitors. *J Clin Invest* 1990; 86:385-391.

113. Urlesberger B, Zobel G, Zenz W, et al. Activation of the clotting system during extracorporeal membrane oxygenation in term newborn infants. *J Pediatr* 1996; 129:264-268.

114. Brister SJ, Ofosu FA, Buchanan MR. Thrombin generation during cardiac surgery: is heparin the ideal anticoagulant? *Thromb Haemost* 1993; 70:259-262.

115. Ellison N, Edmunds LH Jr, Colman RW. Platelet aggregation following heparin and protamine administration. *Anesthesiology* 1978; 48:65-68.

116. Sobel M, McNeill PM, Carlson PL, et al. Heparin inhibition of von Willebrand factor-dependent platelet function in vitro and in vivo. *J Clin Invest* 1991; 87:1787-1793.

117. Pixley RA, Cassello A, De La Cadena RA, Kaufman N, Colman RW. Effect of heparin on the activation of factor XII and the contact system in plasma. *Thromb Haemost* 1991; 66:540-547.

118. Wachtfogel YT, Harpel, PC, Edmunds, LH Jr, Colman RW. Formation of C1s-C1-

inhibitor, kallikrien-C1-inhibitor and plasmin-alpha 2-plasmin-inhibitor complexes during cardiopulmonary bypass. *Blood* 1989; 73:468-471.

119. Cavarocchi NC, Schaff HV, Orszulak TA, Homburger HA, Schnell WA Jr, Pluth JR. Evidence for complement activation by protamine-heparin interaction after cardiopulmonary bypass. *Surgery* 1985; 98:525-531.

120. Kirklin JK, Chenoweth DE, Naftel DC, et al. Effects of protamine administration after cardiopulmonary bypass on complement, blood elements, and the hemodynamic state. *Ann Thorac Surg* 1986; 41:193-199.

121. Warkentin TE. Heparin-induced thrombocytopenia: a ten-year retrospective. *Annu Rev Med* 1999; 50:129-147.

122. Warkentin TE, Levine MN, Hirsch J, et al. Heparin-induced thrombocytopenia in patients treated with low-molecular-weight heparin or unfractionated heparin. *N Engl J Med* 1995; 332:1330-1335.

123. Dager WE, Gosselin RC, Yoshikawa R, Owings JT. Lepirudin in heparin-induced thrombocytopenia and extracorporeal membranous oxygenation. *Ann Pharmacother* 2004; 38:598-601.

124. Deitcher SR, Topoulos AP, Bartholomew JR, Kichuk-Chrisant MR. Lepirudin anticoagulation for heparin-induced thrombocytopenia. *J Pediatr* 2002; 140:264-266.

125. Gikakis N, Khan MMH, Hiramatsu Y, et al. Effect of factor Xa inhibitors on thrombin formation and complement and neutrophil activation during in vitro extracorporeal circulation. *Circulation* 1996; 94(9 Suppl): II341-346.

126. Hirsh J, Levine MN. Low molecular weight heparin. *Blood* 1992; 79:1-17.

127. Gikakis N, Rao AK, Miyamoto S, et al. Enoxaparin suppresses thrombin formation and activity during cardiopulmonary bypass in baboons. *J Thorac Cardiovasc Surg* 1998; 116:1043-1052.

128. Wolzt M, Weltermann A, Nieszpaur-Los M, et al. Studies on the neutralizing effects of protamine on unfractionated and low molecular weight heparin (Fragmin) at the site of activation of the coagulation system in man. *Thromb Haemost* 1995; 73:439-443.

129. Tollefsen DM, Petska CA, Monafo WJ. Activation of heparin cofactor II by dermatan sulfate. *J Biol Chem* 1983; 258:6713-6716.

130. Gillis S, Merin G, Zahger D, et al. Danaparoid for cardiopulmonary bypass in patients with previous heparin-induced thrombocytopenia. *Br J Haemat* 1997; 98:657-659.

131. Harker LA. Therapeutic inhibition of thrombin activities, receptors, and production. *Hematol Oncol Clin North Am* 1998; 12:1211-1230.

132. Matsuo T, Koide M, Kario K. Application of argatroban, direct thrombin inhibitor, in heparin-intolerant patients requiring extracorporeal circulation. *Artif Organs* 1997; 21:1035-1038.

133. Kawada T, Kitagawa H, Hoson M, Okada Y, Shiomura J. Clinical application of argatroban as an alternative anticoagulant for extracorporeal circulation. *Hematol Oncol Clin North Am* 2000; 14:445-457.

134. Spanier TB, Chen JM, Oz MC, et al. Selective anticoagulation with active site-blocked factor IXA suggests separate roles for intrinsic and extrinsic coagulation pathways in cardiopulmonary bypass. *J Thorac Cardiovasc Surg* 1998; 116:860-869.

135. Despotis GJ, Summerfield MD, Joist JH, et al. Comparison of activated coagulation time and whole blood heparin measurements with laboratory plasma anti-Xa heparin concentration in patients having cardiac operations. *J Thorac Cardiovasc Surg* 1994; 108:1076-1082.

136. Hardy JF, Belisle S, Robitaille D, Perrault J, Roy M, Gagnon L. Measurement of

heparin concentration in whole blood with the Hepcon/HMS device does not agree with laboratory determination of plasma heparin concentration using a chromogenic substrate for activated factor X. *J Thorac Cardiovasc Surg* 1996; 112:154-161.

137. Bull BS, Korpman RA, Huse WM, et al. Heparin therapy during extracorporeal circulation. I. Problems inherent in existing heparin protocols. *J Thorac Cardiovasc Surg* 1975; 69:674-684.

138. Gram J, Janetzko T, Jesperson J, Bruhn HD. Enhanced effective fibrinolysis following the neutralization of heparin in open heart surgery increases the risk of post-surgical bleeding. *Thromb Haemost* 1990; 63:241-245.

139. Fleming GM, Gupta M, Remenapp R, Cooley E, Bartlett RH, Annich GM. Comparison of ACT reference ranges for patients on ECMO using Hemochron® 401 and Hemochron® Response models. Presented at: CNMC Conference; February 22, 2005; Keystone, CO.

140. McManus ML, Kevy SV, Bower LK, Hickey PR. Coagulation factor deficiencies during initiation of extracorporeal membrane oxygenation. *J Pediatr* 1995; 126:900-904.

141. Zapol WM, Snider MT, Hill JD, et al. Extracorporeal membrane oxygenation in severe acute respiratory failure. A randomized prospective study. *JAMA* 1979; 242:2193-2196.

142. Butch SH, Knafl P, Oberman HA, Bartlett RH. Blood utilization in adult patients undergoing extracorporeal membrane oxygenated therapy. *Transfusion* 1996; 36:61-63.

143. Kelton JG, Smith JW, Warkentin TE, et al. Immunoglobulin G from patients with heparin-induced thrombocytopenia binds to a complex of heparin and platelet factor 4. *Blood* 1994; 83:3232-3239.

144. Edmunds LH Jr. Extracorporeal perfusion. In: Edmunds LH Jr, ed. *Cardiac Surgery in the Adult.* New York, NY: McGraw-Hill Inc.; 1997: 259-294.

145. Wenger R, Bavaria JE, Ratcliffe MB, et al. Flow dynamics of peripheral venous catheters during extracorporeal membrane oxygenation with a centrifugal pump. *J Thorac Cardiovasc Surg* 1988; 96:478-484.

146. Lichtor JL. Control of perioperative bleeding: blood component therapy. In: Wechsler AS, ed. *Pharmacologic Management of Perioperative Bleeding.* Southhampton, NY: CME Network; 1996: 19-24.

147. Slack SM, Turitto VT. Fluid dynamic and hemorheologic considerations. *Cardiovasc Pathol* 1993; 2(Suppl):11S-21.

148. Goldsmith HL, Turitto VT. Rheological aspects of thrombosis and haemostasis: basic principles and applications. ICTH-Report—Subcommittee on Rheology of the International Committee on Thrombosis and Haemostasis. *Thromb Haemost* 1986; 55:415-435.

149. Blauth CI, Smith Pl, Arnold JV, Jagoe JR, Wootton R, Taylor KM. Influence of oxygenator type on the prevalence and extent of microembolic retinal ischemia during cardiopulmonary bypass. Assessment by digital image analysis. *J Thorac Cardiovasc Surg* 1990; 99:61-69.

150. Hill JD, Aguilar MJ, Baranco A, de Lanerolle P, Gerbode F. Neuropathological manifestations of cardiac surgery. *Ann Thorac Surg* 1969; 7:409-419.

151. Osiovich HC, Peliowski A, Ainsworth W, Etches PC. The Edmonton experience with venovenous extracorporeal membrane oxygenation. *J Pediatr Surg* 1998; 33:1749-1752.

152. Rich PB, Younger JG, Soldes OS, Awad SS, Bartlett RH. Use of extracorporeal life support for adult patients with respiratory failure and sepsis. *ASAIO J* 1998; 44:263-266.

153. Alpard SK, Zwischenberger JB. Adult extracorporeal membrane oxygenation for

severe respiratory failure. Perfusion 1998; 13:3-15.

154. Corry DC, DeLucia A III, Zhu H, et al. Time course of cytokine release and complement activation after implantation of the HeartMate left ventricular assist device. *ASAIO J* 1998; 44:M347-351.

155. Levin EG, Marzec U, Anderson J, et al. Thrombin stimulates tissue plasminogen activator release from cultured human endothelial cells. *J Clin Invest* 1984; 74:1988-1995.

156. Horwitz JR, Cofer BR, Warner BW, Cheu HW, Lally KP. A multicenter trial of 6-aminocaproic acid (Amicar) in the prevention of bleeding in infants on ECMO. *J Pediat Surg* 1998; 33:1610-1613.

157. Hocker JR, Saving KL. Fatal aortic thrombosis in a neonate during infusion of epsilon-aminocaproic acid. *J Pediat Surg* 1995; 10:1490-1492.

158. Sundaram S, Gikakis N, Hack CE, et al. Nafamostat mesilate, a broad spectrum protease inhibitor, modulates platelet, neutrophil and contact activation in simulated extracorporeal circulation. *Thromb Haemost* 1996; 75:76-82.

159. Mellgren K, Skogby M, Friberg LG, Tengborn L, Wadenvik H. The influence of a serine protease inhibitor, nafamostat mesilate, on plasma coagulation, and platelet activation during experimental Extracorporeal Life Support (ECLS). *Thromb Haemost* 1998; 79:342-347.

160. Sato T, Tanaka K, Kondo C, et al. Nafamostat mesilate administration during cardiopulmonary bypass decreases postoperative bleeding after cardiac surgery. *ASAIO Trans* 1991; 37:M194-195.

161. Keh D, Gerlach M, Kurer I, Falke KJ, Gerlach H. Reduction of platelet trapping in membrane oxygenators by transmembraneous application of gaseous nitric oxide. *Int J Artif Org* 1996; 19:291-293.

162. Mellgren K, Friberg LG, Mellgren G, Hedner T, Wennmalm A, Wadenvik H. Nitric oxide in the oxygenator sweep gas reduces platelet activation during experimental perfusion. *Ann Thorac Surg* 1996; 61:1194-1198.

163. Suzuki Y, Malekan R, Hansen CW 3rd, et al. Platelet anesthesia with nitric oxide with and without eptifibatide during cardiopulmonary bypass in baboons. *J Thorac Cardiovasc Surg* 1999; 117:987-993.

164. Sly MK, Prager MD, Everhart RC, Jessen MC, Kulkarni PV. Inhibition surface-induced platelet activation by nitric oxide. *ASAIO J* 1995; 41:M394-398.

165. Annich GM, Meinhardt JP, Mowery KA, et al. Reduced platelet activation and thrombosis in extracorporeal circuits coated with nitric oxide release polymers. *Crit Care Med* 2000; 28:915-920.

166. Zhang H, Annich GM, Miskulin J, et al. Nitric oxide releasing silicone rubbers with improved blood compatibility: preparation, characterization, and in vivo evaluation. *Biomaterials* 2002; 23:1485-1494.

167. Zhang H, Annich GM, Miskulin J, et al. Nitric oxide-releasing fumed silica particles: synthesis, characterizations, and biomedical application. *J Am Chem Soc* 2003; 125:5015-5024.

168. Cheung PY, Sawicki G, Peliowski A, Etches PC, Schulz R, Radomski MW. Inhaled nitric oxide inhibits the release of matrix metalloproteinase-2, but not platelet activation, during extracorporeal membrane oxygenation in adult rabbits. *J Pediatr Surg* 2003; 38:534-538.

169. Gu YJ, Boonstra PW, Rijnsburger AA, Haan J, van Oeveren W. Cardiopulmonary bypass circuit treated with surface-modifying additives: a clinical evaluation of blood compatibility. *Ann Thorac Surg* 1998; 65:1342-1347.

170. Tsai CC, Deppisch RM, Forrestal LJ, et al. Surface modifying additives for improved

device-blood compatibility. *ASAIO J* 1994; 40:M619-624.

171. Kawahito K, Tasai K, Murata S, et al. Evaluation of the antithrombogenicity of a new microdomain structured copolymer. *Artif Org* 1995; 19:857-863.

172. Rubens FD, Labow RS, Lavallee GR, et al. Hematologic evaluation of cardiopulmonary bypass circuits prepared with a novel block copolymer. *Ann Thorac Surg* 1999; 67:689-696.

173. Larm O, Larsson R, Olsson P. A new non-thrombogenic surface prepared by selective covalent binding of heparin via a modified reducing terminal residue. *Biomatr Med Devices Artif Organs* 1983; 11:161-173.

174. Hsu LC, Tong SD. United States Patent: 4,871,357.

175. Edmunds LH Jr, Stenach N. *The blood-surface interface in cardiopulmonary bypass: Principles and Practice.* 2nd ed. Gravlee GP, Davis RF Kurusz M, Utley JR, eds. City, PA: Lippincott Williams & Wilkins; 1999.

176. Gorman RC, Ziats NP, Gikakis N, et al. Surface-bound heparin fails to reduce thrombin formation during clinical cardiopulmonary bypass. *J Thorac Cardiovasc Surg* 1996; 111:1-11.

177. Muehrcke DD, McCarthy PM, Stewart RW, et al. Complications of extracorporeal life support systems using heparin-bound surfaces. *J Thorac Cardiovasc Surg* 1995; 110:843-851.

178. Videm V, Mollnes TE, Bergh K, et al. Heparin-coated cardiopulmonary bypass equipment. II. Mechanisms for reduced complement activation in vivo. *J Thorac Cardiovasc Surg* 1999; 117:803-809.

179. Videm V, Mollnes TE, Fosse E, et al. Heparin-coated cardiopulmonary bypass equipment. I. Biocompatibility markers and development of complications in a high-risk population. *J Thorac Cardiovasc Surg* 1999; 117:794-802.

180. Wildevuur CR, Jansen PG, Bezemer PD, et al. Clinical evaluation of Duraflo II heparin treated extracorporeal circulation circuits (2nd version). The European Working Group on Heparin Coated Extracorporeal Circulation Circuits. *Eur J Cardiothorac Surg* 1997; 11:616-623.

181. Zucker MB, Vroman L. Platelet adhesion induced by fibrinogen adsorbed onto glass. *Proc Soc Exp Biol Med* 1969; 13:318-320.

182. Salzman EW, Merrill EW, Binder A, Wolf CF, Ashford TP, Austen WG. Protein-platelet interaction on heparinized surfaces. *J Biomed Mater Res* 1969; 31:69-81.

183. Adrian K, Mellgren K, Skogby M, Friberg LG, Mellgren G, Wadenvik H. The effect of albumin priming solution on platelet activation during experimental long-term perfusion. *Perfusion* 1998; 13:187-191.

184. Addonizio VP, Strauss JF, Macarak EJ, Colman RW, Edmunds H Jr. Preservation of platelet number and function with prostaglandin E1 during cardiopulmonary bypass in rhesus monkeys. *Surgery* 1978; 83:619-625.

185. Shigeta I, Gluszko P, Downing SW, et al. Protection of platelets during long-term extracorporeal membrane oxygenation in sheep with a single dose of a disintegrin. *Circulation* 1992; (5 Suppl): II398-404.

4

ECLS and the Systemic Inflammatory Response

Ravi S. Radhakrishnan, M.D. and Charles S. Cox, Jr., M.D.

Introduction

During extracorporeal circulation, blood and individual blood components are continuously exposed to the non-biologic synthetic surfaces of the extracorporeal circuit. After exposure of blood to artificial surfaces, a systemic inflammatory reaction is activated which is believed to be responsible for the "post-perfusion" or "post-pump" syndrome associated with standard cardiopulmonary bypass (CPB).[1-11] This systemic response can lead to widespread organ damage and post-operative morbidity.

ECLS differs from standard CPB used in cardiac surgery mainly by the duration of its use. The majority of open-heart operations utilize an extracorporeal circuit for a few hours, compared to the days or weeks that a patient may be supported with ECLS. Other clinically relevant variables that differentiate ECLS from CPB include: 1) the potential for maintenance of pulmonary blood flow, 2) normothermic perfusion, 3) lack of hemodilution, 4) blood priming solutions, and 5) inflammatory stimuli that may be the reason for initiating ECLS. These variables can affect the ultimate systemic response and organ injury associated with ECLS.

There is an abundance of information concerning the systemic inflammatory and immune responses of patients exposed to short-term CPB for cardiac surgery. There is less information about the effects of prolonged ECLS and the systemic inflammatory response. This chapter reviews systemic responses to short- and long-term extracorporeal circulation and will focus on the role of polymorphonuclear leukocyte (PMN)-endothelial activation and interactions as well as the future of anti-inflammatory strategies applicable to clinical ECLS.

Overview

Clinicians caring for ECLS patients have noted that a "whole body inflammatory response" occurs after the initiation of ECLS. Early investigations focused on the abnormal physiology of altered blood flow patterns and blood-foreign surface interactions.[7,8,12,13] A schematic overview of the factors that contribute to the inflammatory response associated with ECLS is shown in Figure 1. The adverse effects of ECLS were noted primarily in the form of acute lung injury (ALI) and its reduction has become the focus of numerous investigations.[14,15] A number of technical modifications of CPB for cardiac surgery led to a reduction in ALI. These improvements include: changing from gas to membrane oxygenators, blood leukocyte filtration and the avoidance of blood priming solutions, and avoidance of pulmonary vascular distention. Although ALI still occurs to varying degrees, these techniques have decreased the incidence of severe ALI after CPB from approximately 20% to 2% of all cardiac procedures.[7] In contrast, it is common to observe an increase in lung and total body water with chest radiograph opacification after initiating ECLS (Figure 2).[16,17]

An important difference between the majority of ECLS patients and routine CPB patients is the frequent presence of a previous inflammatory stimulus in ECLS patients. Most patients who undergo ECLS are profoundly hypoxic. Others are septic or bacteremic with septic shock as the indication for ECLS; thus, the vascular endothelium is often activated, and the PMNs are up-regulated or "primed" to release

toxic reactive oxygen species and proteolytic enzymes. ECLS initiates the release of a cascade of inflammatory mediators (via blood-foreign surface interactions) such as complement, thromboxane, and tumor necrosis factor (TNFα) that serve to amplify the activated PMN and endothelial response resulting in PMN transendothelial migration, microvascular barrier damage, edema formation, and tissue injury. Altered blood flow also plays an important role in the inflammatory response and ultimate organ injury associated with ECLS.[6,13,18,19] Intestinal mucosal hypoperfusion has been associated with endotoxin lipoplysaccharide (LPS) translocation across the gut during ECLS.[20,21] Reduced

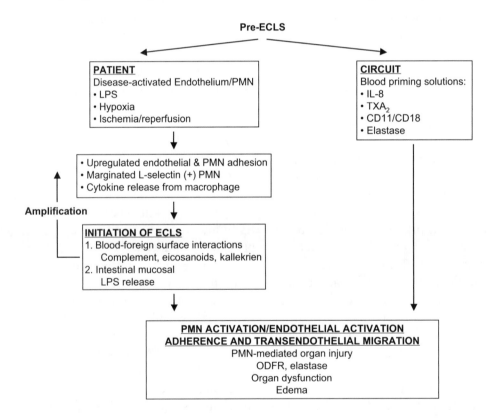

Figure 1. ECLS and the systemic inflammatory response. Both patient and ECLS circuit contribute to the inflammatory response observed with the initiation of ECLS. Disease-activated endothelium and PMNs are further stimulated by the blood-foreign surface interactions and release of pro-inflammatory cytokines and eicosanoids. This amplification of the inflammatory response results in increased PMN adhesion and organ injury. Altered intestinal perfusion and subsequent barrier dysfunction may continue the inflammatory response. PMN-mediated microvascular barrier injury is often manifest by organ edema and ultimately organ dysfunction and/or failure.

pulmonary blood flow during CPB and venoar-terial (VA) ECMO reduces the capillary shear forces which may increase PMN adherence to the pulmonary vascular endothelium, resulting in PMN-mediated tissue injury.[15,22]

Ultimately, the cycle of amplifying inflammatory responses associated with ECLS is broken due to a number of factors: 1) control of inciting stimulus, 2) restoration of tissue perfusion and reversal of hypoxia, 3) passivation of the foreign surface in ECLS circuit, 4) anti-inflammatory properties of heparin, and 5) self-regulation to limit inflammatory response. Non-survivors have sustained irreversible organ injury before and during ECLS and/or the inciting stimulus is never controlled. The factors of endothelial activation, mediator amplification of inflammation, altered blood flow, PMN activation-endothelial interactions, and organ injury will be discussed. Future anti-inflammatory strategies will be aimed at the PMN-endothelial interactions and less at upstream, overlapping, and redundant inflammatory mediators.

Pre-ECLS inflammatory response

As stated above, the inflammatory response to ECLS often begins prior to the initiation of ECLS with the disease process (e.g., sepsis, hypoxia, pulmonary aspiration). These disease processes have their own unique inflammatory response.[23-29] In contrast, the patient undergoing CPB for elective correction of acquired heart disease is usually not critically ill.

In response to ischemia, hypoxia, or inflammatory mediators released from a site of distant inflammation, endothelial cells can change their surface properties allowing adhesion and localization of inflammatory cells.[30] This is referred to as endothelial activation. A major component of endothelial activation by these diverse stimuli is the expression of endothelial adhesion molecules including E-selectin and intercellular adhesion molecule 1 (ICAM-1). These adhesion molecules as well as those expressed on the PMN surface (principally, the $\beta2$ integrins) result in PMN-endothelial adherence and transendothelial migration followed by PMN degranulation, releasing proteolytic enzymes and oxygen derived free radicals (ODFR). This ultimately results in microvascular barrier damage and organ dysfunction.

Hypoxia is the final manifestation of the many conditions treated with ECLS. Hypoxia alone can result in a marked increase in microvascular endothelial permeability in response

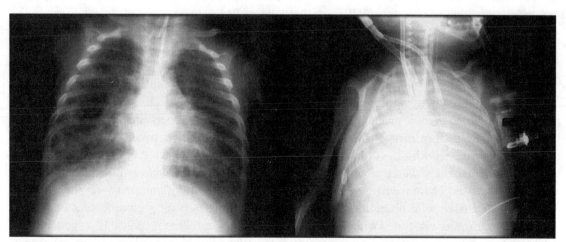

Figure 2. Chest radiographs before and after initiation of ECLS for cardiopulmonary failure. Note the pulmonary opacification and the increase in body wall edema.

to an inflammatory stimulus.[31,32] Numerous studies have shown an increase in endothelial deposition of the complement component C3 after hypoxia. These conditions exist in vivo with the initiation of ECLS for almost any diagnosis. Therefore, it is not surprising that there is a marked increase in vascular endothelial permeability with the initiation of ECLS. Collard et al. have demonstrated in vitro that hypoxia followed by reoxygenation produces intracellular ODFR.[33,34] Further studies link the intracellular ODFR to nuclear factor-κB activation, extracellular epitope expression, and classic complement activation.[35-37] Therefore, hypoxia alone can activate the vascular endothelium, setting the stage for PMN-mediated microvascular barrier injury.

Sepsis or endotoxemia

While sepsis or septic shock is an indication for the initiation of ECLS, ongoing systemic inflammation can exacerbate the usual modest inflammatory response to ECLS alone. Endotoxin (LPS) up-regulates both PMN and vascular endothelial adhesion molecules which results in greater PMN adherence within the microvasculature. Also, endotoxemia produces an increase in pro-inflammatory cytokines that are further exacerbated by the initiation of ECLS. The secondary stimulus of initiating ECLS results in a heightened inflammatory response that is greater than that seen with ECLS or sepsis alone. The microvascular response to ECLS after infusion with LPS has been measured, and there is an increase in the microvascular permeability to protein, resulting in more pronounced edema formation.[38] These data mirror what is observed clinically in patients who develop profound increases in total body water when ECLS is initiated for sepsis. There is growing evidence that the PMN mediates the alterations in microvascular permeability associated with sepsis and ECLS. Future anti-inflammatory strategies with ECLS will focus on altering PMN-endothelial interactions, and less on redundant and overlapping inflammatory mediators.

Extracorporeal circuit

ECLS tubing and the oxygenator contribute to the inflammatory process as well. Finn, Moat, and Elliot have extensively studied the effects of ECLS priming solutions on inflammatory mediator and adhesion molecule up-regulation.[39-43] This group has examined changes in PMN adhesive and secretory function in a mock CPB circuit primed with blood and crystalloid. Using flow cytometry analyses to detect changes in PMN adhesion molecule expression, they demonstrated dramatic changes in PMN expression of the adhesion molecules CD11b/CD18 and L-selectin.[40,41] A rise in CD11b and a fall in L-selectin expression took place in circulating blood. Under flow conditions, L-selectin plays a critical role in the initial tethering of the PMN to the activated endothelium. This is thought to be a prerequisite to the initiation of CD11b/CD18 mediated PMN adhesion to the endothelium. A criticism of these data has been the potentially conflicting findings of simultaneous up- and down-regulation of PMN adhesion molecules that are thought to act in sequence to affect PMN-endothelial adhesion. Finn et al. explain in their analysis of flow cytometry data that at 2 hours of CPB, ~50% of the circulating PMNs have normal L-selectin expression and greatly enhanced CD11b/CD18 expression. This population of cells would be much more likely to adhere to the activated endothelium, especially under conditions of lower blood flow (and shear stress) such as in the pulmonary circulation during reperfusion or VA ECMO. The initial interactions between plasma proteins and biomaterials is depicted in Figure 3. The blood-foreign surface interactions initiate this powerful thrombotic and inflammatory response within minutes. The ensuing complement activation and PMN-cytokine response is responsible for the clinically evident inflammatory response to ECLS initiation.

Finn and others have shown a marked increase in the pro-inflammatory cytokine, IL-8 with in vitro extracorporeal circulation.[41,44] Therefore, a blood-primed extracorporeal circuit is a source of activated PMNs and the PMN chemoattractant, IL-8. Thus, PMNs and these pro-inflammatory cytokines are infused immediately into the systemic and pulmonary circulation. Even with leukocyte depletion, this probably plays a significant role in the augmentation of the systemic inflammatory response syndrome (SIRS) associated with ECLS.[45] These data suggest that future areas of research that could eliminate the need for blood-priming, such as miniature pumps, biocompatible blood substitutes, or specific anti-inflammatory strategies, may minimize the initial inflammatory response to ECLS.

Humoral pathophysiology

Cytokines

Cytokines are polypeptides, produced by a variety of cells, which function as mediators of communication between cells involved in immunity and inflammation.[46] In addition, they are thought to play an essential role in the pathogenesis of shock and multi-organ failure during severe infection.[47,48] The most common cytokines studied in relation to CPB are the ones associated with acute inflammation; specifically, interleukin-1 (IL-l), TNF, interleukin-6 (IL-6), and interleukin-8 (IL-8).

IL-l is predominantly produced by monocytes in response to injury and infection. It is involved in multiple aspects of the acute inflammatory response including fever, synthesis of hepatic acute phase proteins, release of growth factors, alteration in endothelial cell function and permeability, decreased systemic vascular resistance, and loss of body mass.[49] IL-1 also induces production of other cytokines including TNF and IL-6.[50] Extracorporeal circulation during hemodialysis has been shown to stimulate IL-1 production.[51] There are conflicting data on the IL-1 response to short-term CPB. Haeffner-Cavaillon et al. studied IL-1 production in monocytes isolated from 15 patients undergoing CPB.[52] Although no increase in IL-1 activity was observed, a significant increase did occur 24 hours after bypass. The peak in IL-1 production correlated with the peak in body temperature among these patients, which suggests an asso-

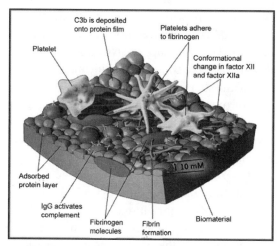

Figure 3. Initial interactions between plasma proteins and biomaterials. When heparinized blood contacts a biomaterial surface, plasma proteins are instantly adsorbed onto the surface to form a dense, thin covering that varies based on different biomaterials and mixtures of plasma proteins. Some adsorbed proteins, including coagulation factor XII, undergo conformational changes to expose reactive domains to circulating blood elements; thus, formation of thrombin and fibrin is initiated through the intrinsic coagulation pathway. Adsorbed IgG triggers complement activation, which is immediately amplified by the alternative pathway. Large amounts of C3b are generated and deposited on the adsorbed protein layer to catalyze activation of downstream complement proteins. During initial contact, fibrinogen is selectively adsorbed onto many biomaterials and expresses reactive sites on α and γ chains that bind αIIbβ3. Thus, within 1-2 minutes, biomaterials initiate powerful thrombotic and inflammatory responses in blood. (Reprinted from Edmunds, H.L. Cardiopulmonary Bypass after 50 Years. *New Engl J Med*, 2004, 351:1603-1606. Copyright ©2004 Massachusetts Medical Society. All rights reserved.)

The figure contains the following labels: C3b is deposited onto protein film; Platelets adhere to fibrinogen; Platelet; Conformational change in factor XII and factor XIIa; Adsorbed protein layer; IgG activates complement; Fibrinogen molecules; Fibrin formation; Biomaterial; 10 mM

ciation between IL-1 and the acute inflammatory response following CPB. In addition, Golej et al. examined the effect of VA vs. venovenous (VV) ECLS on cytokine release and noted an increase in the levels of IL-1 in the bronchoalveolar lavage (BAL) fluid in both the VA and VV groups after 5 hours. They noted a significantly greater increase in the BAL fluid IL-1 levels in the VA group over the VV group.[53] Butler et al. who examined IL-1 production in 20 patients undergoing coronary bypass surgery, reported contrasting results.[54] Plasma levels of IL-6 were significantly elevated above baseline at the end of CPB and peaked 4 hours post-operatively. These levels remained significantly higher than pre-bypass values for 48 hours However, no significant IL-1 response was seen. Two other studies of short-term CPB have also failed to detect circulating levels of IL-1.[42,55] In addition, Fortenberry et al. examined 15 patients before and during ECMO and observed no significant change in serum IL-1 levels.[56]

Primarily-activated macrophages, lymphocytes and Kupffer cells produce TNF, a key cytokine involved in the acute inflammatory response to infection and injury.[48] TNF increases neutrophil adhesion and stimulates neutrophil phagocytosis, degranulation, and superoxide production. TNF also enhances production of other cytokines and may be a factor in the lethal outcome of gram-negative sepsis.[2] Similar to the data on IL-l, evidence for TNF synthesis associated with short-term CPB has been conflicting. Jansen et al. showed a significant increase in TNF levels during CPB, but the increase was associated only with release of the aortic cross-clamp.[57] Plotz reported that TNF concentrations peaked 8 hours after the onset of CPB but quickly fell and remained low throughout the bypass RUN.[58] A study of 19 patients undergoing open cardiac operations failed to detect a change in plasma levels of TNF either in the operative or post-operative period. Another study in adults also failed to demonstrate changes in TNF levels in plasma

or monocyte cultures 24 hours after bypass. In addition, a study of 15 neonates on ECMO for respiratory failure did not reveal a significant change in baseline values of TNF.[52]

Numerous cells including inflammatory and epithelial cells produce IL-6. IL-6 has been identified as one of the key modulators of the hepatic response to injury and inflammation.[59] In vitro, it induces acute phase protein synthesis and has been detected in serum after burn injury and elective operations.[60] IL-6 acts synergistically with IL-1 as a co-stimulator of enhanced T-cell proliferation and may possess additional immunosuppressive effects.[61] Plasma IL-6 levels were shown to significantly increase following short-term CPB irrespective of the type of oxygenator used.[54] Other investigators have also described increases in plasma IL-6 levels following short-term extracorporeal circulation.[55]

IL-8 is a chemoattractant specific for neutrophils and not monocytes.[62] It is also involved in the inflammatory response and has been shown to cause neutrophilia, neutrophil trapping in the lungs, and capillary leak resembling the pathophysiology of the adult respiratory distress syndrome (ARDS).[63] It is also believed that IL-8 is involved in the regulation of neutrophil transendothelial migration, suggesting a significant controlling mechanism for neutrophil-mediated tissue injury.[64] Finn et al. compared IL-8 production in patients undergoing open-heart operations with patients undergoing non-cardiac procedures of similar length and transfusion requirements.[42] All of the CPB patients demonstrated elevations in IL-8 while only 1 patient in the non-cardiac group had a rise in circulating IL-8. Although IL-8 release occurred near the end of bypass, the increase correlated with the duration of bypass. Other investigators have demonstrated an increase in BAL fluid IL-8 levels on ECMO after 5 hours with a greater increase in IL-8 levels in the VA ECMO group as compared with the VV ECMO group.[53] Fortenberry et al. examined 15 neonates with respiratory failure treated with ECMO and demonstrated a significant increase in the serum levels of IL-8 after the initiation of ECMO.[56]

The effect of ECMO on systemic cytokine release was described in an investigation of 9 neonates supported with ECMO.[5] Measurements of IL-l, IL-6, IL-8, and TNF were recorded before, during, and following ECMO. Significant increases in IL-6 and IL-8 occurred during ECMO, while no significant TNF or IL-1 was detected. In another study, Hirthler et al. examined cytokine release in 16 neonates requiring ECMO. Blood samples were obtained at 5 minutes, 1 hour, 12 hours, and 24 hours after the start of ECMO and then daily until decannulation for measurement of IL-l, IL-6, TNF, ODFR, and endotoxin.[6] There was a significant increase in circulating TNF levels at 36 hours of ECMO in all patients. Both IL-1 and IL-6 levels failed to increase during the ECMO course. Interestingly, TNF levels were not elevated in survivors in contrast to non-survivors who had significant elevations after 36 hours. The increase in TNF was also associated with detectable levels of endotoxin and measured elevations of ODFR activity suggestive of sepsis. Yanagi et al. noted an increase in IL-1 and TNFβ, but the magnitude of the increase was not substantially greater than sham-treated animals.[65] Of note, this study used a mini hollow-fiber lung with a blood-free prime. This reduction in blood-foreign-surface interactions and avoidance of initiating the inflammatory cascade with priming may account for these findings. While the available data are limited, these studies suggest that cytokine release is stimulated by both long- and short-term extracorporeal circulation and may also be involved in the acute inflammatory response associated with CPB.

Eicosanoids

Eicosanoids are the derivatives of arachadonic acid metabolism. Membrane peroxidation (or phospholipase A_2 [PLA_2] activation)

provides the arachadonic acid substrate for the synthesis of the pro-inflammatory eicosanoids. Thromboxanes (e.g., TXA_2, TXB_2) can locally regulate ALI. TXB_2 is the stable metabolite of the vasoactive mediator TXA_2. These mediators are of particular importance because ECLS is associated with an increase in circulating TXB_2. TXB_2 as well as other vasoactive and pro-inflammatory eicosanoids affect PMN recruitment and activation, as well as regional perfusion. TXB_2 may influence lung injury by increasing transvascular fluid and protein movement through alterations in the endothelial cytoskeleton, including widening of the interendothelial tight junctions. TXB_2 is a potent vasoconstrictor that can also increase pulmonary capillary pressure, thus augmenting transvascular fluid flux as well as altering regional microvascular perfusion. Both of these actions can increase extravascular lung water, exacerbating lung injury.

An early transient increase in TXB_2 with the initiation of ECLS, with and without previous lung injury, has been demonstrated.[66,67] Indeed, stimulation of TXB_2 synthesis has been observed using in vitro CPB circuits. Bui et al. studied the relationship of ECLS and eicosanoid metabolism in neonates.[68-70] TXB_2 correlated with the pulmonary artery pressure in infants with meconium aspiration syndrome. Based on previous animal data, there was concern that the ECLS circuit induced TXB_2 release and would exacerbate TXB_2-mediated persistent pulmonary hypertension of the newborn and ALI. However, they did not observe an increase in TXB_2 in infants treated with ECLS, and TXB_2 decreased as the lung injury resolved. Similar data were obtained by Dobyns et al.[71] It is difficult to determine from these data the importance of TXB_2 in the pathophysiology of ALI treated with ECLS. Some have suggested that these mediators are epiphenomena of ALI (i.e., markers of ALI which are not causative of ALI). Based on in vivo and in vitro data, we believe that the early TXB_2 release with ECLS exacerbates the initial ALI. Zwischenberger et al. demonstrated this in a sheep model of ALI and ECLS in which there was a characteristic increase in the chemoattractant TXB_2 with an associated increase in pulmonary leukosequestration, lung water, and membrane peroxidation as measured by conjugated diene release.[67] Clinically, most patients recover from this initial phase (characterized by opacification and increased total body water). However, those patients with consistently high TXB_2 release are often those with an exaggerated inflammatory response and poor outcome.[71] Moreover, TXB_2 blockade with TXB_2-receptor antagonists and thromboxane synthase inhibitors has ameliorated PMN-mediated lung injury in animal models. Erez et al. have shown that aspirin markedly reduces serum TXB_2 levels in CPB patients and may play a role in the prevention of pulmonary injury.[72] As with many proximal inflammatory mediators, the eicosanoids exert a significant but not singular influence over the pulmonary response to ECLS. TXB_2 probably plays a role in the initial, early PMN-mediated exacerbation of ALI from which most patients recover.

Complement Activation

The human complement system is composed of 9 different enzyme precursors (C1-C9) which are normally found in plasma and other body fluids. These enzymes are usually inactive, but once activated, they function as important amplifiers of inflammatory reactions. They are produced by a number of cells, including macrophages and vascular endothelial cells, and can be activated by a variety of mechanisms including bound immunoglobulin or the release of hydrolytic enzymes from injured cells or leukocytes. The activated complement fragments are identified by an "a" (i.e., C3a). C3a and C5a stimulate the release of mast cell histamine, cause smooth muscle contraction, and increase vascular permeability.[73] In addition, C5a binds with circulating neutrophil receptors and causes

neutrophil aggregation, particularly in the lung.[74] Several cellular responses follow this interaction, including superoxide generation, chemotaxis, and release of lysosomal enzymes. C3a and C5a production have been associated with a variety of clinical conditions, including pulmonary edema and ARDS.[75]

Activation of the complement system has been extensively studied in both adult and pediatric cardiac patients exposed to short-term extracorporeal circulation. Parker et al. described total serum complement levels in 11 patients who had undergone aortic valvular surgery.[76] Complement levels were significantly reduced at both 4 and 20 hours following surgery. At the time of the report, it was unclear whether this finding was due to an activation or denaturation of the systemic complement. The development of a radioimmunoassay to detect circulating levels of the activated complement components (C3a and C5a) clarified this question. In 1981, Chenowith et al. studied a group of 15 adult patients undergoing CPB.[73] Within 10 minutes of initiating bypass, systemic C3a levels were significantly elevated compared with pre-bypass measurements and continued to increase throughout the duration of CPB. Interestingly, C5a levels showed no significant change. These findings established that it was activation and not denaturation that was responsible for the decrease in total complement levels reported by Parker.[72] The effect of CPB on C3a levels was corroborated in a study of 116 consecutive adult cardiac patients. A significant elevation in C3a was found at the end of bypass, which persisted for 3 hours after operation. In contrast, among patients undergoing closed cardiac procedures without CPB, C3a levels did not change. In addition, elevated C3a levels were associated with the cardiac, pulmonary, renal, and hematological complications documented in post-operative patients.

The effects of short-term CPB on complement activation in children were reported in a prospective study of 30 children undergoing

CPB.[77] Each patient exhibited a rapid increase in C3a levels immediately after the initiation of bypass which peaked after bypass was discontinued. Post-operative complications occurred in 37% and most were associated with significant increases in complement activation. Another study prospectively examined complement activation in 29 children undergoing operation for congenital heart disease.[78] CPB duration ranged from 31-152 minutes. During CPB there were significant increases in the levels of activated C3 and C5. When a comparison was made between patients who developed multi-system organ failure with those that did not, a positive correlation was demonstrated between elevated levels of activated complement and multi-system failure. These data suggest that complement activation may be associated with the adverse systemic effects of short-term CPB. Matsuda linked complement activation during ECLS with increased PMN-endothelial interactions providing more pathophysiological linkage between ECLS-induced complement activation and the PMN-mediated tissue injury.[79]

The effect of ECMO on neonatal complement activation has recently been described. Severe respiratory distress in 5 newborns who were treated with ECMO from 121-309 hours were studied.[80] Immediately following initiation of bypass, plasma C3a levels increased significantly and peaked after 2 hours. There was no change in the levels of C4a or C5a during the entire period of ECMO. Whole complement levels returned to pre-ECMO levels by 24 hours post-bypass. Westfall et al. followed 21 consecutive infants with respiratory failure who required ECMO. Levels of both C3 and C5 decreased (indicating overall complement activation) immediately after initiation of ECMO.[81] By 12 hours on ECMO, the serum complement levels had returned to baseline. Graulich et al. reviewed 6 consecutive neonates and examined C3a, C5a, and sC5b-9 levels. They noted a significant elevation in all 3 components, both in vivo and in vitro. These elevations in serum complement levels peaked after 1 hour and returned to baseline levels after 24 hours.[82] Another study reviewed complement activation associated with ECMO in 10 patients with severe respiratory distress.[58] ECMO duration ranged 55-241 hours Immediately after initiation of ECMO, C3a concentrations increased significantly from pre-bypass levels. These concentrations slowly decreased and by 24 hours of bypass had returned to baseline levels. While most studies have focused on the classical pathway of complement activation, Vallhonrat et al. measured the effect of ECMO on the activation of complement pathways. By measuring C4d levels as a marker of the classical pathway, and Bb as the marker for the alternative pathway, they demonstrated a significant increase in the alternative pathway 1 hour after initiation of ECMO, with levels returning to baseline after 24 hours[83] These results suggest that both short- and long-term extracorporeal circulation cause significant complement activation and that complement levels return to baseline within 24 hours. In addition, the activated components may play a role in the diffuse organ dysfunction seen following short-term bypass; however, the clinical sequelae of complement activation in patients undergoing ECMO remains unclear.

Cellular pathophysiology

PMN-endothelial interactions

A number of studies have investigated the mechanisms of PMN-endothelial interactions after inflammatory stimuli. This work has resulted in the 4-step model of PMN adhesion and transmigration across an endothelial monolayer under flow conditions. Steps 1 and 2 are selectin-mediated, consisting of PMN tethering and rolling in the post-capillary venules.[84-86] Step 3 is PMN adherence, and occurs as PMNs encounter ICAM and the PMN has expressed the β2 integrins.[87-90] Step 4 is transendothelial migration and occurs in the presence of platelet-endothelial cell adhesion molecule 1 (PECAM-1) (Figure 4).

PMN-endothelial interactions have been studied in association with extracorporeal circulation. Initiation of ECLS in vivo is marked by an abrupt decrease in circulating PMNs followed by a leukocytosis. The leukopenia is thought to be due to leukosequestration in the circuit and lungs.[67] L-selectin shedding and CD11/CD18 up-regulation in response to initiating ECLS mark PMN activation in vitro.[40,91] This response has been documented in an in vivo model as well.[56] In vivo, traumatic stress, infection, and other inflammatory processes can increase the number of circulating L-selectin (+) PMNs principally through selective margination of these cells from the bone marrow.[26] The previous pool of circulating PMNs is thought to be the cells that shed the L-selectin adhesion molecules in response to stress. These changes are felt to be in response to blood-foreign surface interactions and soluble mediator release (complement, TXA2, PAF, IL-8) induced by ECLS.

Dreyer et al. have confirmed a CD18-dependent mechanism of pulmonary PMN sequestration and demonstrated up-regulation of pulmonary endothelial ICAM-1 with hypothermic total CPB.[4,87] Friedman et al. have demonstrated 2 important findings regarding the effects of partial pulmonary blood flow and β2-integrin antagonist drug therapy. They noted that maintenance of pulmonary blood flow decreased the lung injury associated with CPB. Moreover, maintaining pulmonary blood flow and β2-integrin antagonism had a synergistic effect on minimizing lung injury.[15] These data have been confirmed using in vitro CPB circuits which demonstrate that polyvinyl chloride (PVC) tubing and priming solutions alone cause CD11b up-regulation and L-selectin shedding.[44]

ECLS, in the setting of a previous inflammatory or hypoxic stimulus, would be expected to result in a marked increase in PMN-endothelial adherence. The endothelium is activated, and the blood-primed circuit infuses a high concentration of pro-inflammatory mediators

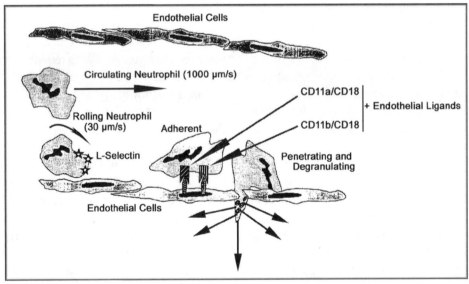

Figure 4. The sequence of PMN-endothelial interactions which leads to PMN adherence and transendothelial migration. These interactions are initiated and controlled by the PMN and endothelial adhesion molecules of the selectin and β-2 integrin families. ECLS and the inflammatory stimuli occurring prior to initiating ECLS result in upregulation of the adhesion molecules which initiate PMN rolling, tethering, adherence, and transendothelial migration. (Reprinted with permission from Elsevier. Elliott MJ. Interaction between neutrophils and endothelium. *Ann Thorac Surg* 1993; 56:1503-1508.)

and activated PMNs. Moreover, the inflammatory response as well as the reduction in pulmonary blood flow with CPB and VA ECLS probably affects pulmonary leukosequestration. Theoretically, maintaining pulmonary blood flow should reduce PMN-endothelial adherence by higher post-capillary venule shear forces.[92] These inflammatory stimuli which increase PMN-endothelial adherence followed by ECLS have been demonstrated in both in vitro and in vivo models.[56,93-95]

Vascular dysfunction

Depending on the site of the vascular bed, there are different responses to the initiation of ECLS and CPB. While data in the ECLS model are limited, there is a large amount of information on the vascular response to CPB. These differential changes in vascular response can be divided into 2 groups of vascular beds: the peripheral vascular bed and the coronary, pulmonary, and mesenteric beds.

In examining the peripheral vascular bed, there is a marked reduction in vascular resistance and abnormal permeability after initiation of CPB.[96] These changes occur due to alterations in vascular smooth muscle tone and by endothelial dysfunction. Peripheral vascular resistance has been shown to decrease after the initiation of CPB.[90,97] The exact mechanism for this dysfunction appears to be multi-factorial, with the release of complement, inflammatory cytokines, and increased nitric oxide (NO) production leading to peripheral vasodilation.[98] In addition, recent data suggest that CPB reduces extracellular signal-related kinase 1/2 (ERK1/2) and p38 activity in peripheral tissue, regulating peripheral vascular dysfunction via a mitogen-activated protein kinase (MAPK) pathway.[99] The coronary,[100] pulmonary,[101] and mesenteric[102] vascular beds show the opposite response: vascular contraction with an increase in vascular resistance after initiation of CPB via activation of MAPK. Also, complement activation has been linked to inhibi-

tion of endothelium relaxation through generation of a membrane attack complex in coronary arteries.[103] Thromboxanes may play a role in the vasoconstriction seen in the pulmonary circulation.[104] Doguet et al. demonstrated an increase in mesenteric endothelial reactivity and subsequent vasoconstriction after CPB and increased reactivity to α-1 adrenergic agonists, suggesting that the risk for mesenteric ischemia may be increased after CPB with the use of vasopressors.[105] Overall, the peripheral vascular bed has a decrease in vascular tone, while the cardiac, pulmonary, and mesenteric vascular beds have a propensity for vasoconstriction, which may lead to further tissue ischemia with the use of CPB.

Vascular dysfunction is also manifested by endothelial cell injury. Various studies have characterized endothelial cell dysfunction in the pulmonary,[106] cardiac,[107] and mesenteric[106] circulation. In the coronary circulation, recent data suggest that endothelial injury is mediated by activation of mitogen-activated protein kinase,[108] the prolonged exposure to potassium, and the generation of ODFR.[107,109] Mesenteric endothelial cells have been shown, in settings of impaired reactivity, such as CPB, to further mediate tissue and endothelial injury by reacting uncharacteristically leading to poor oxygen delivery.[110] In addition, L-arginine has been shown to protect myocardial and mesenteric vascular endothelium from injury by removing ODFR.[111,112] While vascular dysfunction appears to be a multifactorial process, data suggest that complement activation, leukocyte activation/adherence,[113] cytokine and NO production, derangement of the MAPK pathway, and formation of ODFR mediate vascular dysfunction.

Organ edema and dysfunction

Edema formation after the initiation of ECLS is common.[16,114] It is governed by changes in the Starling equation, which result from ECLS. In addition, fluid mobilization and resolution of edema are primary determinants of ECLS duration.[115] Further, edema leads to organ dysfunction. Therefore, edema formation from ECLS and its subsequent resolution are important clinical problems. While edema formation is typically generalized, its functional effects on the heart, lungs, and intestine will be examined.

Edema formation is governed by the Starling equation:[116]

$$Q = K \left[(Pmv - Ppmv) - \sigma(\textstyle\prod mv - \textstyle\prod pmv) \right]$$

where Q is flow, K is microvascular filtration coefficient, P is hydrostatic pressure, $\prod$ is the osmotic pressure, σ is the osmotic reflection coefficient, mv is microvascular, and pmv is perimicrovascular.

Edema during ECLS is increased in various ways as variables in the Starling equation illustrate. Circuit priming with crystalloids causes hemodilution, reducing osmotic pressure in the vessel and leading to myocardial edema and cardiac dysfunction.[117,118] Also, as described above, ECLS and CPB activate many inflammatory mediators, increasing the microvascular filtration coefficient and decreasing the osmotic reflection coefficient through vascular endothelial damage. This vascular endothelial damage and its contribution to organ edema have been demonstrated in coronary,[107] pulmonary,[104,119,120] and intestinal[114,121] microvasculature.

Edema and its effects on organ function have been adequately investigated.[122-125] Studies have shown that myocardial edema causes ventricular dysfunction.[117,126] Studies in the lung have demonstrated the adverse effects of edema on the alveolar-arterial gradient.[127] Examination of the intestine has revealed that intestinal edema leads to decreased intestinal transit[122-125,128] and disruption of intestinal barrier function.[128] Edema has been shown to lead to organ dysfunction in different organ systems. Consequently, understanding the inflammatory response and the formation of organ edema and determining ways to shorten the duration of ECLS to minimize further organ dysfunction is an important goal.

Amplification of the inflammatory response

ECLS alone results in a moderate inflammatory response and concomitant moderate increase in microvascular permeability and edema formation. We have quantified the degree of microvascular barrier injury in the mesenteric circulation using a modification of the Kubes and Granger mesenteric lymphatic fistula technique, since alterations in microvascular permeability have been established as an early marker of organ failure.[27,129,130] These data demonstrate a modest increase in tissue water with the initiation of ECLS that corresponds to an increase in "capillary leak", mathematically described as a decrease in the reflection coefficient (σ in the Starling equation governing transvascular fluid flux).[129] Klein, Demling, and Smith concluded that ECLS contributed very little to the inflammatory response observed clinically in patients who undergo long-term ECLS. [115,119,131,132] In contrast, we noted an exacerbation of the ALI of smoke inhalation after initiating ECLS in a sheep model.[67] The ALI worsened, as evidenced by increased extravascular lung water, increased pulmonary leukosequestration, and increased lipid peroxidation. Indeed, these laboratory findings mimicked the clinical observations of significant increases in total body weight and extravascular lung water after initiation of ECLS in patients with cardiopulmonary compromise from various causes. Using the above-mentioned animal model, a profound increase in microvascular barrier injury after a hemodynamically insignificant dose of endotoxin followed by initiation of ECLS was noted. The pathophysiology of these observations is similar to the "two-hit model" currently described in the critical care literature.[133] The working hypothesis is that the PMN is primed by the initial stimulus of hypoxia, ischemia/reperfusion, or infection ("first hit"), and a second inflammatory stimulus (ECLS with associated complement activation, TXB_2 release, or the "second hit") results in an exaggerated PMN-mediated microvascular barrier injury and edema.[58,119,133-137] Ongoing or severe initial stimuli can result in significant organ dysfunction. Therefore, the prior condition or "inflammatory milieu" of the endothelium and PMN significantly impacts the response to ECLS. Indeed, ECLS may act as an amplifier of the initial inflammatory response. Complement activation, TNFα release, and endotoxemia associated with ECLS can serve to exacerbate PMN-mediated tissue injury.[138-141] For the reasons described above, those patients undergoing elective cardiac procedures usually experience only a minor inflammatory response to ECLS. In contrast, those patients who require emergency initiation of ECLS will often demonstrate an exaggerated inflammatory response.

Intestinal mucosal hypoperfusion

The intestine has been termed the "motor" of multi-organ failure, and numerous studies have examined the relationship between reductions in intestine blood flow and the inflammatory response to injury. Recent work has sought to establish a pathophysiologic link between intestinal hypoperfusion, bacterial translocation, and multi-organ failure or SIRS. A decrease in intestinal mucosal perfusion during normothermic ECLS has been demonstrated.[19,142] In these studies, normothermic ECLS was associated with intestinal mucosal ischemia despite "adequate" global perfusion; there is normal or increased blood flow through the superior mesenteric artery, but the intestinal mucosa remained ischemic (Figure 5). A progressive mucosal acidosis measured by tonometry was demonstrated. Coinciding with these observations are clinical data from

patients undergoing CPB for cardiac surgical procedures. A decrease in gastric mucosal pH was seen and correlated with the degree of decrease with post-operative septic complications.[143] Tao et al. concluded that mucosal ischemia during normothermic CPB resulted from the combination of mucosal hypoperfusion and increased intestinal oxygen consumption (VO_2) (Figure 6). The time course of the mucosal hypoperfusion correlates with the time course of release of TXB_2 and other vasoconstricting mediators. Recent studies of intestinal hypoperfusion/reperfusion in animal models have demonstrated that the mesenteric lymph that drains into the pulmonary circulation up-regulates the endothelial adhesion molecule ICAM-1 and primes PMNs for increased superoxide release.[29] These data support a mechanism of intestinal hypoperfusion and inflammatory mediator release into the pulmonary circulation that contributes to the pulmonary leukosequestration and PMN-mediated lung injury seen with ECLS/CPB. Continued intestinal hypoperfusion could lead to amplification of the initial inflammatory response and worsening of the initial ALI.

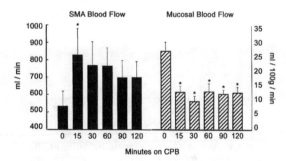

Figure 5. Ileal mucosal blood flow decreases despite supranormal total blood flow through the superior mesenteric artery. The reduction in mucosal blood flow corresponds to the initiation of ECLS and an increase in the circulating concentration of the vasoconstrictor TXA2. (Reprinted with permission from Elsevier. Cox CS, et al. Ileal mucosal hypoperfusion during cardiopulmonary bypass. *Curr Surg* 1992; 49:507-509.)

Resolution and reduction of the inflammatory response

Reversal of inciting stimulus

ECLS is primarily a cardiopulmonary support technique which allows time to complete the therapy for the underlying disease. Persistent pulmonary hypertension is one of the few diseases where ECLS is both a treatment of the underlying cause and is also a cardiopulmonary support technique. In contrast, patients with sepsis and resultant cardiopulmonary failure are only supported with ECLS; treatment of the underlying disease is a separate intervention. Thus, the character and severity of the underlying disease is a primary determinant of the duration and resolution of the inflammatory response. Often, the proinflammatory response known as SIRS is fully manifest despite treatment of the initiating cause of the cardiopulmonary failure. In these circumstances, ECLS offers prolonged support until the inflammatory process has resolved. The initial inflammatory response due to blood contact activation decreases due to "passivation" of the ECLS circuit. Plasma proteins (primarily fibrinogen and albumin) adhere to the ECLS biomaterial surface and are thought to prevent an ongoing inflammatory response. However, these proteins contribute to the thrombogenicity of the surface and potential clot formation within the ECLS circuit.

Ultrafiltration

To combat increased tissue water and edema after CPB, some clinicians have used modified ultrafiltration with success. Naik et al. first described a modified ultrafiltration technique in which filtration was carried out immediately after completion of CPB in a series circuit with the patient, in the absence of the CPB machine.[144] A prospective, randomized, trial with 50 patients demonstrated a significant decrease in blood loss, blood transfusion, and total body water in the modified ultrafiltration group vs. control. In addition, a significant rise in the systolic and diastolic blood pressure was seen.[145] While differing results have been reported, the majority of studies report decreases in total body water, myocardial edema, blood loss, and transfusion requirements; and increases in oxygenation, blood pressure, and contractility.[146] In addition to improvements in clinical indicators, investigators have begun to look at the effect of modified ultrafiltration on serum concentration of inflammatory mediators. Early studies have been equivocal. Dittrich et al. have demonstrated a significant decrease in IL-6 and IL-8 after modified ultrafiltration with more rapid clearance compared to controls.[147] Huang

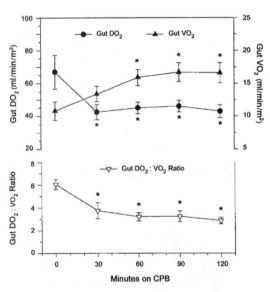

Figure 6. The DO_2:VO_2 relationship in the splanchnic circulation is altered with the initiation of ECLS. There is a decrease in DO_2 despite a stable or increased VO_2 as determined by trans-splanchnic oxygen content measurements. This correlates with the development of ileal mucosal edema. (Reprinted with permission from Elsevier. Tao W, et al. Gut mucosal ischemia during normothermic cardiopulmonary bypass results from blood flow redistribution and increased oxygen demand. *J Thorac Cardiovasc Surg* 1995; 110:819-827.)

et al. have shown that ultrafiltration decreases lung injury, airway resistance, hemodilution, and serum levels of IL-6 and thromboxane B2, with no difference in endothelin-1 levels.[148] Conversely, Pearl et al. have demonstrated no difference in thromboxane B2, leukotriene B4, and endothelin-1 levels with modified ultrafiltration compared with controls, suggesting that changes in these cytokines do not explain improved hemodynamics.[149]

Steroids

Recently, the effect of steroids on the inflammatory response to ECLS has been examined. Lodge et al. confirmed that methylprednisolone does reduce the inflammatory response associated with CPB in a neonatal pig model.[150] Furthermore, they demonstrated that timing of the dose (8 and 1.5 hours prior to initiation of CPB) was important in improving pulmonary compliance, pulmonary vascular resistance, and extracellular fluid accumulation. Griffin et al. showed that dexamethasone given prior and during CPB lowered radiographic lung injury scores.[151] Similarly, Duffy et al. demonstrated improved recovery of left ventricular systolic function after glucocorticoid administration prior to CPB.[152] They also demonstrated significant decreases in IL-6 and increases in IL-10 with steroid administration, possibly via a nuclear factor κB (NFκB) dependent pathway. McBride et al. examined cytokine production after CPB and found that methylprednisolone decreased IL-8 and TNFα, and increased IL-10 serum levels.[153] Varan et al. examined high vs. low dose steroids and showed decreases in IL-6 and IL-8 with no difference between doses.[154] Bourbon et al. examined the levels of IL-6, TNFα, and ODFR after CPB in adults after low and high dose methylprednisolone.[155] They showed significant decreases in IL-6 and TNFα with both low and high dose steroids with no difference between doses. However, ODFR decreased only after high dose steroids.

Heparin

The initiation of ECLS activates an already stimulated or up-regulated inflammatory response (Figure 1). The limitation and reversal of the inflammatory response is probably multifactorial and consists of 1) reversal of the inciting stimulus, 2) passivation of the ECLS circuit with reduction of contact activation of blood elements, and 3) heparin infusion.

Heparin is the primary anticoagulant used in ECLS. Relatively large doses are given prior to ECLS cannulation, and a continuous infusion is administered while on ECLS. Commercial heparin preparations are heterogeneous compounds with molecular weights of 3-30,000 Daltons. The pharmacokinetics of heparin are not completely understood, and most clinical centers measure the biological effects of heparin and not the heparin level. However, heparin serves as a reliable and relatively predictable anticoagulant for ECLS.

Numerous studies in vitro and in vivo have noted beneficial effects of heparin in ALI and inflammatory diseases.[142,156,157] Heparin has also been shown to improve survival in sepsis and endotoxic shock in multiple animal models.[156,158] Further work has elucidated the mechanisms by which heparin may exert a beneficial effect. This phenomenon appears unrelated to its anticoagulative properties. In vitro studies using cultured vascular endothelial cells, show that heparin prevented ODFR-mediated cellular injury.[159] Ex-vivo studies using isolated perfused lungs demonstrated a protective effect of heparin in a model of platelet activating factor (PAF)-induced pulmonary edema.[158] They showed a reduction in lung injury due to heparin–PAF interactions that result in a charge neutralization of PAF. Recent work has demonstrated that heparin decreases PMN-endothelial adhesion by binding to the selectin class of PMN adhesion molecules. These mechanistic studies may help explain the beneficial effects of heparin which have been observed in ECLS animal studies.

While functioning as a clinical anticoagulant, heparin is probably also functioning as a significant anti-inflammatory agent.

Hypothermia

Hypothermia has long been recognized to be organ protective during CPB. Classically, the primary effect of hypothermia was thought to be due to a reduction in oxygen consumption. The role of the PMN in the protective effects of hypothermia has been examined, demonstrating that hypothermia reduces PMN-endothelial adherence.[160,161] Hypothermia has also been shown to decrease the release of L-selectin positive PMNs from the bone marrow. This is a significant finding, as this is potentially the most adherent population of PMNs.[134,137] Recently, Horan et al. examined the effects of mild hypothermia on cytokine levels, complement levels, and coagulation markers and found no significant difference between controls.[162] While the beneficial effects of hypothermia may not be mediated by direct effects on cytokine or complement levels, hypothermia induced during routine CPB procedures, prior to halting flow in the pulmonary circulation, may minimize the adherence and margination of PMNs in the pulmonary microvasculature that would normally occur during normothermic CPB.

Summary

ECLS is used as a long-term support technique for acute cardiopulmonary failure. While it results in hemodynamic stabilization, it can exacerbate an already vigorous inflammatory response to sepsis, hypoxia/reoxygenation, and ischemia/reperfusion. The PMN and vascular endothelium play critical roles in the inflammatory response to ECLS.

A number of factors differentiate long-term ECLS from CPB, and these factors help explain some of the observed differences in the inflammatory response to ECLS as opposed to CPB. Although most centers have moved toward membrane oxygenators for routine CPB, ECLS is initiated in the setting of an activated endothelium with primed PMNs. Crystalloid priming solutions are standard clinical practice for most adult cardiac procedures requiring CPB. In contrast, blood priming is routine for pediatric and neonatal ECLS, and this infuses proinflammatory cytokines and primed PMNs into the circulation. These factors explain, in part, the differing physiologic response to ECLS in these different patient populations. Future study of the SIRS relative to ECLS should occur in models that examine the effects of ECLS in the "primed" or "up-regulated" state and account for the flow characteristics of the circulation being studied (i.e., pulmonary or systemic). Greater understanding of the blood-foreign surface interaction and PMN-endothelial interactions associated with the initiation of ECLS will allow for improvements in equipment design, perfusion techniques, and pharmacologic manipulation of the inflammatory response to ECLS.[25] Studies are currently in progress to evaluate the utility of transient blockade of selectin ligands to inhibit PMN adherence to the activated endothelium during the initiation of ECLS. These studies are importing information gained from other animal models of ischemia/reperfusion and lung injury.[163,164] These and other PMN-specific anti-adhesion therapies may allow true "passivation" of the ECLS circuit and minimization of the inflammatory response associated with ECLS.

References

1. Asimakopoulos G, Taylor KM. Effects of cardiopulmonary bypass on leukocyte and endothelial adhesion molecules. *Ann Thorac Surg* 1998; 66:2135-2144.
2. Boyle EM Jr, Pohlman TH, Cornejo CJ, Verrier ED. Endothelial cell injury in cardiovascular surgery: ischemia-reperfusion. *Ann Thorac Surg* 1996; 62:1868-1875.

3. Butler J, Rocker GM, Westaby S. Inflammatory response to cardiopulmonary bypass. *Ann Thorac Surg* 1993; 55:552-559.

4. Dreyer WJ, Michael LH, Millman EE, Berens KL. Neutrophil activation and adhesion molecule expression in a canine model of open heart surgery with cardiopulmonary bypass. *Cardiovasc Res* 1995; 29:775-781.

5. Fortenberry JD, Bhardwaj V, Bland L, et al. Effects of neonatal extracorporeal membrane oxygenation on neutrophil activation and cytokine levels. *Ped Res* 1994; 35:225A.

6. Hirthler M, Simoni J, Dickson M. Elevated levels of endotoxin, oxygen-derived free radicals, and cytokines during extracorporeal membrane oxygenation. *J Pediatr Surg* 1992; 27:1199-1202.

7. Kirklin JK, George JF, Holman W. The Inflammatory Response to Cardiopulmonary Bypass. In: Gravlee G, Davis RF, Utley JR, eds. Cardiopulmonary Bypass. Philidelphia, PA: Williams and Wilkins; 1993; 233-248.

8. Kirklin JK, Westaby S, Blackstoner EH, Kirklin JW, Chenoweth DE, Pacifico AD. Complement and the damaging effects of cardiopulmonary bypass. *J Thorac Cardiovasc Surg* 1983; 86:845-857.

9. Kleinschmidt S, Wanner GA, Bussmann D, et al. Proinflammatory cytokine gene expression in whole blood from patients undergoing coronary artery bypass surgery and its modulation by pentoxifylline. *Shock* 1998; 9:12-20.

10. Miller BE, Levy JH. The inflammatory response to cardiopulmonary bypass. *J Cardiothorac Vasc Anesth* 1997; 11:355-366.

11. Westaby S. Organ dysfunction after cardiopulmonary bypass. A systemic inflammatory reaction initiated by the extracorporeal circuit. *Intensive Care Med* 1987; 13:89-95.

12. Hornick P, George A. Blood contact activation: pathophysiological effects and therapeutic approaches. *Perfusion* 1996; 11:3-19.

13. Watkins WD, Peterson MB, Kong DL, et al. Thromboxane and prostacyclin changes during cardiopulmonary bypass with and without pulsatile flow. *J Thorac Cardiovasc Surg* 1982; 84:250-256.

14. Dreyer WJ, Michael LH, Millman EE, Berens KL, Geske RS. Neutrophil sequestration and pulmonary dysfunction in a canine model of open heart surgery with cardiopulmonary bypass. Evidence for a CD18-dependent mechanism. *Circulation* 1995; 92:2276-2283.

15. Friedman M, Wang SY, Sellke FW, Cohn WE, Weintraub RM, Johnson RG. Neutrophil adhesion blockade with NPC 15669 decreases pulmonary injury after total cardiopulmonary bypass. *J Thorac Cardiovasc Surg* 1996; 111:460-468.

16. Anderson HL 3rd, Coran AG, Drongowski RA, Ha HJ, Bartlett RH. Extracellular fluid and total body water changes in neonates undergoing extracorporeal membrane oxygenation. *J Pediatr Surg* 1992; 27:1003-1007; discussion 1007-1008.

17. Underwood MJ, Pearson JA, Waggoner J, Lunec J, Firmin RK, Elliot MJ. Changes in "inflammatory" mediators and total body water during extra-corporeal membrane oxygenation (ECMO). A preliminary study. *Int J Artif Organs* 1995; 18:627-632.

18. Cox CS Jr, Zwischenberger JB, Fleming RYD, et al. Ileal Mucosal Hypoperfusion during Cardiopulmonary Bypass. *Curr Surg* 1992; 49:507-509.

19. Tao W, Zwischenberger JB, Nguyen TT, et al. Gut mucosal ischemia during normothermic cardiopulmonary bypass results from blood flow redistribution and increased oxygen demand. *J Thorac Cardiovasc Surg* 1995; 110:819-828.

20. Ohri SK. Systemic inflammatory response and the splanchnic bed in cardiopulmonary bypass. *Perfusion* 1996; 11:200-212.

21. Ohri SK, Bjarnason I, Pathi V, et al. Effects of cardiopulmonary bypass on gut blood

flow, oxygen utilization, and intramucosal pH. *Ann Thorac Surg* 1994; 57:1193-1199.

22. Jones DA, Smith CW, McIntire LV. Leucocyte adhesion under flow conditions: principles important in tissue engineering. *Biomaterials* 1996; 17:337-347.

23. Caplan MS, Hsueh W, Sun XM, Gidding SS, Hageman JR. Circulating plasma platelet activating factor in persistent pulmonary hypertension of the newborn. *Am Rev Respir Dis* 1990; 142:1258-1262.

24. Fransen E, Maessen J, Dentener M, Senden N, Geskes G, Buurman W. Systemic inflammation present in patients undergoing CABG without extracorporeal circulation. *Chest* 1998; 113:1290-1295.

25. Giroir BP. Mediators of septic shock: new approaches for interrupting the endogenous inflammatory cascade. *Crit Care Med* 1993; 21:780-789.

26. Maekawa K, Futami S, Nishida M, et al. Effects of trauma and sepsis on soluble L-selectin and cell surface expression of L-selectin and CD11b. *J Trauma* 1998; 44:460-468.

27. Nieuwenhuijzen GA, Knapen MF, Oyen WJ, Hendriks T, Corsten FH, Goris RJ. Organ damage is preceded by changes in protein extravasation in an experimental model of multiple organ dysfunction syndrome. *Shock* 1997; 7:98-104.

28. VanderMeer TJ, Wang H, Fink MP. Endotoxemia causes ileal mucosal acidosis in the absence of mucosal hypoxia in a normodynamic porcine model of septic shock. *Crit Care Med* 1995; 23:1217-1226.

29. Zallen G, Moore EE, Johnson J, et al. Posthemorrhagic mesenteric lymph primes circulating neutrophils and provokes lung injury. *Proc Am Assoc Acad Surg* 1998; 32:185A.

30. Cain BS, Meldrum DR, Sezman CH, et al. Surgical implications of vascular endothelial physiology. *Surgery* 1997; 122:516-526.

31. Ali MH, Schlidt SA, Hynes KL, Marcus BC, Gewertz BL. Prolonged hypoxia alters endothelial barrier function. *Surgery* 1998; 124:491-497.

32. Gupta N, Jacobs DL, Miller TA, Smith GS, Dahms TE. Hypoxia-reoxygenation potentiates zymosan activated plasma-induced endothelial injury. *J Surg Res* 1998; 77:91-98.

33. Collard CD, Agah A, Stahl GL. Complement activation following reoxygenation of hypoxic human endothelial cells: role of intracellular reactive oxygen species, NF-kappaB and new protein synthesis. *Immunopharmacology* 1998; 39:39-50.

34. Collard CD, Vakeva A, Bukusoglu C, et al. Reoxygenation of hypoxic human umbilical vein endothelial cells activates the classic complement pathway. *Circulation* 1997; 96:326-333.

35. Tennenberg SD, Clardy CW, Baily WW, Solomkin JS. Complement activation and lung permeability during cardiopulmonary bypass. *Ann Thorac Surg* 1990; 50: 597-601.

36. Graulich J, Sonntag J, Marcinkowski M, et al. Complement activation by in vivo neonatal and in vitro extracorporeal membrane oxygenation. *Mediators Inflamm* 2002; 11:69-73.

37. Paparella D, Yau TM, Young E. Cardiopulmonary bypass induced inflammation: pathophysiology and treatment. An update. *Eur J Cardiothorac Surg* 2002; 21:232-244.

38. Cox CS Jr, Allen SJ, Butler D, Sauer H, Frederick J. Extracorporeal circulation exacerbates microvascular permeability after endotoxemia. *J Surg Res* 2000; 91:50-55.

39. Elliott MJ, Finn AH. Interaction between neutrophils and endothelium. *Ann Thorac Surg* 1993; 56:1503-1508.

40. Finn A, Moat N, Rebuck N, Klein N, Strobel S, Elliot M. Changes in neutrophil CD11b/CD18 and L-selectin expression and release of interleukin 8 and elastase in paediatric cardiopulmonary bypass. *Agents Actions* 1993; 38 Spec No:C44-46.

41. Finn A, Morgan BP, Rebuck N, et al. Effects of inhibition of complement activation using recombinant soluble complement receptor 1 on neutrophil CD11b/CD18 and L-selectin expression and release of interleukin-8 and elastase in simulated cardiopulmonary bypass. *J Thorac Cardiovasc Surg* 1996; 111:451-459.

42. Finn A, Naik S, Klein N, Levinsky RJ, Strobel S, Elliott M. Interleukin-8 release and neutrophil degranulation after pediatric cardiopulmonary bypass. *J Thorac Cardiovasc Surg* 1993; 105:234-241.

43. Finn A, Rebuck N, Moat N. Neutrophil activation during cardiopulmonary bypass. *J Thorac Cardiovasc Surg* 1992; 104:1746-1748.

44. el Habbal MH, Smith LJ, Elliott MJ, Strobel S. Cardiopulmonary bypass tubes and prime solutions stimulate neutrophil adhesion molecules. *Cardiovasc Res* 1997; 33:209-215.

45. Allen SM. Leucocyte depletion in cardiothoracic surgery. *Perfusion* 1996; 11:270-277.

46. Dinarello CA. The physiological and pathological effects of cytokines. In: The Proceedings of the Second International Workshop on Cytokines; December 10-14, 1989; Hilton Head Island, SC. Progress in leukocyte biology v. 10B 1990; xxxvi: 460.

47. Dinarello CA. Interleukin-1 and the pathogenesis of the acute-phase response. *N Engl J Med* 1984. 311:1413-1418.

48. Movat HZ. Tumor necrosis factor and interleukin-1: role in acute inflammation and microvascular injury. *J Lab Clin Med* 1987. 110: 668-681.

49. Dinarello CA. Biology of interleukin 1. *Faseb J* 1988. 2:108-115.

50. Tosato G, Jones KD. Interleukin-1 induces interleukin-6 production in peripheral blood monocytes. *Blood* 1990; 75:1305-1310.

51. Lonnemann G, Koch KM, Shaldon S, Dinarello CA. Studies on the ability of hemodialysis membranes to induce, bind, and clear human interleukin-1. *J Lab Clin Med* 1988; 112:76-86.

52. Haeffner-Cavaillon N, Roussellier N, Ponzio O, et al. Induction of interleukin-1 production in patients undergoing cardiopulmonary bypass. *J Thorac Cardiovasc Surg* 1989; 98:1100-1106.

53. Golej J, Winter P, Schoffmann G, et al. Impact of extracorporeal membrane oxygenation modality on cytokine release during rescue from infant hypoxia. *Shock* 2003; 20:110-115.

54. Butler J, Chong GL, Baigrie RJ, Pillai R, Westaby S, Rocker GM. Cytokine responses to cardiopulmonary bypass with membrane and bubble oxygenation. *Ann Thorac Surg* 1992; 53:833-838.

55. Markewitz A, Faist E, Lang S, Endres S, Hultner L, Reichart B. Regulation of acute phase response after cardiopulmonary bypass by immunomodulation. *Ann Thorac Surg* 1993; 55:389-394.

56. Fortenberry JD, Bhardwaj V, Niemer P, Cornish JD, Wright JA, Bland L. Neutrophil and cytokine activation with neonatal extracorporeal membrane oxygenation. *J Pediatr* 1996; 128:670-678.

57. Jansen NJ, van Oeveren W, van den Broek L, et al. Inhibition by dexamethasone of the reperfusion phenomena in cardiopulmonary bypass. *J Thorac Cardiovasc Surg* 1991; 102:515-525.

58. Plotz FB, van Oeveren W, Bartlett RH, Wildevuur CR. Blood activation during neonatal extracorporeal life support. *J Thorac Cardiovasc Surg* 1993; 105:823-832.

59. Nijsten MW, de Groot ER, ten Duis HJ, Klasen HJ, Hack CE, Aarden LA. Serum levels of interleukin-6 and acute phase responses. *Lancet* 1987; 2:921.

60. Shenkin A, Fraser WD, Series J, et al. The serum interleukin 6 response to elective surgery. *Lymphokine Res* 1989 8:123-127.

61. Van Snick J. Interleukin-6: an overview. *Annu Rev Immunol* 1990; 8:253-278.

62. Yoshimura T, Matsushima K, Oppenheim JJ, Leonard EJ. Neutrophil chemotactic factor produced by lipopolysaccharide (LPS)-stimulated human blood mononuclear leukocytes: partial characterization and separation from interleukin 1 (IL 1). *J Immunol* 1987; 139:788-793.

63. Rot A. Some aspects of NAP-1 pathophysiology: lung damage caused by a blood-borne cytokine. In: Westwick J, Lindley IJD, Kunkel SL, eds. *Chemotactic Cytokines*. New York, NY: Plenum Press; 1991; 127-135.

64. Huber AR, Kumkel SL, Todd RF 3rd, Weiss SJ. Regulation of transendothelial neutrophil migration by endogenous interleukin-8. *Science* 1991; 254:99-102.

65. Yanagi F, Terasaki H, Matsukawa A, Ohkawara S, Morioka T, Yoshinaga M. Cytokine generation in rabbits during extracorporeal lung assist with a mini hollow fiber lung. *Artif Organs* 1996; 20:209-217.

66. Kobinia GS, LaRaia PJ, D'Ambra MN, et al. Effect of experimental cardiopulmonary bypass on systemic and transcardiac thromboxane B2 levels. *J Thorac Cardiovasc Surg* 1986; 91:852-857.

67. Zwischenberger JB, Cox CS Jr, Minifee PK, et al. Pathophysiology of ovine smoke inhalation injury treated with extracorporeal membrane oxygenation. *Chest* 1993; 103:1582-1586.

68. Bui KC, Hammerman C, Hirschl R, et al. Plasma prostanoids in neonatal extracorporeal membrane oxygenation. Influence of meconium aspiration. *J Thorac Cardiovasc Surg* 1991; 101:612-617.

69. Bui KC, Hammerman C, Hirschl RB, et al. Plasma prostanoids in neonates with pulmonary hypertension treated with conventional therapy and with extracorporeal membrane oxygenation. *J Thorac Cardiovasc Surg* 1991; 101:973-983.

70. Bui KC, Martin G, Kammerman LA, Hammerman C, Hill V, Short BL. Plasma thromboxane and pulmonary artery pressure in neonates treated with extracorporeal membrane oxygenation. *J Thorac Cardiovasc Surg* 1992; 104:124-129.

71. Dobyns EL, Wescott JY, Kennaugh JM, Ross MN, Stenmark KR. Eicosanoids decrease with successful extracorporeal membrane oxygenation therapy in neonatal pulmonary hypertension. *Am J Respir Crit Care Med* 1994; 149:873-880.

72. Erez E, Erman A, Snir E, et al. Thromboxane production in human lung during cardiopulmonary bypass: beneficial effect of aspirin? *Ann Thorac Surg* 1998; 65:101-106.

73. Chenoweth DE, Cooper SW, Hugli TE, Stewart RW, Blackstone EH, Kirklin JW. Complement activation during cardiopulmonary bypass: evidence for generation of C3a and C5a anaphylatoxins. *N Engl J Med* 1981; 304:497-503.

74. Williams JJ, Yellin SA, Slotman GJ. Leukocyte aggregation response to quantitative plasma levels of C3a and C5a. *Arch Surg* 1986; 121:305-307.

75. Hosea S, Brown E, Hammer C, Frank M. Role of complement activation in a model of adult respiratory distress syndrome. *J Clin Invest* 1980; 66:375-382.

76. Parker DJ, Cantrell G, Stroud R, Karp R, Digerness SB. Changes in serum complement and immunoglobulins following cardiopulmonary bypass. *Surgery* 1972; 71:824-827.

77. Meri S, Aronen M, Leijala M. Complement activation during cardiopulmonary bypass in children. *Complement* 1988; 5:46-54.

78. Seghaye MC, Duchateau J, Grabitz RG, et al. Complement activation during cardiopulmonary bypass in infants and children. Relation to postoperative multiple system organ failure. *J Thorac Cardiovasc Surg* 1993; 106:978-987.

79. Matsuda T, Itoh S, Anderson J. Endothelial injury during extracorporeal circulation: neutrophil-endothelium interaction induced by complement activation. *J Biomed Mater Res* 1994; 28:1387-1395.

80. Darling EM, Harris WE, Cooper ES, et al. Complement Activation during long term Extracorporeal Membrane Oxygenation in Neonates. *J Extr-Corp Tech* 1988; 20:20-24.

81. Westfall SH, Stephens C, Kesler K, Connors RH, Tracy TF Jr, Weber TR. Complement activation during prolonged extracorporeal membrane oxygenation. *Surgery* 1991; 110:887-891.

82. Graulich J, Sonntag J, Marcinkowski M, et al. Complement activation by in vivo neonatal and in vitro extracorporeal membrane oxygenation. *Mediators Inflamm* 2002; 11:69-73.

83. Vallhonrat H, Swinford RD, Ingelfinger JR, et al. Rapid activation of the alternative pathway of complement by extracorporeal membrane oxygenation. *Asaio J* 1999; 45:113-114.

84. Abbassi O, Kishimoto TK, McIntire LV, Anderson DC, Smith CW. E-selectin supports neutrophil rolling in vitro under conditions of flow. *J Clin Invest* 1993; 92:2719-2730.

85. Jones DA, Abbassi O, McIntire LV, McEver RP, Smith CW. P-selectin mediates neutrophil rolling on histamine-stimulated endothelial cells. *Biophys J* 1993; 65:1560-1569.

86. Jones DA, Smith CW, Picker LJ, McIntire LV. Neutrophil adhesion to 24-hour IL-1-stimulated endothelial cells under flow conditions. *J Immunol* 1996; 157:858-863.

87. Dreyer WJ, Burns AR, Phillips SC, Lindsey ML, Jackson P, Kukielka GL. Intercellular adhesion molecule-1 regulation in the canine lung after cardiopulmonary bypass. *J Thorac Cardiovasc Surg* 1998; 115:689-698; discussion 698-699.

88. Gopalan PK, Smith CW, Lu H, Berg EL, McIntire LV, Simon SI. Neutrophil CD18-dependent arrest on intercellular adhesion molecule 1 (ICAM-1) in shear flow can be activated through L-selectin. *J Immunol* 1997; 158:367-375.

89. Lawrence MB, Smith CW, Eskin SG, McIntire LV. Effect of venous shear stress on CD18-mediated neutrophil adhesion to cultured endothelium. *Blood* 1990; 75:227-237.

90. Wang JH, Sexton DM, Redmond HP, Watson RW, Croke DT, Bouchier-Hayes D. Intercellular adhesion molecule-1 (ICAM-1) is expressed on human neutrophils and is essential for neutrophil adherence and aggregation. *Shock* 1997; 8:357-361.

91. Gillinov AM, Bator JM, Zehr KJ, et al. Neutrophil adhesion molecule expression during cardiopulmonary bypass with bubble and membrane oxygenators. *Ann Thorac Surg* 1993. 56:847-853.

92. Konstantopoulos K, McIntire LV. Effects of fluid dynamic forces on vascular cell adhesion. *J Clin Invest* 1996; 98:2661-2665.

93. Butler J, Parker D, Pillai R, Westaby S, Shale DJ, Rocker GM. Effect of cardiopulmonary bypass on systemic release of neutrophil elastase and tumor necrosis factor. *J Thorac Cardiovasc Surg* 1993; 105:25-30.

94. Larson DF, Bowers M, Schechner HW. Neutrophil activation during cardiopulmonary bypass in paediatric and adult patients. *Perfusion* 1996; 11:21-27.

95. Graulich J, Walzog B, Marcinkowski M, et al. Leukocyte and endothelial activation in a laboratory model of extracorporeal membrane oxygenation (ECMO). *Pediatr Res* 2000; 48:679-684.

96. Ruel M, Khan TA, Voisine P, Bianchi C, Sellke FW. Vasomotor dysfunction after

cardiac surgery. *Eur J Cardiothorac Surg* 2004; 26:1002-1014.

97. Stamler A, Wang SY, Aguirre ED, Johnson RG, Sellke FW. Cardiopulmonary bypass alters vasomotor regulation of the skeletal muscle microcirculation. *Ann Thorac Surg* 1997; 64:460-465.

98. Reilly PM, Wilkins KB, Fuh KC, Haglund U, Bulkley GB. The mesenteric hemodynamic response to circulatory shock: an overview. *Shock* 2001; 15:329-343.

99. Khan TA, Bianchi C, Araujo EG, et al. Cardiopulmonary bypass reduces peripheral microvascular contractile function by inhibition of mitogen-activated protein kinase activity. *Surgery* 2003; 134:247-254.

100. Cain AE, Tanner DM, Khalil RA. Endothelin-1--induced enhancement of coronary smooth muscle contraction via MAPK-dependent and MAPK-independent [Ca(2+)](i) sensitization pathways. *Hypertension* 2002; 39:543-549.

101. Yamboliev IA, Hedges JC, Mutnick JL, Adam LP, Gerthoffer WT. Evidence for modulation of smooth muscle force by the p38 MAP kinase/HSP27 pathway. *Am J Physiol Heart Circ Physiol* 2000; 278: H1899-1907.

102. Ohanian J, Cunliffe P, Ceppi E, Alder A, Heerkens E, Ohanian V. Activation of p38 mitogen-activated protein kinases by endothelin and noradrenaline in small arteries, regulation by calcium influx and tyrosine kinases, and their role in contraction. *Arterioscler Thromb Vasc Biol* 2001; 21:1921-1927.

103. Stahl GL, Reenstra WR, Frendl G. Complement-mediated loss of endothelium-dependent relaxation of porcine coronary arteries. Role of the terminal membrane attack complex. *Circ Res* 1995; 76:575-583.

104. Shafique T, Johnson RG, Dai HB, Weintraub RM, Sellke FW. Altered pulmonary microvascular reactivity after total cardio-

pulmonary bypass. *J Thorac Cardiovasc Surg* 1993; 106:479-486.

105. Doguet F, Litzler PY, Tamion F, et al. Changes in mesenteric vascular reactivity and inflammatory response after cardiopulmonary bypass in a rat model. *Ann Thorac Surg* 2004; 77:2130-2137.

106. Sinclair DG, Haslam PL, Quinlan GJ, Pepper JR, Evans TW. The effect of cardiopulmonary bypass on intestinal and pulmonary endothelial permeability. *Chest* 1995; 108:718-724.

107. Sellke FW, Shafique T, Ely DL, Weintraub RM. Coronary endothelial injury after cardiopulmonary bypass and ischemic cardioplegia is mediated by oxygen-derived free radicals. *Circulation* 1993; 88:II395-400.

108. Khan TA, Bianchi C, Ruel M, Voisine P, Sellke FW. Mitogen-activated protein kinase pathways and cardiac surgery. *J Thorac Cardiovasc Surg* 2004; 127:806-811.

109. Sellke FW, Friedman M, Dai HB, et al. Mechanisms causing coronary microvascular dysfunction following crystalloid cardioplegia and reperfusion. *Cardiovasc Res* 1993; 27:1925-1932.

110. Vallet B. Vascular reactivity and tissue oxygenation. *Intensive Care Med* 1998; 24:3-11.

111. Kronon MT, Allen BS, Halldorsson A, Rahman S, Wang T, Ilbawi M. Dose dependency of L-arginine in neonatal myocardial protection: the nitric oxide paradox. *J Thorac Cardiovasc Surg* 1999; 118:655-664.

112. Andrasi TB, Soos P, Bakos G, et al. L-arginine protects the mesenteric vascular circulation against cardiopulmonary bypass-induced vascular dysfunction. *Surgery* 2003; 134:72-79.

113. Boyle EM Jr, Pohlman TH, Johnson MC, Verrier ED. Endothelial cell injury in cardiovascular surgery: the systemic inflammatory response. *Ann Thorac Surg* 1997; 63:277-284.

114. Cox CS Jr, Allen SJ, Butler D, Sauer H, Frederick J. Extracorporeal circulation exacerbates microvascular permeability after endotoxemia. *J Surg Res* 2000; 91:50-55.

115. Kelly RE Jr, Phillips JD, Foglia RP, et al. Pulmonary edema and fluid mobilization as determinants of the duration of ECMO support. *J Pediatr Surg* 1991; 26:1016-1022.

116. Starling EH. On the absorption of fluids from the connective tissue spaces. *J Physiol Lond* 1896; 19:312-326.

117. Mehlhorn U, Geissler HJ, Laine GA, Allen SJ. Myocardial fluid balance. *Eur J Cardiothorac Surg* 2001; 20:1220-1230.

118. Foglia RP, Partington MT, Buckberg GD, Leaf J. Iatrogenic myocardial edema with crystalloid primes: Effects on left ventricular compliance, performance, and perfusion. *Surg Forum* 1978; 29:312-315.

119. Smith EE, Naftel DC, Blackstone EH, Kirklin JW. Microvascular permeability after cardiopulmonary bypass. An experimental study. *J Thorac Cardiovasc Surg* 1987; 94:225-233.

120. Royston D, Minty BD, Higenbottam TW, Wallwork J, Jones GJ. The effect of surgery with cardiopulmonary bypass on alveolar-capillary barrier function in human beings. *Ann Thorac Surg* 1985; 40:139-143

121. Cox CS Jr, Brennan M, Allen SJ. Impact of hetastarch on the intestinal microvascular barrier during ECLS. *J Appl Physiol* 2000; 88:1374-1380.

122. Barden RPT, WD, Ravdin IS, Frank IL. The influence of the serum protein on the motility of the small intestine. *Surg Gyn & Ob* 1938; 66:819-821.

123. Barden RP, Ravdin IS, Frazier WD. Hypoproteinemia as a factor in the retardation of gastric emptying after operations of the billroth I or II types. *Am J Roent and Rad Therapy* 1937; 38:196-202.

124. Mecray PM, Barden RP, Ravdin IS. Nutritional edema: its effect on the gastric emptying time before and after gastric operations. *Surgery* 1937; 1:53-64.

125. Ravdin IS. Hypoproteinemia and its relation to surgical problems. *Ann Surg* 1940; 112:576-583.

126. Davis KL, Mehlhorn U, Laine GA, Allen SJ. Myocardial edema, left ventricular function, and pulmonary hypertension. *J Appl Physiol* 1995; 78:132-137.

127. Gilbert TB, Barnas GM, Sequeira AJ. Impact of pleurotomy, continuous positive airway pressure, and fluid balance during cardiopulmonary bypass on lung mechanics and oxygenation. *J Cardiothorac Vasc Anesth* 1996; 10:844-849.

128. Moore-Olufemi SD, Xue H, Attuwayvi BO, et al. Resuscitation-induced gut edema and intestinal dysfunction. *J Trauma* 2005; 58:264-270.

129. Cox CS Jr, Allen SJ, Brennan M. Analysis of intestinal microvascular permeability associated with cardiopulmonary bypass. *J Surg Res* 1999; 83:19-26.

130. Kubes P, Granger DN. Nitric oxide modulates microvascular permeability. *Am J Physiol* 1992; 262:H611-615.

131. Demling RH, Hicks RE, Edmunds LH Jr. Changes in extravascular lung water during venovenous perfusion. *J Thorac Cardiovasc Surg* 1976; 71:291-294.

132. Kazzi NJ, Schwartz CA, Palder SB, Whittlesey GC, Klein MD, Brans YW. Effect of extracorporeal membrane oxygenation on body water content and distribution in lambs. *ASAIO Trans* 1990; 36:817-820.

133. Patrick DA, Moore FA, Moore EE, Barnett CC Jr, Silliman CC. Neutrophil priming and activation in the pathogenesis of postinjury multiple organ failure. *New Horiz* 1996; 4:194-210.

134. Cocks RA, Chan TY, Rainer TH. Leukocyte L-selectin is up-regulated after mechanical trauma in adults. *J Trauma* 1998; 45:1-6.

135. DePuydt LE, Schuit KE, Smith SD. Effect of extracorporeal membrane oxygenation

on neutrophil function in neonates. *Crit Care Med* 1993; 21:1324-1327.

136. Stahl RF, Fisher CA, Kucich U, et al. Effects of simulated extracorporeal circulation on human leukocyte elastase release, superoxide generation, and procoagulant activity. *J Thorac Cardiovasc Surg* 1991; 101:230-239.

137. van Eeden SF, Kitagawa Y, Klut ME, Lawrence E, Hogg JC. Polymorphonuclear leukocytes released from the bone marrow preferentially sequester in lung microvessels. *Microcirculation* 1997; 4:369-380.

138. Hill GE, Whitten CW, Landers DF. The influence of cardiopulmonary bypass on cytokines and cell-cell communication. *J Cardiothorac Vasc Anesth* 1997; 11:367-375.

139. Klebanoff SJ, Vada MA, Harlan JM, et al. Stimulation of neutrophils by tumor necrosis factor. *J Immunol* 1986; 136:4220-4225.

140. Kubo H, Graham L, Doyle NA, Quinlan WM, Hogg JC, Doerschuk CM. Complement fragment-induced release of neutrophils from bone marrow and sequestration within pulmonary capillaries in rabbits. *Blood* 1998; 92:283-290.

141. Laidler J, Paes ML, Wheeler J, et al. Detection of circulating TNF-alpha after elective cardiopulmonary bypass. *Perfusion* 1991; 6:51-54.

142. Cox CS Jr, Zwischenberger JB, Traber DL, Traber LD, Haque AK, Herndon DN. Heparin improves oxygenation and minimizes barotrauma after severe smoke inhalation in an ovine model. *Surg Gynecol Obstet* 1993; 176:339-349.

143. Fiddian-Green RG, Baker S. Predictive value of the stomach wall pH for complications after cardiac operations: comparison with other monitoring. *Crit Care Med* 1987; 15:153-156.

144. Naik SK, Knight A, Elliott MJ. A successful modification of ultrafiltration for

cardiopulmonary bypass in children. *Perfusion* 1991; 6:41-50.

145. Naik SK, Knight A, Elliott M. A prospective randomized study of a modified technique of ultrafiltration during pediatric open-heart surgery. *Circulation* 1991; 84(5 Suppl):III422-431.

146. Chew MS. Does modified ultrafiltration reduce the systemic inflammatory response to cardiac surgery with cardiopulmonary bypass? *Perfusion* 2004; 19 (Suppl 1): S57-60.

147. Dittrich S, Aktuerk D, Seitz S, et al. Effects of ultrafiltration and peritoneal dialysis on proinflammatory cytokines during cardiopulmonary bypass surgery in newborns and infants. *Eur J Cardiothorac Surg* 2004; 25:935-940.

148. Huang H, Yao T, Wang W, et al. Continuous ultrafiltration attenuates the pulmonary injury that follows open heart surgery with cardiopulmonary bypass. *Ann Thorac Surg* 2003; 76:136-140.

149. Pearl JM, Manning PB, McNamara JL, Saucier MM, Thomas DW. Effect of modified ultrafiltration on plasma thromboxane B2, leukotriene B4, and endothelin-1 in infants undergoing cardiopulmonary bypass. *Ann Thorac Surg* 1999; 68:1369-1375.

150. Lodge AJ, Chai PJ, Daggett CW, Ungerleider RM, Jaggers J. Methylprednisolone reduces the inflammatory response to cardiopulmonary bypass in neonatal piglets: timing of dose is important. *J Thorac Cardiovasc Surg* 1999; 117:515-522.

151. Griffin MP, Wooldridge P, Alford BA, McIlhenny J, Ksenich RA. Dexamethasone therapy in neonates treated with extracorporeal membrane oxygenation. *J Pediatr* 2004; 144:296-300.

152. Duffy JY, Nelson DP, Schwartz SM, et al. Glucocorticoids reduce cardiac dysfunction after cardiopulmonary bypass and circulatory arrest in neonatal piglets. *Pediatr Crit Care Med* 2004; 5:28-34.

153. McBride WT, Allen S, Gormley SM, et al. Methylprednisolone favourably alters plasma and urinary cytokine homeostasis and subclinical renal injury at cardiac surgery. *Cytokine* 2004; 27:81-89.

154. Varan B, Tokel K, Mercan S, Donmez A, Aslamaci S. Systemic inflammatory response related to cardiopulmonary bypass and its modification by methyl prednisolone: high dose versus low dose. *Pediatr Cardiol* 2002; 23:437-441.

155. Bourbon A, Vionnet M, Leprince P, et al. The effect of methylprednisolone treatment on the cardiopulmonary bypass-induced systemic inflammatory response. *Eur J Cardiothorac Surg* 2004; 26:932-938.

156. Griffin MP, Gore DC, Zwischenberger JB, et al. Does heparin improve survival in experimental porcine gram-negative septic shock? *Circ Shock* 1990; 31:343-349.

157. Zapata-Sirvent RL, Hansbrough JF, Greenleaf GE, Grayson LS, Wolf P. Reduction of bacterial translocation and intestinal structural alterations by heparin in a murine burn injury model. *J Trauma* 1994; 36:1-6.

158. Darien BJ, Fareed J, Centgraf KS, et al. Low molecular weight heparin prevents the pulmonary hemodynamic and pathomorphologic effects of endotoxin in a porcine acute lung injury model. *Shock* 1998; 9:274-281.

159. Hiebert LM, Liu JM. Heparin protects cultured arterial endothelial cells from damage by toxic oxygen metabolites. *Atherosclerosis* 1990; 83:47-51.

160. Le Deist F, Menasche P, Kucharski C, Bel A, Piwnica A, Bloch G. Hypothermia during cardiopulmonary bypass delays but does not prevent neutrophil-endothelial cell adhesion. A clinical study. *Circulation* 1995; 92:II354-358.

161. Menasche P, Peynet J, Haeffner-Cavaillon N, et al. Influence of temperature on neutrophil trafficking during clinical cardiopulmonary bypass. *Circulation* 1995; 92:II334-340.

162. Horan M, Ichiba S, Firmin RK, et al. A pilot investigation of mild hypothermia in neonates receiving extracorporeal membrane oxygenation (ECMO). *J Pediatr* 2004; 144:301-308.

163. Mulligan MS, Miyasaka M, Suzuki Y, et al. Anti-inflammatory effects of sulfatides in selectin-dependent acute lung injury. *Int Immunol* 1995; 7:1107-1113.

164. Palma-Vargas JM, Toledo-Pereyra L, Dean RE, Harkema JM, Dixon RA, Kogan TP. Small-molecule selectin inhibitor protects against liver inflammatory response after ischemia and reperfusion. *J Am Coll Surg* 1997; 185:365-372.

5

Principles and Practice of Venovenous ECMO

James D. Fortenberry, M.D., F.C.C.M., F.A.A.P., Robert Pettignano, M.D., F.A.A.P., F.C.C.M., M.B.A., and Francine Dykes, M.D.

Introduction

ECMO requires the diversion of blood from a major systemic vessel through a gas exchange device (membrane oxygenator) and back to a major blood vessel. The venoarterial (VA) approach has served as the primary mode of cannulation for both cardiac and respiratory failure since the advent of extracorporeal support. VA support utilizes a central vein for drainage and an artery for return. VA cannulation thus provides direct cardiovascular support. Venovenous (VV) cannulation provides an alternative means of extracorporeal support for patients with severe respiratory failure who do not require cardiac support. VV cannulation utilizes a major vein for blood drainage and a vein for return of oxygenated blood to the right heart. The VV approach, while not providing direct circulatory support, replaces pulmonary gas exchange and theoretically offers indirect cardiac support without ligation of a major artery. While originally an experimental technique[1], the use of VV ECMO increased significantly over the past decade in neonatal, pediatric, and adult respiratory failure patients requiring extracorporeal support. This chapter reviews the types of VV ECMO, advantages and disadvantages of this approach, general indications, clinical experience, and practical management issues.

Types of VV ECMO

VV ECMO is performed using two general approaches to cannulation and delivery of flow, with either two separate drainage and return cannulas (two-site VV ECMO) or a single double lumen catheter (DLVV ECMO) (Table 1).

Table 1. Types of VV ECMO cannulation and directional flow (additional cannulas can be added for augmented drainage).

I. Continuous
A. Two-site VV: 2 separate placement sites with single lumen cannulas
1. Internal jugular drainage to femoral or saphenous vein return
2. Femoral or saphenous drainage to internal jugular vein return
3. One or both saphenous veins drainage to femoral vein return (ECCO$_2$R)
B. Single-site VV: 1 double lumen cannula in internal jugular vein
II. Tidal flow
A. Single lumen in internal jugular vein

Continuous flow two-site VV ECMO

Continuous flow VV ECMO provides support via simultaneous drainage of deoxygenated blood and return of oxygenated blood. Initial experience with VV ECMO required the cannulation of two separate venous sites. The two veins most commonly used for cannulation were the jugular and femoral veins. During two-site VV ECMO, blood was typically drained out of the right atrium (RA) through an internal jugular venous cannula and returned to the femoral vein. More recently, the predominant circulation path in two-site VV ECMO is drainage from catheters in the femoral vessels (and cephalad jugular vein, if used) and return to a catheter in the RA. The two-site VV ECMO approach is the primary mode used in pediatric and adult patients with severe respiratory failure (Figure 1).

Continuous flow one-site VV ECMO

The development of various sizes of double lumen catheters has allowed VV ECMO to be performed using a single vein as both the drainage and return sites for blood (Figure 2) in infants and children. In neonates ≤4 kg, a double lumen cannula can be placed into the internal jugular vein, avoiding use of the femoral vein. Blood is drained from the RA through one port, circulated through the membrane oxygenator, and returned to the RA via a second port in the double lumen catheter. A key to the success of DLVV ECMO is the design of the double lumen cannula, which minimizes recirculation. These aforementioned forms of VV ECMO provide continuous flow ECMO support, generally requiring flows of approximately 120-150 cc/kg/min for adequate patient oxygenation. DLVV ECMO is the predominant form of VV ECMO employed in neonates.

Tidal flow ECMO

In contrast to continuous flow, tidal flow ECMO is a much less utilized technique, offering the theoretical benefits of requiring a single site with a single lumen catheter, and decreased recirculation. Tidal flow ECMO uses a pump that allows blood flow to alternate bi-directionally, in a tidal pattern. The key element is a combination of reservoirs with an alternating tubing clamp system connected to the cannula. Blood initially drains from the patient to a "venous" reservoir and is pumped through the oxygenator. Oxygenated blood is then returned from an "arterial" reservoir to the patient after clamp changes. In contrast to continuous flow, tidal flow ECMO can have significant hemodynamic consequences. While the venous clamp is open, blood is drained from the patient, leading to hypovolemia. Conversely, when the arterial

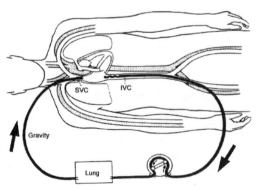

Figure 1. Schematic representation of two-site VV ECMO support.

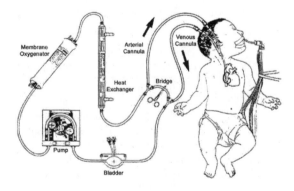

Figure 2. Schematic representation of one-site VV ECMO support using a DLVV cannula.

clamp is opened, intravascular volume is replenished, potentially causing volume overload. As a result, cardiac output can vary widely over a few cycles as right ventricular filling changes. Tidal flow support has not been widely used in clinical practice. Tidal flow VV ECMO support requires equipment not available for clinical use in the U.S. and is therefore not widely used there. The largest human experience with tidal flow VV developed in France, where it has been utilized for both neonatal and pediatric patients.[2,3]

Extracorporeal carbon dioxide removal

In certain settings such as severe upper or lower airway obstruction, patient oxygenation is adequate but CO_2 retention, high intrathoracic pressures, or barotrauma become problematic. Consequently, when CO_2 is removed primarily by VV ECMO, spontaneous breathing decreases and the requirement for respirator support is reduced.[4,5] Gattinoni and Kolobow developed the methodology for extracorporeal carbon dioxide removal (ECCO$_2$R) in animals and then applied it clinically.[4-7] Either continuous or tidal flow VV ECMO can also be used at low flow rates (30 ml/kg/min) to remove CO_2 from the blood. During ECCO$_2$R, the patient's lungs provide the primary source of oxygenation, and thus, the technique is dependent to some degree on pulmonary gas exchange. The patient is left on low frequency, small tidal volume ventilation aimed at maintaining optimal lung inflation. The ECMO circuit allows for efficient removal of arterial CO_2, minimizing the need for excessive ventilatory effort and decreasing barotrauma. This technique may be used for patients who require extracorporeal support for severe lower or upper airway obstruction, as in severe status asthmaticus, where CO_2 removal is more problematic than oxygenation. ECCO$_2$R can also allow for invasive techniques such as bronchoscopy and surgical airway intervention to be performed safely.

Historical development of VV ECMO

VV ECMO was first described by Kolobow in an animal model in 1969.[1] The successful use of VV ECMO for neonatal patients with respiratory failure was first reported in 1982 using a two-site approach.[8] Unfortunately, neonates undergoing femoral vein cannulation for two-site ECMO often had venous and/or arterial circulatory compromise to the cannulated limb.[8,9] Disadvantages of the two-site VV ECMO approach in the neonate include the longer operative time required for placement of cannulas in separate surgical sites, problems with the groin wound, and subsequent swelling of the leg, however, many of the problems attributed to two-site VV support were overcome with the development of double lumen catheter which required the use of only the internal jugular vein.[10,11] The original VV cannula, consisted of two thin-walled, steel tubes located inside each other. It was inflexible with the potential to lacerate vascular or cardiac structures. Later modifications produced a flexible, thin-walled cannula with two channels of unequal size that provided optimal venous drainage and return flows with decreased potential for perforation.

Comparison of VV and VA ECMO

VV and VA ECMO differ significantly (Table 2). These differences illustrate both advantages and disadvantages of VV ECLS. Most of the major risks inherent to VA bypass apply equally to VV ECMO since instrumentation, systemic anticoagulation, and long-term perfusion are required; however, VV ECMO provides several safety advantages over VA cannulation. Most importantly, VV ECMO avoids instrumentation and ligation of the carotid artery. The advent of VV cannulas and the use of percutaneous VV cannulation techniques may allow for shorter cannulation times with decreased long-term morbidity, such as ligation of the jugular vein. Additionally, use of a double lumen catheter could provide significant time-savings from cannulating one instead of multiple vessels.

The potential for direct ischemic lung injury from decreased pulmonary blood flow during VA ECMO is also eliminated with the use of VV ECMO, as VV support provides well oxygenated blood to the lungs. This could contribute to decreased pulmonary inflammation; recent animal studies suggest diminution of bronchoalveolar cytokine response with VV cannulation compared to VA.[12]

VV cannulation has potential advantages for the brain. VA cannulation requires ligation of the carotid artery that potentially is permanent. VV cannulation routes possible thromboemboli arising from the ECMO circuit to the pulmonary rather than the systemic and cerebral circulation as seen with VA support. During VV ECMO, blood entering the cerebral circulation is not as highly oxygenated nor is it under as much pressure as during VA ECMO. This could decrease

the risk of cerebral reperfusion injury, particularly in infants with cerebral autoregulation altered by prior insult.[13] Studies have shown varying effects of VA and VV ECMO on cerebral blood flow.[13-15] However, both a recent human infant study[14] and a neonatal lamb study[15] using continuous laser doppler flow found persistent decreased cerebral blood flow velocities in VA compared to VV cannulation. The decline in cerebral blood flow with VA support is thought to be related to decrease in cardiac output, increase in cerebral vascular resistance, and diminished vascular pulsatility.

The primary disadvantage of VV ECMO is that it does not provide direct circulatory support. Maximum achievable oxygen delivery in some cases may be inadequate to meet demand. Oxygenation may be lower than on VA ECMO because of the mixing of ECMO return blood with desaturated systemic venous blood. Refractory hypotension or increased metabolic rate, as with sepsis, accentuate these problems on VV

Table 2. Comparison of features for VA and VV ECMO.

	VA ECMO	VV ECMO
Cannulation site(s)	Internal jugular vein, right atrium, or femoral vein plus right common carotid, axillary, or femoral artery, or aorta (directly)	Internal jugular vein alone, jugular-femoral, femoro-femoral, sapheno-saphenous vein, or right atrium (directly)
Usual arterial oxygen tension (P_aO_2) achieved	60-150 torr	45-80 torr
Indicator(s) of oxygenation sufficiency	"Mixed" venous saturation or P_aO_2 and calculated oxygen consumption	Cerebral venous saturation; O_2 difference "across the membrane"; patient P_aO_2, pre-membrane saturation trend
Cardiac effects	Decreased preload, increased afterload; CVP varies, pulse pressure low; coronary oxygenation provided by left ventricular blood; "cardiac stun" possible	Negligible effects; CVP and pulse pressure unaffected; may improve coronary oxygenation; may reduce right ventricular afterload
Oxygen delivery capacity	High	Moderate, improves with additional drainage (including cephalad drain)
Circulatory support	Partial to complete	No direct effect, but improved delivery of oxygen to coronary and pulmonary circulation can improve cardiac output
Effect on pulmonary circulation	Moderately to markedly decreased	Unchanged or improved with oxygenated blood
Presence of right-to-left shunt	Decreased hemoglobin saturation of blood in aorta	Increased hemoglobin saturation of blood in aorta
Presence of left-to-right shunt	Potential pulmonary congestion and systemic hypoperfusion	Potential pulmonary congestion and systemic hypoperfusion
Recirculation	None	Major impact on oxygen delivery

CVP = central venous pressure

ECMO. The problem can also be exacerbated by recirculation, a disadvantage unique to VV ECMO.

While not providing direct cardiac support, VV ECMO does offer a variety of advantageous circulatory effects relative to VA ECMO. VV support does not decrease right ventricular preload, pulmonary blood flow, left atrial return, or left ventricular output, since the volume of blood drained from and returned to the central venous system is equal. In contrast, VA ECMO decreases right ventricular preload and pulmonary blood flow, and it increases left ventricular afterload.[16-19] The absence of a change in left ventricular afterload with VV support may eliminate the isolated left ventricular "stun" syndrome seen in a subset of VA-supported patients.[19] Occasionally, however, some patients placed on VV ECMO manifest symptoms consistent with right ventricular stun. These patients develop severe pulmonary hypertension with right ventricular dilation. The dilated right ventricle can cause bowing of the ventricular septum into the left ventricle, reducing filling, and compromising cardiac output. Careful management of preload, myocardial contractility, and afterload can reverse this problem without the need for conversion to VA support.

Echocardiographic studies demonstrate that patients managed on VV ECMO have normal cardiac function.[17] VV ECMO may indirectly improve cardiac performance by increasing mixed venous oxygen content returning to the pulmonary circulation. Compared to VA ECMO, the oxygen saturation of the blood delivered to the pulmonary artery is higher because oxygenated blood is delivered to the RA, not the aorta. The higher mixed venous oxygen saturation in the pulmonary arteries may decrease pulmonary vascular resistance and right ventricular afterload. In addition, avoidance of increased left ventricular afterload with improved oxygen delivery to the coronary arteries may improve myocardial performance.

Another cardiovascular advantage of VV perfusion is that it preserves physiologic pulsatility. When compared to non-pulsatile flow, pulsatile flow decreases vascular resistance, decreases afterload, and improves organ perfusion. Differences in pulsatile and non-pulsatile flow could also produce differing effects on renal function. However, experimental animal studies show comparable effects of VV and VA support on blood pressure, renal blood flow, and plasma renin activity.[19]

VV ECMO is also more dependent on optimal venous drainage (e.g., maximum venous cannula size and appropriate position) than VA support because of the inefficiency imposed by recirculation. VV ECMO may also require separate surgical sites if two-site VV support is being provided, as opposed to the placement of both catheters in the neck for VA ECMO. This disadvantage is obviously minimized with use of a DLVV cannula. Finally, interpretation of blood gas data is conceptually different with VV ECMO compared to VA, requiring some re-education for teams whose experience is limited to VA ECMO.

Reported clinical experience

The ELSO Registry data reflect the sharp rise in VV ECLS use in patients with acute respiratory failure (ARF) (Figure 3). VV support has routinely been used in the majority (60-70%) of adults with ARF receiving ECMO. However, VV use in neonates and children has grown steadily from absence of use in 1988 to ~30% of neonatal ECMO cases reported in 2003. Similarly, VV use in pediatric cases has risen from 18% in 1988 to ~40% of all cases in 2003. Experience with the use of VV ECMO specifically related to ARF can be categorized by age.

Neonatal respiratory failure

Andrews et al. first reported successful clinical use of VV ECMO in human neonates in 1983.[20] In 1985, the successful support of 11 neonates with VV ECMO using the internal jugular vein for drainage and an iliac vein for return was reported.[7] Although survival was comparable to neonatal VA support, enthusiasm for VV in neonates was limited by the complications with femoral vein cannulation. Development of DLVV cannulas[8,9] resulted in a slow increase in the use of VV ECLS. Cornish et al. in 1993 reported the successful use of VV ECMO in 17 neonates[21] and suggested that the perceived limitations of VV ECMO be reconsidered. In this series, the average dopamine infusion dose was 16 mcg/kg/min prior to VV ECMO, and no patient required conversion to VA support for hemodynamic instability.

Anderson et al. in 1993 compared conventional VA ECMO with DLVV ECMO in 243 neonates.[22] When compared to neonates on VA ECMO, patients treated with DLVV ECMO had better survival (95% vs. 87%), shorter ECMO runs (100 vs. 132 hours) and fewer neurological complications. However, DLVV patients were generally more stable prior to cannulation, and the authors suggested that the variance in outcomes could potentially be attributed to a difference in severity of illness between treatment groups. Single-center neonatal experience also supported the initial use of VV support.[23] VV was successfully initiated in 57 of 63 neonates, although 5 later required conversion to VA.

Increased VV use was also shown in the ELSO Registry data. From 1991-98, VV use increased from 1-32% of all neonatal ECMO cases (Figure 3).[24] Preferential use of VV ECMO was reported in neonates with congenital diaphragmatic hernia;[25] this was confirmed by other single-center experiences.[26] VV support was provided in 14% of 2628 neonatal CDH cases in the ELSO Registry (1990-98)[27] with 17% of the VV requiring conversion to VA. Neurologic complications were markedly lower with VV ECMO. VV ECMO use has also been extended to selected "elective" neonatal cases requiring complex tracheal reconstruction.[28]

Development of percutaneous cannulation techniques has further advanced the ability to provide neonatal VV support. Reickert et al.[29] described percutaneous cannulation in neonates using a 12F double lumen catheter in patients

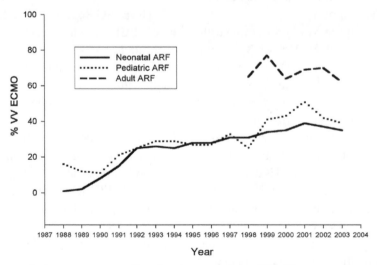

Figure 3. VV cannulation as a percent of total patients receiving ECMO support, by year. Results are demonstrated for each age category. Data obtained from the ELSO Registry Report of the Extracorporeal Life Support Organization: International Summary. ELSO, Ann Arbor, MI, July, 2004.

>3 kg. Eleven of 20 patients were cannulated without "exposure-assistance" or complete open placement. Improvements in catheter design and function[30] continue to result in greater use of VV. Several reports have also described use of the umbilical vein as an alternative vessel for reinfusion[31], but double lumen cannulas have generally made this approach unnecessary.

Overall, VV support has been used in ~22% of all neonatal ECMO cases from 1988-2003.[32] While preferential use of VV is desired, superiority to VA cannulation has not been proven in a prospective fashion. ELSO Registry data has demonstrated a higher survival rate (91% vs. 81%) and a lower rate of major neurological complications for VV.[33] However, when patients treated with VV ECMO are compared to VA ECMO patients matched for maturity, weight, and severity of illness, differences in outcome between these two types of ECMO are not statistically significant.[34]

Clinical experience with tidal flow VV ECMO has also been reported in neonates. Survival in a series of 107 neonates supported with tidal flow VV ECMO was 85%.[10] The nature and frequency of complications were similar to that reported for neonates treated with VA ECMO. Although the FiO_2 requirement was decreased in these patients compared to pre-bypass levels, the FiO_2 was higher than typically used during VA or continuous flow VV ECMO.

Pediatric respiratory failure

Pediatric experience with VV support is more difficult to evaluate given the heterogeneity of diseases treated. Single-center experience with VV as an alternative in pediatric ARF[35] was first reported in 1991. In a large series,[36] 53 of 128 ECMO children with ARF received VV support.[35] However, these series still used VA support for the majority of pediatric ARF patients. A more recent single-center report describes the primary use of VV support for pediatric ARF.[37,38] VV ECMO was used in 82%

of pediatric ARF patients requiring ECMO with 81% survival. Successful use of VV ECMO has also been described for specific pediatric disease processes, including pediatric trauma patients[39] with ARF and children with acute pulmonary hemorrhage.[40]

ELSO Registry experience supports the increased use of VV techniques for pediatric ARF, increasing from 11 to 39% of all ECMO cases from 1990-2003 (Figure 3). Overall, VV support represented ~31% of all pediatric ARF ECMO cases from 1988-2003.[32] Comparison of outcomes between pediatric patients with ARF on VV or VA ECMO is difficult, especially in the absence of randomized trials. In retrospective single-center reports, VV patients have improved survival. However, VA patients had higher severity of illness scores, lower PaO_2 oxygenation, and greater vasopressor needs prior to ECMO, suggesting a tendency to select VA for sicker patients. Zahraa et al. evaluated the ELSO Registry for pediatric ARF data prior to 1998 and found no statistically significant difference in survival between patients receiving VV (60.1%) or VA (55.8%).[41]

Adult respiratory failure

ELSO Registry data indicate that a majority of adult ARF patients have received VV cannulation (Figure 3). Of adult patients with ARF, 68% of 584 reported to the ELSO Registry from 1988-2003 were placed on VV ECMO. It is likely that concerns over carotid artery ligation in adults and the ease of femoral cannulation techniques have encouraged its use in this age group. ECMO survival for adult ARF has been lower than for neonates and children,[42] but survival is likely related to adult co-morbidities rather than cannulation method. Previous randomized adult ECMO trials found no benefit of ECMO compared to standard therapy. This has been attributed to reliance on VA support[43] or from excessive bleeding complications.[44] Gattinoni et al. reported better outcomes in adults using ECCO R techniques in association with lung rest, which has become a standard approach in ECMO protocols elsewhere.[46] In the University of Michigan report on the world's largest single-center adult ECMO experience,[47] 77% of 255 adult ECMO ARF patients received initial VV support, and 53% of VV patients survived to discharge. The CESAR trial in the U.K. is preferentially employing VV cannulation techniques for patients randomized to ECMO; results from this study are forthcoming.

Principles of VV ECMO

Continuous flow ECMO is the most common form of VV ECMO presently in use; the discussion below addresses the details of patient management for this form of ECMO.

Patient Selection

In the past, VV cannulation has been reserved for patients who were hemodynamically stable and had only moderate respiratory failure. Some centers do not consider VV support for neonates with congenital diaphragmatic hernia (CDH) or in pediatric patients who require vasopressor support. However, substantial success has been documented for VV cannulation for ARF in all age groups. VV cannulation can now be considered the primary cannulation approach in all patients with ARF meeting accepted general criteria for ECMO. The only specific exclusion criteria for neonates is the inability to insert a DLVV cannula and the inability to adequately support gas exchange. In the child or adult, inability to obtain adequate venous access or to adequately support gas exchange once on VV support merits the use of VA support.

Decisions about the use of VV ECMO for ARF patients with associated significant circulatory compromise are less straightforward. VV ECMO does not provide direct circulatory support and may not support patients with inadequate cardiac performance. However, as noted

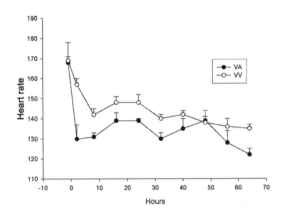

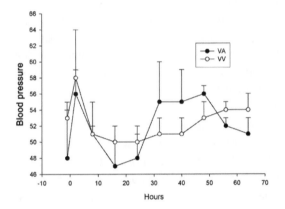

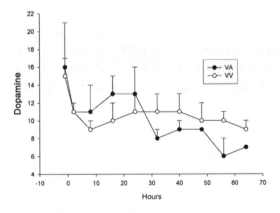

Figure 4. Mean heart rate (A), blood pressure (B), and dopamine requirements (C) in a comparison group of neonates receiving either VV or VA support. Vital sign improvements were similar between groups, and dopamine was weaned in a similar fashion with both VV and VA support. (Modified from Cornish JD, Clark RH. *ECMO: Extracorporeal Cardiopulmonary Support in Critical Care.* 1995: 87-109.)

previously, both neonates[21,48] and children[36] with significant circulatory compromise requiring substantial doses of vasopressors and inotropes have been shown to tolerate VV cannulation effectively. Mean arterial pressure (MAP) typically improves and VV support often allows weaning of inotropes in neonatal respiratory failure (Figure 4). Similar improvements were reported in a case series of pediatric patients with respiratory failure who required vasopressors prior to cannulation for VV ECMO.[36] Pettignano et al. found a rapid decline in the need for vasopressor support with the initiation of VV ECMO (Figure 5). This improvement is likely associated with decreased intrathoracic pressures with lung rest, improved oxygenation, and reversal of acidosis. Weaning may be accomplished more readily than in VA ECMO patients due to the improved coronary blood flow and decreased cardiac afterload.

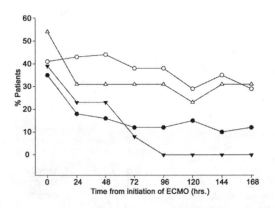

Figure 5. Percent of pediatric VV and VA ECMO patients requiring inotropes and vasopressors, by hour. In this series, 24 of 68 VV ECMO children required vasopressors (epinephrine, norepinephrine, dopamine >10 mcg/kg/min) and 28 required inotropes (dobutamine, milrinone, dopamine <10 mcg/kg/min) prior to cannulation. Inotrope/pressor requirements did not increase, and VV patients were weaned in a manner similar to VA patients. Legend: inotropes: open circle-VV, open triangle-VA; vasopressors: closed circle-VV, closed triangle-VA.[37]

Presently, absolute criteria do not exist for determining suitability of ARF patients for VV support. Roberts et al. recommended that VV cannulation be used in all cases of neonatal ARF except where double lumen cannulation is impossible or when septic shock is refractory to inotropic support prior to ECMO (inotrope score >100).[48] VV support should be considered for both pediatric and adult patients unless appropriately sized venous cannulas cannot be placed, the patient is in refractory shock despite maximal pressor support, or cardiac arrest is imminent. VV support is generally not recommended for patients with myocardial failure following cardiac surgery, recent and severe cardiac arrest, or with refractory rhythm disturbances associated with systemic hypotension. While the experience with VV has been quite encouraging, selection of the appropriate mode of ECMO still requires a careful assessment of the patient's clinical condition.

For patients in which the choice of support is uncertain, an alternative approach is to isolate both the right common carotid artery and the internal jugular vein; venous access can then be obtained and VV support initiated. VV support can continue if the patient's oxygenation and MAP improve over the subsequent 15-30 minutes. If the patient does not improve or worsens on ECMO, the carotid artery can be cannulated, both lumens of the venous cannulas used for venous drainage, and the patient converted to VA support.

Principles of gas exchange during VV ECMO

Effects of recirculation on oxygen delivery

A sound understanding of the concept of recirculation is critical to the successful application of VV ECMO and to the appropriate interpretation of blood gas results obtained on VV support. The source of blood for oxygenation by VV ECMO arises from the same venous capacitance source to which it is returned after oxygenation. A portion of blood that has just been oxygenated in the circuit will thus flow directly from the re-infusion site and be taken up by the venous drainage catheter, instead of being delivered to the patient's circulation. This amount of redundant flow is defined as the recirculation fraction (Figure 6).

Mathematically, recirculation fraction (R) can be estimated as:

$$R = \frac{SpreOx - SVO_2}{SpostOx - SVO_2}$$

where SpreOx is the oxygen saturation of the blood entering the oxygenator, SpostOx is the oxygen saturation of the blood exiting the oxygenator, and SVO_2 is the true mixed venous oxygen saturation in the patient. This calculation is more precise if oxygen content rather than oxygen saturation is used, but for clinical purposes the difference is small. If increased amounts of highly oxygenated blood return from the oxygenator, SpreOx increases and becomes closer to SpostOx; R increases as less desaturated blood/minute is made available to the oxygenator.

Unfortunately, it is impossible to measure actual mixed venous oxygen saturation during VV ECMO since oxygenated blood from the ECMO circuit has been added to the blood in the pulmonary artery. Approximations of the SVO_2 during VV ECMO may be obtained by sampling blood from another major vein not affected by recirculation (e.g., from the inferior vena cava (IVC) when the RA has been cannulated directly, or from a cephalad catheter in the right internal jugular vein).

Factors that affect recirculation

Calculation of a specific recirculation fraction is less important than understanding the factors that alter it. The four primary factors af-

fecting recirculation are the ECMO pump flow, venous catheter position, native cardiac output, and right atrial blood volume. The impact of pump flow on recirculation is straightforward. If pump flow is higher, the drainage of blood from the RA back into the ECMO circuit increases, and streaming of oxygenated blood from the return catheter to the venous drainage catheter is more likely to occur (Figure 6). Recirculation fraction increases in a relatively linear fashion with increasing pump flow. Oxygen delivery to the patient first increases and then decreases as pump flow increases beyond optimal flow and minimal recirculation (Figure 7). The reason for the decreased effective oxygen delivery is that the recirculation percentage limits the amount of oxygen delivered to the patient. Effective pump flow may be described by the equation:

Effective Pump Flow =
Total Pump Flow - (Total Pump Flow x Recirculation Fraction)

At some maximal flow, the recirculation fraction is 100%, and effective flow again becomes zero. The ideal pump rate is one that provides the highest effective pump flow at the lowest rpm of the pump, yielding the least degree of tubing wear and hemolysis.

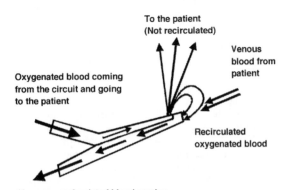

Figure 6. Schematic diagram of the principles of recirculation in VV support (illustrated for a DLVV catheter).

Optimal flow is not fixed as there are at least three other factors that affect recirculation fraction: catheter position, cardiac output and right atrial volume. If the tip of the drainage and infusion catheters are directed at each other from close range, the recirculation fraction will be high. When using a double lumen catheter, if the catheter is positioned either high in the superior vena cava (SVC) or low in the IVC, outflow from the catheter will tend to remain within the confines of the vessel and return to the catheter before it can reach the RA. This phenomenon may explain why there might be an unexpected fall in the patient's arterial oxygen saturation with catheter position changes. Changes in catheter position can occur with increased or decreased lung inflation, increasing edema of the neck at the site of anchoring sutures, a change in the patient's position, or patient movement.

Cardiac output also affects recirculation. If the oxygenated blood delivered to the RA

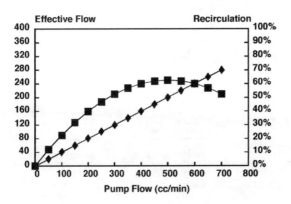

Figure 7. The change in effective pump flow and recirculation compared with set pump flow in VV support. The change in effective pump flow (■) and recirculation(♦) compared with set pump flow in VV support. Note that as pump flow is increased, recirculation increases linearly. Effective pump flow initially increases, then plateaus, then decreases. This is due the to effects of increased recirculation on limiting the amount of oxygen provided to the patient and thus the effective oxygen delivery. This is an idealized curve; the actual curve will vary with catheter size and position.

by the circuit is moved rapidly into the right ventricle and then to the lungs, left heart, and body, it is less accessible to the drainage catheter for return to the ECMO pump. In contrast, during cardiac standstill, all of the oxygenated blood flowing into the RA drains back into the ECMO circuit, since there is no forward flow. Improved cardiac output can improve overall oxygenation by decreasing recirculation. For related reasons, right atrial intravascular volume also influences recirculation. Oxygenated blood is more likely to be drained directly back into the ECMO circuit if it is delivered to the RA with decreased volumes of deoxygenated blood than if the oxygenated blood is diluted in a larger volume of desaturated blood in a normal RA. Thus, increasing intravascular volume can immediately decrease recirculation and allow for more effective oxygen delivery. The immediate benefits of decreasing recirculation must be weighed against the overall effect of increasing extravascular lung water.

Since VV ECMO provides no direct circulatory support, it can be difficult to achieve the same level of oxygen delivery during VV as during VA ECMO. However, when the recirculation fraction is minimal and cardiac output is supported, oxygen delivery can be similar to that seen with VA. Oxygenation is optimized when the hemoglobin concentration is approximately 15 g/dl, when recirculation fraction is low, and when the venous drainage catheter is large enough to achieve ~120-140 ml/kg/min flow.

Oxygen delivery from the circuit to the patient can be significantly increased by the use of a second drainage catheter in a site not subject to recirculation such as a catheter inserted in a cephalad direction in the internal jugular vein to the level of the jugular venous bulb. Increased oxygen delivery results from decreased recirculation. A second catheter also provides cerebral venous decompression. The cephalad catheter can provide as much as half the venous return to the ECMO circuit. Since the blood draining from the jugular venous bulb has a low mixed venous saturation, the amount of oxygen that can be added to the blood as it passes through the membrane lung is increased. In Pettignano's series,[36] 55 of 68 VV ECMO patients received more than one drainage cannula, including 46 with cephalad catheters. Similar success in obtaining adequate flow and blood/oxygen delivery was reported in another series with a three-cannula VV technique.[49] While theoretically appealing, review of the ELSO Registry did not reveal an outcome benefit with routine cephalad jugular drainage cannulas in VV ECMO for neonatal ARF.[50]

Measurement of oxygenation on VV ECMO

At present, there is no simple direct measure of oxygenation during VV ECMO. Mixed venous oxygen saturation readings from a pulmonary artery cannot be interpreted because the oxygen delivered to the patient from the ECMO circuit is injected into the venous system. There are, however, several indirect ways to estimate oxygen sufficiency which are more useful in combination than with any single measurement taken by itself.

Pre-oxygenator venous saturation readings do not reflect changes in the patient's true mixed venous saturation. This measure is strongly influenced by the recirculation fraction. When catheter recirculation is high, blood sampled from the pre-oxygenator site will have a high saturation even if the patient's mixed venous saturation is dropping and oxygen delivery is inadequate. The pre-oxygenator saturation value, taken in combination with an invasive or non-invasive arterial saturation reading, yields useful information about the changing balance of recirculation and systemic oxygen delivery. For example, if the pre-oxygenator saturation rises and the patient's arterial oxygen saturation falls, the recirculation fraction has increased. Alternatively, if the pre-oxygenator saturation falls and the patient's arterial oxygen saturation rises, the recirculation fraction has decreased. Increases in the patient's saturation with no change or a slight increase in pre-oxygenator saturation generally indicate improvement in the patient's lung function and cardiac output. The pre-oxygenator saturation increases because the patient's mixed venous saturation is increasing. The patient's arterial saturation improves because the respiratory system is adding oxygen to the pulmonary blood and the mixed venous saturation is higher. A summary of VV ECMO blood gas interpretation is provided in Table 3.

Table 3. VV ECMO scenario chart

Patient arterial oxygen saturation	Cephalad catheter oxygen saturation (if available)	Venous drainage oxygen saturation	Interpretation	Management
Increasing	Increasing or stable	Increasing or stable	Oxygenation improving	Wean ECMO flow
Decreasing	Decreasing or stable	Decreasing or stable	Oxygenation worsening	Check catheter position and pump flow, try to increase flow
Decreasing	Stable but with decreased flow	Increasing	Increased recirculation probably due to loss of cephalad catheter flow	Evaluate catheter position, adjust head position, add or subtract shoulder roll, apply gentle traction to catheter
Decreasing	Decreasing or stable with good flow	Increasing	Increased recirculation probably due to changing catheter position	Evaluate cardiac output and catheter position, consider giving volume
Decreasing but stable (with increased PaCO$_2$)	Increasing with increase flow	Stable	Poor ventilation	Adjust sweep gas flow or mix; if off ECMO, adjust ventilator support
Stable (with decreased PaCO$_2$)	Decreasing with decreased flow	Increasing	Over ventilation	Adjust sweep gas flow or mix; if off ECMO, adjust ventilator support
Decreasing and decreased BP	Decreasing and decreased flow	Increasing	Evaluate for compromised cardiac output	Consider pericardial effusion if pulse pressure is decreased

Another approach is to use a measure of venous saturation not affected by recirculation as an approximation of "true" mixed venous saturation. Blood drawn from a catheter in the IVC, or from a catheter draining blood from the jugular venous bulb, can provide this information. Oxygen saturation can be continuously monitored from a cephalad drainage cannula to provide continuous and accurate readings of jugular venous oxygenation and help with an estimate of oxygen sufficiency. Changes in jugular venous oxygenation have been correlated with changes in systemic pH.[51] Unfortunately, these values are not very sensitive to changes in the patient's cardiopulmonary status since cerebral blood flow in VV ECMO appears to be preserved even in patients with life-threatening cardiopulmonary failure.

Circuit and patient management on VV ECMO

Conceptually, VV ECMO is quite simple. In practice, it exemplifies the advantage of careful attention to detail.

Patient preparation

The usual intensive care support and monitoring procedures are followed as well as ECMO evaluation and testing protocols based on age and disease process including cranial ul-trasound, echocardiogram, coagulation studies, and others. Communication between the ECMO physician, the referring hospital and physician, the bedside staff, and support services such as the blood bank, OR, and laboratory must be maintained on an ongoing and continual basis. The family must be advised of the risks and benefits of ECMO and any changes in their child's status.

In addition, patients with severe ARF are at risk for cardiovascular collapse. Intravascular volume and acid-base balance should be normalized to the extent possible. Inotropic use should be optimized. Electrolyte concentrations should be checked and adjusted as required. Particular attention should be paid to ionized calcium, potassium, and magnesium concentrations. Hemoglobin concentration should be measured and optimized.

Priming the VV ECMO circuit

Circuit blood priming practices vary between ECMO centers, but some general approaches exist. Fresh units of packed red blood cells (PRBCs) <5 days old are preferred. An appropriate albumin concentration, osmotic pressure, procoagulant/anticoagulant factor balance and electrolyte concentrations are all important in priming. The components for circuit prime blood used at our center are presented in Table 4. This mixture results in a circuit sodium con-

Table 4. Egleston Children's ECMO Center components for prime blood.

1. Begin with ~2 units of fresh, CMV negative, packed RBCs
2. Irradiate units immediately prior to delivery to the floor
3. To each unit of packed RBCs add:
   a. 40 ml 25% albumin
   b. 25 ml THAM
   c. 10 meq $NaHCo_3$
   d. 100 units (as 1.0 ml) heparin
4. Mix well (by rocking)
5. Add 3 ml 10% calcium gluconate
6. Mix again

centration of ~136 mEq/l, potassium of 3.5-6.5 mEq/l (depending on the age of the blood), total protein of 4.0 g/dl, albumin concentration ~3.0 g/dl, osmolarity of ~280 mOsm/l, and a hematocrit of 45-55%. If washed PRBCs are used and resuspended to a hematocrit of 75-85%, the same quantities of additives may be used as those listed in Table 4, even if the volume of each unit is <250 ml. However, the potassium concentration may be quite low (1.5-2.5 mEq/l) in the final washed cell prime. Potassium concentration should be measured, adjusted, and circuit electrolytes repeated before the patient is connected to the circuit. Hypokalemia may result in significant dysrhythmias and, thus, a false but perceived failure of VV ECMO. Bolus administration of potassium rapidly into the circuit or directly into patient can result in cardiac arrest.

Circuit ionized calcium levels are also measured once blood is circulating in the primed circuit. Typically, it will be necessary to add calcium gluconate to the circuit and repeat circuit blood gas, potassium, and ionized calcium concentrations before connecting the patient to the circuit. Failure to measure and normalize the ionized calcium concentration and to adequately pressurize the VV circuit may result in secondary hypotension[52] seen upon initiation of VV support. Initiation of ECMO in a patient that has been hyperventilated or has metabolic alkalosis can also accentuate a drop in ionized calcium concentration. The blood-primed circuit should be circulated, filtered, and warmed before the patient is connected to the circuit.

Some centers also pressurize the ECMO circuit prior to cannulation using fluids to achieve high post-membrane pressures (generally 100 mm Hg at a pump rate of 200 ml/min) as a means of achieving adequate circuit volume as the patient goes on ECMO. This practice, known as "hyperpriming", lacks specific evidence of benefit, but theoretically aids in decreasing the hypotension occasionally seen with VV support. Hypotension is distinctly uncommon with use of this technique.

Table 5. Catheter sizes for VV cannulation based on patient weight.

Patient weight (kg)	Venous drain (right internal jugular/ saphenous/femoral)	Arterialized venous return if not double lumen (right internal jugular/femoral)	Additional venous drain (if used)
2.0 - ≤3.0	12F double lumen	N/A	10F cephalad (arterial catheter)
3.0 - ≤6.5	14-15F double lumen	N/A	10-12F cephalad (arterial catheter)
6.5 - ≤12	18F double lumen	14 F	14F cephalad (arterial catheter)
12 - ≤15	18F double lumen + additional drain	15 F	15-17F cephalad or femoral
15 - ≤20	18F double lumen + additional drain 21F	15-17 F	19F cephalad or femoral
20 - ≤30	21-23F	17-19 F	19-21F cephalad or femoral
30 -≤ 60	23-27F	19 F	21-23F femoral
>60	27-29F	21 F	23 F femoral

Catheter choices are guidelines only and are based on general use at Children's Healthcare of Atlanta at Egleston. Double lumen catheters provide both venous drainage and venous return. Cephalad catheters are placed in the right internal jugular vein. Arterial catheters are the catheter type used in cephalad position.

Patient cannulation

VV cannulation can now be performed in all age and weight range due to the diversity of catheter sizes available (Table 5). Neonates formerly presented difficulty with VV cannulation because of limb perfusion problems associated with extremity cannulation and the absence of small DLVV catheters. Advances in catheter construction have now made double lumen catheters as small as 12F available for use. Availability of DLVV catheters of up to 21F in size has allowed for percutaneous DLVV catheterization in many patients. Larger DLVV catheters (23-27F) are currently under evaluation for Food and Drug Administration (FDA) approval. While this theoretically requires catheterization of only a single vessel in many patients, VV flow and oxygenation considerations can make cannulation of an additional drainage vessel in combination with the DLVV cannula advantageous. Optimal cannula locations and flow patterns vary according to patient size.

For neonates, the standard technique employs a DLVV cannula advanced through the right internal jugular vein to the level of the mid RA. Based on center preference, a cephalad-directed internal jugular vein catheter can be placed to augment flow. Simultaneous venous drainage from a 10F or 12F cephalad-directed internal jugular catheter may extend the useful weight range of the 14F DLVV cannula up to 4.5 kg. Cephalad-directed venous catheters can access one-third to one-half of total drainage, providing better venous return to the circuit and augmenting oxygen delivery.

Ideally, the tip of the double lumen catheter should be in the lower third of the RA. This placement assures that all of the venous side holes are in the atrium. It is possible to perforate the SVC if a side hole remains in the vessel. In infants, the junction of the IVC and the RA is approximately 0.5 centimeter above the diaphragm; thus, the catheter may be considered to be in optimal position if its

tip is visible on chest radiograph ~1 centimeter above the diaphragm. Unfortunately, this relationship changes regularly with alterations in ventilator settings on ECMO even if the catheter is properly secured in the vessel by suture to the skin of the neck and behind the ear. Prior to cannulation, the patient's lungs are often maximally inflated. With lung rest on ECMO support and lower MAP, lung volume falls, and the diaphragm rises. If the catheter position in the chest does not change secondary to the rise in the diaphragm, then the heart will rise on the catheter, moving the catheter toward or into the IVC. This may result in increased recirculation fraction and falling arterial saturation. Traction on the circuit tubing connected to the catheter will move it in the cephalad direction enough for correction. It is rarely necessary to re-open the incision and reposition the catheter. The reverse situation with cannula position can occur as lung healing brings improved compliance and higher mean lung volumes. Releasing traction on the circuit tubing can restore optimal cannula position. A chest radiograph is recommended if there is any question regarding catheter's position. In general, it is best not to try to reposition a catheter that is functioning well.

Radial orientation or rotation of the DLVV cannula is also important. These catheters are designed with venous and arterial side holes positioned opposite each other. The arterial or return side holes will be directed toward the tricuspid valve if the catheter is secured to the neck (usually just behind the ear) with the red-labeled arm of the "Y" (arterial return) directed up or anterior to the venous arm. This orientation will further help to minimize recirculation.

For large children and adults, the surgical approaches that have been most widely used require cannulation of both the internal jugular vein and of one or two of the femoral, saphenous, or iliac vessels. European ECMO programs have typically employed drainage of blood from the femoral vessels and return of blood to the patient through the internal jugular vein (femoro-atrial flow). This approach, being used more widely in adult patients, has a marked advantage of minimizing recirculation. On the other hand, venous drainage is a limiting factor that could affect total oxygen delivery. Many U.S. programs previously utilized a large bore cannula in the right internal jugular vein for drainage to the ECMO circuit and a smaller catheter in the groin for arterialized return (atrio-femoral flow). This approach may result in a higher recirculation fraction than the European method, but the greater flow achievable may compensate and allow for higher pump flows for total respiratory support using "rest" ventilator settings.

A prospective comparison of atrio-femoral and femoro-atrial flow performed in adult VV ECMO patients questioned these assumptions.[53] Using a modified bridge to allow conversion between the two directions, investigators found that femoro-atrial bypass achieved higher maximal flow and higher mixed venous oxygen saturations than the atrio-femoral direction. Femoro-atrial bypass also required less flow to maintain an equivalent mixed venous saturation, implying decreased recirculation.

Egleston's preference for two-site VV ECMO in older children, adolescents, and adults is to utilize a femoral vein for drainage and the internal jugular vein for return to provide femoro-atrial flow. A second venous drainage site is obtained in most cases using either an additional femoral drain or a cephalad jugular cannula. Rarely-used alternatives to saphenous or femoral cannulation include a subclavian vein, the left internal jugular vein, and direct cannulation of the RA via thoracotomy.

Patient management on ECMO

Identifying the optimal flow to allow for adequate oxygenation and to minimize recirculation is of paramount importance. Once cannulated, VV flow is initiated at 10-15 ml/kg/min and advanced over 10-15 minutes to a maximum of 140-150 ml/kg/min. Determi-nation of this maximal flow rate is helpful to establish the highest flow rates that can be obtained with the patient and circuit. Flow is then decreased, while monitoring the patient's pulse oximeter, until an optimal flow for adequate oxygenation is observed. Because of the effects of recirculation, this will often not be the highest attainable flow. Oxygen saturations greater than 88-90% are generally accepted, but occasionally lower saturations are tolerated. Oxygenation is more difficult to monitor in the VV ECMO patient. VV oxygenation can be assessed to some degree by monitoring several values: the trend in pre-oxygenator saturation, changes in pulse oximeter saturation which reflect arterial oxygenation but not tissue sufficiency, jugular venous oxygen saturation in the blood drained from a cephalad catheter if present, and total oxygen uptake across the oxygenator assuming no initial pulmonary contribution to gas exchange. These measures are helpful but not specific in assessing adequate oxygenation. Trends and acute changes can be more beneficial than absolute values, and must also be evaluated in the context of patient physical examination and acid-base balance. Ventilator settings are reduced for lung rest. This typically includes a low rate, tidal volume (and peak inspiratory pressure [PIP]), and inspired oxygen concentration, while maintaining a longer inspiratory time and adequate peak end expiratory pressure (PEEP) to prevent complete expiratory collapse.

Most of the details of patient management are not different for VV ECMO vs. VA ECMO patients. Care of the skin, careful monitoring for the development of decubitus breakdown (especially over the occipital ridge and the sacral prominence), oral hygiene, perineal cleansing, and other conventional nursing care is practiced. Increasing efforts to minimize sedation in order to decrease drug accumulation and allow more precise monitoring of neurologic status are being practiced. Neuromuscular block is also increasingly avoided or, if used, a daily break is employed. Physical examination may be augmented by cranial ultrasonography as needed in neonates.

Nutritional support of the neonate on VV ECMO has typically been provided almost exclusively using total parenteral nutrition. However, recent experience suggests that enteral nutrition can be safely provided on neonatal VV ECMO.[54] In the pediatric and adult ECMO patient, where concerns for bowel ischemia are diminished, experience also favors use of continuous enteral feeds to provide full nutritional support. Enteral nutrition in children on both VV and VA support has been shown to be well tolerated and to provide sufficient caloric intake in a cost-effective manner.[55] Similar tolerance of enteral feeding has been reported in adult VV ECMO patients as well.[56]

For a patient who is not at increased risk of bleeding, typical parameters include the maintenance of a platelet count >100,000/mm^3, prothrombin time in the normal range for the given age, fibrinogen concentration >100 mg/dl, and the activated coagulation time (ACT, using the Hemochron system) at 200-220 seconds. In patients who are at a higher risk of bleeding complications, parameters are adjusted to maintain fibrinogen concentration >150 mg/dl and ACT in the range of 180-200 seconds.

Fluid management on ECMO

Volume overload is frequently encountered in patients requiring either VA or VV support. The deterioration in renal function observed with non-pulsatile flow during VA ECMO has led to the recommendation of the routine use of hemofiltration. Despite preservation of pulsatile flow, VV ECMO has been associated with a similar decline in renal function in neonates.[57] During the first 48 hours of VV ECMO, urine output is often less than 1cc/kg/hr even in patients with normal blood pressure and serum albumin, and with a significantly positive fluid balance. After 96 hours of ECMO, renal func-

tion usually returns to normal. The cause of this decline in renal function remains unclear, but could be a result of circuit stimulation of vasoactive substances that reduce renal blood flow. Early institution of continuous hemofiltration can be helpful in alleviating volume overload and managing fluids on ECMO while avoiding high doses of diuretics. The volume status must be monitored carefully with this technique because of the possibility that significant intravascular depletion could affect the ability to maintain desired VV pump flow.

Discontinuation of ECMO

VV ECMO offers an additional advantage over VA ECMO; a patient can have a "trial off" VV ECMO by discontinuing oxygen to the membrane oxygenator without actually decannulating the patient. Discontinuing oxygen to a VA ECMO circuit simply produces a large shunt and does not allow accurate assessment. In one approach to trial off ECMO, VV pump flow is decreased progressively as the oxygenation improves generally to a minimum of 40 ml/kg/min (minimum total flow of 200 cc/min) as tolerated. An alternative approach to discontinuing VV support involves weaning membrane oxygenator FiO_2 rather than pump flow. However, post-membrane oxygenation is not significantly diminished by this technique even with minimal fractions due to the high oxygenator efficiency. An "oxygen challenge" can be performed to determine native pulmonary contribution by simply increasing the patient's ventilator oxygen fraction to 1.0 and evaluating arterial dissolved oxygen tension (a PaO_2 >100 is considered adequate). If the ECMO patient responds to increased ventilator FiO_2 with an adequate increase in PaO_2 and is stable at minimal pump flow with good gas exchange, ventilator support is increased to acceptable and expected post-ECMO settings and an arterial blood gas obtained. If this first arterial blood gas is acceptable, one can turn off the gas flow to the membrane oxygenator and "cap" (connect the gas inlet and outlet ports with rubber tubing) the gas inlet and outlet ports. Blood exiting the "capped" oxygenator can remain well oxygenated for 10-20 minutes, and a repeated blood gas determination should be delayed until post-oxygenator circuit blood is the same color as venous drainage blood. The patient can then be decannulated if blood gas values, over a period of 1-2 hours, show acceptable gas exchange on reasonable ventilator settings.

Pulmonary vascular tone may also need to be assessed in neonates prior to decannulation. This is particularly important in neonates who had severe pulmonary hypertension before initiation of ECMO and in neonates with CDH. In patients with echocardiographic evidence of persistent pulmonary hypertension, a delay in decannulation for at least 24 hours should be considered with reevaluation to minimize the possibility of rebound hypertension off ECMO.

Summary

VV ECMO support offers a means of extracorporeal support for patients with primary acute respiratory failure. Its use provides potential advantages and safety over VA support, including decreased cardiac effects and avoidance of carotid artery sacrifice. VV support can be tolerated even in patients requiring significant vasopressor support due to secondary cardiovascular insufficiency prior to cannulation. Understanding the concept of recirculation and its causes is critical to management of VV ECMO. Growing use of VV support in neonates and children, as noted in the ELSO Registry, supports its efficacy.

References

1. Kolobow T, Zapol W, Pierce J. High survival and minimal blood damage in lambs exposed to long term (1 week) veno-venous pumping with a polyurethane chamber roller pump with and without a membrane blood oxygenator. *Trans Am Soc Artif Intern Organs* 1969; 15:172-177.

2. Chevalier JY, Durandy Y, Batisse A, Mathe JC, Costil J. Preliminary report: extracorporeal lung support for neonatal acute respiratory failure. *Lancet* 1990; 335:1364-1366.

3. Chevalier JY, Couprie C, Larroquet M, Renolleau S, Durandy Y, Costil J. Venovenous single lumen cannula extracorporeal lung support in neonates. A five year experience. *ASAIO J* 1993; 39:M654-658.

4. Gattinoni L, Kolobow T, Tomlinson T, et al. Low-frequency positive pressure ventilation with extracorporeal carbon dioxide removal (LFPPV-ECCO2R): an experimental study. *Anesth Analg* 1978; 57:470-477.

5. Kolobow T, Borelli M, Spatola R, Tsuno K, Prato P. Single catheter venous-venous membrane lung bypass in the treatment of experimental ARDS. *ASAIO Trans* 1987; 33:561-564.

6. Kolobow T. An update on adult extracorporeal membrane oxygenation- extracorporeal CO_2 removal. *ASAIO Trans* 1988; 34:1004-1005.

7. Kolobow T, Borelli M, Spatola R, Tsuno K, Prato P. Single catheter veno-venous membrane lung bypass in the treatment of experimental ARDS. *ASAIO Trans* 1988; 34:35-38.

8. Andrews AF, Nixon CA, Cilley RE, Roloff DW, Bartlett RH. One- to three-year outcome for 14 neonatal survivors of extracorporeal membrane oxygenation. *Pediatrics* 1986; 78:692-698.

9. Klein MD, Andrews AF, Wesley JR, et al. Venovenous perfusion in ECMO for newborn respiratory insufficiency. A clinical comparison with venoarterial perfusion. *Ann Surg* 1985; 201:520-526.

10. Zwischenberger JB, Toomasian JM, Drake K, Andrews AF, Kolobow T, Bartlett RH. Total respiratory support with single can-

nula venovenous ECMO: double lumen continuous flow vs. single lumen tidal flow. *ASAIO Trans* 1985; 31:610-615.

11. Andrews AF, Zwischenberger JB, Cilley RE, Drake KL. Venovenous extracorporeal membrane oxygenation (ECMO) using a double lumen cannula. *Artif Organs* 1987; 11:265-268.

12. Golej J, Winter P, Schoffman G, et al. Impact of extracorporeal membrane oxygenation modality on cytokine release during rescue from infant hypoxia. *Shock* 2003; 20:110-115.

13. Short BL, Walker LK, Gleason CA, Jones MD, Jr., Traystman RJ. Effect of extracorporeal membrane oxygenation on cerebral blood flow and cerebral oxygen metabolism in newborn sheep. *Pediatr Res* 1990; 28:50-53.

14. Fukuda S, Aoyama M, Yamada Y, et al. Comparison of venoarterial versus venovenous access in the cerebral circulation of newborns undergoing extracorporeal membrane oxygenation. *Pediatr Surg Int* 1999; 15:78-84.

15. Hunter CJ, Blood AB, Bishai JM, et al. Cerebral blood flow and oxygenation during venoarterial and venovenous extracorporeal membrane oxygenation in the newborn lamb. *Pediatr Crit Care Med* 2004; 5:475-481.

16. Strieper MJ, Sharma S, Dooley KJ, Cornish JD, Clark RH. Effects of venovenous extracorporeal membrane oxygenation on cardiac performance as determined by echocardiographic measurements. *J Pediatr* 1993; 122:950-955.

17. Martin GR, Chauvin L, Short BL. Effects of hydralazine on cardiac performance in infants receiving extracorporeal membrane oxygenation. *J Pediatr* 1991; 118:944-948.

18. Martin GR, Short BL, Abbott C, O'Brien AM. Cardiac stun in infants undergoing extracorporeal membrane oxygenation. *J Thorac Cardiovasc Surg* 1991; 101:607-611.

19. Ingyinn M, Rais-Bahrami K, Evangelista R, et al. Comparison of the effect of venovenous versus venoarterial extracorporeal membrane oxygenation on renal blood flow in newborn lambs. *Perfusion* 2005; 19:163-170.

20. Andrews AF, Klein MD, Toomasian RI, Roloff D, Bartlett RH. Venovenous extracorporeal membrane oxygenation in neonates with respiratory failure. *J Pediatr Surg* 1983; 18:339-346.

21. Cornish JD, Heiss KF, Clark RH, Strieper MJ, Boecler B, Kesser K. Efficacy of venovenous extracorporeal membrane oxygenation for neonates with respiratory and circulatory compromise. *J Pediatr* 1993; 122:105-109.

22. Anderson HL, Snedecor SM, Otsu T, Bartlett RH. Multicenter comparison of conventional venoarterial access versus venovenous double-lumen catheter access in newborn infants undergoing extracorporeal membrane oxygenation. *J Pediatr Surg* 1993; 28:530-535.

23. Osiovich HC, Peliowski A, Ainsworth W, Etches PC. The Edmonton experience with venovenous extracorporeal membrane oxygenation. *J Pediatr Surg* 1998; 3:1749-1752.

24. Roy BJ, Rycus P, Conrad SA, Clark RH. The changing demographics of neonatal extracorporeal membrane oxygenation patients reported to the ELSO Registry. *Pediatrics* 2000; 106:1334-2338.

25. Heiss KF, Clark RH, Cornish JD, et al. Preferential use of venovenous extracorporeal membrane oxygenation for congenital diaphragmatic hernia. *Pediatr Surg* 1995; 30:416-419.

26. Kugleman A, Gangitano E, Pincros J, Tantivit P, Taschuk R, Durand M. Venovenous versus venoarterial extracorporeal membrane oxygenation in congenital diaphragmatic hernia. *J Pediatr Surg* 2003; 38:1131-1136.

27. Dimmitt RA, Moss LR, Rhine WD, Benitz WE, Henry MC, Vanmeurs KP. Venoarterial versus venovenous extracorporeal membrane oxygenation in congenital diaphragmatic hernia: the

Extracorporeal Life Support Organization Registry, 1990-1999. *J Pediatr Surg* 2001; 36:1199-1204.

28. Hines MH, Hansell DR. Elective extracorporeal support for complex tracheal reconstruction in neonates. *Ann Thorac Surg* 2003; 76:175-178.

29. Reickert CA, Schreiner RJ, Bartlett RH, Hirschl RB. Percutaneous access for venovenous extracorporeal life support in neonates. *J Pediatr Surg,* 1998; 33:365-369.

30. Rais-Bahrami K, Walton DM, Sell JE, Rivera O, Mikesell GT, Short BL. Improved oxygenation with reduced recirculation during venovenous ECMO: comparison of two catheters. *Perfusion* 2002; 17:415-419.

31. Kato J, Nagaya M, Norihiro N, Tanaka S. Venovenous extracorporeal membrane oxygenation in newborn infants using the umbilical vein as a reinfusion route. *J Pediatr Surg* 1998; 33:1446-1448.

32. Extracorporeal Life Support Registry, University of Michigan, July 2004.

33. Zwischenberger JB, Nguyen TT, Upp JR, Jr., et al. Complications of neonatal extracorporeal membrane oxygenation. Collective experience from the Extracorporeal Life Support Organization. *J Thorac Cardiovasc Surg* 1994; 107:838-849.

34. Gauger PG, Hirschl RB, Delosh TN, Dechert RE, Tracy T, Bartlett RH. A matched pairs analysis of venoarterial and venovenous extracorporeal life support in neonatal respiratory failure. *ASAIO J* 1995; 41:M573-M579.

35. Adolf V, Heaton J, Steiner R, et al. Extracorporeal membrane oxygenation for nonneonatal respiratory failure. *J Pediatr Surg* 1991; 26:326-330.

36. Swaniker F, Kolla S, Moler F, et al. Extracorporeal life support outcome for 128 pediatric patients with respiratory failure. *J Pediatr Surg* 2000; 35:197-202.

37. Pettignano R, Fortenberry JD, Heard ML, et al. Primary use of the venovenous approach for extracorporeal membrane oxygenation in pediatric acute respiratory failure. *Pediatr Crit Care Med* 2003; 4:291-298.

38. Dalton H. Venovenous extracorporeal membrane oxygenation: an underutilized technique? *Pediatr Crit Care Med* 2003; 4:385-386.

39. Fortenberry JD, Meier AH, Pettignano R, Heard M, Chambliss CR, Wulkan M. Extracorporeal life support for posttraumatic acute respiratory distress syndrome at a children's medical center. *J Pediatr Surg* 2003; 38:1221-1226.

40. Kolovos NS, Schuerer DJ, Moler FW, et al. Extracorporal life support for pulmonary hemorrhage in children: a case series. *Crit Care Med* 2002; 30:577-580.

41. Zahraa JN, Moler FW, Annich GM, Maxvold NJ, Bartlett RH, Custer JR. Venovenous versus venoarterial extracorporeal life support for pediatric acute respiratory failure: are there differences in survival and acute complications? *Crit Care Med* 2000; 28:521-523.

42. Bartlett RH, Roloff DW, Custer JR, Younger JG, Hirschl RB. Extracorporeal life support: The University of Michigan experience. *JAMA* 2000; 283:904-908.

43. Zapol WM, Snider MT, Hill JD, et al. Extracorporeal membrane oxygenation in severe acute respiratory failure: a randomized prospective study. *JAMA* 1979; 242:2193-2196.

44. Morris AH, Wallace CJ, Menlove RL, et al. Randomized clinical trial of pressure-controlled inverse ratio ventilation

and extracorporeal CO2 removal for adult respiratory distress syndrome. *Am J Respir Crit Care Med* 1994; 149:295-305.

45. Gattinoni L, Pesenti A, Mascheroni D, et al. Low frequency positive pressure ventilation with extracorporeal CO_2 removal in severe acute respiratory failure. *JAMA* 1986; 256:881-886.

46. Linden V, Palmer K, Reinhard J, et al. High survival in adult patients with acute respiratory distress syndrome treated by extracorporeal membrane oxygenation, minimal sedation, and pressure supported ventilation. *Intensive Care Med* 2000; 26:1630-1637.

47. Hemmila M, Rowe S, Boules T, et al. Extracorporeal life support for severe acute respiratory distress syndrome in adults. *Ann Surg* 2004; 240:595-607.

48. Roberts N, Westrope C, Pooboni SK, et al. Venovenous extracorporeal membrane oxygenation for respiratory failure in inotrope dependent neonates. *ASAIO J* 2003; 49:568-571.

49. Ichiba S, Peek GJ, Sosnowski AW, Brennan KJ, Firmin RK. Modifying a venovenous extracorporeal membrane oxygenation circuit to reduce recirculation. Ann Thorac Surg 2000; 69:298-299.

50. Skarsgard ED, Salt DR, Lee SK. Venovenous extracorporeal membrane oxygenation in neonatal respiratory failure: does routine, cephalad jugular drainage improve outcome? *J Pediatr Surg* 2004; 39:672-676.

51. Pettignano R, Labuz M, GauthierTW, Huchkaby J, Clark RH. The use of cephalad cannulae to monitor jugular venous oxygen content during extracorporeal membrane oxygenation. *Crit Care* 1997; 1:95-99.

52. Meliones JN, Moler FW, Custer JR, Dekeon MK, Chapman RA, Bartlett RH. Normalization of priming solution ionized calcium concentration improves hemodynamic stability of neonates receiving venovenous ECMO. *ASAIO J* 1995; 41:884-888.

53. Rich PB, Awad SS, Crotti S, Hirschl RB, Bartlett RH, Schreiner RJ. A prospective comparison of atrio-femoral and femoro-atrial flow in adult venovenous extracorporeal life support. *J Thorac Cardiovasc Surg* 1998; 116:628-632.

54. Hanekamp M, Spoel M, Sharman-Koendjbiharie I, Peters JW, Albers MJ, Tibboel D. Routine enteral nutrition in neonates on extracorporeal membrane oxygenation. *Ped Crit Care Med* 2005; 6:275-279.

55. Pettignano R, Heard M, Davis R, Labuz M, Hart M. Total enteral nutrition versus total parenteral nutrition during pediatric extracorporeal membrane oxygenation. *Crit Care Med* 1998; 26:358-363

56. Scott LK, Boudreaux K, Thaljeh F, Grier LR, Conrad SA. Early enteral feedings in adults receiving venovenous extracorporeal membrane oxygenation. *J Parenteral Enteral Nutr* 2004; 28:295-300.

57. Roy BJ, Cornish JD, Clark RH. Venovenous extracorporeal membrane oxygenation affects renal function. *Pediatrics* 1995; 95:573-578.

6

ECLS Equipment and Devices

Douglas R. Hansell, B.S., R.R.T.

Introduction

The equipment used for ECLS is in large part borrowed from the OR. Heart-lung bypass pumps and devices have been modified to meet the needs of ECLS. A key component of the ECLS system is the oxygenator. The development and evolution of ECLS are discussed elsewhere in this text. Early efforts using bubble oxygenators revealed sequelae associated with hemolysis and platelet consumption. Theodore Kolobow developed a silicone membrane gas exchange device in 1963 as a way to decrease these sequelae. This "membrane oxygenator" remains in use more than 40 years later as the predominant gas exchange device for prolonged ECLS. However, many centers in the U.S. and abroad are using hollow fiber gas exchange devices in an effort to further reduce blood/surface interaction and resistance, again in an effort to improve patient outcomes. Heparin-bonded circuits, new gas exchange devices, sophisticated computer controlled and servo-regulated pump systems are all a part of the ongoing efforts to provide safer care and to improve patient outcome.

ECMO physics

ECMO systems move blood through tubing, provide gas exchange through an artificial lung, and warm the blood back to body temperature before returning the blood to the patient. The laws of physics govern all these processes.

Poiseuille's Law, which governs the movement of gas or fluid through a tube, states that, at a constant driving pressure, flow will vary directly with the pressure and the fourth power of the radius of the tube, and inversely with the length of the tube and the viscosity. Therefore, the smaller the diameter, and the longer the tube the greater the pressure required to move a given volume.

In nature, almost everything moves along a gradient. The greater the gradient, the more rapid the movement. If you put a drop of dye in a beaker of water, the molecules of dye will disperse until the concentration is constant. The more concentrated the dye, the more rapidly it will disperse. This principle guides the application of the countercurrent exchange which is used to maximize the gradient whenever possible. In the gas exchange device, sweep gas flows in a direction opposite to the blood flow. The PO_2 of the gas entering the gas exchange device will be at its greatest (approximately 760 mm Hg) at the point the blood exiting the device is at its highest (approximately 550 mm Hg). As oxygen is extracted from the sweep gas during the transit through the device the diffusion gradient is maintained as the blood entering the gas exchange device (with a PO_2

of approximately 50 mm Hg) is matched with a gas with a PO_2 of approximately 300 mm Hg. This process is mirrored with CO_2 in the gas exchange device.

ECMO circuitry

ECMO systems are designed to provide temporary cardiac and pulmonary support to patients that are incapable of maintaining adequate tissue oxygen delivery. This is done by pumping the blood, delivering oxygen, and removing CO_2.

The ECMO circuit is made from PVC tubing. Tubing sizes range from ¼-inch inside diameter for the neonatal patient to ⅜-inch or ½-inch for pediatric and adult patients. Each ECMO center designs a circuit that best meets the needs of their institution (Figures 1 & 2). Monitoring probes and infusion ports are placed in a variety of positions. There are a few simple rules when designing an ECMO circuit.

First the shorter the circuit length, the better. Resistance within a tube increases with length. Also, as the ECMO circuit length increases, the total foreign surface area in which the blood comes in contact also increases, the

priming volume and potential for heat loss also increases. The tubing should be just long enough to reach from pump to patient and allow for safe patient transport when necessary. Secondly, the fewer connectors, the better. Every connector in the circuit introduces the potential for turbulent flow. These areas of turbulent flow are where clots form. Additionally, the manufacturer should complete every connection whenever possible. When the circuit manufacturer makes the connection, it is chemically sealed, decreasing the likelihood of a connector coming apart under high-pressure conditions.

Surface coatings

The body recognizes the circuit, as well as the other components that make up the delivery system, as a foreign substance. The blood reacts to contact with this surface by activating platelets, complements, and other inflammatory mediators (Chapter 4).[1,2] One of the techniques used to reduce this response is to add albumin to the prime; this lays down a protein coating on the internal surfaces of the circuit and reduces the inflammatory response.

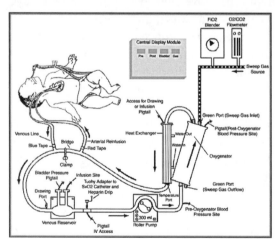

Figure 1. ECMO circuit designed for a membrane gas exchange device and roller pump. Courtesy, Children's Hospitals & Clinics, Minneapolis, MN.

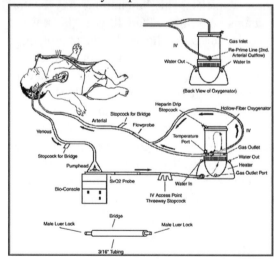

Figure 2. EMCO circuit configured for a hollow fiber gas exchange device and centrifugal pump. Courtesy, Children's Hospitals & Clinics, Minneapolis, MN.

Activation of the complement system and the subsequent release of inflammatory mediators contribute to the development of acute respiratory distress syndrome (ARDS) and other organ dysfunction. Consequently, several manufacturers have developed surface bonding materials designed to minimize complement, platelet, and inflammatory mediator activation. These surfaces are also designed to be less thrombogenic.

While there are several coatings commercially available the one most commonly used is the Carmeda BioActive Surface (CBAS, Carmeda; Stockholm, Sweden). Carmeda covalently bonds heparin molecules to the plastic while antithrombin binding site remains exposed to the blood.[3] When using a centrifugal pump system and a hollow fiber gas exchange device, the entire circuit can be coated from venous to arterial cannula (i.e., "tip to tip"). While some systemic heparinization is still required, some centers delay the initiation of the heparin infusion for up to 12 hours when using Carmeda circuits. When initiated, the heparin doses are lower. Also, a number of investigators have documented reduced activation of platelets and the complement system.[4-7] While this is an attractive concept, there are no convincing studies that show a reduction in morbidity or mortality in the ECMO population. In a study by Svenmarker et al., the use of heparin-coated circuits reduced the mean length of hospital stay from 7.8 ±2.5 to 7.3 ±1.8 days (P=0.040) and post-operative ventilation time from 9.7 ±9.2 to 8.2 ±8.5 hours (P=0.018), blood loss at 8 hours post-surgery from 676 ±385 to 540 ±245 ml (P=0.001), proportion of patients exposed to allogenous blood transfusions 39.2 vs. 23.9% (P=0.001), post-operative coagulation disturbances 4.4 vs. 0.4% (P=0.006), neurological deviations 9.4 vs. 3.9% (P=0.021), and atrial fibrillation 26.4 vs. 18.0% (P=0.041). No effects were found with respect to perioperative platelet count, post-operative fever, and 5-year survival.[8]

ECMO cannulas

The ECMO cannula is one of the major limiting factors in providing optimal ECMO flow. Since resistance to flow increases as the internal diameter of the tube decreases, as large a cannula as possible is placed to ensure adequate flows. Typically, pump flows are maintained at 60-120 ml/kg/min, and a cannula that is too small can adversely affect the ability to provide adequate support. As the flow through the arterial cannula is driven actively by the ECMO pump, the resistance is less critical than on the venous side. However, it remains advantageous to create as little resistance as possible to reduce the potential for hemolysis, circuit rupture, and to reduce the ECMO system afterload (the latter is especially important when using centrifugal pumps).

The dual lumen venovenous (VV) cannula (Figure 3) was developed to provide a simple means of providing VV support. This cannula, inserted via the right internal jugular vein, is advanced to the right atrium (RA) (Figure 4) to ensure effective delivery of oxygenated blood to the RA. Currently available in sizes up to 18F, larger VV cannulas are being developed.

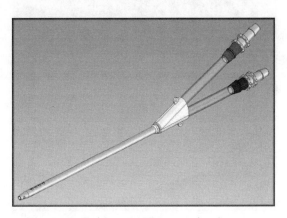

Figure 3. OriGen DLVV cannula. Courtesy, Origen Biomedical.

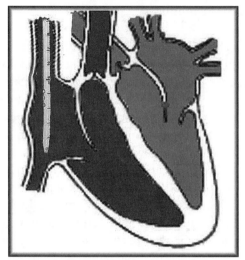

Figure 4. Correct positioning of the DLVV cannula. Courtesy, OriGen Biomedical.

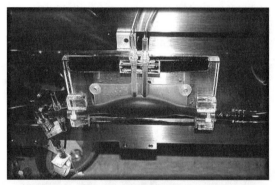

Figure 5. The 30 ml bladder. Courtesy, The author.

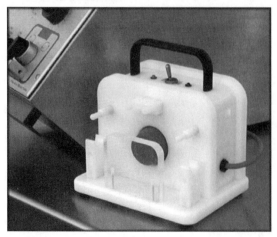

Figure 6. The bladder controller. Courtesy, OriGen Biomedical.

The cannula size, measured in French units (F), describes the external diameter; the wall thickness and length of the cannulas must also be considered. While cannulas manufactured by different companies may be the same size (e.g., 10F) the inside diameter may be quite different. The M number, which describes flow-pressure characteristics based upon length, internal diameter, and side hole placement, provides a measure of resistance through various sizes of cannulas (Table 1).[9]

Bladder holder/pump controller

The bladder (Figure 5) serves as a reservoir from which the ECMO pump draws blood. This reservoir also keeps negative pressure from pulling the vessel wall into the cannula and reduces the likelihood of trauma to the vena cava. A potential problem with the bladder, especially at low pump flows, is clots that may form at the apex and base of the bladder due to the disruption of laminar flow. If venous return is inadequate, the pump can exert enough negative pressure on the blood to cause cavitation. Cavitation is the action of air being pulled out of solution. To reduce or stop pump flow in the event venous return is insufficient, a servo-regulation mechanism consisting of either a pressure sensitive switch or a pressure monitoring system, is used. This is not necessary with a centrifugal pump.

The bladder holder may serve as part of the pump controller, as with the OriGen bladder controller ("Bladder Box") (OriGen Biomedical, Austin, TX), or it may be a holder that merely serves as a support for the bladder. Most centers mount the holder as low on the pump console as possible to maximize gravity drainage, and servo-regulation occurs via a pressure-monitoring device. These servo-regulation mechanisms are built in to the latest generation of perfusion systems available from a variety of manufacturers (e.g., Stockert and Jostra). Figure 6

The Bladder Box (Figure 6) serves as a servo-regulation and safety device and is manufactured by OriGen. This device consists of two components: a holder and controller box. The bladder is placed in the holder, which has a pressure sensitive switch installed along the back wall. A cable connects this switch to the controller. If blood flowing out of the bladder exceeds the flow into the bladder, the bladder will collapse. As the bladder collapses, the pres-sure on the switch is released and the controller, which is connected to the roller pump, will sound an alarm and stop the pump. Once the bladder pressure increases and compresses the switch, pump resumes flow.

The later generation perfusion systems have pressure modules available that monitor circuit pressures via pressure transducers and regulate the roller pump. These pump controllers elimi-nate the need for bladder box servo-regulation.

Table 1. M Numbers for various ECLS cannulas.

Manufacturer	Length (cm)	Size (F)	M Number
Arterial cannulas			
Bio-Medicus	25	8	4.40
Bio-Medicus	25	10	4.00
Bio-Medicus	25	12	3.55
Bio-Medicus	25	14	3.25
Bio-Medicus	37	17	3.05
Bio-Medicus	37	19	2.80
Bio-Medicus	37	21	2.60
DLP	17	17	2.95
DLP	17	21	2.60
Elecath	8	8	4.55
Elecath	12	10	4.10
Elecath	12	12	3.85
Elecath	12	14	3.60
Elecath	12	16	3.40
Venous cannulas			
Bio-Medicus	25	8	4.35
Bio-Medicus	25	10	3.90
Bio-Medicus	25	12	3.55
Bio-Medicus	25	14	3.35
Bio-Medicus	50	17	3.40
Bio-Medicus	50	19	3.15
Bio-Medicus	50	21	2.90
Bio-Medicus	50	29	2.30
DLP	52	21	3.05
Elecath	12	8	4.45
Elecath	12	10	3.90
Elecath	12	12	3.80
Elecath	12	14	3.70
Elecath	12	16	3.30
Double lumen cannulas			
OriGen	12	Drainage	4.66
		Infusion	3.85
OriGen	15	Drainage	4.30
		Infusion	3.53
OriGen	18	Drainage	4.09
		Infusion	3.42

The pressure control module is connected to the bladder, and serves as a pressure regulator and limits flow. A minimum bladder pressure limit is set, and as the bladder pressure falls to the limit, the module alarms and the pump either slows if there is partial loss of venous return or stops if there is complete loss of venous return.

Both systems are used in centers worldwide, and selection of the system is often a matter of operator preference and institutional finances. While both systems provide for safer operation of the roller pump, the OriGen bladder controller merely serves as an on/off switch and causes abrupt changes in flow. The phenomenon known as "bladder chatter" is the sound of the pressure switch clicking off and on. The pressure control module system reduces flow rather than stopping the pump if there is reduced venous return. Both provide monitoring and regulation. The newer pressure-controlled perfusion systems are so effective at regulating flow that a number of centers have opted to eliminate the bladder.

Another device used to regulate venous flow is the Better-Bladder (Circulatory Technology Inc., Oyster Bay, NY). The Better-Bladder is a section of standard tubing with a thin-walled, sausage-shaped balloon, sealed within a clear rigid housing. The pressure of the blood flowing through the tubing is transmitted across the balloon to the chamber and monitored, via a pressure port, by a transducer. Mounted perpendicular to the floor, the Better-Bladder does not have the clotting issues associated with conventional bladder systems. Additionally, it may be mounted anywhere on the venous limb of the circuit, as the pressure drop is relative to the pressure limits set on the servo-regulating device.[10]

Pumps

The heart of the ECMO system is the blood pump. The pump pulls the blood either from a venous reservoir or directly from the patient, and then pushes it through the oxygenator back to the patient. Two types of pumps are used: the vortex or centrifugal pump, and the occlusive or roller pump.

Vortex or centrifugal pump

The centrifugal pump consists of a polycarbonate cone built around several smaller diameter cones (Figure 7). These cones are attached to a magnetic disc that, when attached to a controller, spins at an adjustable rate. As the disc spins it creates a constrained vortex that creates a negative pressure in the pump head. This pulls the blood into the pump and directs it out at the top of the vortex, similar to the way a tornado sucks up debris and blows it out the top.

Because the cones impart energy to the blood flowing into the pump head, flow provided is dependent upon pump preload (blood volume available from patient), pump afterload (restriction to the outflow to patient), the size of the biohead, and the pump speed. Therefore, flow may be variable at a set RPM and measuring actual flow with a flow probe, electromagnetic or Doppler, is important.

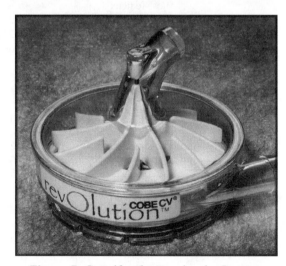

Figure 7. Centrifugal pump head. Courtesy, Cobe Cardiovascular.

Advantages of the centrifugal pump

The centrifugal pump has superior blood handling characteristics compared with the roller pump due to the reduced energy required to move a volume of blood. At higher liter flows (i.e., higher rpm) less mechanical energy is required than with the roller pump. Additionally, the pump does not usually exert excessive negative pressure on the blood which can cause cavitation, nor can it generate excessive positive pressure in the system. However, sudden loss of inflow at a high rpm can lead to red blood cell damage. Additionally, the centrifugal pump is able to trap small amounts of air in the constrained vortex of blood within the pump head.

Disadvantages of the centrifugal pump

While the centrifugal pump's inability to exert excessive negative pressure or generate excessive positive pressure in the system enhances its safety, those limitations are a disadvantage when one wishes to maintain a set flow. Anything that increases resistance to the outflow of the pump will reduce flow to the patient. A rise in patient systemic vascular resistance (SVR) or blood pressure, a kink in the arterial cannulas, or compressing the chest cavity as you roll the patient may cause a profound reduction in the pump output. Likewise, a drop in blood pressure or SVR, hypovolemia, or kinking of the venous return line will also cause a reduction in pump output. Moreover, due to the higher rpm required and the heat generated by the pump, indices of hemolysis have been reported to be significantly higher at low flows (0.3 lpm) with centrifugal pumps than roller pumps.[11]

Occlusive or roller pump

The roller pump works by compressing the tubing, thereby pushing the blood through the raceway (Figure 8). While the roller moves the blood along with positive displacement, blood from the venous reservoir is pulled into the tubing by negative pressure. A DC motor powers the central axis either directly or with a belt drive system. Belts may require adjusting or replacement and a direct drive system may be more susceptible to failure in the event of a fluid spill in the raceway housing. Roller pumps, like centrifugal pumps, may be operated manually in case of a power failure.

The output of the roller pump is dependent upon the size of the raceway tubing, the occlusion pressure of the rollers, pump rpm, and the supply of blood available. With roller pumps, one must adjust the size of the tubing to provide adequate pump output. Larger diameter tubing reduces rpm and wear on the tubing. To that end, differing raceway diameters are used for neonatal, pediatric, and adult patients. For neonates and small pediatric patients weighing <14 kg, a ¼-inch interior diameter tubing is used. This tubing will deliver approximately 9.7 ml/rpm (using a 6-inch roller head). Patients weighing 15-30 kg require a ⅜-inch interior diameter

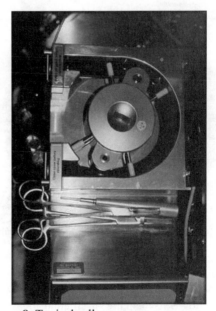

Figure 8. Typical roller pump.

tubing, delivering ~22 ml/rpm. Patients weighing >30 kg require a ½-inch interior diameter tubing, delivering approximately 39 ml/rpm. The lpm indicator must be set appropriately for the diameter of the tubing used. The display on the pump is based on the rpm of the roller. This may be set automatically by selecting the tubing size in a menu on the roller head in the latest generation of roller systems, or by setting manually in older systems.

The roller pump applies direct and repeated pressure on the tubing. This action can occur as frequently as 120 or more times per minute for periods of ≥300 hours in larger patients. Therefore, the tubing used must be resistant to the creasing and possible erosion. In "Super Tygon" tubing, (Saint-Gobain Performance Plastics Corporation, Valley Forge, PA) the plasticizers are laid down in longer chains than standard tubing, providing this durability. Occlusion must be set appropriately to ensure that the proper volume is moving through the tubing with each revolution. The methods for setting occlusion vary.

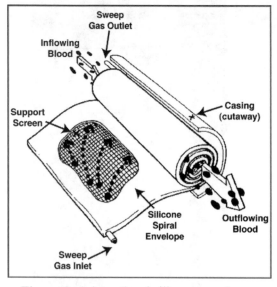

Figure 9. Schematic of silicone membrane oxygenator.

Advantages of the roller pump

The main advantage of the roller pump is the constant flow provided by volume displacement. Another advantage is reduced hemolysis at the low flows used in neonates.

Disadvantages of the roller pump

The roller pump will continue to rotate independent of the amount of blood available in the venous reservoir or the pressure in the circuit. The use of servo-regulation mechanisms to regulate pump flow has overcome this shortcoming for circuit volumes or pressures that reach unsafe levels.

Gas exchange devices

Silicone membrane oxygenator

Currently Medtronic manufactures the only oxygenator approved for long-term use in the U.S. The oxygenator is a membrane lung made of a thin silicone rubber sheath with a plastic screen spacer inside (Figure 9). This silicone sheet is wound around a polycarbonate core. Encased in a silicone rubber sleeve, the configuration allows blood to pass on one side of the membrane and sweep gas to flow in the opposite direction on the other side. This maximizes gas exchange across the membrane. The membrane is very efficient. Several methods are used to regulate CO_2. CO_2 may be added either as a carbogen mixture or as pure CO_2, to the sweep gas to raise the circuit PCO_2 to normal physiologic levels (35-45 torr), or may be regulated by altering the minute ventilation or sweep flow across the lung. With the addition of CO_2, continuous monitoring of post-oxygenator blood gases is recommended to ensure that the pH and PCO_2 are in target range. This oxygenator is available in sizes ranging from 0.4 m² to 4.5 m². The size is selected based on the patient size and the total anticipated blood flow requirements (Tables 2 and 3). The maximal blood flow is equal to 1.5 times the oxygenator membrane surface area, while the maximal sweep gas flow is limited to 3 times the oxygenator membrane surface area. For example, a 0.8 m² oxygenator has a maximum rated blood flow of 1.2 lpm, and a maximum rated sweep gas flow of 2.4 lpm. Two primary indicators of membrane lung function are the pre- to post-membrane pressure difference, or trans-membrane pressure, and the ability to exchange gas.

The pressure generated by flow across the oxygenator gives important information about the patient, circuit, and oxygenator function; therefore, it is important that the specialist monitors both pre- and post-membrane pressures. A rise in both pre- and post-oxygenator pressure signifies an increase in resistance after the oxygenator. Potential causes include arterial cannula kink or patient hypertension/hypervolemia. A drop in both pressures signifies a loss of pump flow, possibly due to loss of pump occlusion or hypotension/hypovolemia. An increase in the difference between the pre- and post-membrane (transmembrane) pressures will signify an increase in the resistance inside the oxygenator. The most likely cause is clot formation. All oxygenators have maximal blood phase and transmembrane pressure limitations.

Hollow fiber oxygenators

The use of hollow fiber oxygenators (HFOs) for long-term support is gaining acceptance in the ECMO community. In the U.S. there are currently no HFOs approved for long-term use. In fact, the devices used in the U.S. are approved for less than 8 hours of continuous use. This is because the hollow fibers are actually microporous. That is, they are capillary tubes with tiny holes through which gas exchange takes place. This construction makes the devices susceptible to plasma leak and early failure.[12] This failure is reported to occur more rapidly when patients are receiving IV lipids.[13]

Despite this, a growing number of ECMO centers have incorporated these devices into their ECMO systems. Experience has shown that the devices can function for 72 hours and longer. There are a number of advantages cited. The first rationale is the ease of priming. An experienced practitioner can prime and "de-

Table 2. Medtronic oxygenator specifications.

Model No.	0800	1500	2500	4500	MiniMax	Maxima
Type	SM	SM	SM	SM	HF	HF
Surface area (m²)	0.8	1.5	2.5	4.5	0.8	2.3
Priming volume (ml)	100	175	455	665	149	480
Max. gas flow (lpm)	2.4	4.5	7.5	13.5	na	na
Max. blood flow (lpm)	1.2	1.8	4.5	6.5	2.3	7.0
Max. patient weight (kg)	11	19	70	≥ 96	20	100
Blood port diameter (in.)	1/4	1/4	3/8	3/8	1/4	3/8

SM = silicone membrane, HF = hollow fiber.

Table 3. Guidelines for selecting oxygenator.

Membrane surface area (m²)	0.8	1.5	2.5	4.5
Max. blood flow (lpm)	0.9	1.4	4.0	6.0
Max. patient weight (kg)	9	14	<40	<60

Ensure that you do not exceed the specifications of the oxygenator; therefore, leave some room for increased patient requirements or reduced oxygenator function. For patients ≥60 kg consider parallel oxygenators.

bubble" the HFO in <5 minutes. Second, there is the advantage of bioactive coating. The HFO is available with coatings that reduce the incidence of clotting making the device especially appealing in the post-operative and trauma patient. Third, there is improved gas exchange with less surface area. The reduced surface area produces less platelet activation especially when combined with bioactive coatings. Finally, extremely low resistance is another advantage. The pressure drop across the silicone membrane is often between 100-150 mm Hg. The typical pressure drop across the hollow fiber devices is 10–20 mm Hg. Less resistance yields less disruption of red blood cells.

There are a number of hollow fiber gas exchange devices that combine the advantages of a solid membrane device with the hollow fiber device by using capillary tubes constructed of "membranes". One commonly used material is polymethylpentene. This material may be heparin-bonded and has superior burst characteristics (>1,500 mm Hg). The Medos HiLite 7000LT (MEDOS Medizintechnik AG, Stolberg, Germany) has a priming volume of 275 ml and is rated for blood flows of 7 lpm. Peek et al. have reported the satisfactory use of this device for adult ECMO.[14] It is unclear whether these devices will be available in the U.S.

Pathophysiology of membrane gas exchange devices

As is true for our patients' lungs, the membrane gas exchange device is subject to alterations in function brought on by edema, embolism, and atelectasis. These conditions alter the proximity of blood on one side of the membrane to the gas on the other side causing ventilation perfusion mismatch. Also, like the human lung, the devices are more efficient at exchanging CO_2 than oxygen.

Alterations on the gas side of the membrane may include collapse of the gas phase (atelectasis) or condensation (edema); this can

occur if the sweep gas flow rate is too low. In this case, the CO_2 level in the post-oxygenator blood gradually increases. Oxygen exchange does not drop until a profound loss of surface area occurs.

Alterations on the blood phase of the membrane primarily consist of embolic events. This leads to a high ratio of ventilation to perfusion (V/Q) and a drop in post-membrane PaO_2. CO_2 transfer will be unaffected until the available surface area lost is large. The other indication that significant emboli are present is a rise in the pre- to post-membrane pressure gradient.

ECMO heat exchanger/heater

Given the large surface area in which the blood is exposed to as it moves through the circuit, a great deal of heat is lost during extracorporeal circulation. While hypothermia is routinely used in the OR, normothermia is usually the goal in ECMO. All ECMO systems use a heat exchanger, either post oxygenator or integrated in the oxygenator. Medtronic and Gish manufacture the most commonly used heat exchangers. ECMO heat exchangers consist of stainless steel tubes enclosed in a clear, hollow polycarbonate core. The blood runs inside the stainless steel tubes and water warmed to 37-40°C flows outside the tubes, warming it. Stainless steel is used in ECMO applications due to the tendency of aluminum to corrode with long-term exposure to blood products. The heat exchanger also serves a secondary purpose. When placed after the oxygenator it serves as a bubble trap.

The ECMO heater must be able to warm the blood back to slightly higher than desired body temperature and should be limited to a maximum temperature of around 42°C to avoid blood hemolysis, and bubble formation. Additionally, it should provide water flow at low pressures, typically around 3-4 psi. This ensures that any leak in the heat exchanger will result in blood flowing into the water bath and not the reverse. Many heaters provide a microprocessor-controlled temperature sensor and regulation mechanisms. The operator may set the desired blood temperature, and the heater will warm the water bath accordingly. Like most applications in ECMO, the flow of warmed water through the heat exchanger runs countercurrent to the blood flow to maintain the widest gradient possible. This ensures optimal transfer of heat into the blood. Cincinnati Sub-Zero (Cincinnati, Ohio) manufactures heaters designed for ECMO applications across a range of patient sizes. From the heat exchanger, the blood returns to the patient.

Bridge

The final component of the circuit is a bridge between the arterial and venous limbs of the circuit. This bridge provides a bypass if the patient requires isolation from the circuit for any reason, allowing flow to continue through the circuit and reducing the risk of the circuit clotting. The bridge remains clamped unless needed. The specialist unclamps or "flashes the bridge" for brief periods each hour to ensure that the line remains patent. An innovative stopcock bridge is becoming more common in the ECMO community. This bridge is incorporated into the circuit using leur lock connectors instead of "Y" tubing connectors. The bridge remains flushed with heparinized solution and the stopcocks remain closed to the circuit. This configuration reduces the hazards associated with flashing the bridge (e.g., sudden changes in blood pressure, cerebral blood flow) while continuing to provide the safety benefits of a bridge.

Safety and monitoring devices

Additional equipment attached to the ECMO system consists of monitors and safety devices. Failure of any of the many components required for extracorporeal support could lead to a fatality. It is imperative that the systems are monitored, not only for adequate function, but for signs of failure as well. The most important monitoring device remains the ECMO specialist. Only through diligence, attention to detail, and constant monitoring of the ECMO system and patient can one reduce the risk of failure or respond quickly to the failures that are bound to occur with such a complex system. The devices described below are attached to the ECMO system. The patient monitoring devices (e.g., ECG, pulse oximeter) are also important in determining the effectiveness of our therapeutic intervention.

In-line blood gas and saturation monitors

Arterial and venous blood gas samples are frequently evaluated to monitor the effectiveness of cardiopulmonary support. The ability to continuously monitor pH, oxygen saturation, and PCO_2 on the venous and arterial side of the ECMO system provides valuable data to the clinician.

Most centers monitor the venous blood for oxygen saturation. In venoarterial (VA) ECMO this directly reflects the effectiveness of oxygen delivery, with the goal being an SvO_2 around 70-75%. Monitors use either a dual wavelength device or an indwelling catheter. The dual wavelength monitor is very similar to a pulse oximeter, using red and infrared wavelengths. These waves are transmitted across the blood path, and oxygen saturation is calculated based on the light absorbed in the blood. Alternatively, indwelling fiber-optic catheter can be used to measure venous saturation. Inserted into the circuit blood stream via a rotating hemostatic valve, the tip serves as a reflective spectrophotometer. Reflected light is measured at the optical module and converted to electrical signals that display the calculated percent saturation. Either device provides excellent monitoring capability and alarms for low and high saturations.

In CPB applications, continuous arterial and venous pH, blood gas, and oxygen saturation monitoring are becoming standard. A flow-through cell inserted in the circuit is commonly used containing a semipermeable membrane that allows gas and ions to pass out of the blood to a sensor. This sensor contains pH, oxygen, and CO_2 microsensors connected to a fiber optic light cable. The intensity of each signal returning to the sensor is proportional to the hydrogen ions, oxygen, and CO_2 present in the blood. Arterial bicarbonate and venous oxygen saturation are calculated and, along with pH, PCO_2, and PO_2, are displayed on the monitor. Alterations in pump flow, membrane oxygenator function, and patient status are reflected in the oxygen and CO_2 levels. Early signs of a failing oxygenator, disconnected sweep gas line, increased patient metabolic demands, or the need to suction the VV ECMO patient are readily reflected in the parameters displayed with this monitor.

Flow measurement devices

Transonic flow measurement devices provide accurate quantitation of pump flow. This is useful when shunts such as hemofiltration devices are placed in the ECMO system. Volume flow is measured by ultrasonic transit time. A flow tube is positioned between transducers that generate wide beams of ultrasound. The flowmeter derives an accurate measure of the ultrasound wave's travel time from one transducer to the other, resulting from the motion of the liquid. This transit time is a measure of flow. The Transonic HT109 (Transonic Systems, Ithaca, NY) uses a reusable, clip-on flow sensor and has alarms for high and low flow. It may be used as a bubble detector as well.

Bubble detectors

Bubble detectors are often used to detect and warn the operator that air has entered the ECMO system. This is a critical problem, especially in VA ECMO where air can enter into the arterial system and flow directly to the cerebral circulation. Bubble detectors use either ultrasound or infrared technology. Ultrasound transducers send a signal through the tubing to a receiver. The signal passing through fluid becomes the reference. Alterations in this signal are interpreted as air and an alarm sounds. Bubbles as small as 300-600 µl can trigger this alarm. It should be noted that a rapid infusion of a liquid of a different density (e.g., platelets) might also trigger this alarm. Infrared sensors use absorbed light as the reference. Bubbles passing through the fluid will alter the light absorbed and trigger the alarm. Air volumes as small as 500 µl are detectable with infrared technology.

ACT analyzers

Since blood that is in contact with an artificial surface will clot, heparin is infused to reduce the coagulability. To ensure that the clotting time is maintained within an acceptable range, a small sample of blood is withdrawn from the circuit hourly and an activated clotting time (ACT) is measured. Heparin or other anticoagulation therapy is adjusted based on the ACT results. The ACT is performed at the bedside using a variety of devices such as the Hemochron 801 (ITC, Edison, NJ) or ACT Plus (Medtronic, Inc. Minneapolis, MN). New devices on the market include the Hemochron Signature Plus. Some of the newer devices include the ability to record data, lock-out unauthorized users, and ensure compliance with Clinical Laboratory Improvement Amendments (CLIA) and/or the College of American Pathologists (CAP) regulations.

A recent phenomenon within ELSO centers is the use of an array of devices with different methods of measuring the ACT. The challenge that ECMO centers face is the determination of a standard ACT range. In the past, as most centers used similar devices, the ECMO community as a whole considered an ACT range of 180–220 seconds a reasonable standard. The varieties of devices now used have made it un-feasible to establish a widely accepted standard. A positive result of this problem is an increased awareness of the many factors that affect coagulation status. We are no longer monitoring the anticoagulation status of the patient; rather, we are monitoring the patient's coagulation state.

Conclusion

ECMO systems provide oxygen delivery and CO_2 removal for patients unable to sustain adequate gas exchange, or cardiac support for patients in cardiac failure. The devices utilized to provide this life-saving technology must achieve this as simply and safely as possible.

References

1. Plotz FB, vanOeveren W, Bartlett RH, Wildevuur CR. Blood activation during neonatal extracorporeal life support. *J Thorac Cardiovasc Surg* 1993; 105:823-832.
2. Westfall SH, Stephens C, Kesler K, Connors RH, Tracy TF, Jr., Weber TR. Complement activation during prolonged extracorporeal membrane oxygenation. *Surgery* 1991; 110:887-891.
3. Larm O, Larsson R, Olsson P. A new non-thrombogenic surface prepared by selective covalent binding of heparin via a modified reducing terminal residue. *Biomater Med Devices Artif Organs* 1992; 2-3:161-173.
4. Plotz FB, van Oeveren W, Hultquist KA, Miller C, Bartlett RH, Wildevuur CR. A heparin-coated circuit reduces complement activation and the release of leukocyte inflammatory mediators during extracorporeal circulation in a rabbit. *Artif Organs* 1992; 16:366-370.
5. Whittelsley GC, Kundu SK, Salley SO, Nowlen TT, Klein MD. Is heparin necessary for extracorporeal circulation? *ASAIO Trans* 1988; 34:823-826.
6. Toomasian JM, Hsu LC, Hirschl RB, Heiss KF, Hultquist KA, Bartlett RH. Evaluation of Duraflo II heparin coating in prolonged extracorporeal membrane oxygenation. *ASAIO Trans* 1988; 34:410-414.
7. Mollnes TE, Videm V, Gotze O, Harboe M, Oppermann M. Formation of C5a during cardiopulmonary bypass: inhibition by precoating with heparin. *Ann Thorac Surg* 1991; 52:92-97.
8. Svenmarker S, Haggmark S, Jansson E, et al. Use of heparin-bonded circuits in cardiopulmonary bypass improves clinical outcome. *Scand Cardiovasc J* 2002; 36:241-246.
9. Montoya JP, Merz SI, Bartlett RH. A standardized system for describing flow/pressure relationships in vascular access devices. *ASAIO Trans* 1991; 37:4-8.
10. Tamari Y, Lee-Sensiba K, King S, Hall MH. An improved bladder for pump control during ECMO procedures. *J Extra Corpor Technol* 1999; 31:84-90.
11. Tamari Y, Lee-Sensiba K, Leonard EF, Parnell V, Tortolani. The effects of pressure and flow on hemolysis caused by Bio-Medicus centrifugal pumps and roller pumps. Guidelines for choosing a blood pump. *J Thorac Cardiovasc Surg* 1993; 106:997-1007.
12. Palder SB, Shaheen KW, Whittlesey GC, Nowlen TT, Kundu SK, Klein MD. Prolonged extracorporeal membrane oxygenation in sheep with a hollow-fiber oxygenator and a centrifugal pump. *ASAIO Trans* 1988; 34:820-822.
13. Knoch M, Kollen B, Dietrich G, Muller E, Mottaghy K, Lennartz H. Progress in venovenous long-term bypass techniques for the treatment of ARDS. Controlled clinical trial with the heparin-coated bypass circuit. *Int J Artif Organs* 1992; 15:103-108.
14. Peek G, Killer H, Reeves R, Sosnowski AW, Firmin RK. Early experience with a polymethyl pentene oxygenator for adult extracorporeal life support. *ASAIO J* 2002 48:480-482.

7

Vascular Access for Extracorporeal Support

Thomas Pranikoff, M.D. and Michael H. Hines, M.D.

Introduction

The establishment and maintenance of adequate vascular access is essential for ECLS. Cannulation techniques vary depending on the type of support needed, patient age and size, and clinical situation. This chapter will review general principles and elaborate on some specific situations commonly encountered when obtaining vascular access.

Principles

Patient management prior to ECLS

Management of patients prior to ECLS can be quite challenging. The decision of what location to use to cannulate the patient (e.g., ICU, OR, ER) needs to be well thought out. Adequate monitoring and nursing care are essential. The ability to transport the patient safely with adequate ventilation and hemodynamic support should be considered. The required equipment, including cannulas, surgical instruments, and ECMO circuit and components, as well as OR and ECLS personnel, must be available.

The procedure should be explained to the family and consent obtained. Meanwhile, blood and platelets should be ordered from the blood bank. The patient should be anesthetized to facilitate safe cannulation, avoid anxiety and

discomfort, and reduce the likelihood of air embolus. Generally, a combination of narcotic (fentanyl) and paralytic (rocuronium) is used. After the vessels have been surgically exposed or a guidewire has been placed for percutaneous access, the patient is systemically heparinized (100 units/kg) and 3 minutes are allowed for adequate anticoagulation before the cannulas are placed into the vascular system.

Type of support

There are two principal modes of extracorporeal support: venovenous (VV) bypass, which provides respiratory support alone, and venoarterial (VA) bypass, which provides both cardiac and respiratory support. A comparison of VV and VA bypass is shown in Table 1.

VA bypass removes blood from the systemic venous circulation, usually from the right atrium via the right internal jugular vein, and returns the blood to the systemic arterial circulation in the aortic arch via the right common carotid artery. In VV bypass, blood is also drained from the venous circulation and returned to the venous circulation either through a single double lumen catheter in the right atrium via the jugular vein or by using two cannulas in the jugular and femoral veins. Most cases of respiratory failure can be managed with VV bypass if cardiac function is adequate. This may be difficult to determine when the patient is severely hypoxemic and on high pressure ventilation, as both conditions depress cardiac function and may increase the need for inotropic support. After ECLS is initiated and airway pressures are decreased, cardiac output increases and inotropic support can usually be weaned. VV bypass offers several advantages over VA bypass: avoiding arterial cannulation eliminates the potential for arterial embolization and ischemia, arterial ligation or repair is unnecessary, blood flow is preserved and oxygenation of pulmonary circulation is improved, and there are no hemodynamic effects; in particular, there is no increase in afterload.

Cannula considerations

During ECLS, it is important to use a drainage (venous) cannula with the largest lumen and shortest length possible, since venous drainage is only achieved by gravity siphon. In this system, if preload is adequate, the limiting factor in determining maximum flow is cannula resistance, which is directly proportional to the length and inversely proportional to the fourth power of the luminal radius. This simple relationship becomes more complicated for devices that are not uniform in shape. Cannula size is reported according to its outer diameter in current practice; however, identically sized cannulas may vary in their inner diameter because of differences in wall thickness. A simple method to describe the pressure-flow characteristics of vascular cannulas has been developed. Catheters are tested for their pressure-flow relationship and an "M-number" is determined which represents a resistive factor that can be used to approximate the expected flow at a specific pressure difference.[1,2] The M-number and flow values expected for a typical ECLS situation using a pressure gradient of 100 cm H_2O siphon are shown in Table 2.

Venous cannulas generally have both end and side holes to allow flow even if the end of the cannula is occluded. Arterial cannulas generally have only end holes to prevent arterial injury. The cannula should resist kinking while remaining flexible and thin-walled to offer the least resistance possible. Wire-wound cannulas such as Bio-Medicus (Medtronic, Minneapolis, MN) are very resilient to kinking, while the thin-walled double lumen cannulas are more prone to kink.

Table 1. Comparison of VV and VA bypass.

	Venoarterial (VA)	Venovenous (VV)
Cannulation Site	V: IJ, FV, RA A: RCCA, Ax, Fem, Ao	IJ, FV, saphenous v., RA
PaO₂	60-150 mm Hg	45-80 mm Hg
Indicator of O₂ adequacy	SvO_2, PvO_2	PaO_2, cerebral SvO_2, transmembrane $DavO_2$
Cardiac Effects	↓preload, ↑afterload, ↓pulse pressure, LV blood → coronary O_2	negligible
O₂ delivery capacity	High	moderate
Circulatory support	Partial to complete	No <u>direct</u> effect
Pulmonary circulation **R→L shunt**	↓SaO₂ in aorta	↑SaO₂ in aorta
L→R shunt	May cause pulmonary congestion and systemic hypoperfusion	May cause pulmonary congestion and systemic hypoperfusion

Table 2. Commonly used ECLS cannulas.

Venous Cannulas (Single Lumen):

Manufacturer	Size (F)	Length (cm)	M#	Flow @ 100cmH$_2$O
Biomedicus	8	25	4.35	0.5
	10	25	3.9	0.9
	12	25	3.55	1.5
	14	25	3.35	2.0
	15	50	3.65	1.3
	17	50	3.4	1.9
	19	50	3.15	2.6
	21	50	2.9	3.2
	23	50	2.65	5.0
	25	50	2.55	6.0
	27	50	2.4	6.5
	29	50	2.3	8.0
DLP	17	53	3.3	2.2
	21	53	3.05	3.0
	28	65	2.5	5.5
RMI	18	52	3.2	2.5
	20	52	3.0	3.0
	28	52	2.3	8.0

Venous Cannulas (Double Lumen):

Manufacturer	Size (F)	Length (cm)	M# (V)	Flow @ 100cmH$_2$O	M# (A)
Origen	12	8	3.9	0.9	4.7
	15	8	3.5	1.6	4.3
	18	15	3.4	1.9	3.8
Jostra	12		4.1	0.8	4.6
	15		3.6	1.4	4.6
Kendall	14	10	3.5	1.6	5.1

Arterial Cannulas:

Manufacturer	Size (F)	Length (cm)	M#	Flow @ 100cmH$_2$O
Biomedicus	8	25	4.40	0.5
	10	25	4.00	0.9
	12	25	3.55	1.5
	14	25	3.25	2.4
	15	37	3.30	2.2
	17	37	3.05	3.0
	19	37	2.80	3.8
	21	37	2.60	5.0
	23	38	2.40	6.5
DLP	8	23	4.5	0.4
	14	23	3.3	2.2
	16	23	3.0	3.0
	17	17	2.95	3.2
	21	17	2.65	5.0
RMI	18	15	3.0	3.0
	20	25	3.0	3.0
	20	15	2.8	3.8
	22	25	3.1	2.9

Vascular access for ECLS in the neonate is particularly challenging due to the small vessel size. The route of access depends on the method used. VA bypass is indicated if both cardiac and pulmonary support are required, or in neonates where access for VV support can not be obtained (e.g., the vein is too small). For VA access, the preferred site for venous drainage is the right atrium via the right internal jugular vein, and the aortic arch via the right common carotid artery is preferred for arterial infusion. The internal jugular vein and carotid artery are relatively large in the neonate and usually simple to cannulate. For VV access, a double lumen cannula is placed into the right atrium via the right internal jugular vein. This technique is limited by the size of the vein, because the smallest cannula currently available is 12F.

Selection of cannulation technique

VA bypass requires arterial ligation to prevent leakage around the cannula when placed by cutdown and possible distal embolization from flow past the cannula. In infants and small children the carotid artery is usually safe to ligate distally without major sequelae.[3] The incidence of neurologic impairment was similar for ECMO survivors after carotid ligation and conventionally managed babies in the U.K. Collaborative ECMO Trial.[4] Schumacher et al. found that the right hemisphere is more commonly involved when brain lesions are seen after carotid artery ligation.[5] However, this lateralization was not found in another study of 74 infants after carotid artery ligation.[6] VV bypass can be performed either using this technique of vein ligation or without vessel ligation via a percutaneous or semi-open technique. While jugular vein ligation is usually well tolerated, there is evidence that vein ligation may produce high venous pressure which can lead to cerebral ischemia.[7] Percutaneous access utilizes the Seldinger technique to place the cannula. Because the size of the vessel in relation to the cannula is unknown, vessel disruption is a risk. For this reason, the semi-open technique is preferred.[8] This technique requires a small incision to visualize the size of the vein as an aid to select the correct cannula size. Cannula insertion can also be visualized through this incision if desired. With this technique, vessel ligation is not performed. This has several advantages: cephalad flow into the cannula increases the amount of deoxygenated blood available to enter the bypass circuit, the vessel may remain patent after decannulation (and can be recannulated if needed), and the risk of the cannula kinking at the vessel is reduced because the vessel is not fixed to the cannula with a ligature that the cannula can pivot on. An adjustment of cannula depth is also much simpler when this technique is used.

Cannulation for neonatal ECLS

Open technique for VA or VV[9]

Pre-operative: Vascular cannulation and decannulation are performed in the neonatal ICU under adequate sedation and neuromuscular blockade. Neuromuscular blockade is especially important in preventing the potentially lethal complication of an air embolus during introduction of the venous cannula. The instruments and sterile procedures used are identical to those used in the OR. Heparin sodium (100 units/kg) is drawn up for subsequent administration. Lo-

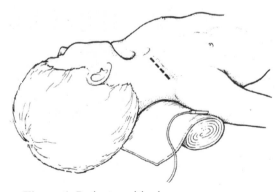

Figure 1. Patient positioning.

cal anesthesia is administered by infiltration of 1% lidocaine.

Operation: The patient is placed supine with the head turned to the left. A roll is placed transversely beneath the shoulders. Special attention is paid to ensure that the endotracheal tube is positioned to prevent kinking under the drapes during the procedure. A piece of suction tubing split lengthwise and placed over the tube at the connector can be used to prevent kinking. The chest, neck, and right side of the face are aseptically prepared and draped.

Incision (Figure 1): A transverse cervical incision approximately 2-3 centimeters in length is made one finger's breadth above the clavicle over the lower aspect of the right sternocleidomastoid muscle.

Exposure of the carotid sheath (Figure 2): The platysma muscle and subcutaneous tissues are divided with electrocautery and the sternocleidomastoid muscle is exposed. Dissection is continued bluntly between the sternal and clavicular heads of the muscle. The omohyoid muscle will be seen superiorly. It may be necessary to divide the omohyoid muscle tendon

to expose the carotid sheath. Two alternating self-retaining retractors are placed.

Dissection of the vessels (Figure 3): The carotid sheath is opened and the internal jugular vein, common carotid artery, and vagus nerve are identified and isolated. Dissection is progressed proximally and distally along the vessels, dissecting the vein first. Special care should be taken while dissecting the vein to avoid vessel spasm, which makes subsequent introduction of a large venous cannula difficult. Manipulation of the vein therefore should be minimized. There is often a branch on the medial aspect of the internal jugular vein which must be ligated. Ligatures of 2-0 silk are placed proximally and distally around the internal jugular vein. The common carotid artery lies medial and posterior to the internal jugular vein and has no branches, which makes its dissection proximally and distally safe. Ligatures of 2-0 silk are also placed around the carotid artery. Once vessel dissection is completed, heparin (100 units/kg) is administered intravenously and 3 minutes are allowed for circulation. During this period, papaverine is instilled into the

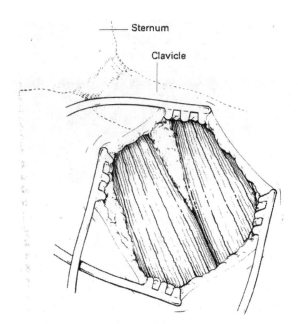

Figure 2. Superficial dissection.

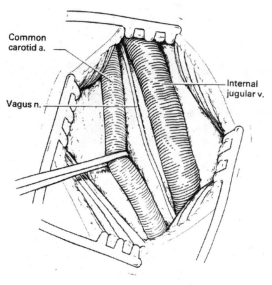

Figure 3. Deep dissection with exposed internal jugular vein, common carotid artery, and vagus nerve.

125

wound to enhance vein dilatation. The vagus nerve should be identified.

Arteriotomy/venotomy (Figure 4): For VA bypass, the arterial cannula is selected (most commonly 10F) and marked with a 2-0 silk ligature at a point that will allow the tip of the cannula to lie at the ostium of the brachiocephalic artery (~2.5 centimeters) and left uncut. The venous cannula (usually 12-14F) is similarly marked at a point equal to the distance from the venotomy to the right atrium (~6 centimeters). An obturator is placed into the venous cannula to prevent blood from flowing out through the side holes during introduction into the vessel. The common carotid artery is ligated distally. Proximal control is obtained with the use of an angled ductus clamp. A transverse arteriotomy is made near the distal ligature. Full thickness stay sutures of 6-0 polypropylene are placed on the proximal edge of the artery to prevent subintimal dissection during cannula insertion. Following arterial cannulation, a venotomy is performed in similar fashion. Gentle retraction of the caudal ligature around the vein precludes the need for a ductus clamp during venotomy

and venous cannulation. Stay sutures are also not routinely necessary for venous cannulation.

Cannula placement (Figure 5): The cannulas are carefully placed into the artery and vein and secured using 2 circumferential 2-0 silk ligatures. A small piece of silastic vessel loop can be left inside the ligatures to protect the vessels from injury during decannulation when the ligatures are sharply divided. The ends of the marking ligatures are tied to the most distal circumferential ligature for extra security. Immediately after each cannula is secured, the cannula is carefully de-aired via back-bleeding and filling with heparinized saline. For VV bypass, the double-lumen cannula is placed into the venotomy and the tip advanced to the mid-right atrium. It is crucial to maintain the arterial reinfusion (red) port anteriorly to minimize recirculation of reinfused blood while securing the cannula.

Wound closure (Figure 6): The wound is irrigated with saline and hemostasis obtained. The skin is closed with continuous monofilament suture. The wound is dressed with gauze. The

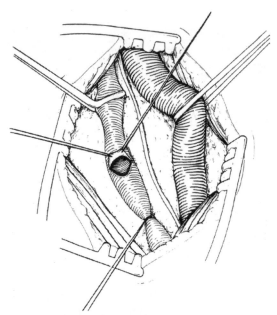

Figure 4. Carotid artery ligated distally and proximal arteriotomy.

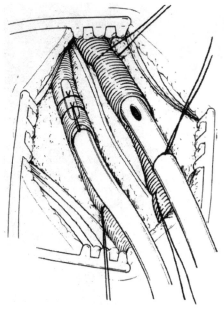

Figure 5. Arterial cannula secured. Venous cannula being inserted.

cannula is sutured to the skin with several 2-0 silk sutures. Special attention should be directed to affixing the cannulas securely to the bed.

Semi-open technique for VV[10]

Incision and vein exposure (Figure 7): A transverse cervical incision 1.5-2 centimeters in length is made 2 centimeters above the right clavicle between the heads of the sternocleido-mastoid muscle. The platysma is divided with electrocautery and the anterior surface of the internal jugular vein is exposed with minimal dissection. The vessel is observed and either a 12F or 15F OriGen VV ECMO cannula (OriGen Biomedical Inc., Austin, Texas) is selected.

Guidewire placement (Figure 8): The cannula skin exit position is selected so that the cannula will lie behind the right ear when the head is returned to the midline. The needle/catheter are placed through the skin 2 centimeters superior to the incision and into the internal jugular vein to enter either under the skin flap or just inside the incision. The needle is removed and a 0.035-inch diameter guidewire is advanced and the catheter is withdrawn. A Teflon guiding obturator is placed over the guidewire into the vessel and right atrium. The skin exit is slightly enlarged with a scalpel.

Cannula placement (Figure 9): Heparin (100 units/kg) is administered and 3 minutes are allowed for circulation. The selected cannula is advanced over the Teflon obturator into the vein under direct vision to confirm entrance into the vein. The arterial (red) port of the cannula must be directed anteriorly to allow the arterial blood to be directed towards the tricuspid valve and minimize recirculation. The tip of the cannula is placed 6-9 centimeters from the skin incision.

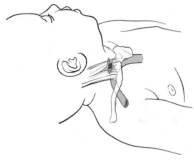

Figure 7. Superficial dissection exposing anterior surface of internal jugular vein.

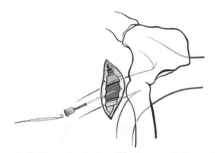

Figure 8. Introducer needle inserted through superior skin flap into vein.

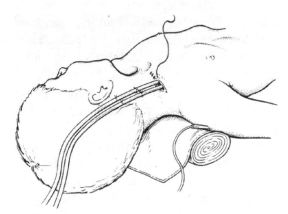

Figure 6. Cannulas secured to skin. Wound closed.

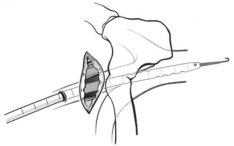

Figure 9. Cannula, dilator, and guidewire inserted into vein under direct vision.

Wound closure and cannula fixation (Figure 10): The relatively low venous pressure allows adequate hemostasis around the venotomy site without any ligature. This prevents kinking of the thin-walled cannula which often occurs at the area of a ligature if used around the vessel. Repositioning of the cannula only requires removing the skin sutures, repositioning the cannula, and replacing skin sutures. The cannula is fixed to the skin with several 2-0 silk sutures. The incision is closed with a monofilament suture.

Decannulation: After weaning of ECLS has occurred and the decision to come off ECLS has been made, decannulation can be performed by removing the skin sutures, pulling the cannula, and holding pressure on the catheter exit site for 5 minutes or until bleeding stops. Care must be taken to remove the entire cannula rapidly to prevent air from entering the side holes while the end of the cannula remains in the vessel.

Cannulation for pediatric ECLS

Pediatric patients >10 kg have bypass needs similar to adults. Their vessels are larger and more options for access are available. VV bypass is used preferentially for respiratory support. VA bypass is reserved for cardiac support, including post-operative patients who fail to wean from car-

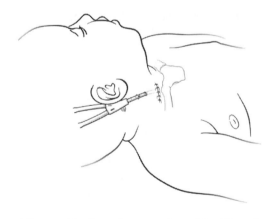

Figure 10. Cannula secured to skin. Wound closed.

diopulmonary bypass (CPB) after heart surgery. Children who are not yet old enough to walk have very small femoral vessels which are not suitable for bypass access. For this reason, in this group (<10 kg), either a double lumen cannula in the jugular vein for VV bypass, or single cannulas in the jugular vein and carotid artery for VA bypass must be used. Occasionally, a small child with respiratory failure has a jugular vein which is too small to allow a double lumen cannula large enough for adequate flow on VV bypass, and instead must be placed on VA bypass.

VV bypass

As described above, VV bypass in children <10 kg can be achieved using a double lumen cannula either placed by a modified Seldinger technique, as described above, or entirely percutaneous if the vein is judged to be adequate to receive the cannula. Children >10 kg usually have veins that are large enough to utilize a two-cannula technique by placing cannulas in the femoral and jugular veins.[11] The selection of cannulas is, again, based on two criteria: the largest cannula that the vein will accept and a large enough drainage cannula to allow for adequate flow (100 cc/kg/min) which may be estimated by the M-number. The decision of which cannula to use for drainage and reinfusion has two considerations. The jugular vein cannula will often allow more drainage. If the end of this cannula is in the atrium and pre-load is adequate, it can drain until the atrium collapses around the cannula and the pump flow is interrupted by servo-regulation. Flow is thought to be higher in this situation because the atrium is spherical in shape compared to the cylindrical shape of the femoral or iliac veins. However, if pump blood is reinfused into the femoral vein, recirculation is often significant. This may be due to the direction of blood draining into the right atrium from the inferior vena cava which is directed preferentially into the jugular cannula before mixing occurs. Rich et al. showed that draining blood from the femoral cannula and reinfusing into the jugular cannula results in higher arterial saturation (i.e. higher oxygen delivery), in spite of lower achievable total flow, because recirculation is minimal.[12] This method of bypass is preferable and utilizes a femoral cannula that reaches the intrahepatic vena cava, which is large and does not collapse.

VA bypass

For cardiac failure, most pediatric patients are cannulated through the neck using the jugular vein and carotid artery by cutdown, as described previously for the open technique for VA cannulation for neonatal ECLS. For patients placed on bypass after cardiac surgery, surgeons may utilize the cannulation sites in the chest that were used for CPB.

Cannulation for adult ECLS

VV bypass

Cannulation for adult VV bypass uses 2 cannulas placed in the jugular and femoral veins. These cannulas can be placed safely by a percutaneous method.[13] A large cannula (23-29F) should be placed for drainage and a somewhat smaller cannula (21-23F) for venous reinfusion. It is especially important for the drainage cannula to have side holes, in addition to an end hole, to maximize flow and allow flow to continue if the end becomes obstructed. An adult-size double lumen cannula is under development and will be available for use soon. Recirculation is a problem which can be solved, as described in the section on pediatric cannulation, by draining from the femoral vein and returning to the right atrium.

VA bypass

VA bypass in adults can be achieved using several different cannulation schemes. Jugular vein to carotid artery bypass as used in newborns has been successful and works well, especially

for combined cardiac and pulmonary support. It provides good perfusion to all branches of the aortic arch and distal aorta, but it increases afterload by increasing aortic pressure. Jugular vein to femoral artery bypass provides adequate distal perfusion, but this can fail to perfuse the aortic arch in situations where the native cardiac function is good. If the blood ejected from the left ventricle is desaturated because of pulmonary dysfunction, the aortic arch may not receive well-oxygenated pump blood and the result will be hypoxemia in the upper half of the body. This can be solved by adding an additional perfusion cannula to the venous circulation (jugular or femoral vein) to create venoarteriovenous (VAV) bypass.[14] This increases oxygenation of the right ventricular blood much like VV bypass and provides the hemodynamic support of VA bypass. The increased afterload from VA bypass may prevent the failing left ventricle from ejecting blood, resulting in high left atrial pressure and pulmonary edema. This can be managed by draining blood from the left atrium into the venous side of the bypass circuit either from direct cannulation of the left atrium by thoracotomy or by catheter-based balloon atrial septostomy.

Arterial cannulation may be performed either percutaneously or by direct cutdown of the vessel. With either method, if the cannula is large enough to diminish flow, distal ischemia may result. Several methods of managing this have been described. Placement of a distal perfusion catheter can be used with the open technique by placing a connector with a side port and placing small tubing directed into the vessel distally at the cutdown site. With the percutaneous technique, an arterial line can be placed into either the dorsalis pedis or posterior tibial artery by cutdown and the distal pressure measured. If the pressure is <50 mm Hg, the catheter can be perfused by a line from the perfusion limb of the circuit.[15]

Decannulation can be performed in a manner similar to that previously described for the vein (direct pressure for percutaneously placed line, ligation of the jugular vein for cutdown placement). Arterial decannulation is more complicated. Direct pressure may be all that is needed for percutaneously-placed arterial cannulas. The larger the cannula in relation to the artery, the more likely that a pseudoaneurysm or arterial stenosis will result. An alternative to this method is venous patch angioplasty, a technique that is used for removing arterial cannulas placed by cutdown. In this technique, the vessel is controlled by a clamp and the cannula is removed. A diamond-shaped patch of vein is then sutured into the defect, which both closes the hole and prevents stricture at the repair site.

Transthoracic cannulation

There are circumstances when cervical or thoracic access for VA extracorporeal support is either not possible or practical, particularly in patients who have failed to wean from CPB or who have undergone post-sternotomy resuscitation. In these circumstances, direct cannulation of the arterial and venous system is performed using techniques and cannulas that are standard for CPB. Purse-string sutures are placed in the ascending aorta and usually directly in the right atrium and brought through snares that allow the suture to be tightened around the cannula and secured, preventing leaking of blood around the cannula, and in the case of the venous side, preventing air from entering into the system. While cannulas placed in the OR are usually lightly secured to the drapes or left lying on the field, it is critical to secure the cannulas in a more stable manner when providing more prolonged extracorporeal support, particularly for safety during transport. In general, this involves suturing the cannula to the chest wall and closing the wound with an artificial dressing, with the cannulas exiting between the suture line between the material and the skin. If the patient awakens and starts to move or attempts to breathe or

cough, the sternal edges can separate and put tension on the cannulas, risking dislodgement. This can be prevented by either using continuous neuromuscular blockade or by using 1 or 2 heavy sutures or sternal wires to bridge the distance between the sternal edges. This has been found to provide adequate stabilization of the support apparatus, and is often preferable to paralytics.

Cannulation problems

Cannulation of patients for ECMO can be quite challenging and problems are frequently encountered. By adequately preparing the patient, complications can usually be avoided. Proper training and support of the surgeon performing these procedures will allow most of these problems to be managed without adverse outcomes.

Threading the venous catheter

An inability to thread the venous catheter may occur because the vein is too small, the catheter is too big, or there is a left-sided superior vena cava without an innominate vein. The clavicle or first rib can sometimes obstruct if the patient's head is hyperextended or hyperrotated; therefore, one should attempt to reposition the head. There may also be severe mediastinal shift with diaphragmatic hernia, pneumothorax, or effusion.

Vein division

Especially in small newborns, it may be difficult to introduce the venous cannula and during attempts to do this, the vein may become divided. This makes further attempts to introduce the cannula even more difficult. Vascular control is the primary goal, and is best accomplished with a vascular clamp. Once done, a guide wire may be helpful to introduce the cannula. Placing stay sutures will help to provide traction during cannula placement. A ligature should be placed around the vein to tie in the cannula. At decannulation, a purse-string suture may be used to control bleeding.

Proximal vein lost in mediastinum

During a difficult venous cannulation in which the cannula does not thread easily, sudden loss of resistance may be due to division of the vein which may then invert into the mediastinum. Bleeding may be controlled by direct finger pressure. If the vein end can be retrieved with forceps, cannulation may be performed as described above for vein division. If no other suitable vein is available, median sternotomy and access via a thoracic approach may be needed. If other access is available, control can usually be achieved by suturing the fascia to cover the hole where the vein was lost and applying direct pressure.

Lack of venous return

If there is no flow after placement of the cannula, the cannula and circuit tubing should be examined for kinking. Chest radiography or fluoroscopy should be used to assess the position of the venous cannula, which should be repositioned or replaced as needed.

Intrathoracic vein perforation

Sudden cessation of flow with hemodynamic instability may be the result of intrathoracic vessel perforation. This situation requires immediate median sternotomy and vascular repair, with subsequent open cannulation.

Summary

Vascular access for ECLS requires a thorough understanding of the patient's needs for bypass, and the specific solution according to age and size. Understanding these principles will allow the surgeon to provide access for most clinical situations in a logical manner. Providing access is usually straightforward, but can be challenging and may require management of vascular complications.

References

1. Montoya JP, Merz SI, Bartlett RH. A standardized system for describing flow/pressure relationships in vascular access devices. *ASAIO Trans* 1991; 37:4-8.

2. Sinard JM, Merz SI, Hatcher MD, Montoya JP, Bartlett RH. Evaluation of extracorporeal perfusion catheters using a standardized measurement technique--the M-number. *ASAIO Trans* 1991; 37:60-64.

3. Streletz LJ, Bej MD, Graziani LJ, et al. Utility of serial EEGs in neonates during extracorporeal membrane oxygenation. *Pediatr Neurol* 1992; 8:190-196.

4. UK Collaborative ECMO Trial Group. UK collaborative randomised trial of neonatal extracorporeal membrane oxygenation. *Lancet* 1996; 348:75-82.

5. Schumacher RE, Barks JD, Johnston MV, et al. Right-sided brain lesions in infants following extracorporeal membrane oxygenation. *Pediatrics* 1988; 82:155-161.

6. Lazar EL, Abramson SJ, Weinstein S, Stolar CJ. Neuroimaging of brain injury in neonates treated with extracorporeal membrane oxygenation: lessons learned from serial examinations. *J Pediatr Surg* 1994; 29:186-191.

7. Walker LK, Short BL, Traystman RJ. Impairment of cerebral autoregulation during venovenous extracorporeal membrane oxygenation in the newborn lamb. *Crit Care Med* 1996; 24:2001-2006

8. Peek GJ, Firmin RK, Moore HM, Sosnowski AW. Cannulation of neonates for venovenous extracorporeal life support. *Ann Thorac Surg* 1996; 61:1851-1852.

9. Pranikoff T, Hirschl RB. Neonatal extracorporeal membrane oxygenation. In: Carter

DC, Russell RCG, eds. *Rob and Smith's Operative Surgery.* 5th ed. London, England: Butterworth-Heinemann; 1995.

10. Pranikoff T, Hirschl RB. Neonatal extracorporeal membrane oxygenation. In: Carter DC, Russell RCG, eds. *Rob and Smith's Operative Surgery.* 6th ed. London, England: Butterworth-Heinemann; 2005.

11. Foley DS, Swaniker F, Pranikoff T, Bartlett RH, Hirschl RB. Percutaneous cannulation for pediatric venovenous extracorporeal life support. *J Pediatr Surg* 2000; 35:943-947.

12. Rich PB, Awad SS, Crotti S, Hirschl RB, Bartlett RH, Schreiner RJ. A prospective comparison of atrio-femoral and femoro-atrial flow in adult venovenous extracorporeal life support. *J Thorac Cardiovasc Surg* 1998; 116:628-632.

13. Pranikoff T, Hirschl RB, Remenapp R, Swaniker F, Bartlett RH. Venovenous extracorporeal life support via percutaneous cannulation in 94 patients. *Chest* 1999; 115:818-822.

14. Miskulin J, Annich G, Grams R, Boules T, McGillicuddy J, Hirschl R, Bartlett R. Venous-arteriovenous cannulation for adult ECMO patients with cardiogenic shock. Presented at: 14th Annual ELSO Conference; September 10-12, 2004; Chicago, IL.

15. Bartlett RH, personal communication.

8

Emergencies During ECLS and Their Management

Brittany B. DeBerry, M.D., James Lynch, B.S., R.R.T., Dai H. Chung, M.D., and
Joseph B. Zwischenberger, M.D.

Introduction

The success or failure of ECMO therapy is highly dependent upon the prompt recognition and management of complications as they emerge. Complications during ECMO are the rule, not the exception.[1,2] It is the nature of long-term heart-lung bypass for potentially catastrophic complications to arise unexpectedly and emergently. An understanding of the physiology of ECMO, familiarity with the ECMO circuit, and the attainment of a certain level of confidence in managing patients on ECMO prepare us to deal with the majority of the problems encountered with ECLS.
The proper training of ECMO personnel, coupled with the valuable knowledge acquired from experience, is crucial to the success of an ECMO program. In addition to experienced physicians, ECMO team personnel include a nurse with extensive ICU experience, a respiratory therapist, and a perfusionist. Each center uses different combinations of ECMO personnel at any given time, and some centers have demonstrated the cost-effective and safe use of a single-trained ECMO specialist both to manage patients and to monitor the ECMO circuit. Regardless of how many trained personnel are involved with the management of ECMO patients, extensive and thorough didactic courses for the ECMO specialist, including simulated patient care situations to address common complications, are essential to prepare each team member to deal with each potential complication.

The complications encountered during ECMO can be classified as mechanical or patient-related. Any mechanical component of the ECMO apparatus may fail; therefore, constant system checks and monitoring are done in an effort to prevent most complications from becoming disastrous. Although patient complications span the entire field of critical care medicine, they are often related to systemic heparinization and include intracranial hemorrhage (ICH), gastrointestinal (GI) hemorrhage, and cannula site bleeding.

As of January 2005, 29,908 neonatal, pediatric, or adult ECMO cases have been reported to the ELSO Registry with an overall survival rate of 76%.[1] There was an average of 2.7 complications per case as reported by the ELSO Registry. These complications are divided into the following categories: mechanical, hemorrhagic, neurologic, renal, cardiovascular, pulmonary, infectious, and metabolic. Despite nationwide dissemination of ECMO experience, increasing complication rates have been reported. This increase has been attributed to several factors: 1) an increase in complexity of the patient's clinical conditions, largely due to expanded entry criteria; 2) an increased number of ECMO centers with fewer case experiences per program; 3) less reluctance to report complications; and 4) changes in the data form to capture an increasing number of minor complications.

Mechanical complications

Mechanical complications in neonatal and pediatric respiratory ECMO patients are listed in Table 1. There were 18,044 mechanical complications reported in 22,346 cases of neonatal and pediatric respiratory ECMO, or an average of 0.81 mechanical complications per case.[3] For all age groups (including adults) the most common mechanical complication reported remains clots in the various components of the circuit, representing nearly 53% and 28% of all reported mechanical complications in neonates and pediatric respiratory patients, respectively. In pediatric ECMO, oxygenator failure was reported significantly more frequently than in neonates (13.7 vs. 5.7%). Other commonly encountered complications included cannula problems, tubing rupture, and pump malfunction. The entire circuit, which includes bladder box, connectors,

electrical components, carbogen or CO_2 tanks, blenders, and circuit monitoring equipment, is subject to mechanical failure. The management of common mechanical complications is outlined in Table 2.

Thrombosis

Clots in the circuit are the most common mechanical complication during ECMO.[1,2] Since the initial development of ECMO, a dilemma has existed: higher systemic anticoagulation (activated clotting time [ACT] >250 seconds) decreases thrombosis but increases bleeding, while lower systemic anticoagulation (ACT <250 seconds) increases thrombosis but decreases bleeding. Despite vigilant heparin management, formation of clots in the circuit cannot be completely avoided, especially with prolonged ECMO support. The development of very small clots in the circuit is not preventable and may represent no significant danger to patients. However, major clots can lead to oxygenator failure or a consumptive coagulopathy, as well as the potential for pulmonary

Table 1. Neonatal and pediatric respiratory mechanical complications. (ELSO Registry, January 2005)

Complications	Neonatal N=19,701		Pediatric N=2,934	
	Reported n (%)	Survived n (%)	Reported n (%)	Survived n (%)
Oxygenator failure	1129 (6)	621 (55)	401 (13)	179 (45)
Raceway rupture	67 (1)	41 (61)	20 (1)	7 (35)
Other tubing rupture	140 (1)	104 (74)	108 (4)	51 (47)
Pump malfunction	346 (2)	235 (68)	89 (3)	43 (48)
Heat exchanger failure	175 (1)	121 (69)	18 (1)	7 (39)
Clots:				
Oxygenator	3605 (18)	2429 (67)	202 (7)	106 (52)
Bridge	2166 (11)	1474 (68)	129 (4)	68 (53)
Bladder	3194 (16)	2233 (70)	169 (6)	88 (52)
Hemofilter	492 (3)	213 (43)	93 (3)	40 (43)
Other	946 (5)	561 (59)	216 (7)	111 (51)
Air in circuit	1026 (5)	735 (72)	58 (2)	30 (52)
Cracks:				
Pigtail connectors	612 (3)	438 (72)	29 (1)	16 (55)
Cannula problems	2205 (11)	1531 (69)	409 (14)	200 (49)

or systemic emboli. The extracorporeal circuit presents a large foreign surface for activation of neutrophils, lymphocytes, and platelets, which can lead to the release of inflammatory mediators and oxygen free-radical activation.[4-8] In order to overcome the difficulty of maintaining systemic heparinization, heparin-coated Carmeda systems (Medtronic, Minneapolis, MN) were trialed at a few centers with disappointing results.[9,10] Several animal models have been used to further investigate the advantage of using the Carmeda-coated systems in order to reduce the amount of systemic anticoagulation required for the patient. Most studies have shown that with the Carmeda-coated system, minimal clotting can be achieved with lower heparin doses;[11] however, its ultimate benefit to clinical use is unknown.

Cannula problems

Cannulas must be inserted with great care to avoid vascular injury during insertion. The potential vascular injuries during cannula insertion include tearing of the internal jugular vein and/or superior vena cava with loss of venous control resulting in massive intrathoracic bleeding as well as intimal dissection of the common carotid artery preventing proper cannula placement and potentially leading to lethal aortic dissection.

The venous catheter can be misdirected into the subclavian vein or across the foramen ovalis, resulting in flow obstruction. Anatomic variations of the right atrium (aneurysmal atrial septum or redundant eustachian valve) can also interfere with venous return. Even after appropriate venous cannula placement, cannula obstruction due to kinking is a common problem; therefore, adequate flow is extremely dependent on patient neck positioning and cannula fixation.

Problems with arterial cannulation can also arise from the catheter being inserted too far into the ascending or descending aorta or from being misplaced into the subclavian artery. A cannula in the ascending aorta can cause increased afterload to left ventricular outflow and may contribute to left ventricular failure and cardiac stun. In addition, the cannula can be improperly placed across the aortic valve, causing aortic insufficiency. Finally, the cannula can be inserted against the left ventricular endothelium with the potential for left ventricle disruption or

Table 2. Management of mechanical complications.

Complications	Management
Tubing rupture	Stop pump flow and repair/replace damaged tubing
Air in circuit	
Venous	Aspirate air, identify source
Arterial	Stop ECMO flow, clamp arterial and venous lines, check for the sources of air entry, and repair or change component or circuit
Oxygenator failure	Aspirate air, if detected Repair or replace oxygenator
Power failure	Hand crank until power available Battery pack or hospital emergency power supply
Decannulation	Apply direct pressure Stop pump flow, increase ventilator settings Surgical hemostasis; replace volume

perforation. The placement of a cannula in the descending aorta can compromise coronary and cerebral blood flow as well as cause streaming of hyperoxygenated blood from the ECMO circuit without adequate mixing. The distance from the orifice of the innominate artery to the take-off of the right subclavian artery can be remarkably short (1-1.5 centimeters). If the arterial cannula is pulled out to the point at which the arterial infusion selectively enters the right subclavian artery, the right upper extremity can be infused with the entire post-oxygenator blood flow while the rest of the body is hypoxic and cyanotic. Pulse oximeter monitoring on the right upper extremity may not indicate the true state of blood flow and oxygen delivery to the rest of the body.

Proper cannula positioning during venovenous (VV) ECMO is crucial due to the potential problems of recirculation with inadequate cannula position. Several catheters have recently been developed with balloons and other devices to help prevent this problem while on VV ECMO.[12,13] A chest radiograph shows relative location but cannot indicate physiologic performance or complications relative to vessel integrity. The use of echocardiography to confirm cannula location has been recommended by some to assess cannula position to decrease the number of operations for cannula repositioning.[14,15] Although echocardiographs can be very helpful, their use during cannulation requires coordination and experience by the cannulating team as well as the echocardiographer.

Air embolism

The ECMO circuit is designed to pump blood safely and efficiently, but with most roller and centrifugal pumps a large bolus of air can circulate rapidly and is often fatal. Air in the circuit represents 4% of all complications reported and can range from a few small bubbles seen in the bladder to a complete venous airlock. Venous airlock usually results from dislodgment of the venous cannula so that one or more of the side holes in the cannula is outside the vessel.[16] Massive airlock requires the patient to come off ECMO support with either removal of the air or repriming and replacing the entire ECMO circuit. For small amounts of air in the venous line, the air can be moved to the venous reservoir by sequentially raising the venous line and then aspirating the air out of the circuit.

There are several potential sources of an air embolus. One possible source arises when the partial pressure of oxygen in the blood is very high or supersaturated, as seen post-oxygenator, where oxygen can easily be forced out of solution. Hitting the membrane or operating the circuit in a low ambient pressure environment (such as in-flight in a non-pressurized cabin) may produce foam in the top of the oxygenator. Operating the pump with a clamp on the venous side of the circuit with the bladder in the priming mode or with the outlet arm of the bladder kinked (as can occur during "walking" of the raceway) can generate a markedly negative pressure in the blood path and pull large amounts of gas out of solution (cavitation). This is precisely the problem the bladder box system is designed to avoid.

The most dramatic air embolus occurs when a small tear develops in the membrane of the oxygenator, allowing blood to leak into the gas path of the oxygenator. The blood gradually moves down to the gas exhalation port where it may either be blown out in small drops or accumulate and form a clot. If this clot obstructs the egress of gas, backpressure will develop inside the gas path of the oxygenator. When the gas pressure exceeds that of the blood, a large bolus of air crosses the membrane and enters the blood path. As it flows out of the membrane to the heat exchanger (and the arterial line filter, if it is used), the gas trapping capacity of these two devices (~45 ml for each) may be rapidly exceeded, and the air embolus will flow via the arterial line toward the patient's arterial circulation.

Prevention and rapid response when air embolism is recognized is imperative. Several preventive measures to eliminate the most common causes of an air embolus include keeping the post-membrane PO_2 <600 mm Hg, monitoring the toggle switches on the bladder box to ensure proper functioning, strictly prohibiting placement of extraneous clamps on the circuit, and adherence to precautions with regard to the procedure for "walking the raceway". Lightly occluding the gas exhalation port of the membrane with your finger as a part of the hourly circuit check will alert the practitioner when there is blood rather just water being expelled. However, fully occluding the gas exhalation port even briefly can cause a precipitous rise in the gas phase pressure across the membrane, risking a membrane rupture and/or development of an air embolus.

Strict adherence to the hourly protocol and general vigilance for problems permit the prompt recognition and appropriate response to an air embolus. If a bolus of air is seen, immediately stop ECMO flow by clamping the venous and arterial lines and opening the bridge. The patient should be hand-bagged to achieve acceptable oxygen saturation while the problem in the circuit is identified and corrected. If the air is flowing toward the arterial cannula, a clamp is immediately placed on the arterial tubing close to the patient to prevent an air embolus from entering the patient. If, however, air has already entered the patient, additional protective measures should be taken. Once the patient is off ECMO, the head is lowered relative to the body as much as possible in order to move any air pockets away from the cerebral circulation. Using a sterile catheter-tipped syringe, all air is aspirated out of the arterial cannula. High dosages of inotropic drugs may be necessary if any air has entered the coronaries and caused acute cardiac decompensation. Once the patient has been stabilized, the cause of the air leak should be identified and corrected. If a hyperbaric chamber facility is available, its immediate use should also be considered.

Membrane oxygenator failure

The majority of ECMO centers use Medtronic membrane lung oxygenators. Overall, oxygenator failure represents only 5.7% of mechanical complications in neonatal respiratory ECMO patients; however, it represents a significantly higher percentage of mechanical complications in pediatric (13.7%) as well as adult (18%) patients.[3] Although the exact criteria used for documenting oxygenator failure from each center are not well defined, this category of mechanical complications represents the second most frequently encountered mechanical complication in ECMO patients. Some centers report failure when decreased oxygen or CO_2 transfer occurs. Other centers monitor pre- and post-oxygenator pressure gradients, platelet count, plasma-free hemoglobin, and fibrin split products to demonstrate when the oxygenator may be causing a consumptive coagulopathy. A failing membrane should be changed immediately after recognition to prevent an air/blood leak. Other signs of membrane failure include deterioration in gas exchange (decreasing PO_2 or decreasing CO_2 transfer), platelet consumption, or increasing pre-membrane pressures with stable post-membrane pressures. A double-diamond tubing arrangement with dual connectors, both pre- and post- oxygenator, allows in-line replacement of the oxygenator without interrupting ECMO flow.

Tubing rupture

Initially, polyvinyl chloride (PVC) tubing required advancing the raceway every 24 hours to prevent tubing fatigue and possible rupture. Since the availability of Super Tygon (S65HL) (Norton Performance Plastics, Inc., Akron, OH) raceway tubing, the complication of tubing rupture has become virtually non-existent in neonatal cases (1%) and is seldom seen in pediatric patients (4.4%). With prolonged ECMO support, the raceway should be advanced approximately every 10-14 days for neonates with ¼-inch Super Tygon tubing and every 4-6 days in older patients with ⅜-inch Super Tygon tubing. Occasionally, the tubing of the circuit must be repaired while the patient is on ECMO because a connection has come loose or there is damage to the tubing. Tubing may be easily cut with the jaws of a tubing clamp if the tubing becomes too close to the hinged joint of the clamp or it may be pierced by penetrating towel clamps or crack from fatigue (usually seen at the main or in the raceway).

Other circuit components

Proper functioning of the heat exchanger to maintain normal physiologic body temperature is imperative during ECMO support. Whenever a heat exchanger malfunction occurs (<1%), it can rapidly lead to significant hypothermia, especially in neonates. Defective heat exchangers have also been responsible for aluminum particle emboli;[17] however, redesign has eliminated this problem. Pump failure has also become less common as direct and belt drive pumps have been manufactured specifically with long-term extracorporeal support in mind. The majority of programs continue to use roller pumps for neonatal ECMO and the centrifugal pump for older pediatric (>30 days) and adult patients.

Occasionally the pump cuts out; this is a manifestation of inadequate venous return to the pump. Figure 1 outlines a management protocol to address this problem. All causes of inadequate venous return must be considered. Hypovolemia can be easily corrected with intravascular volume expansion. The circuit must also be checked to rule out any kinks or obstructions that cause inadequate venous return. Likewise, the venous catheter placement should be confirmed by chest radiograph or echocardiography. Echocardiography can also ensure that cardiac tamponade

is not the cause of the obstruction to venous return. If these maneuvers do not uncover the etiology, placement of an additional venous drainage catheter may be necessary.

Replacement or repair of equipment

The management response algorithm for replacement of malfunctioning equipment, especially if the circuit is squirting blood or pumping air, is illustrated in Figure 2. Upon recognition of the problem, the patient must be immediately taken off ECMO support by the placement of a tubing clamp on the venous line first, opening the bridge, and then lastly clamping the arterial line (Very Bad Accident). The pump is turned off to allow correction of the problem in the circuit. The only exception to this sequence of clamp placement is with the detection of a massive air embolism, in which the arterial line should be clamped first. The patient should be hand-bagged with 100% oxygen

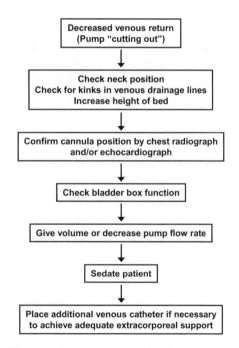

Figure 1. Management of inadequate venous return.

or placed on ventilator settings to ensure adequate respiratory support. After clamping either side, the damaged equipment part is quickly replaced. In the case of damaged tubing, the involved segment is prepped with Betadine and replaced with a piece of sterile connector or tubing. After these are joined together, a careful search for air in the circuit is made. All extraneous clamps are removed from the circuit, and the pump is allowed to recirculate, looking again for any evidence of air. Once completed, the patient is placed back on ECMO.

If repair necessitates the removal of a large segment of tubing such as the raceway, then a replacement piece should be inserted where the damaged portion was removed. This is performed by making the connection to one of the loose ends while the clamps are still in place. The replacement piece is filled with fluid from its free end, holding it upright in a vertical position. It is easiest to do this with a large syringe and an 18-gauge needle or small feeding tube placed well into the piece of tubing, touching the inside tubing wall. Fluids that froth easily, such as albumin or fresh frozen plasma (FFP), should be avoided for this purpose. When the insertion segment is filled, the connection is made and the procedure completed as described above.

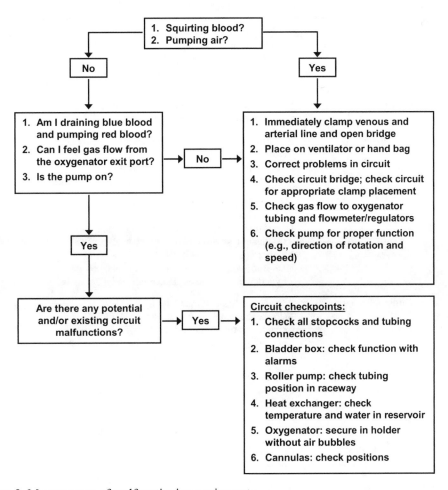

Figure 2. Management of malfunctioning equipment.

Patient complications

Patient complications can manifest as dysfunction in virtually all other organ systems (Table 3). The January 2005 ELSO Registry report of patient complications during ECMO revealed 43,193 or an average of 1.44 complications per case. The overall incidence of patient-related complications is nearly twice that of mechanical circuit-related events but has decreased compared to a few years ago. These complications include surgical or cannula site bleeding, intracranial infarct or bleed, hemolysis, renal insufficiency requiring dialysis or hemofiltration, hypertension, seizures, electrolyte abnormalities, pneumothorax, cardiac dysfunction or arrhythmias, gastrointestinal hemorrhage, and infection. Despite advances in hemostatic agents, such as tissue glues and sealant,[18] bleeding remains the most devastating and difficult problem encountered. The management of patient-related complications is summarized in Table 4.

Surgical hemorrhage

Bleeding is the most common complication of ECMO, largely due to the requirement for systemic heparinization. A small to moderate amount of bleeding is frequently seen at the

Table 4. Management of patient complications.

Complications	Management
Surgical hemorrhage	Use electrocautery and topical hemostatic agents Judicious use of platelets and FFP Consider systemic anticoagulant agents (Amicar) Monitor previous invasive procedure sites
Hematologic	Monitor for clots in the circuit or membrane Careful titration of heparin with tight ACT parameters
Neurologic	Perform daily cranial ultrasound during first week Treat hypertension if present Avoid hypoxia, acidosis, and hypercarbia Discontinue ECMO when intracranial bleed increases
Renal	Monitor daily weight and fluid balance Maintain total fluid intake 80-100 ml/kg/day Use of diuretics for hypervolemia; minimize excessive fluid administration Monitor creatinine and BUN Hemofiltration/dialysis for: hypervolemia, hyperkalemia, acidosis, azotemia
Cardiopulmonary	Avoid hypertension; treat with hydralazine Increase the pump flow or consider VA ECMO Consider inotropic support Rule out hypoxia as a cause of cardiac dysfunction Left-to-right shunt may occur due to PDA
Metabolic/infection	Monitor calcium due to citrate in the blood Consider inadequate tissue perfusion if acidosis present Prophylactic antibiotics Surveillance cultures for early signs of sepsis
Gastrointestinal	Consider liver cholestasis if direct hyperbilirubinemia present Consider early enteral feedings Prophylactic treatment for gastritis

Table 3. Neonatal and pediatric respiratory failure complications. (ELSO Registry, January 2005)

Complications	Neonatal N=19,701		Pediatrics N=2,934	
	Reported n (%)	Survived n (%)	Reported n (%)	Survival n (%)
Hemorrhagic				
Gastrointestinal	342 (1)	157 (46)	118 (4)	30 (25)
Cannula site	1218 (6)	823 (68)	277 (9)	30 (25)
Surgical site	1209 (6)	554 (46)	459 (16)	217 (47)
Hemolysis	2366 (12)	159 3(67)	259 (9)	108 (42)
DIC	282 (1)	109 (39)	88 (3)	24 (27)
Neurological				
Brain death	196 (1)	0 (0)	176 (6)	0 (0)
Seizures:				
Clinical	2112 (10)	1309 (62)	211 (7)	72 (34)
EEG	143 (1)	68 (48)	40 (1)	15 (38)
CNS infarct	1702 (9)	933 (55)	95 (3)	39 (41)
CNS hemorrhage	1144 (6)	526 (46)	143 (5)	39 (27)
Renal				
Creatinine 1.5-3.0	1547 (8)	835 (54)	289 (10)	81 (28)
Creatinine >3.0	298 (2)	105 (35)	142 (5)	39 (27)
Dialysis required	679 (3)	278 (41)	534 (18)	169 (32)
Hemofiltration required	2601 (13)	1442 (55)	438 (15)	182 (42)
CAVHD required	128 (1)	41 (32)	92 (3)	26 (28)
Cardiovascular				
Inotropes on ECLS	1602 (13)	1602 (62)	1267 (43)	555 (44)
CPR required	464 (2)	199 (43)	172 (6)	32 (19)
Myocardial stun	1096 (6)	653 (60)	30 (1)	9 (30)
Arrhythmia	788 (4)	426 (54)	236 (8)	80 (4)
Hypertension	2477 (12)	1821 (74)	347 (12)	205 (59)
PDA	1074 (6)	659 (62)	9 (1)	3 (30)
Tamponade	108 (1)	42 (48)	44 (2)	15 (34)
Pulmonary				
Pneumothorax	1198 (6)	724 (60)	386 (13)	157 (41)
Pulmonary hemorrhage	853 (4)	384 (45)	132 (5)	42 (32)
Infectious				
Culture-proven	1280 (7)	704 (55)	610 (21)	283 (46)
WBC <1,500	85 (1)	37 (44)	96 (3)	32 (33)
Metabolic				
Glucose <40	591 (3)	352 (60)	26 (1)	6 (23)
Glucose >240	687 (4)	381 (55)	264 (9)	98 (37)
pH <7.2	584 (3)	201 (34)	129 (4)	32 (25)
pH >7.6	1195 (6)	892 (75)	54 (2)	37 (69)
Hyperbilirubinemia	1625 (8)	1069 (66)	93 (3)	26 (28)

DIC: disseminated intravascular coagulation
CNS: central nervous system
EEG: electroencephalogram
CAVHD: continuous arteriovenous hemodialysis
WBC: white blood cell
PDA: patent ductus arteriosus

neck cannulation site. Neck bleeding can be minimized by the liberal use of electrocautery at the time of surgical dissection, delaying systemic anticoagulation until completion of vessel exposure, and thorough hemostasis after cannulation with the use of a topical hemostatic agent. The standard practice of securing the ECMO cannulas with two silk ties over a vessel loop also minimizes the risk for excessive bleeding from the venotomy or arteriotomy sites.

Despite all these preventive measures, bleeding from the surgical wound frequently occurs. A key step in managing bleeding complications includes determining whether there is a significant amount of bleeding. A small volume of bleeding from minor surface oozing is quite common, but when a large amount of bleeding is noted (i.e., >10 cc/hr in a neonate), potentially catastrophic complications such as major vascular injury or displacement of the cannula out of the vessels may be imminent or may have already occurred. Neck wound bleeding most often occurs from a small vessel and can be controlled with finger pressure at the site, management of the heparin infusion rate, decreasing the ACT to 180-220 seconds, and maintaining the platelet count at >125,000/μl. Topical placement of hemostatic agents (e.g., Gelfoam thrombin, Oxycel, fibrin glue) can be helpful. If significant bleeding persists despite the treatment strategies outlined above, surgical exploration of the neck wound should not be delayed. Surgical re-exploration with evacuation of the clot and liberal use of cautery and hemostatic agents are helpful in achieving hemostasis.

Significant bleeding that is not attributable to the neck incision may represent a great risk and must be aggressively identified. A decreasing hemoglobin, tachycardia, hypotension, or a rise in the PaO_2 on venoarterial (VA) ECMO suggest the presence of acute bleeding. Intracranial, GI, intrathoracic, abdominal, and retroperitoneal bleeding have all been observed in patients on ECMO. Therefore, sudden changes

such as seizures, dilated pupils, cardiac tamponade with narrowed pulse pressure, abdominal distension, bloody stool, or blood nasogastric tube aspirate warrant immediate investigation by ultrasound or computed tomography (CT) scan when appropriate.

Patients who have undergone invasive procedures are at an increased risk for bleeding. For example, a patient who has undergone a congenital diaphragmatic hernia (CDH) repair is at an increased risk for post-operative bleeding. Procedures such as thoracostomy, suprapubic bladder aspiration, paracentesis, lumbar puncture, or vascular access, which are often considered routine for non-ECMO patients, present considerable risks for bleeding in ECMO patients. Initial management of bleeding includes lowering the ACT parameters (180-220 seconds) and ensuring the platelet count is >125,000 μl. Re-exploration of an operative site allows more direct control of potential bleeding sites; however, in general, bleeding is due to generalized oozing from systemic heparinization rather than from a surgical source. Occasionally, briefly discontinuing the heparin infusion should be considered to allow for hemostasis in spite of the increased risk of development of clots in the circuit, particularly in the membrane oxygenator.

When surgical procedures, such as diaphragmatic hernia repair, are performed immediately before or on ECMO, the following protocol for patient management is recommended in an effort to minimize bleeding complications. Pre-operatively, the platelet count should be >125,000/μl and the ACT 180-220 seconds. At the start of the operation, one unit of platelets and 10 cc/kg of FFP in neonates may be infused. Packed red blood cells (PRBCs) should be available for immediate infusion, if necessary. All tissues, including skin, are cut with electrocautery. Dissection is performed slowly with meticulous hemostasis and ligation of all identifiable vessels. A generous amount of topical hemostatic agent (e.g., fibrin glue, Gelfoam thrombin) should also be used. Operative field hemostasis must be confirmed prior to fascial and skin closures. Because of the risk for bleeding on ECMO, some centers favor repair of CDH after ECMO;[19] however, the ideal timing for CDH repair should be based on individual surgical and institutional experience.

When bleeding occurs into the intrathoracic, abdominal, or retroperitoneal cavity, it should be effectively drained and/or explored. Allowing such bleeding to tamponade is rarely successful and can often lead to profound hemodynamic decompensation. Several causes for hemodynamic deterioration and their appropriate management are described in Table 5. Blood loss should be replaced on a volume-for-volume basis. In the event that the bleeding continues despite blood product replacement and conservative management, a more aggressive approach to re-explore any wound or surgical site is usually necessary. If the bleeding presented with tamponade and hemodynamic decompensation, consideration should be given to leaving the wound open for delayed closure.

GI bleeding may be due to a mild gastritis and may respond to the above measures plus saline lavage, antacids, and/or H_2 blocker. In extreme cases, vasopressin may be used. Esophageal bleeding may be treated similarly, or balloon tamponade may be applied. A recommended strategy for the treatment of bleeding is summarized in Figure 3.

Heparin-bonded, non-thrombogenic circuits were developed to provide ECMO support with minimal or no systemic heparin administration. The use of heparin-bonded circuits also appears to decrease platelet, leukocytes, complement, and kinin system activation.[20] Despite initial enthusiasm for this new technology in patients with active bleeding, coagulopathy, or undergoing major operations while on ECMO, the experiences reported have been mixed.[10,21-24]

Both aminocaproic acid (Amicar) and aprotinin have been recommended as drugs to decrease bleeding and ICH complications during ECMO.[25-29] Wilson et al. reported that Amicar, an inhibitor of fibrinolysis, administered just prior to or after cannulation (100 mg/kg

Table 5. Differential diagnosis of cardiopulmonary decompensation during ECMO.

Etiology	Clinical findings	Diagnosis and management
Pericardial tamponade	VA: ↑PaO_2, ↓flow and perfusion VV: ↓PaO_2 and ↓tissue perfusion	Echocardiogram Pericardiocentesis or open window
Tension hemothorax and/or pneumothorax	VA: ↑PaO_2, ↓flow and perfusion VV: ↓PaO_2 and ↓tissue perfusion	Chest radiograph Needle or tube thoracostomy
Acute hypoxia	Oxygenator failure Disconnected sweep O_2	Check oxygenator for gas exchange or membrane leak Check O_2 tank and connection
Cardiac ischemia, electrolyte imbalance	Arrhythmia, labile HR ↓BP and tissue perfusion	Support CO with inotropes, fluids Correct electrolytes
Massive hemorrhage	Pallor or cyanosis, labile HR, ↓Hct, ↓BP, and ↓tissue perfusion	Cranial ultrasound Echocardiogram Ultrasound chest and/or abdomen
Sepsis	Shock, poor perfusion, DIC	Sepsis work-up Adjust antibiotics, pressors, fluids

DIC: disseminated intravascular coagulation

bolus, then 30 mg/kg/hr infusion) significantly decreased the incidence of ICH and other bleeding complications in high-risk neonates.[26] In contrast, Horwitz et al. reported that the incidence of significant ICH and overall transfusion requirements did not decrease in a multi-center trial when using Amicar for 72 hours in neonatal ECMO (excluding CDH patients).[30] There were no major thrombotic complications related to Amicar use in this study. Recently, Downward et al. reported a significant reduction in surgical site bleeding with the use of Amicar, but no change in the rate of ICH.[31]

Aprotinin is a naturally occurring protease inhibitor derived from the bovine lung which inhibits fibrinolysis and coagulation and has platelet-preserving properties.[20,28,29] Aprotinin has been shown to decrease bleeding during open heart surgery.[32] Brunet et al. reported that an aprotinin infusion (2×10^6 Kallikrein Inhibitor Units [KIU] loading dose, then 5×10^5 KIU/hr)

added to heparin stopped life-threatening bleeding in 2 adult patients during prolonged extracorporeal CO_2 removal.[25] Bleeding stopped a few hours after aprotinin infusion in both cases, but in the second patient, relapse immediately occurred when administration was discontinued; bleeding stopped again after restarting the aprotinin infusion. Further clinical trials are required to determine the safety and efficacy of aprotinin during prolonged ECMO. Other anticoagulant agents such as Nafamostat mesilate (a synthetic protease inhibitor) and Transexamic acid (a plasminogen inhibitor) have recently been reported to minimize the incidence of bleeding complications in ECMO patients.[33,34]

Neurologic complications

ICH remains a devastating complication for pediatric patients requiring ECMO support, occurring in 6% of patients <30 days and in

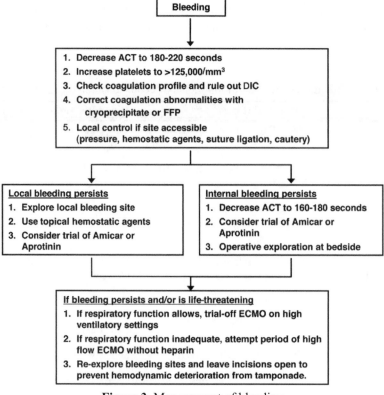

Figure 3. Management of bleeding.

5% in pediatric patients reported to the ELSO Registry. As a rule, the appearance of a new ICH or enlargement of a pre-existing bleed is an indication to discontinue ECMO support. Factors that increase the pressure gradient between the blood vessel lumen in the germinal matrix and the surrounding brain tissue increase the likelihood of small-vessel rupture and potential hemorrhage. Hypoxia may also directly injure brain capillary endothelial cells and lead to significant intracranial bleeding. In general, factors contributing to ICH in critically ill neonates include hypoxia, hypercapnia, acidosis, ischemia, hypotension, sepsis, coagulopathy, thrombocytopenia, venous hypertension, seizures, birth trauma, and rapid infusions of colloid or hypertonic solution. Premature infants are at greatest risk for experiencing ICH on ECMO. Recently, Hardart et al. reported that post-conceptual age was the best age-related predictor of ECMO-related ICH in premature infants (<37 weeks gestational age).[35]

During ECMO, patients are exposed to additional factors that may increase the risk of ICH. These factors include ligation of the right common carotid artery and internal jugular vein, systemic heparinization, thrombocytopenia, coagulopathy, and systolic hypertension.[35-37] Daily cranial ultrasound, especially during the first week on ECMO, can aid in the early diagnosis of ICH.[38] For VA ECMO support, ligation of the right common carotid artery and internal jugular vein is generally performed for cannula placement. This practice can decrease regional cerebral blood flow while simultaneously increasing cerebral venous pressure promoting ICH.[39] Schumacher et al. reported right-sided ICH lesions in 8 of 69 infants following ECMO support.[39] Others have not shown a higher incidence of right-sided CNS lesions with right common carotid arterial ligation.[40] Blood flow to the right cerebral hemisphere is usually preserved after right carotid artery ligation by collateral circulation via the external carotid artery and the anterior communicating artery

of the Circle of Willis. Non-invasive vascular studies have demonstrated adequate cerebral blood flow occurs during ECMO as well as early after decannulation[41,42] and in late follow-up.[43-45] Electroencephalographic (EEG) monitoring has also been utilized during neonatal ECMO and experience shows a lack of consistently lateralized abnormal tracings before, during, and after ECMO.[46] A few centers reconstruct the common carotid artery at decannulation, but that can also be associated with increased complications such as carotid dissection, thrombosis, emboli, or late stenosis.[47-52]

In addition to the obvious increased risk of intracranial bleeding from systemic heparinization, the ECMO circuit also exposes the patient's blood to a large surface area of foreign material, creating the setting for ongoing blood-surface interactions. Thrombocytopenia requiring platelet transfusions, altered platelet function, and activation of complement and white blood cells (WBCs) occur during extracorporeal circulation.[53-56] This list of potentially detrimental factors that may increase the risk and/or extent of ICH must be balanced against the cardiovascular stabilization and reversal of hypoxia, hypercapnia, and acidosis afforded by ECMO. Heparin infusion rates must be carefully adjusted to prevent large variations in the degree of anticoagulation, and hypertension must be avoided whenever possible and rapidly treated when present. Prior to the initiation of ECMO support, head ultrasound is mandatory for all patients to identify those in whom significant ICH is already present.

Patients on VV ECMO have a much lower rate of major neurologic complications when compared to VA ECMO patients. The incidence of seizures and associated survival rates (6% and 89% for VV vs. 13% and 61% for VA, respectively) or cerebral infarction (9% and 69% for VV vs. 14% and 46% for VA, respectively) are improved with VV; these favorable results for VV ECMO have had a substantial impact on overall survival;[1,2] however, no difference in neurologic outcomes has been proven.[57] Additionally, use of the cephalic jugular drainage for VV bypass can provide augmented venous flow and potentially prevent cerebral venous hypertension.[58]

Although better survival and neurologic complication rates on VV ECMO may be associated with lower severity of illness than in VA ECMO patients, the overall success of the technique persists. In a retrospective analysis of neonatal ECMO, birth weight and gestational age were the most significant correlates with the incidence of ICH.[36] Most programs have avoided the use of ECMO in infants <34 weeks gestation because of the high incidence of ICH. More importantly, post-conceptual age should be used to evaluate premature neonates for potential ECMO, rather than simply their postnatal age.[35] Modification of current ECMO technique may soon allow successful ECMO even in small premature infants. Bui et al. showed that the survival of moribund premature infants may be 50% or greater with ECMO using improved indications and technology.[59] Differentiation between pre-existing deficits and those secondary to ECMO remains difficult. However, some infants at high-risk for brain damage (low Apgar scores, perinatal cardiac arrest, profound hypoxia, and prolonged fetal distress) have normal neurodevelopmental outcome, so definitive predictors of outcome remained undetermined.

In the program at Galveston, ECMO is discontinued in patients when ICH is associated with profound clinical deterioration including flaccidity and fixed pupils. Patients without clinical signs of ICH (ultrasound diagnosis only) are maintained at lower ACT parameters (180-220 seconds) with platelet counts kept >125,000/μl. Repeat cranial ultrasound examinations are performed and ECMO is discontinued if ICH progresses or when the patient can be supported on mechanical ventilation, even if higher ventilator pressures are necessary.

Hematologic complications

Thrombocytopenia is expected during the use of ECMO as platelets are activated and aggregate in the extracorporeal circuit and preferentially are then sequestered in the lung, liver, and spleen.[6,53] Thrombocytopenia is a result of decreased production, increased consumption, sequestration or removal to extravascular sites, and dilution. In addition, hypoxia has been shown to be a factor in the inhibition of platelet production by blood-forming organs. Thrombocytopenia can occur up to 4 days after the termination of ECMO for the treatment of neonatal respiratory failure; therefore, platelet counts need to be measured frequently during this period.[53] Severe antecedent hypoxia has also been correlated with the development of thrombocytopenia after ECMO. Furthermore, severe coagulation factor deficiencies often pre-exist in patients requiring ECMO, contributing to their potential bleeding problems.[60]

Instability of previously well-controlled coagulation parameters (ACT, platelet count, fibrinogen) may be an early predictor of a bleeding event.[61,62] Hemolysis is a complication often related to the ECMO membrane and/or circuit.[63] Clots in the circuit or membrane may also promote coagulopathy by activation of complement, WBCs, platelets, or coagulation factors that cause erythrocytes to adhere and lyse on the fibrin strands. These theories are reinforced by data that show decreased plasma-free hemoglobin levels after membrane and circuit change-out.[64]

A recommended algorithm managing hemolysis is outlined in Figure 4. Recently, silicone rubber, ultrathin, hollow fiber membrane has been shown to produce significantly less hemolysis and improved gas exchange for long-term ECMO due to its nonporous characteristics.[65] This extracapillary-type ECMO oxygenator was developed for pediatric applications and demonstrated a higher gas transfer rate, lower blood flow resistance, and less hemolysis when compared to conventional silicone, coil-type ECMO membrane oxygenators. This type of membrane oxygenator may significantly minimize hemolysis complications, which are routinely encountered particularly with prolonged ECMO support.

Renal insufficiency

Oliguria during ECMO is common, especially during the first 24-48 hours. An ultrasound of the kidneys is commonly performed to exclude major anatomic anomalies that could be responsible for renal insufficiency refractory to diuretics such as furosemide. Sell et al.[66] reported the use of continuous hemofiltration for renal failure during ECMO. The apparatus is easily added in-line to the ECMO circuit and allows a removal of excess volume and solutes while retaining the proteins and cellular components of the intravascular space. The classic indications for dialysis are the same for its use on ECMO: hypervolemia, hyperkalemia,

acidosis, and azotemia. Hyperkalemia and hypervolemia are easily managed with continuous hemofiltration, but azotemia is more difficult to manage due to chronic hemolysis and occult GI bleeding.

Cardiopulmonary complications

Systemic hypertension is a common and potentially serious complication of ECMO. Sell et al.[67] reported that 38 of 41 newborns (93%) treated with ECMO developed systolic blood pressures >90 mm Hg. 44% of those with hypertension developed detectable ICH, and 27% developed clinically significant ICH. Utilization of a medical management protocol using hydralazine, nitroglycerine, and captopril decreased the incidence of clinically significant ICH from 50%, prior to protocol therapy, to 9% following protocol therapy. Boedy et al.[68] also reviewed the incidence of hypertension during ECMO by determining blood pressure measurements from indwelling aortic catheters in 31 in-

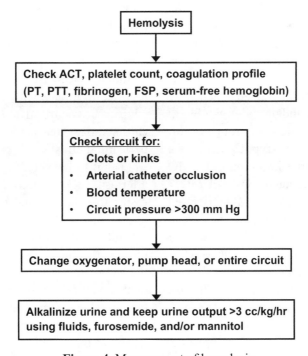

Figure 4. Management of hemolysis.

fants placed on ECMO. Systemic hypertension, defined as systolic blood pressures >100 mm Hg for ≥ 4 consecutive hours, occurred in 18 of the 31 neonates. There was no evidence of increased plasma renin activities in hypertensive infants when compared with pre-ECMO controls or with the normotensive infants. Sodium and colloid loads were also not significantly different between hypertensive and normotensive neonates. Additionally, the duration of ECMO support was not found to be associated with development of hypertension (mean time on ECMO at onset of hypertension was 43.8 ±38.5 hours; range, 1-142 hours). Interestingly, their data indicated that hypertension did not seem to predispose neonates to an increased incidence of ICH. At Galveston, hydralazine is used (0.1 mg/kg IV) for systolic blood pressure >90 mm Hg with effective control of blood pressure.

It is unusual to have catastrophic hemodynamic deterioration while a patient is on VA bypass. Immediate evaluation should focus on venous catheter displacement, adequacy of systemic volume status, and the possibility of circuit failure. Major cardiac dysfunction is usually not appreciated during VA bypass with full flow (120 ml/kg/min). In infants, some degree of cardiac depression is fairly common early in the course of ECMO, particularly with severely asphyxiated patients.[69,70] Coronary arterial and abdominal organ blood flow is predominantly derived from the left ventricle during ECMO.[71] Hypocalcemia is a frequent occurrence after initiation of ECMO and can contribute to hypotension on ECMO.[72] "Stunned myocardium" after ECMO is defined as left ventricular shortening fraction decreasing by ≥25% with initiation of ECMO and returning to normal after 48 hours on ECMO.[69,70] This syndrome may occur despite relief of hypoxia. Underlying congenital heart disease can also be masked by respiratory failure in 2% of ECMO cases.[73] VA bypass is preferred over VV support when the patient presents with labile or unstable hemodynamics.

If cardiac arrest, dysrhythmia, or a drop in cardiac output secondary to severe myocardial dysfunction occurs, the initial treatment while on VA ECMO is to increase the pump flow. This may require the addition of blood volume to the circuit. The cause of the acute event can then be identified and treated. Treatment may include the administration of standard cardiac medications, anti-arrhythmic agents, inotropic agents, and/or correction of electrolyte abnormalities. If the pump flow cannot be increased sufficiently to compensate for a significant fall in cardiac output, or if the patient is on VV ECMO, this event must be handled much the same as a cardiac arrest in any other non-ECMO patient. The most common cause of cardiac dysfunction in ventilated neonates remains hypoxia from respiratory causes rather than cardiac failure. First, check the ECMO circuit, oxygenator, and endotracheal tube; listen for breath sounds; and hand ventilate the patient. Assess the infant for the development of a tension hemothorax or pneumothorax. The reason the desired ECMO flows cannot be achieved may be that venous return to the heart is being impeded by accumulating blood or air in the chest or pericardium.[74] The differential diagnosis of cardiopulmonary decompensation and its management are shown in Table 5. Decreased survival rates have been reported in infants with cardiovascular events such as myocardial stun, arrhythmia, and cardiac arrest, but not with hypertension and pericardial effusion.[75]

Right-to-left shunting via the patent ductus arteriosus (PDA) is frequently seen with severe respiratory failure and persistent pulmonary hypertension of the newborn (PPHN). With resolution of pulmonary hypertension, flow through the ductus reverses (left-to-right), and the PDA usually closes within 24 hours. The ductus may remain patent with significant left-to-right shunting and may lead to pulmonary edema resulting in decreased systemic blood flow and oxygenation. In an animal study, a considerable left-to-right shunt via the ductus during VA ECMO has been shown to reduce cerebral blood flow and oxygenation.[76] Likewise, if renal failure occurs and a previous hypoxic or ischemic insult cannot be identified, then the possibility of decreased renal perfusion during ECMO from a PDA must be considered. A PDA on ECMO may present with any of the following: a decreased PaO_2, an increased $PaCO_2$, decreased peripheral perfusion, acidosis, and/or increasing ECMO flow and volume requirements. The clinical diagnosis may be confirmed using doppler echocardiography. Some centers have tried using IV indomethacin to treat PDA while on ECMO; however, many clinicians discourage this practice because of the effect on platelet function, which increases the risks of bleeding. Once the diagnosis is established, diuretics are used while maintaining ECMO flow until the PDA closes. Neonates with left-to-right ductal shunt will experience prolonged ECMO bypass time, possibly because of interactions with pulmonary and renal function.[77] Recently, a successful non-invasive transcatheter closure of PDA was reported;[78] however, surgical ligation is associated with bleeding complications and is rarely necessary.[75]

Intrathoracic complications

Pericardial tamponade and tension hemothorax or pneumothorax all have a similar pathophysiology of increasing intrapericardial pressure and decreasing venous return (Figure 5). With decreased venous return to the heart, the pulmonary blood and native cardiac output are decreased, and the relative contribution of the extracorporeal circuit to peripheral perfusion is increased. Therefore, peripheral perfusion is initially maintained by the non-pulsatile flow of the ECMO. The peripheral PaO_2 may increase while the patient may exhibit decreased perfusion with a narrowed pulse pressure, along with a decrease in oxygen delivery as evidenced by a drop in SvO_2. The triad of increased PaO_2,

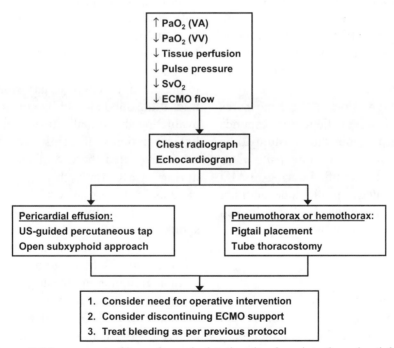

Figure 5. Management of hemodynamic deterioration from intrathoracic etiology.

poor peripheral perfusion, and decreased venous return with progressive hemodynamic deterioration is consistently associated with tension pneumothorax (Figure 5).[74]

The diagnosis of tension hemothorax and pneumothorax is best confirmed by chest radiograph. A persistent drop in hemoglobin despite transfusion, along with thoracic opacity, may suggest the presence of significant hemothorax. Pericardial tamponade may be suggested on plain chest radiograph by enlargement of the cardiac silhouette. However, an echocardiogram can identify a pericardial effusion as well as document the degree of hemodynamic compromise.

For emergency treatment of both tension hemothorax and pneumothorax, and cardiac tamponade, the placement of a percutaneous drainage catheter is recommended. For cardiac tamponade, the placement of an angiocatheter into the pericardium using ultrasound guidance can accomplish initial relief of hemodynamic decompensation. A guide wire may then be passed using modified Seldinger technique to place a multi-holed drainage tube. A 5F pediatric feeding tube, peritoneal dialysis catheter, or other type of catheter may be successfully used for this purpose. For hemothorax or pneumothorax, an angiocatheter or chest tube may be used for emergent decompression. If these measures are unsuccessful or the patient only responds transiently, an emergency thoracostomy tube is necessary. As noted, any time a site of abnormal bleeding is identified during ECMO, the immediate strategy must include modification of the anticoagulation regimen followed by surgical exploration if bleeding persists.

Infection

Sepsis is both an indication for and a complication of ECMO. Based on recent ELSO Registry data, infants uncommonly demonstrate positive culture-proven sepsis (6%). However, in pediatric, cardiac, and adult ECMO patients, the incidence of septic complications during ECMO with positive cultures ranges from 10-22% with <50% survival. In general, patients requiring ECMO support for sepsis have a much poorer overall outcome. Septic patients also have a greater frequency of other complications such as seizures, GI tract bleed, and renal dysfunction; the prognosis is poor, especially for those with fungal infections.[79,80] All ECMO patients should receive prophylactic antibiotic coverage against gram positive organisms, and frequent surveillance cultures must be obtained to closely monitor patients.

Gastrointestinal complications

Traditionally, patients were not fed and instead maintained on total parental nutrition (TPN) while on ECMO. Direct hyperbilirubinemia due to cholestasis was found to be common;[81] however, it typically resolves without sequelae and is probably related to hemolysis as well as cholestasis. Biliary calculi have been reported in 2 of 121 patients in post-ECMO follow-up.[82] The hemolysis, TPN, diuretics, and prolonged fasting associated with ECMO may predispose patients to the development of biliary stones. Biliary tract ultrasound should be considered when evaluating abdominal pain or jaundice in post-ECMO patients. Recently, several centers have advocated the use of enteral feedings during ECMO for both pediatric and adult patients.[83,84] Hanekamp et al. recently reported that the gut hormone levels show normal responses after the introduction of enteral feeding on ECMO in neonates, comparable with those in non-ECMO age-matched controls, further strengthening the argument for use of enteral nutrition even in the most severely ill neonates on ECMO.[85] Patients on either VV or VA ECMO can tolerate enteral nutrition without complications.[83,85,86]

Failure to wean

There are no strict guidelines on the exact duration of ECMO support. Each case requires an ongoing assessment of risk and benefit. With the emergence of more complicated etiologies for cardiopulmonary failure requiring ECMO support, prolonged ECMO runs are becoming more common. In general, after 2-3 weeks of ECMO support without significant pulmonary improvement, diuretics and/or a hemofilter are used to remove additional fluid. Ventilator support is increased to the maximal acceptable pressures along with inspired oxygen. An echocardiogram is repeated to determine the presence of a PDA with predominant left-to-right shunt and to, once again, rule out congenital heart disease such as total anomalous pulmonary venous return. A trial off ECMO is then attempted with maximum tolerable ventilator settings. If the trial off ECMO is unsuccessful, then cardiac catheterization and/or open lung biopsy should be considered to identify potentially irreversible conditions such as congenital pulmonary lymphangiectasia, alveolar capillary dysplasia, or cyanotic congenital heart disease. If no correctable lesions are found, a decision must be made to discontinue ECMO support or to continue indefinitely if there is a perceived potential for improvement or objective signs of improvement without any complications. A recommended management response in the case of failure to wean off ECMO is outlined in Figure 6.

Summary

Complications during ECMO frequently occur and range from minor to potentially fatal. They can be classified as mechanical- or patient-related complications. Any component of the circuit can fail, and constant checks and monitoring can prevent most problems from becoming serious. Bleeding related to systemic heparinization is the most common and frequently serious complication during ECMO. The appropriate management of these clinical problems requires thorough knowledge of the patients' underlying pathophysiology and of the ECMO circuit, as well as clinical experience.

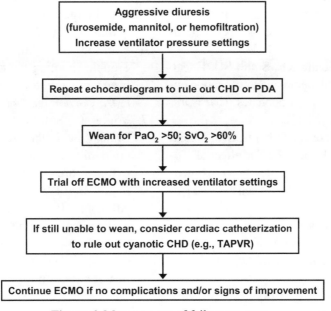

Figure 6. Management of failure to wean.

References

1. Upp JR Jr, Bush PE, Zwischenberger JB. Complications of neonatal extracorporeal membrane oxygenation. *Perfusion* 1994; 9:241-256.

2. Zwischenberger JB, Nguyen TT, Upp JR Jr, et al. Complications of neonatal extracorporeal membrane oxygenation. Collective experience from the Extracorporeal Life Support Organization. *J Thorac Cardiovasc Surg* 1994; 107:838-848; discussion 848-839.

3 ELSO Data Registry Report: International Summary. Ann Arbor, MI: University of Michigan, January 2005.

4. Cavarocchi NC, England MD, Schaff HV, et al. Oxygen free radical generation during cardiopulmonary bypass: correlation with complement activation. *Circulation* 1986; 74: III 130-133.

5. Eberhart RC. Interactions of blood and artificial surfaces: In search of "heparin-free" cardiopulmonary bypass. In: Arensman RM, Cornish JD, Eds. *Extracorporeal Life Support.* Boston, MA: Blackwell Scientific Publications; 1993: 105-125.

6. Robinson TM, Kickler TS, Walker LK, Ness P, Bell W. Effect of extracorporeal membrane oxygenation on platelets in newborns. *Crit Care Med* 1993; 21:1029-1034.

7. DePuydt LE, Schuit KE, Smith SD. Effect of extracorporeal membrane oxygenation on neutrophil function in neonates. *Crit Care Med* 1993; 21:1324-1327.

8. Bergman P, Belboul A, Friberg LG, al-Khaja N, Mellgren G, Roberts D. The effect of prolonged perfusion with a membrane oxygenator (PPMO) on white blood cells. *Perfusion* 1994; 9:35-40.

9. Rossaint R, Slama K, Lewandowski K, et al. Extracorporeal lung assist with heparin-coated systems. *Int J Artif Organs* 1992; 15:29-34.

10. Muehrcke DD, McCarthy PM, Stewart RW, et al. Complications of extracorporeal life support systems using heparin-bound surfaces. The risk of intracardiac clot formation. *J Thorac Cardiovasc Surg* 1995; 110:843-851.

11. Murphy JA, Savage CM, Alpard SK, Deyo DJ, Jayroe JB, Zwischenberger JB. Low-dose versus high-dose heparinization during arteriovenous carbon dioxide removal. *Perfusion* 2001; 16:460-468.

12. Okamoto T, Ichinose K, Tanimoto H, et al. Preliminary experiment with a newly developed double balloon, double lumen catheter for extracorporeal life support vascular access. *ASAIO J* 2003; 49:583-588.

13. Rais-Bahrami K, Walton DM, Sell JE, Rivera O, Mikesell GT, Short BL. Improved oxygenation with reduced recirculation during venovenous ECMO: comparison of two catheters. *Perfusion* 2002; 17:415-419.

14. Irish MS, O'Toole SJ, Kapur P, et al. Cervical ECMO cannula placement in infants and children: recommendations for assessment of adequate positioning and function. *J Pediatr Surg* 1998; 33:929-931.

15. Rais-Bahrami K, Martin GR, Schnitzer JJ, Short BL. Malposition of extracorporeal membrane oxygenation cannulas in patients with congenital diaphragmatic hernia. *J Pediatr* 1993; 122:794-797.

16. Faulkner SC, Chipman CW, Baker LL. Trouble shooting the extracorporeal membrane oxygenator circuit and patient. *J Extra Corpor Technol* 1993; 24:120-129.

17. Vogler C, Sotelo-Avila C, Lagunoff D, Braun P, Schreifels JA, Weber T. Aluminum-containing emboli in infants treated with extracorporeal membrane oxygenation. *N Engl J Med* 1988; 319:75-79.

18. Atkinson JB, Gomperts ED, Kang R, et al. Prospective, randomized evaluation of the efficacy of fibrin sealant as a topical hemostatic agent at the cannulation site in neonates undergoing extracorporeal membrane oxygenation. *Am J Surg* 1997; 173:479-484.

19. Sigalet DL, Tierney A, Adolph V, et al. Timing of repair of congenital diaphragmatic hernia requiring extracorporeal membrane oxygenation support. *J Pediatr Surg* 1995; 30:1183-1187.

20. Plotz FB, van Oeveren W, Bartlett RH, Wildevuur CR. Blood activation during neonatal extracorporeal life support. *J Thorac Cardiovasc Surg* 1993; 105:823-832.

21. Chen YS, Ko WJ, Lin FY, Huang SC, Wang SS, Tu YK. New application of heparin-bonded extracorporeal membrane oxygenation in difficult neurosurgery. *Artif Organs* 2001; 25:627-632.

22. Bianchi JJ, Swartz MT, Raithel SC, et al. Initial clinical experience with centrifugal pumps coated with the Carmeda process. *ASAIO J* 1992; 38:M143-146.

23. Tsuno K, Terasaki H, Otsu T, Okamoto T, Sakanashi Y, Morioka T. Newborn extracorporeal lung assist using a novel double lumen catheter and a heparin-bonded membrane lung. *Intensive Care Med* 1993; 19:70-72.

24. Toomasian JM, Hsu LC, Hirschl RB, Heiss KF, Hultquist KA, Bartlett RH. Evaluation of Duraflo II heparin coating in prolonged extracorporeal membrane oxygenation. *ASAIO Trans* 1988; 34:410-414.

25. Brunet F, Mira JP, Belghith M, et al. Effects of aprotinin on hemorrhagic complications in ARDS patients during prolonged extracorporeal CO2 removal. *Intensive Care Med* 1992; 18:364-367.

26. Wilson JM, Bower LK, Fackler JC, Beals DA, Bergus BO, Kevy SV. Aminocaproic acid decreases the incidence of intracranial hemorrhage and other hemorrhagic complications of ECMO. *J Pediatr Surg* 1993; 28:536-540; discussion 540-531.

27. Feindt P, Volkmer I, Seyfert U, Huwer H, Kalweit G, Gams E. Activated clotting time, anticoagulation, use of heparin, and thrombin activation during extracorporeal circulation: changes under aprotinin therapy. *Thorac Cardiovasc Surg* 1993; 41:9-15.

28. Spannagl M, Dietrich W, Beck A, Schramm W. High dose aprotinin reduces prothrombin and fibrinogen conversion in patients undergoing extracorporeal circulation for myocardial revascularization. *Thromb Haemost* 1994; 72:159-160.

29. Wachtfogel YT, Kucich U, Hack CE, et al. Aprotinin inhibits the contact, neutrophil, and platelet activation systems during simulated extracorporeal perfusion. *J Thorac Cardiovasc Surg* 1993; 106:1-9; discussion 9-10.

30. Horwitz JR, Cofer BR, Warner BW, Cheu HW, Lally KP. A multicenter trial of 6-aminocaproic acid (Amicar) in the prevention of bleeding in infants on ECMO. *J Pediatr Surg* 1998; 33:1610-1613.

31. Downard CD, Betit P, Chang RW, Garza JJ, Arnold JH, Wilson JM. Impact of AMICAR on hemorrhagic complications of ECMO: a ten-year review. *J Pediatr Surg* 2003; 38:1212-1216.

32. Dietrich W, Barankay A, Dilthey G, et al. Reduction of homologous blood requirement in cardiac surgery by intraoperative aprotinin application--clinical experience in 152 cardiac surgical patients. *Thorac Cardiovasc Surg* 1989; 37:92-98.

33. Nagaya M, Futamura M, Kato J, Niimi N, Fukuta S. Application of a new anticoagulant (Nafamostat Mesilate) to control hemorrhagic complications during extracorporeal membrane oxygenation--a preliminary report. *J Pediatr Surg* 1997; 32:531-535.

34. van der Staak FH, de Haan AF, Geven WB, Festen C. Surgical repair of congenital diaphragmatic hernia during extracorporeal membrane oxygenation: hemorrhagic complications and the effect of tranexamic acid. *J Pediatr Surg* 1997; 32:594-599.

35. Hardart GE, Hardart MK, Arnold JH. Intracranial hemorrhage in premature neonates treated with extracorporeal membrane

oxygenation correlates with conceptional age. *J Pediatr* 2004; 145:184-189.

36. Cilley RE, Zwischenberger JB, Andrews AF, Bowerman RA, Roloff DW, Bartlett RH. Intracranial hemorrhage during extracorporeal membrane oxygenation in neonates. *Pediatrics* 1986; 78:699-704.

37. Hardart GE, Fackler JC. Predictors of intracranial hemorrhage during neonatal extracorporeal membrane oxygenation. *J Pediatr* 1999; 134:156-159.

38. Khan AM, Shabarek FM, Zwischenberger JB, et al. Utility of daily head ultrasonography for infants on extracorporeal membrane oxygenation. *J Pediatr Surg* 1998; 33:1229-1232.

39. Schumacher RE, Barks JD, Johnston MV, et al. Right-sided brain lesions in infants following extracorporeal membrane oxygenation. *Pediatrics* 1988; 82:155-161.

40. Campbell LR, Bunyapen C, Holmes GL, Howell CG Jr., Kanto WP Jr. Right common carotid artery ligation in extracorporeal membrane oxygenation. *J Pediatr* 1988; 113:110-113.

41. Raju TN, Kim SY, Meller JL, Srinivasan G, Ghai V, Reyes H. Circle of Willis blood velocity and flow direction after common carotid artery ligation for neonatal extracorporeal membrane oxygenation. *Pediatrics* 1989; 83:343-347.

42. Lohrer RM, Bejar RF, Simko AJ, Moulton SL, Cornish JD. Internal carotid artery blood flow velocities before, during, and after extracorporeal membrane oxygenation. *Am J Dis Child* 1992; 146:201-207.

43. Towne BH, Lott IT, Hicks DA, Healey T. Long-term follow-up of infants and children treated with extracorporeal membrane oxygenation (ECMO): a preliminary report. *J Pediatr Surg* 1985; 20:410-414.

44. Taylor GA, Short BL, Fitz CR. Imaging of cerebrovascular injury in infants treated with extracorporeal membrane oxygenation. *J Pediatr* 1989; 114:635-639.

45. Lott IT, McPherson D, Towne B, Johnson D, Starr A. Long-term neurophysiologic outcome after neonatal extracorporeal membrane oxygenation. *J Pediatr* 1990; 116:343-349.

46. Streletz LJ, Bej MD, Graziani LJ, et al. Utility of serial EEGs in neonates during extracorporeal membrane oxygenation. *Pediatr Neurol* 1992; 8:190-196.

47. Spector ML, Wiznitzer M, Walsh-Sukys MC, Stork EK. Carotid reconstruction in the neonate following ECMO. *J Pediatr Surg* 1991; 26:357-359; discussion 359-361.

48. Baumgart S, Streletz LJ, Needleman L, et al. Right common carotid artery reconstruction after extracorporeal membrane oxygenation: vascular imaging, cerebral circulation, electroencephalographic, and neurodevelopmental correlates to recovery. *J Pediatr* 1994; 125:295-304.

49. Moulton SL, Lynch FP, Cornish JD, Bejar RF, Simko AJ, Krous HF. Carotid artery reconstruction following neonatal extracorporeal membrane oxygenation. *J Pediatr Surg* 1991; 26:794-799.

50. Desai SA, Stanley C, Gringlas M, et al. Five-year follow-up of neonates with reconstructed right common carotid arteries after extracorporeal membrane oxygenation. *J Pediatr* 1999; 134:428-433.

51. Levy MS, Share JC, Fauza DO, Wilson JM. Fate of the reconstructed carotid artery after extracorporeal membrane oxygenation. *J Pediatr Surg* 1995; 30:1046-1049.

52. Cheung PY, Vickar DB, Hallgren RA, Finer NN, Robertson CM. Carotid artery reconstruction in neonates receiving extracorporeal membrane oxygenation: a 4-year follow-up study. Western Canadian ECMO Follow-Up Group. *J Pediatr Surg* 1997; 32:560-564.

53. Anderson HL III, Cilley RE, Zwischenberger JB, Bartlett RH. Thrombocytopenia in neonates after extracorporeal membrane

oxygenation. *ASAIO Trans* 1986; 32:534-537.

54. Vallhonrat H, Swinford RD, Ingelfinger JR, et al. Rapid activation of the alternative pathway of complement by extracorporeal membrane oxygenation. *ASAIO J* 1999; 45:113-114.

55. Graulich J, Sonntag J, Marcinkowski M, et al. Complement activation by in vivo neonatal and in vitro extracorporeal membrane oxygenation. *Mediators Inflamm* 2002; 11:69-73.

56. Peek GJ, Firmin RK. The inflammatory and coagulative response to prolonged extracorporeal membrane oxygenation. *ASAIO J* 1999; 45:250-263.

57. Van Meurs KP, Nguyen HT, Rhine WD, Marks MP, Fleisher BE, Benitz WE. Intracranial abnormalities and neurodevelopmental status after venovenous extracorporeal membrane oxygenation. *J Pediatr* 1994; 125:304-307.

58. Finer NN, Tierney AJ, Ainsworth W. Venovenous extracorporeal membrane oxygenation: the effects of proximal internal jugular cannulation. *J Pediatr Surg* 1996; 31:1391-1395.

59. Bui KC, LaClair P, Vanderkerhove J, Bartlett RH. ECMO in premature infants. Review of factors associated with mortality. *ASAIO Trans* 1991; 37:54-59.

60. McManus ML, Kevy SV, Bower LK, Hickey PR. Coagulation factor deficiencies during initiation of extracorporeal membrane oxygenation. *J Pediatr* 1995; 126:900-904.

61. Hirthler MA, Blackwell E, Abbe D, et al. Coagulation parameter instability as an early predictor of intracranial hemorrhage during extracorporeal membrane oxygenation. *J Pediatr Surg* 1992; 27:40-43.

62. Stallion A, Cofer BR, Rafferty JA, Ziegler MM, Ryckman FC. The significant relationship between platelet count and haemorrhagic complications on ECMO. *Perfusion* 1994; 9:265-269.

63. Kawahito S, Maeda T, Motomura T, et al. Hemolytic characteristics of oxygenators during clinical extracorporeal membrane oxygenation. *ASAIO J* 2002; 48:636-639.

64. Steinhorn RH, Isham-Schopf B, Smith C, Green TP. Hemolysis during long-term extracorporeal membrane oxygenation. *J Pediatr* 1989; 115:625-630.

65. Motomura T, Maeda T, Kawahito S, et al. Development of silicone rubber hollow fiber membrane oxygenator for ECMO. *Artif Organs* 2003; 27:1050-1053.

66. Sell LL, Cullen ML, Whittlesey GC, Lerner GR, Klein MD. Experience with renal failure during extracorporeal membrane oxygenation: treatment with continuous hemofiltration. *J Pediatr Surg* 1987; 22:600-602.

67. Sell LL, Cullen ML, Lerner GR, Whittlesey GC, Shanley CJ, Klein MD. Hypertension during extracorporeal membrane oxygenation: cause, effect, and management. *Surgery* 1987; 102:724-730.

68. Boedy RF, Goldberg AK, Howell CG Jr, Hulse E, Edwards EG, Kanto WP Jr. Incidence of hypertension in infants on extracorporeal membrane oxygenation. *J Pediatr Surg* 1990; 25:258-261.

69. Martin GR, Short BL, Abbott C, O'Brien AM. Cardiac stun in infants undergoing extracorporeal membrane oxygenation. *J Thorac Cardiovasc Surg* 1991; 101:607-611.

70. Holley DG, Short BL, Karr SS, Martin GR. Mechanisms of change in cardiac performance in infants undergoing extracorporeal membrane oxygenation. *Crit Care Med* 1994; 22:1865-1870.

71. Kinsella JP, Gerstmann DR, Rosenberg AA. The effect of extracorporeal membrane oxygenation on coronary perfusion and regional blood flow distribution. *Pediatr Res* 1992; 31:80-84.

72. Meliones JN, Moler FW, Custer JR, et al. Hemodynamic instability after the initiation

of extracorporeal membrane oxygenation: role of ionized calcium. *Crit Care Med* 1991; 19:1247-1251.

73. Palmisano JM, Moler FW, Custer JR, Meliones JN, Snedecor S, Revesz SM. Unsuspected congenital heart disease in neonates receiving extracorporeal life support: a review of ninety-five cases from the Extracorporeal Life Support Organization Registry. *J Pediatr* 1992; 121:115-117.

74. Zwischenberger JB, Bartlett RH. Extracorporeal circulation for respiratory or cardiac failure. *Semin Thorac Cardiovasc Surg* 1990; 2:320-331.

75. Becker JA, Short BL, Martin GR. Cardiovascular complications adversely affect survival during extracorporeal membrane oxygenation. *Crit Care Med* 1998; 26:1582-1586.

76. van Heijst AF, van der Staak FH, Hopman JC, Tanke RB, Sengers RC, Liem KD. Ductus arteriosus with left-to-right shunt during venoarterial extracorporeal membrane oxygenation: effects on cerebral oxygenation and hemodynamics. *Pediatr Crit Care Med* 2003; 4:94-99.

77. Tanke R, Daniels O, Van Heyst A, Van Lier H, Festen C. The influence of ductal left-to-right shunting during extracorporeal membrane oxygenation. *J Pediatr Surg* 2002; 37:1165-1168.

78. Brown KL, Shekerdemian LS, Penny DJ. Transcatheter closure of a patent arterial duct in a patient on veno-arterial extracorporeal membrane oxygenation. *Intensive Care Med* 2002; 28:501-503.

79. Douglass BH, Keenan AL, Purohit DM. Bacterial and fungal infection in neonates undergoing venoarterial extracorporeal membrane oxygenation: an analysis of the registry data of the extracorporeal life support organization. *Artif Organs* 1996; 20:202-208.

80. Meyer DM, Jessen ME, Eberhart RC. Neonatal extracorporeal membrane oxygenation complicated by sepsis. Extracorporeal Life Support Organization. *Ann Thorac Surg* 1995; 59:975-980.

81. Walsh-Sukys MC, Cornell DJ, Stork EK. The natural history of direct hyperbilirubinemia associated with extracorporeal membrane oxygenation. *Am J Dis Child* 1992; 146:1176-1180.

82. Almond PS, Adolph VR, Steiner R, Hill CB, Falterman KW, Arensman RM. Calculous disease of the biliary tract in infants after neonatal extracorporeal membrane oxygenation. *J Perinatal* 1992; 12:18-20.

83. Scott LK, Boudreaux K, Thaljeh F, Grier LR, Conrad SA. Early enteral feedings in adults receiving venovenous extracorporeal membrane oxygenation. *JPEN J Parenter Enteral Nutr* 2004; 28:295-300.

84. Piena M, Albers MJ, Van Haard PM, Gischler S, Tibboel D. Introduction of enteral feeding in neonates on extracorporeal membrane oxygenation after evaluation of intestinal permeability changes. *J Pediatr Surg* 1998; 33:30-34.

85. Hanekamp MN, Spoel M, Sharman-Koendjbiharie M, et al. Gut hormone profiles in critically ill neonates on extracorporeal membrane oxygenation. *J Pediatr Gastroenterol Nutr* 2005; 40:175-179.

86. Pettignano R, Heard M, Davis R, Labuz M, Hart M. Total enteral nutrition versus total parenteral nutrition during pediatric extracorporeal membrane oxygenation. *Crit Care Med* 1998; 26:358-363.

9

Referral and Transport of ECMO Patients

Robert J. DiGeronimo, M.D., Cody L. Henderson, M.D., and Peter H. Grubb, M.D.

Introduction

Determination of appropriate timing for referral and transport of patients who are candidates for ECMO remains extremely challenging. The use of ECMO has expanded over the past two decades beyond neonatal respiratory failure. Currently, ECMO is accepted as a rescue modality to support a variety of etiologies of reversible cardiopulmonary failure in both children and adults including acute respiratory distress syndrome (ARDS), trauma, cardiac failure, and, in some cases, as a bridge to transplant. Advances in critical care medicine coupled with this expanded role for ECMO have complicated our ability to define criteria for ECMO. It is more difficult to identify which patients ultimately will not respond to conventional management and when these patients should be considered for referral to an ECMO center. Thus, a common goal for both non-ECMO and ECMO centers alike is early recognition and safe transfer of those patients who might benefit from ECMO, reducing not only mortality but morbidity.[1]

In the neonatal population, the widespread dissemination of adjunctive therapies such as high frequency ventilation (HFV), surfactant, and inhaled nitric oxide (iNO) to non-ECMO centers has raised concerns that their use may be delaying referral for ECMO because of ill-defined failure criteria.[2-4] Boedy et al. in 1990 was the first to describe the idea that there exists a "hidden" mortality associated with ECMO referral.[5] They reported that 12% of 158 outborn neonates referred to their center for ECMO died either before, during, or shortly after transport to their hospital. The University of Michigan additionally reported that 10% of their non-neonatal referrals for ECMO between 1988 and 1990 either died during conventional transport or were denied transport because of cardiorespiratory instability.[6] This "hidden" mortality is difficult to quantify for the ECMO community as a whole since these data are not reported. However, the experience of an unstable patient dying during the transport process is nearly universal among ECMO centers. Until improved modes of conventional transport become widely available and more reliable criteria are established to identify pre-ECMO patients, the safe movement of critically ill patients to ECMO centers will remain problematic.

Recent advances in inter-hospital transport have enhanced our ability to safely move ECMO candidates. These advances include the use of iNO,[7] HFV,[8,9] and circulatory assist devices other than ECMO.[10-12] Another alternative method of transporting unstable patients who meet ECMO criteria is to perform mobile ECMO. This approach has been adopted by several centers in the U.S., to include Wilford Hall Medical Center (WHMC), Arkansas Children's Hospital (ACH), and the University of Michigan Medical Center (UMMC), as well as the Karolinska Hospital in Sweden, and the Virchow-Klinikum in Germany.[4,6,13-15] Development of a mobile ECMO program should only be seriously considered by regional ECMO programs whose referral population would potentially benefit from having this capability. The personnel and equipment necessary to safely perform transport ECMO, as well as the distances often involved in moving these patients, are significantly different than those required for conventional transport. It is essential that those centers that develop mobile ECMO programs continue to encourage early referral and transport by conventional means as the safest and often most rapid alternative for ECMO candidates.

This chapter will discuss the process of ECMO referral, including advances in conventional transport, as well as give an overview of experience and requirements for performing inter- and intra-hospital mobile ECMO transport.

Referral and transport for ECLS

The most important factor in optimizing ECMO referral is early identification of patients failing conventional therapy. Guidelines should be established by each regional ECMO center, along with their referring hospitals, to determine the appropriate timing of transfer for individual disease processes specific for neonates, children, and adults.[16] The stability of the patient, distance, availability of transportation, experience, and capability of the transport team are all critical factors that need to be taken into consideration when deciding the timing for ECMO referral. Non-ECMO centers in remote locations should have a lower threshold for transporting a patient eligible for ECMO, compared to a center in close proximity where only a short ground transport to the receiving ECMO institution would be necessary. Known fetal conditions that may require ECMO, such as

congenital diaphragmatic hernia (CDH), preferentially should be delivered at an ECMO center given the uncertainty of accurately predicting severity of illness prenatally.

Recent advances in the medical management of patients with neonatal respiratory failure have resulted in fewer patients being referred for and treated with ECMO.[2,3,17] High frequency mechanical ventilation techniques have reduced the use of ECMO for pulmonary failure in neonates and have increasingly become available in centers without ECMO capability. The wider application of this technology, coupled with the overall reduction in ECMO availability, has created situations where patients who meet ECMO criteria while on HFV are unable to be moved to an ECMO center using conventional transport ventilation. Wilson et al. in 1996 noted that at least 6 neonatal patients referred for ECMO over a 3-year period to their institution were unable to be converted from HFV to mechanical ventilation for transport and subsequently died.[2]

The inability to transition from HFV to conventional ventilation has spurred efforts to adapt this modality for use in transport. Successful inter-hospital transports of neonatal and adult patients using high frequency techniques such as high frequency jet ventilation (HFJV) have been recently reported. A number of issues require consideration before moving a potential ECMO candidate with this technique.[18,19] The requirement for an in-line conventional ventilator in addition to the HFJV increases both bulk and weight of the equipment needed to support the patient during transport.[4] The increased gas and power consumption may require additional compressed gas cylinders and battery support to ensure safe transfer of the patient. The combination of these factors limits the practical range of HFJV as an option for transport, especially when relying on rotary aircraft. High frequency oscillatory ventilation (HFOV), while widely used in both ECMO and non-ECMO centers, has not been successfully adapted for inter-hospital transport in part because of limitations imposed by the bulk of the device and high gas consumption rates. Therefore, it is unlikely that HFOV or HFJV will be a viable option for routine use in transport in the near future.

Alternative HFV devices that are under investigation for use during transport include the Duotron Transporter and VDR-3C Percussinator (Percussionaire Corporation, Sandpoint, Idaho), which are both high frequency flow interrupters. The Duotron Transporter has the capability to deliver both high frequency and conventional ventilation, weighs ~3 pounds, and is pneumatically driven with low gas consumption. A recent report describes use of the Duotron Transporter in over 800 patients.[8] The majority of these patients were neonates with respiratory failure, and a number of them were successfully converted from HFOV for transport to ECMO centers.[20] During transport, patients were able to maintain stable oxygenation and often improve ventilation and pH balance. Additional experience has been reported as well for the VDR-3C Percussinator for neonatal transport of patients already on HFV at the time of referral.[9]

The widespread availability of iNO has also decreased the need for ECMO.[21,22] As with the increased use of HFV in non-ECMO centers, the need to move iNO responders approaching or meeting ECMO criteria, or patients who have demonstrated significant rebound pulmonary vasoconstriction following attempts to wean iNO, has created a requirement for transportable iNO systems.[23] The American Academy of Pediatrics statement on the use of iNO addresses these issues and strongly recommends that centers, which offer iNO without the availability of ECMO, establish appropriate criteria for treatment failure and mechanisms for timely referral in collaboration with a regional ECMO center.[24] Concerns for transport team safety given the potential for accumulation of NO and other nitrogen oxides in the confines of the aircraft cabin have been investigated and a number of commercially available transport

systems are currently approved for use by the FAA.[25,26] A sizeable experience using in-flight iNO in newborns with hypoxemic respiratory failure has been recently reported.[7] In this report, the authors discuss their experience of having transported 25 term newborns while using iNO therapy ($\leq$20 ppm for all transports). The mean age at transport was 3.2 days, and the average duration of transport was 1.6 hours. Diagnoses included CDH (10), persistent pulmonary hypertension (PPHN) (6), meconium aspiration syndrome (MAS) (4), sepsis (4), and non-CDH pulmonary hypoplasia (1). All patients had severe hypoxemia as assessed by an A ratio (0.10 $\pm$0.01), and had sustained or improved oxygenation with iNO therapy during transport. All patients survived the transport to the receiving institution. Presently, most ECMO centers that manage neonates with respiratory failure have the capability to routinely transport infants on iNO.

Recent success has been reported with transporting older children and adult patients with primary cardiac failure assisted by mechanical circulatory support devices other than ECMO.[10-12] The use of ventricular assist devices (VADs) has rapidly expanded because of their ability to provide perioperative support in cases of relatively isolated ventricular dysfunction. However, children usually need more complete cardiorespiratory support, as their heart failure is often complicated by hypoxemia, pulmonary hypertension, and/or right ventricular failure.[27] ECMO still remains the most common method of mechanical circulatory support for children in the U.S., as the lack of an oxygenator in the circuit and overall size of VADs have limited the use of these devices in smaller patients.[27] Recently, however, several centers have described the successful use of VADs in a number of pediatric cardiac patients including neonates.[27-30] The use of VADs offers several potential advantages over ECMO including the delivery of pulsatile flow and a decreased requirement for anticoagulation. Both of these factors may benefit patients who require extended extracorporeal support while awaiting cardiac recovery and/or transplantation.[27,28] Continued experience and adaptation of VAD technology over time, especially in neonatal and pediatric cardiac patients, may ultimately lessen the need for ECMO support in this population. Additionally, VADs may play a future role in providing an adjunct for the stabilization and transport of critically ill patients referred for ECMO.

Transport of patients on ECLS

Despite advances in technology and the changing demographics of the referral population, a significant number of patients still fail maximal medical therapy and ultimately require ECMO.[3,17] While the majority of these patients can be successfully moved to an ECMO center in a timely manner, a number of patients remain that either miss their window of opportunity or rapidly become too unstable for transport with existing modalities. Additionally, there are a number of medical centers both in the U.S. and abroad located in relatively remote geographic areas that do not have a regional ECMO center for consultation and/or early referral. In an effort to decrease the morbidity and mortality of this population of patients, WHMC and other institutions have developed the capability for mobile ECMO transport. Bartlett et al. published the first successful use of mobile ECMO to transport 2 patients in 1977, 1 of whom survived to discharge.[31] Because of the geographic diversity of its military and civilian population, WHMC began performing neonatal ECMO transports in November 1985. The ACH mobile ECMO program has been in existence since 1991 and ACH remains one of the few centers with extensive experience in this area. Several European ECMO centers also have recognized a need for ECMO transport and have recently published their experiences.[14,15]

The difficulty and expense of developing and maintaining an ECMO transport team can-

not be overestimated. As previously discussed, centers must critically evaluate the need for such a capability based on their pattern of referral. An inherent problem with ECMO transports is the major delays involved from the time of the initial referral until the arrival of the ECMO team, supplies, and eventual cannulation of the patient. Reported delays range from 2-24 hours, and are often even greater for long-distance transports.[14,15,32,33] Patients must remain stable enough to survive until the transport team can arrive and place them on ECMO. An additional problem with mobile ECMO, especially with longer distance transports, is the shortage of personnel and/or aircraft at the time of the request resulting in an inability to perform the transport. When the limitations unique to ECMO transport are combined with traditional ECMO criteria, it becomes clear that mobile ECMO is not a substitute for early referral and conventional transport. At WHMC an estimated 40% of patients referred to us for consideration of ECMO transport have traditionally been accepted and transported.[13]

Inter-hospital transport on ECMO

Inter-hospital transport can be classified as either local, regional, or long-distance based on the distances involved in moving the patient. The categorization of mobile ECMO transports in this manner can be extremely useful in helping to define the resources and personnel required to safely accomplish them. As a general guideline, transports are defined as: 1) local when <150 miles and performed by ground, 2) regional for distances of 150-1,000 miles requiring either rotary or fixed wing aircraft, and 3) long-distance for >1,000 miles and generally requiring jet aircraft capability.

Patient selection

The criteria by which patients are accepted for ECMO transport by WHMC and other facilities are similar to those defined for ECMO as outlined in other chapters of this text for patients with reversible respiratory and/or cardiac failure and will, therefore, not be detailed here. Those centers involved in performing mobile ECMO have also previously reported their own institution-specific guidelines.[4,6,13] In addition to those candidates meeting standard ECMO criteria who are too unstable for conventional transport, there exists another subset of patients eligible for mobile ECMO. This is that group of patients who have already been placed on ECMO and require additional therapies such as cardiac surgery or transplantation that are unavailable at the referral institution. We use the term "extra-institutional transfers" to describe this group.[13] These patients are often placed on ECMO because of rapid onset of cardiopulmonary failure before a definitive diagnosis is made. Some examples are: patients with congenital heart disease (e.g., critical aortic stenosis or total anomalous pulmonary venous return), congenital lung dysplasias (e.g., congenital surfactant protein deficiency, pulmonary lymphangectasia, or alveolar capillary dysplasia), or older children and adults with severe ARDS.[34-38] Additionally, patients placed on ECMO for primary cardiac failure following acute myocarditis, cardiomyopathy, or coronary artery bypass surgery may be candidates for bridge to transplantation. Since the majority of these patients will be unable to wean from ECMO for transport, moving them while on ECMO remains the only option if transplantation is to be considered.

While patients can be successfully bridged to transplant on ECMO, the morbidity and mortality associated with this process remains high. Many patients ultimately do not survive prolonged bypass while awaiting organ availability.[39-41] Given this and the tremendous resources required to transport these patients, the use of mobile ECMO as a bridge to transplant needs to be carefully evaluated. Transplant centers offering ECMO as a bridge to transplant will remain the best judge of the utility of ECMO in this setting, and should therefore consider having the capability to perform ECMO transport when needed for this purpose.

Background and experience

As previously discussed in the introduction to this chapter, a number of centers in addition to WHMC have the capability to routinely perform mobile ECMO and have previously published their experience.[4,6,13-15] A summary of the international mobile ECMO experience to date representing a combined 424 patients and overall survival of 63% is presented in Table 1. The original focus of the WHMC mobile ECMO program was the transport of neonatal patients with respiratory failure.[42] Cornish et al. published our initial experience detailing the successful transport of 13 neonates on ECMO in 1991 over distances ranging from 17-1,400 miles.[33] Survival to discharge for these patients was 31% (compared to 79% for the neonatal ECMO population). No patients died during transport and only minor equipment problems occurred. The authors postulated that the decreased survival in the transport group was caused by delayed referral and the moribund condition at the time of cannulation. Eleven of these original transports involved long-distance air transports. Since the publication by Cornish et al. in 1991, WHMC has performed an additional 23 neonatal transports for respiratory failure with an 87% survival.

In 1993, WHMC expanded its ECMO transport program to include pediatric patients and reconfigured the transport cart to accommodate patients up to adult-size. In total, we have successfully conducted 60 mobile ECMO transports (47 neonatal and pediatric transports) with an overall survival to discharge of 67%. This compares favorably to our overall ECMO survival of 78%. The majority of these transports have been for respiratory failure, with a survival of 70% in neonates and 67% for pediatric patients (Table 1). All of our transports have utilized ground vehicles for local transports or fixed-wing aircraft for regional and long-distance transports.

Both ACH and UMMC have used a combination of ground, helicopter, or fixed-wing aircraft for their inter-hospital transport of ECMO patients. The advantages and disadvantages of these different modes of transportation are outlined in Table 2. In addition to both local and regional transports, WHMC currently maintains the ability to perform long-distance ECMO transport in efforts to make ECMO available to critically ill military and civilian children living in remote locations where this modality is not available, and conventional transport is unfeasible. Our unique access to large military aircraft outfitted to support aeromedical transports including "trans-oceanic flights" makes such transports possible. Since the institution of our mobile ECMO program, nearly half of our transports have involved distances >1,000 miles and several have involved distances >6,500 miles.

UMMC's program was originally developed to transport adults on ECMO and was later expanded to include neonates and children.[6,43] In 2002, Foley et al. published the UMMC experience; 100 pediatric and adult patients (with severe respiratory or cardiac instability) were transported on ECMO to their center from 1990-99.[6] A diagnosis of ARDS was seen in 78%, with an overall survival to discharge of 66% (60% adult and 78% pediatric). Patients with primary cardiac failure had a 57% survival rate. Their median transport distance was 44 miles (range 2-790), with 80% of these being performed exclusively by ground. Since this publication, UMMC has successfully transported an additional 90 patients on ECMO with an overall survival of 62% (Table 1).[44] This has included 11 regional transports between 150-1,000 miles as well as 1 long-distance transport of >1,000 miles. The UMMC experience continues to primarily involve the transport of children and adults with respiratory failure (87% of their total 190 patients) (Table 1).

Table 1. International mobile ECMO experience.

ECMO Center	Patient Category	n	Total patients (%)	Survival to discharge (%)
Wilford Hall	Neonatal respiratory	36	60	70
San Antonio, TX, U.S.A.	Pediatric respiratory	9	15	67
	Cardiac*	5	8	40
	Extra-institutional	10	17	70
Arkansas Children's	Neonatal respiratory	30	23	86
Little Rock, AR, U.S.A.	Pediatric respiratory	69	51	53
	Cardiac#	34	25	56
	Adult respiratory	1	<1	100
University of Michigan	Neonatal respiratory	3	2	33
Ann Arbor, MI, U.S.A.	Pediatric respiratory	56	29	77
	Cardiac#	22	12	59
	Adult respiratory	109	57	56
Karolinska	Neonatal respiratory	15	52	80
Stockholm, Sweden	Pediatric respiratory	7	24	57
	Adult respiratory	7	24	71
Virchow-Klinikum	Pediatric respiratory	1	88	100
Berlin, Germany	Adult respiratory	7	12	75

* Pediatric cardiac patients only.
# Includes pediatric and adult cardiac patients combined.

Of interest, UMMC has successfully transported a significant percentage of their patients on venovenous (VV) support; 64% of adults were transported on VV as compared to 28% of pediatric respiratory failure referrals.[45] Survival was also better in the VV subgroup for both adults (69% vs. 25%) and pediatric (93% vs. 69%) patients.[45] UMMC follows the same threshold for using VV ECMO for transport as per their in-house ECMO criteria, (i.e., primarily selecting those patients for VV with good cardiac output and adequate hemodynamics).[44,45] This approach differs from both that of WHMC and ACH, which almost exclusively have used venoarterial (VA) support to transport patients on ECMO. Both centers' patient populations differ from UMMC given their relatively greater proportion of neonatal and pediatric respiratory failure patients relative to adults. The primary use of VA also reflects the concern with the feasibility of safely converting patients from VV to VA support outside of the hospital should hemodynamic instability develop; especially during high risk, regional and long-distance air transports,

which represent the predominance of transports performed by both WHMC and ACH. [46]

Since the inception of its mobile ECMO program, ACH has transported a total of 134 patients on ECMO, with an overall survival of 73% (Table 1).[47] The majority of their transports have been regional and performed via helicopter, with a smaller percentage involving fixed-wing aircraft or exclusive ground transport.[46] ACH also has the most extensive experience in transporting both children and adults with primary cardiac failure on ECMO, having moved 34 patients (25% of their ECMO transports) (Table 1). Children represent the majority of these cardiac patients (82%), and survival is significantly better in children vs. adults (61% vs. 33%, respectively).[47] Survival for the ACH cardiac subgroup was 59% overall, significantly lower than for their patients with respiratory failure, which similarly reflects both the WHMC and UMMC experience (Table 1). This increased mortality in patients transported on ECMO with cardiac failure is consistent with the increased mortality seen in the ELSO data for cardiac support as a

Table 2. Choice of vehicles for inter-hospital transport of patients on ECMO.

Attribute	Ground Ambulance	Helicopter	Fixed-wing Aircraft
Availability	Excellent	Weather-dependent	Variable
Convenience	Door-to-door	Door-to-door (potentially)	2 airports, 2 ambulances, 4 patient transfers
Safety	Excellent	Good	Good
Space for multiple attendants	Ample	Limited	Variable
Vibration	Little	Severe	Moderate
Noise	Little	Loud	Moderate-loud
Pressurization	Not necessary	Not available	Available and necessary
Distance to referring hospital	0-200 miles	50-450 miles	>350 miles
Ability to divert in transport	Excellent	Good	Poor
Cost	Low	High	High
Weight	Virtually unlimited	Limited by aircraft, distance, temperature	Limited by aircraft, distance
Loading	Relatively easy	Limited by aircraft configuration	Varies by aircraft

whole. Mortality rates for cardiac patients transported with mobile ECMO likely reflect both the greater difficulty of moving these patients and the frequent non-reversibility of their underlying cardiac disease.

Personnel and equipment

At WHMC, a multi-disciplinary approach to ECMO transport is used, involving our neonatologists, pediatric surgeons, pediatric intensivists, cardiologists, and ECMO coordinators to determine the utility of ECMO based on the age and underlying disease of the patient in each individual case. A detailed history and evaluation to rule out contraindications to ECMO needs to be obtained from the referring center. In general, this involves excluding underlying irreversible disease processes (except for cases involving bridge to transplant), irreversible neurologic injury, or uncontrolled bleeding. Durations of mechanical ventilation >7-10 days are considered a relative contraindication for ECMO. Once accepted as a candidate for ECMO, every effort is made to stabilize the patient and move

them via conventional transport to our hospital. If this is not possible, our ECMO transport protocol is activated, and the likelihood of the patient surviving until our mobile ECMO team can arrive and initiate bypass is assessed. Verbal consent is obtained from the families of all patients accepted for transport prior to departure of the team (followed by written consent after arrival), with an explanation of the risks and benefits of ECMO, as well as those unique to performing transport on ECMO.

The referring hospital is sent a list of blood products required for circuit priming and initial ECMO support. For those patients who must be moved extended distances, additional blood products need to be ready for use during the return transport as well. A circuit is pre-primed with saline prior to leaving the ECMO center in an effort to decrease the time at the referral hospital. Since most referring centers are unfamiliar with an ECMO cannulation, it is essential to bring all supplies required to initiate and maintain ECMO for the duration of the transport. All of the equipment is pre-packaged and stored in 3 portable rolling containers. Our

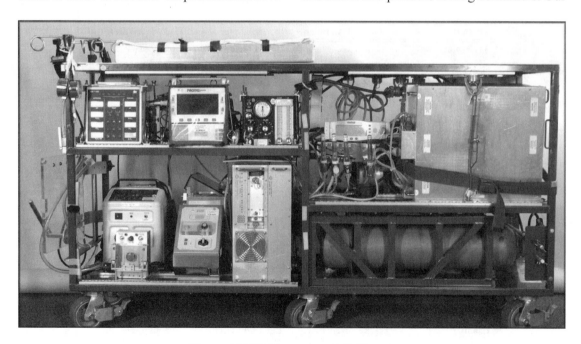

Figure 1. WHMC transport ECMO cart.

transport cart is shown in Figure 1. This cart is designed to fit into the back of a standard ambulance and can accommodate neonatal through adult-sized patients (cart dimensions: 84" x 20" x 52.5"; 740 pounds). It has a removable bassinette tray bolted to the top which can be replaced with a pad to carry larger patients. The cart is designed so that all necessary ECMO equipment is secured to the 2 shelves below the patient. This equipment includes a Stöckert roller pump (Cobe Cardiovascular, Arvada, CO), Seabrook water heater (Cincinnati Sub-Zero, Cincinnati, OH), OriGen bladder box, Model BB, (OriGen Biomedical, Austin, TX), cardiorespiratory monitor, MVP-10 ventilator (Bio-Med Inc., Guilford, CT), 3 uninterruptible power sources, and in-line saturation monitor CDI 400 (Terumo/Sarns/CDI, Ann Arbor, MI). The latter provides continuous arterial and venous blood gases from the ECMO circuit, as well as venous saturation. Standard manometers are used to monitor pre- and post-membrane pressures. Also housed on the transport cart are 3 "Q" tanks containing medical air, oxygen, and carbogen. All of the above equipment has been tested by the Air Force Research Laboratory at Brooks Air Force Base, San Antonio, Texas, and meets or exceeds all U.S. Air Force (USAF) airworthiness standards for aeromedical equipment. The USAF requirements meet or exceed FAA standards (Table 3). For certification, all transport equipment must maintain its proper function when subjected to extremes of temperature, vibration, and other conditions that may occur in-flight. Equipment must also pass electromagnetic interference (EMI) testing so that its use does not interfere with aircraft navigational and control systems.

For those transports that involve moving a patient that has already been placed on ECMO at the referring center, we are often able to successfully transfer the existing ECMO circuit to our transport cart. This procedure involves having the patient off bypass for 30-60 seconds while the raceway is transferred between pumps,

and avoids having to prime a new circuit. Upon arrival back to WHMC, we routinely reverse this process and transfer the circuit from the transport cart to our standard ECMO unit, with the final maneuver, again, being the transfer of the raceway between pumps.

We are only able to perform this procedure if the referral center's circuit is compatible with our transport equipment. In those cases when there is an incompatibility, new circuits are used. Additionally, if the circuit is old and has clots that would place the patient at increased risk during transport (which also factors in the distance and time required for transport), then a new circuit is used.

In the absence of this practice, patients would be exposed to up to 2 circuit changes in a relatively short time period. The obvious advantages of this practice are avoiding exposure to a new circuit(s) and blood products (with the associated inflammatory response), shortening the transport, and fewer blood products and circuit supplies used. In addition, the patient is much less likely to require additional blood products during transport and is less likely to have bleeding complications.

We have not had any significant complications with transports involving this approach, having reserved its use for mainly local and/or short regional transports, and would not recommend it for long-distance transports. The theoretical concern would be related to transporting a patient with an existing circuit that was compromised, thereby increasing the potential risks for complications during transport.

The WHMC ECMO transport team is individually tailored for specific transports. For long-distance air transports where multiple shifts of personnel are needed, essential personnel generally includes at least 2 ECMO physicians, 2 neonatal/pediatric ICU/adult ICU fellows, 1 staff surgeon, 2 patient nurses, 2 ECMO coordinators, and 1 respiratory therapist. Vehicles required for ground ECMO transport include an ambulance and 2 large vans to carry transport

Table 3. USAF and FAA standards.

Agency	FAA	USAF
Baseline performance assessment	No information	When the device first arrives, the assigned Integrated Product Team members conduct a review validating the device functions as advertised and as expected. The assessment familiarizes evaluation personnel with operation and characteristics of the device, noting design weaknesses and potential safety hazards relating to the aeromedical environment and human factors such as man-machine interface and potential for operator error. During this phase, baseline performance measurements are taken for later comparison to test data.
Electrical safety	Test parameters not similar to USAF	MIL-STD-810E
Vibration testing	RTCA/DO-160E Section 8	MIL-STD-810E
Electromagnetic interference testing	RTCA/DO-160E Section 20 & 21	MIL-STD-46ID
Radiated emissions	Section 21	*RE 102*
Radiated susceptibility	Section 20	*RS 103*
Conducted emissions	Section 21	*CE 102*
Conducted susceptibility	Section 20	*CS 101, CS 114, CS 115 & CS 116*
Environmental testing	RTCA/DO-160E Section 4, 5 & 6	MIL-STD-810E
Humidity operation	Section 6	*94 ±4% Rh, 85°F ±3.6°F (29.5°C ±2°C) for 4 hrs.*
Hot temperature operation	Section 4	*120°F ±3.6°F (49°C ±2°C) for 2 hrs.*
Cold temperature operation	Section 4	*32°F ±7.2 (0°C ±4°C) for 2 hrs.*
Hot temperature storage		*140°F ±3.6°F (60°C ±2°C) for 6 hrs.*
Cold temperature storage		*40°F ±3.6°F (-40°C ±2°C) for 6 hrs.*
Altitude testing	RTCA/DO-160E Section 4	Performance check at 15,000 feet above sea level, barometric pressure of 429.0 mm Hg. Ascent and descent rate is 5,000 ft/min.
Rapid decompression testing	RTCA/DO-160E Section 4	This protocol involves a chamber flight ascending to 8,000 ft then decompressing to 45,000 ft in 60 sec. while observing equipment performance and potential safety hazards. The chamber is then returned to ground level, where an equipment performance check is accomplished to verify operational ability. This procedure is repeated for a 7 sec. and 1 sec. rapid decompression.
Airborne performance	No information	Aeromedical evacuation crewmembers evaluate the medical equipment during actual aircraft flights to validate laboratory findings and assess human factors (human factors assessment additionally guided by MIL-STD-1472D) during in-flight operation.

The table above is a comparison of the Environmental Conditions and Test Procedures for Airborne Equipment between the USAF and FAA. The FAA uses Radio Technical Commission for Aeronautics (RTCA) standards and documents to test airborne equipment for airworthiness. RTCA is a not-for-profit corporation that develops consensus-based recommendations regarding communications, navigation, surveillance and air traffic management (CNS/ATM) system issues. RTCA functions as a Federal Advisory Committee. Its recommendations are used by the FAA as basis for policy, program, and regulatory decisions; and by the private sector as the basis for development, investment, and other business issues (www.rtca.org/aboutrtca.asp). Airborne equipment encompasses any equipment that is used onboard the aircraft and does not make any special distinction if it is a medical equipment.

Whenever Original Equipment Manufacturer (OEM) makes a claim that their equipment has been FAA-certified, it is in the best interest of the USAF to verify for the Environmental Qualification Form (EQF). The EQF provides the necessary information regarding which environmental tests were conducted and, where applicable, the appropriate environmental category of the equipment being tested. Environmental category pertains to the minimum standard environmental test conditions. OEMs are also encouraged to use the nameplate marking system. This nameplate marking system is a supplemental and optional method of identifying the environmental test results.

personnel and equipment. For all air transports, it is important to remember that ground transport is also required to move the patient to and from the airport; the logistics of this should be carefully planned to minimize time outside of the hospital. WHMC uses a variety of USAF fixed-wing aircraft with aeromedical capability, and the aircraft chosen depends on availability and distance of the transport. To minimize complications related to atmospheric pressure with air transport, we routinely maintain cabin pressure at an altitude of ≤5,000 feet. The FAA allows medical transport aircraft to fly up to pressures of 10,000 feet, but the majority of air transport services fly at an altitude between 5-10,000 feet.

The neonatal transport cart utilized by ACH is shown (Figure 2). This cart features a conventional CPB roller pump (Stockert-Sorin, Irvine, CA) positioned at the extreme right of a 3 pump base. The position of the pump head to the far right allows platform space to secure monitors. The pump is rotated 90° to allow easy access to raceway tubing. Incorporated into the pump base are 2 extension masts located on

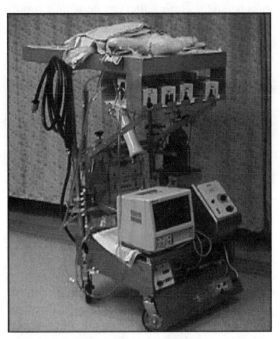

Figure 2. ACH transport ECMO cart.

the back corners of the base. Both masts are reduced in height to facilitate loading into the aircraft. A computer-aided perfusion system (CAPS) servo-regulates the roller pump and is attached to one of the masts. The CAPS is positioned as close to the base as possible and between both masts to lower the center of gravity and maximize stability. The right side of the pump is free of accessory equipment to allow securing of the pump against an inner wall for transport in the mobile ECMO vehicle. To allow use of the ECMO pump in different modes of transport, components of the ECMO circuitry and pump are positioned to allow safe loading into a standard 36-inch cargo door. Infants are placed in a custom-designed cradle for transport. The plastic cradle has a steel brace bolted to it and is attached to the top of the masts and stabilized with securing clamps. One side of the cradle drops, allowing access to the patient and cannulation site. Cradles in 2 sizes are available for infants and children up to 20 pounds, while larger patients are transported on a stretcher and moved in conjunction with the pump. All ECMO equipment, including the water heater and monitors, are connected via a power column inside the pump base. The ECMO pump has 2 available sources of power (AC or battery) built into the pump base. The equipment is transported in 7 separate packs organized for each phase of transport. The team typically consists of 4 persons including 2 physicians (1 surgeon and 1 neonatologist, intensivist, or cardiologist), 1 surgical assistant, and 1 ECMO coordinator.[4]

Since the majority of the UMMC ECMO transports are done by ground, they use a custom-built critical care ambulance. Unique features of this vehicle include a seating capacity for 6 crew members in back and 2 in front, 2-4 kW electrical generators, a 110-volt electrical invertor, 4 M-tanks of oxygen, an 800 pound capacity hydraulic lift, and a 250 gallon diesel fuel tank allowing for extended range.[6] UMMC places the majority of their required

ECMO supplies in several large travel packs that are easily transportable. While UMMC has traditionally used a standard roller pump (Cobe Cardiovascular, Arvada, CO) in their circuit for mobile ECMO, they more recently have changed to using centrifugal pumps for all patients over 10 kg (Biomedicus 550, Eden Prairie, MN) and for air transport of those under 10 kg (Medtronic Biopump, Minneapolis, MN). A roller pump is still used exclusively for ground transport of children under 10 kg.[6,45] An example of the UMMC transport circuit configuration using a centrifugal pump is shown (Figure 3). The use of the centrifugal pump allows for simplification and miniaturization of the circuit, and with its active suction, eliminates the need for gravity drainage. Potential disadvantages of this system are hemolysis if suction is excessive, reverse flow if power fails, and difficult manual operation in the event of power failure.[6] An additional concern with the use of centrifugal pumps during air transport is its potential for excessive electromagnetic interference (EMI). For all transports, UMMC utilizes a combination of ECLS personnel to include at least 2 physicians, 2 ECLS specialists to prime and operate the circuit, and additional support personnel as required.[6]

Potential complications

To date, the number of life-threatening complications or deaths reported by major centers routinely performing ECMO transport has been

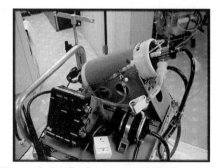

Figure 3. UMMC transport ECMO cart.

remarkably limited given the high-risk nature of this process. UMMC has had two patient deaths during ECMO transport from causes unrelated to ECMO.[44] They have additionally reported 17 minor transport-related complications that occurred during their most recent published experience of 100 cases.[6] The most common problem was related to temporary failure by the electrical power supply to the circuit. There were 10 episodes of failure of the ambulance power supply and 4 incidents of failure of the circuit battery that resulted in a transient period of manual operation of the pump until power was restored. Minor circuit tubing or connector leakage also occurred in a small number of cases, as well as several isolated incidents of membrane lung thrombosis and leakage, circuit tubing rupture, and circuit hypocarbia (attributed to excessive lung surface area). None of these incidents resulted in an adverse outcome.[6]

Both WHMC and ACH have reported minor problems similar to the UMMC experience, with the loss of power to the transport cart and pump being one of the more frequent problems.[4,32,33] By definition, all ECMO transports require a period when the cart's battery system must supply power to the circuit to safely move the patient to and from the airport after leaving the hospital. Additionally, the battery must provide back-up should the power supply in the ambulance or aircraft fail during transport. To address this problem, WHMC has designed its battery supply to provide uninterrupted power to our equipment for up to 4 hours from each individual unit (2 additional units are routinely included for each transport). The availability of a reliable power source, appropriate converters, and extension cords specific for each transport is essential for the safety of ECMO transports. Despite the potential for increased bleeding complications in neonatal patients that are heparinized and transported on ECMO, neither WHMC nor ACH have reported an increased incidence of intracranial hemorrhage when compared to non-transported ECMO cases.[13,32]

The two European centers performing ECMO transport also have reported a low rate of complications. Roissant et al.[14] reported damage to a membrane stopcock requiring changing of the membrane lung, while Linden et al.[15] reported three ambulance compressor and helicopter electric circuit malfunctions that occurred during transport. None of these events resulting in any adverse patient effects.

Intra-hospital transport on ECMO

The capability to safely transport a patient on ECMO for a diagnostic or interventional procedure within the hospital is a necessity for all ECMO centers. Common destinations include radiology for computerized tomography or other specialized imaging, the cardiac catheterization lab, or the OR. Centers that utilize ECMO as an adjunct to their pediatric cardiac surgery programs are more likely to perform these types of transports. ACH recently reviewed their experience with 62 intra-hospital ECMO transports.[4] The most common reason for these transports was to further evaluate possible structural abnormalities in patients with congenital heart disease. Several children had suspected abnormalities of the pulmonary veins or arteries that could not be adequately evaluated with echocardiography. A number of these patients eventually required transport back to the OR while on ECMO for repair or palliation of their underlying heart disease, including the need for transplant in those with unresolved cardiogenic shock. In addition, Seib et al. reported cardiac catheterization in children on ECMO with severe ventricular dysfunction requiring atrial septostomy for left heart decompression at ACH.[48]

DesJardins published a series in 1999 of 15 children with known congenital heart disease who underwent cardiac catheterization while on ECMO.[49] Of these patients, 2 were placed on ECMO prior to cardiac surgery, while the remaining 13 were begun post-operatively. In 8 patients, catheterization was done to evaluate the anatomy of the pulmonary or coronary arteries beyond what

could be determined with echocardiography. The remainder had a variety of indications for catheterization including the need for an interventional procedure, assessment of hemodynamic status following failure to wean off ECMO, and ruling out possible pulmonary venous obstruction. Successful vascular access was achieved in all patients, either with wiring over existing access or by placing new percutaneous lines including 5 femoral artery and 6 femoral vein catheters. While the majority of the patients underwent the procedure without significant complications, 1 patient died due to severe retroperitoneal hemorrhage following arterial trauma.

A relatively more common indication for intra-hospital ECMO transport at many institutions, including WHMC, is the need to obtain more specialized diagnostic imaging than is routinely available at the bedside. Lidegran et al. recently published a study reviewing the transport of 112 patients on ECMO over a 6-year period, including neonatal, pediatric, and adult patients, for computerized tomography scans.[50] The main indications for CT were for further evaluation of suspected underlying disease processes and/or complications that occurred while on ECMO support. Overall, 57% of the studies revealed findings that affected treatment, including the discovery of CNS, thoracic, and abdominal pathology. To accomplish these transports, this group used a standard ECMO cart (Stockert SIII, Stockert Instruments; Munich, Germany) modified with the addition of a portable gas supply. Patients were not removed from their hospital beds for transport. Instead, they remained in their hospital bed and were carefully moved along with the ECMO equipment that was on a separate cart. Given the relative close proximity of the radiology suite, total time outside of the ICU was less than 60 minutes and there were no reported complications associated either with the transports or the examinations themselves.

When performing in-house ECMO transports at WHMC, we routinely use our transport cart as previously described for inter-hospital cases, transferring the existing circuit to and from the cart. As with any mobile ECMO transport, extreme care must be taken to monitor the patient and ensure the cannulas are secure at all times, particularly when moving the patient between beds. Prior to leaving the ICU, efforts are made to secure the transport route, and inspect the receiving area to assess the adequacy of space for the procedure. Plans are discussed with ancillary personnel who may be unfamiliar with ECMO to lessen potential complications and/or delays. The accompanying team of ECMO personnel should include at minimum a circuit specialist, the patient's nurse, a respiratory therapist, and an ECMO physician. All necessary emergency equipment and supplies should be transported with the patient and the surgical team should be notified and available if needed. Given careful preparation and these precautions, intra-hospital ECMO transport can be safely performed when necessary.

Summary

In summary, the timing and referral for transport of those patients needing ECMO remains a complicated and difficult process given the current diversity of indications for ECLS. Regional ECMO centers need to continue to work closely with their non-ECMO referral base to establish guidelines and encourage the safest possible transport of ECMO candidates to their institution. The collective experience reported by ECLS centers with mobile ECMO programs has demonstrated the feasibility of transporting ECMO patients both between and within hospitals. Mobile ECMO provides a life-saving option for the inter-hospital transport of those patients with a predicted high mortality that cannot be moved with conventional technology. Transport on ECLS, however, remains an extremely labor-intensive and risk-laden modality that should not take the place of timely referral to an ECMO center. The individual centers with mobile ECMO programs need to continually reassess the need for this resource, while at the same time investigating alternative means to transport critically ill patients meeting ECMO criteria.

References

1. Kanto WP, Bunyapen C. Extracorporeal Membrane Oxygenation: Controversies in selection of patients and management. *Clin Perinatol* 1998; 25:123-135.

2. Wilson JM, Bower LK, Thompson JE, Fauza DO, Fackler JC. ECMO in evolution: The impact of changing patient demographics and alternative therapies on ECMO. *J Pediatr Surg* 1996; 31:1116-1123.

3. Roy BJ, Rycus P, Conrad SA, Clark RH. The changing demographics of neonatal extracorporeal membrane oxygenation patients reported to the Extracorporeal Life Support Organization (ELSO) registry. *Pediatrics* 2000; 106:1334-1338.

4. Taylor BJ, Moss MM, Heulitt MJ. Referral and transport of ECMO patients. In: Zwischenberger JB et al, ed. *ECMO: Extracorporeal Cardiopulmonary Support in Critical Care*. 2nd ed. Ann Arbor, MI: Extracorporeal Life Support Organization, 2000: 645-658.

5. Boedy RF, Howell CG, Kanto WP. Hidden mortality rate associated with extracorporeal membrane oxygenation. *J Pediatr* 1990; 117:462-464.

6. Foley DS, Pranikoff T, Younger JG, et al. A review of 100 patients transported on extracorporeal life support. *ASAIO J* 2002; 48:612-619.

7. Kinsella JP, Griebel J, Schmidt JM, Abman SH. Use of inhaled nitric oxide during interhospital transport of newborns with hypoxemic respiratory failure. *Pediatrics* 2002; 109:158-161.

8. Honey G, Bleak T, Karp T, Null D. Use of the Duotron Transporter® HFV during neonatal transport. *Adv Neonatal Care*. In press.

9. Villareal D, Vijay D, Cleary J. Transport high frequency using the VDR-3C Percussinator. In: Annual ECMO/New Technologies Conference; 1999; Keystone, CO.

10. McBride LR, Lowdermilk GA, Fiore AC, et al. Transfer of patients receiving advanced mechanical circulatory support. *J Thorac Cardiovasc Surg* 2000; 119:1015-1020.

11. Reiss N, el-Banayosy A, Posival H, et al. Transport of hemodynamically unstable patients by a mobile mechanical circulatory support team. *Artif Organs* 1996; 20:959-963.

12. Mestres CA, Sanchez-Martos A, Rodriguez-Ribo A, et al. Long-distance transportation of patients with a paracorporeal ventricular assist device. *Int J Artif Organs* 1998; 21:425-428.

13. Wilson BJ, Heiman HS, Butler TJ, Negaard KA, DiGeronimo RJ. A 16-year neonatal/pediatric extracorporeal membrane oxygenation transport experience. *Pediatrics* 2002; 109:189-193.

14. Rossaint R, Pappert D, Gerlach H, et al. Extracorporeal membrane oxygenation for transport of hypoxaemic patients with severe ARDS. *Br J Anesth* 1997; 78:241-246.

15. Lindén V, Palmér K, Reinhard J, et al. Inter-hospital transportation of patients with severe acute respiratory failure on extracorporeal membrane oxygenation- national and international experience. *Intensive Care Med* 2001; 27:1643-1648.

16. Bergman KA, Geven WB, Molendijk A. Referral and transportation for neonatal extracorporeal membrane oxygenation. *Eur J Emerg Med* 2002; 9:233-237.

17. Hintz SR, Sutter DM, Sheehan AM, Rhine WD, Van Meurs KP. Decreased use of neonatal extracorporeal membrane oxygenation (ECMO): How new treatment modalities have affected ECMO utilization. *Pediatrics* 2000; 106:1339-1343.

18. Scuderi J, Elton CB, Elton DR. A cart to provide high frequency jet ventilation during transport for neonates. *Respir Care* 1992; 37:129-136.

19. Allen PD, Turner DT, Brink MJ. Ground transport of an infant on high-frequency jet ventilation: a case presentation. *Neonatal Network* 1995; 14:39-43.

20. Null D, Primary Children's, UT, personal communication, 2004.

21. Inhaled nitric oxide in full-term and nearly full-term infants with hypoxic respiratory failure. The Neonatal Inhaled Nitric Oxide Study Group. *N Engl JMed* 1997; 336:597-604.

22. Davidson D, Barefield ES, Kattwinkel J, et al. Inhaled nitric oxide for the early treatment of persistent pulmonary hypertension of the term newborn. A randomized, double-masked, placebo-controlled, dose-response, multicenter study. The I-NO/PPHN Study Group. *Pediatrics* 1998; 101:325-334.

23. Davidson D, Barefield ES, Kattwinkel J, et al. Safety of withdrawing inhaled nitric oxide therapy in persistent pulmonary hypertension of the newborn. *Pediatrics* 1999; 104:231-236.

24. Committee on Fetus and Newborn, American Academy of Pediatrics. Use of Inhaled Nitric Oxide. *Pediatrics* 2000; 106:344-345.

25. Dhillon JS, Kronick JB, Singh NC, Johnson CC. A portable nitric oxide scavenging unit designed for use on neonatal transport. *Crit Care Med* 1996; 24:1068-1071.

26. Qureshi MA, Shah NJ, Hemmen CW, Thill MC, Kruse JA. "Exposure of intensive care unit nurses to nitric oxide and nitrogen dioxide during therapeutic use of inhaled nitric oxide in adults with acute respiratory distress syndrome." *Am J Crit Care* 2003; 12:147-153.

27. Duncan BW. Mechanical circulatory support for infants and children with cardiac disease. *Ann Thorac Surg* 2002; 73:1670-1677.

28. Throckmorton AL, Allaire PE, Gutgesell HP, et al. Pediatric circulatory support systems. *ASAIO J* 2002; 48:216-221.

29. Konertz W, Hotz H, Schneider M, et al. Clinical experience with the MEDOS-HIA-VAD system in infants and children. *Ann Thorac Surg* 1997; 63:1138-1144.

30. Ishino K, Loebe M, Uhleman F, et al. Circulatory support with paracorporeal pneumatic ventricular assist device (VAD) in infants and children. *Euro J Cardiothorac Surg* 1997; 11:965-972.

31. Bartlett RH, Gazzaniga AB, Fong SW, et al. Extracorporeal membrane oxygenator support for cardiopulmonary failure. Experience in 28 cases. *J Thorac Cardiovasc Surg* 1977; 73:375-386.

32. Heulitt MJ, Taylor BJ, Faulkner SC, et al. Interhospital transport of neonatal patients on extracorporeal membrane oxygenation: Mobile-ECMO. *Pediatrics* 1995; 95:562-566.

33. Cornish JD, Carter JM, Gerstmann DR, Null DM. Extracorporeal membrane oxygenation as a means of stabilizing and transporting high risk neonates. *ASAIO Transactions* 1991; 37:564-568.

34. Finer NN. Neonatal selection criteria for ECMO. In: Zwischenberger JB et al, ed. *ECMO: Extracorporeal Cardiopulmonary Support in Critical Care.* 2nd ed. Ann Arbor, MI: Extracorporeal Life Support Organization, 2000: 358.

35. Butler TJ, Yoder BA, Seib P, Lally KP and Smith VC. ECMO for left ventricular assist in a newborn with aortic stenosis. *Pediatr Cardiol* 1994; 15:38-40.

36. Cassidy J, Smith J, Goldman A, et al. The incidence and characteristics of neonatal irreversible lung dysplasia. *J Pediatr* 2002; 141:426-428.

37. Tibballs J, Chow CW. Incidence of alveolar capillary dysplasia in severe idiopathic persistent pulmonary hypertension of the newborn. *J Paediatr Child Health* 2002; 38:397-400.

38. Hamvas A, Nogee LM, Mallory GB, et al. Lung transplantation for treatment of infants with surfactant protein B deficiency. *J Pediatr* 1997; 130:231-239.

39. Fiser WP, Yetman AT, Gunselman RJ, et al. Pediatric arteriovenous extracorporeal membrane oxygenation (ECMO) as a bridge to cardiac transplantation. *J Heart Lung Transplant* 2003; 22:770-777.

40. Goldman AP, Cassidy J, de Leval M, et al. The waiting game: bridging to paediatric heart transplantation. *Lancet* 2003; 362:1967-1970.

41. Levi DL, Marelli D, Plunkett M, et al. Use of assist devices and ECMO to bridge pediatric patients with cardiomyopathy to transplantation. *J Heart Lung Transplant* 2002; 21:760-770.

42. Cornish JD, Gerstmann DR, Begnaudd MJ, Null DM, Ackerman NR. In-flight use of extracorporeal membrane oxygenation for severe neonatal respiratory failure. *Perfusion* 1986; 1:281-287.

43. Anderson H, Steimle C, Shapiro M, et al. Extracorporeal life support for adult cardiorespiratory failure. *Surgery* 1993; 114:161-172.

44. Wyrick P, University of Michigan, personal communication, 2005.

45. Remenapp R, University of Michigan, personal communication, 2005.

46. Fiser R, University of Arkansas, personal communication, 2005.

47. Taylor B, University of Arkansas, personal communication, 2005.

48. Seib PM, Faulkner SC, Erickson CC, et al. Blade and balloon arterial septostomy for left heart decompression in patients with severe ventricular dysfunction on extracorporeal membrane oxygenation. *Catheter Cardiovasc Interv* 1999; 46:179-186.

49. DesJardins SE, Crowley DC, Beekman RH, Lloyd TR. Utility of cardiac catheterization in pediatric cardiac patients on ECMO. *Catheter Cardiovasc Interv* 1999; 46:62-67.

50. Lidegran M, Palmér K, Jorulf H, and Lindén V. CT in the evaluation of patients on ECMO due to acute respiratory failure. *Pediatr Radiol* 2002; 32:567-574.

10

The ELSO Registry

Steven A. Conrad, M.D., Ph.D. and Peter T. Rycus, M.P.H.

Introduction

Extracorporeal life support (ECLS) is an extraordinary therapy applied in selected critically ill patients with severe cardiopulmonary failure. In order to document and share the experience gained during the growth of ECLS, the Extracorporeal Life Support Organization (ELSO) maintains a data registry that tracks the application and outcome of ECLS. ELSO is a consortium of health care professionals who employ extracorporeal circulation for support of severe cardiopulmonary failure. Approximately 110 institutions are active members of ELSO and contribute ongoing data to the Registry. The Registry contains data collected on over 30,000 cases since 1976. The vast majority of ECLS cases performed in the U.S., and a rapidly growing number performed internationally, are recorded in the database.

Formal reporting of the data accumulated in the Registry takes place twice annually, in the form of the collective experience (the International Summary) as well as center-specific reports. The International Summary provides an in-depth descriptive summary of all cases reported to the Registry at the time of its publication and is distributed to all member institutions. The center-specific reports, provided to individual centers, include detailed information on cases performed at that institution, as well as benchmarks of the individual center against the summary data.

While the overall goal of the Registry is to provide a collective history of the progress of ECLS, there are many uses and functions of the Registry.

- Summary of cumulative experience
- Ad hoc queries to support patient care
- Support for research papers
- Support for the Food and Drug Administration approval of devices
- Benchmarking by individual centers

The origins of the Registry precede the founding of ELSO. Established by a small group of centers to exchange information about a growing technology and record its progress, data entry began in 1984 and includes information collected since 1976. When ELSO was formed in 1989, development and maintenance of a registry was one of its chartered functions. The initial focus of the Registry was on neonatal data, since pediatric and adult ECLS were not in widespread use at that time. As the application of ECLS broadened to include pediatric and adult patients, as well as for support in cardiac failure, three additional databases were created.

History of the Registry

The Registry is maintained at the ELSO office in Ann Arbor, near the campus of the

University of Michigan Medical Center. The structure and implementation of the Registry has changed since its initial deployment in order to accommodate changes in the demographics of ECLS, as well as advances in computer information technology.

Original implementation

From its inception as a computer database in 1988 until 1999, the Registry was implemented as four individual databases in the dBase database format using Microsoft FoxPro: a neonatal respiratory database, a pediatric respiratory database, a neonatal/pediatric cardiac database, and an adult cardiac/respiratory database. Four different forms were used in data collection. These databases were comprised primarily of free-text fields, resulting in complex data entry, high requirements for data storage, and deficient capabilities for search and retrieval. Although there was considerable congruity between the four databases, each had a different number of data items on their respective data submission forms.

The original Registry structure performed exceptionally well and has supported both research and patient care. As the applications of ECLS have increased in both number and scope, the limitations of the database in its original structure became evident. A specific search, for example, would typically require a manual examination of free-text fields to detect alternate entries, followed by construction of a complex query which had to be executed across multiple tables. Searches often had to be repeated on the different databases and compiled manually.

Re-engineered Registry features

To support the continued growth of the Registry, a re-engineering of the database was authorized by the ELSO Steering Committee in 1997 and was completed in late 1998. The goals and features of the new Registry include the following:

- Conversion from four databases to a single registry database structure to store all ECLS cases, eliminating the a-priori division into categories (above) for which a given case may not be mutually, exclusively classified (e.g., a case with both cardiac and respiratory components)
- Restructuring from a single-table (flat-file) structure to a multi-table normalized data structure with established integrity rules
- Implementation of validation rules to reduce data entry errors
- Use of an extensible, industry-accepted database query language for all data access (Structured Query Language [SQL])
- Development of a single, uniform data entry form for all ECLS cases
- Elimination of all but a few essential free-text data fields to provide consistency of ECLS data through the use of pre-defined data categories and classifications
- Adoption of standardized hierarchical classification systems for diagnoses (ICD-9-CM), and surgical procedures current procedural terminology (CPT), to allow data retrieval based on any desired range of specificity
- Electronic data submission with e-mail and Internet-based delivery, enhancing data validation and eliminating manual data entry

Database implementation

The re-engineered Registry was written as a Microsoft Access database composed of two database files. Patient data were stored in a back-end database which is accessed through forms, code tables, and reports using a linked front-end database. The back-end ran on a Microsoft NT Server platform and was accessible over a local area network to provide flexibility and multi-user capability for data entry. This platform used the NT security model for both database and web security.

The dual-file configuration was instrumental for migrating the back-end data portion of the database to a high-performance ODBC-compliant database server (Microsoft SQL Server) in 1999 to provide for an increase in performance, reliability, and security. The front-end Access application was maintained and re-linked to the new database with minimal modification, and continues to be used for internal data entry and updates.

The traditional paper entry form was discontinued on implementation of the Microsoft Access database and was rewritten as a Microsoft Word electronic form. It is filled in directly in Microsoft Word, optionally printed, and submitted via e-mail to the ELSO Registry office. The Microsoft Access application imports the data directly from the form, thus eliminating the need for manual entry and the risk of data entry errors. To further reduce errors, the Microsoft Word form provides limited data validation prior to its submission to ELSO.

Web-based Internet deployment

Migration to Microsoft SQL Server enabled the development of a Web-based application for external data entry and retrieval, now entering its final implementation. Registry case reports are now completed with a Web-based form using a secure, encrypted Internet connection which enters data directly into the ELSO Registry database (Figure 1). This assures availability of the most current information and facilitates entry from international centers. Security and data protection are enhanced through the use of role-based authorization, allowing assignment of sensitive functions only to specific individuals.

Registry addenda

The Registry contains information of interest regarding the general aspects of ECLS, but does not include more specialized data which are important for some ECLS applications. For example, the use of ECLS for cardiac support, specialized information includes descriptions of complex congenital cardiac abnormalities and specifics on cardiac surgical procedures. These data are unique to cardiac support, and no standardized classification systems adequately document such situations. In 1998, ELSO authorized the development of a cardiac addendum to the Registry which would be capable of recording additional case-specific data. Because of the relational structure of the re-engineered Registry, incorporation of the cardiac addendum data could be accomplished without changes to the existing database structure. Data collection could then be performed through the use of addendum data sheets in combination with the existing form, rather than creating a new, separate cardiac ECLS data form. Classification systems for anatomical description and evolving surgical procedures are being developed to support data collection and retrieval.

Registry data summary

Data have been collected from 1976 to present from 132 domestic and international centers. The data include a rapidly expanding number

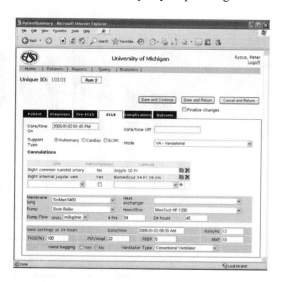

Figure 1. Web-based data entry form.

of entries in the non-neonatal age group, with adults being the most rapidly growing category of patients. The number of centers has remained relatively constant over the past several years (Figure 2). The Registry data are published semi-annually as the ELSO International Summary and are distributed to active centers. A manuscript form of the International Summary is published periodically in the ASAIO Journal, most recently in 2005 for the data collection period through December 2004.[1] Active centers also receive center-specific reports, which provide both detailed and summary information specific to the individual center. This enables a center to compare its progress with that of the entire Registry.

A summary of data collected through December 2004 is presented in Table 1. The total number of cases was 29,908, with 76% of patients surviving ECLS and 66% surviving to discharge home or transfer to other institutions. Table 1 provides the numbers of cases performed and survival according to age group and type of support. The highest survival is neonatal respiratory support (77% to discharge). For this report, neonatal is defined as age ≤30 days, pediatric >30 days to <18 years, and adults ≥18 years of age.

Neonatal respiratory failure

The number of neonatal respiratory support cases performed annually has declined from its peak in 1992 after stabilizing in 2000 (Figure 3). This decline most likely represents the application of alternative therapies which successfully averted the need for ECLS. The widespread use of exogenous surfactant administration began in the early 1990s, has increased in frequency, and is responsible for a large percentage of the decline. Additionally, the availability of inhaled nitric oxide (iNO) for pulmonary artery vasodilatation, combined with improvements in ventilator management, especially high frequency oscillatory ventilation (HFOV), have reduced the requirement for ECLS.

Roy et al.[2] recently reviewed the changing demographics of neonatal patients undergoing extracorporeal support for respiratory failure over the 10-year period 1988-1997. The percentage of ECMO-treated neonates with congenital diaphragmatic hernia (CDH) increased from 18% to 26% and the percentage with respiratory distress syndrome decreased from 15% to 4%. The use of surfactant, HFOV, and iNO increased from none in 1988 to 36%, 46%, and 24%, respectively, in 1997.

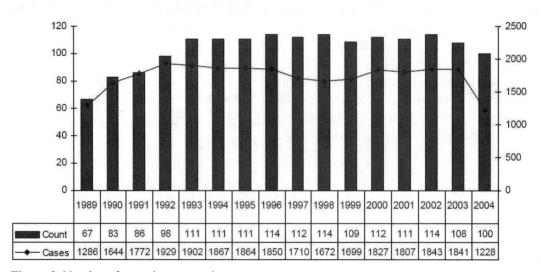

	1989	1990	1991	1992	1993	1994	1995	1996	1997	1998	1999	2000	2001	2002	2003	2004
Count	67	83	86	98	111	111	111	114	112	114	109	112	111	114	108	100
Cases	1286	1644	1772	1929	1902	1867	1864	1850	1710	1672	1699	1827	1807	1843	1841	1228

Figure 2. Number of reporting centers by year.

Table 1. Overall ECLS outcomes (through 2004).

	Total patients	Survived ECLS		Survived discharge/transfer	
		n	(%)	n	(%)
Neonatal					
Respiratory	19,463	16,623	85	14,942	77
Cardiac	2,344	1,351	58	896	38
eCPR	174	109	63	72	41
Pediatric					
Respiratory	2,883	1,847	64	1,608	56
Cardiac	3,059	1,778	58	1,312	43
eCPR	332	161	50	124	39
Adult					
Respiratory	1,025	610	60	542	53
Cardiac	499	228	46	159	32
eCPR	139	68	49	51	37
Total	29,908	22,775	76	19,706	66

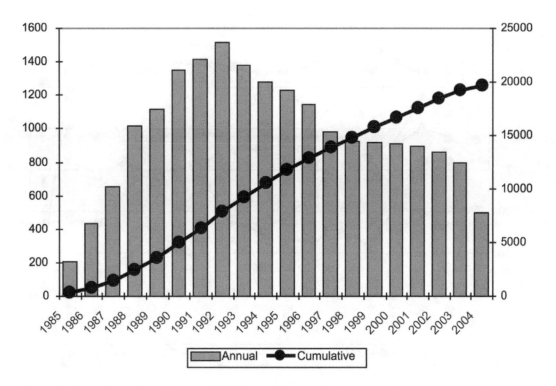

Figure 3. Annual number of neonatal ECLS cases for respiratory support.

Historically ELSO has tracked criteria determined by centers as the basis for initiating ECLS, including $aADO_2$, oxygenation index, acute deterioration, failure of maximal therapy, barotrauma, and cardiac arrest or failure. It was recognized that these criteria are not mutually exclusive, are highly subjective, and have been applied inconsistently across centers. Because of difficulty in interpreting trends, these criteria have been removed from the database and have been replaced by pre-ECLS physiologic parameters such as ventilator settings, hemodynamics, and blood gases.

Diagnosis-specific annual survival rates have not changed significantly over the past decade (Figure 4). Cumulative survival rates are the highest for meconium aspiration syndrome (94%) and lowest for CDH (52%). Survival rates for major neonatal diagnoses and average duration of support are given in Table 2.

The Registry tracks a large set of pre-defined mechanical or equipment-related and patient-related complications (Table 3). In general, complications are recorded if they require intervention or result directly in morbidity. Cerebral infarction and hemorrhage, serious patient-related complications, occurred in 8.6% and 5.8% of neonates, respectively. Hemorrhagic complications are fairly common and include bleeding from cannulation sites (6.2%), other surgical sites (6.1%), and the GI tract (1.7%). Hemolysis (plasma hemoglobin >50 mg/dl) was reported in 12% of cases. The most common mechanical complications is clotting in the circuit, with an 18.3% incidence. Tubing rupture occurred in 0.3% of cases, and oxygenator failure was reported in 5.7%.

Venoarterial (VA) remains the most common support mode for neonatal respiratory failure, but the incidence of venovenous (VV) support is increasing. Historically, >75% of patients have been supported in the VA configuration, but in 2004 this fell to <60%.

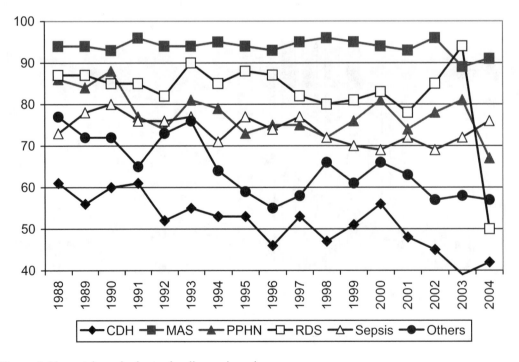

Figure 4. Neonatal survival rates by diagnosis and year.

Table 2. Survival and support duration in neonatal ECLS by diagnosis (through 2004).

Diagnosis	Total cases	Avg. run time (hrs)	Survival (%)
CDH	4,629	233	52
MAS	6,663	129	94
PPHN/PFC	2,996	145	78
RDS	1,388	133	84
Sepsis	2,396	138	75
Pneumonia	268	211	59
Air leak syndrome	97	167	72
Other	1,264	170	64

Table 3. Complications of ECLS in neonatal respiratory support (through 2004).

Complication	Incidence (% reported)	Survival (%)
Mechanical		
Oxygenator failure	5.7	55
Pump malfunction	1.8	68
Raceway rupture	0.3	61
Cannula problems	11.2	69
Clots	18.3	67
Air in circuit	5.2	72
Patient-related		
Intracranial hemorrhage	5.8	46
Intracranial infarction	8.6	55
Seizures	10.7	62
Cannulation site bleeding	6.2	68
Surgical site bleeding	6.1	46
GI bleeding	1.7	46
Hemolysis	12.0	67
Pulmonary hemorrhage	4.3	45
Culture-proven infection	6.5	55
Hyperbilirubinemia	8.2	66

Pediatric respiratory failure

The application of ECLS in pediatric respiratory support is expanding, with over 200 cases/yr being reported since 1995 (Figure 5). The most common diagnoses leading to the application of ECLS for respiratory support are provided in Table 4. Survival rates have been increasing over the past decade, from 30% survival prior to 1986, to presently over 50%. Pneumonia caused by various infectious etiologies continues to be the most common diagnosis with 61% survival. Pediatric acute respiratory distess syndrome (ARDS), primarily due to non-operative conditions or post-traumatic injury, has a 51% reported survival. Over 700 patients experienced a diverse set of other causes for acute respiratory failure (ARF) and had a 54% overall survival.

The most common mode of support for pediatric ECLS is VA, but the use of VV is increasing. Since 1976, 30% of reported cases have been initiated on VV support, but in the past year, this has risen to >35%. The use of a double-lumen catheter for VV access is also increasing.

Bleeding complications are higher in the pediatric group than in the neonatal group (Table 5). A 9% incidence of cannulation site bleeding was reported, with a 16% rate of bleeding from other surgical sites. Hemolysis occurred less frequently (9% vs. 12% in neonates), as did intracranial hemorrhage (5% vs. 6%). Mechanical complications are common. The incidence of clotting in the circuit was lower (7% vs. 18%), but a higher incidence of oxygenator failure occurred (15% vs. 6%). Infectious complications were frequent, with a 21% incidence of culture-proven infection.

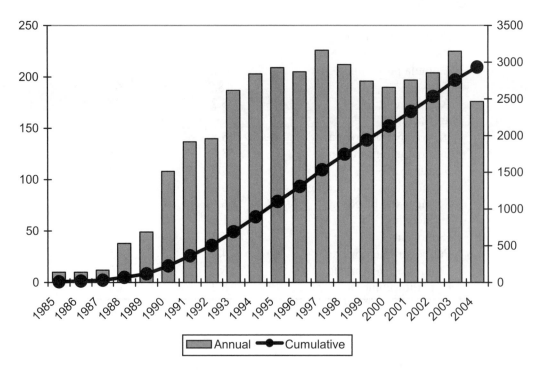

Figure 5. Annual and cumulative pediatric ECLS cases for respiratory support.

Adult respiratory failure

The most rapidly growing application of ECLS is for adult respiratory failure (Figure 6). The number of adult cases remained small until 1994, at which time a significant increase began and has continued. Earlier numbers were small most likely because earlier randomized, controlled trials suggested no significant benefit in this age group.[3,4] However, continued poor results with conventional ventilatory management prompted a resurgence of interest in adult ECLS. Supported by improvements in tech-nique, including experience with VV ECLS and percutaneous cannulation, recent experience has led to better results with fewer complications than previously reported.

Survival has consistently improved each year for the past decade. Cumulative overall survival for all diagnoses is 54%. Unlike the pediatric group, ARDS is the most common diagnosis leading to ECLS in adults (Table 6), with survival rates of 51% for both non-trauma or surgical etiologies and for trauma or surgi-cally-related ARDS. The highest survival is seen with viral pneumonia (63%).

Table 4. Survival and support duration in pediatric ECLS by diagnosis (through 2004).

Diagnosis	Total cases	Avg. run time (hrs)	Survival (%)
Viral pneumonia	747	318	63
Bacterial pneumonia	309	265	55
Pneumocystis pneumonia	22	371	41
Aspiration pneumonia	170	279	65
ARDS, post-op/trauma	72	223	63
ARDS, other	286	294	52
Other respiratory failure	608	244	47
Other	720	200	54

Table 5. Complications of ECLS in pediatric respiratory support (through 2004).

Complication	Incidence (% reported)	Survival (%)
Mechanical		
Oxygenator failure	13.7	45
Pump malfunction	3.0	48
Raceway rupture	0.7	35
Cannula problems	13.9	49
Clots	6.9	52
Air in circuit	2.0	52
Patient-related		
Intracranial hemorrhage	4.9	27
Intracranial infarction	3.2	41
Seizures	7.2	34
Cannulation site bleeding	9.4	61
Surgical site bleeding	15.6	47
GI bleeding	4.0	25
Hemolysis	8.8	42
Pulmonary hemorrhage	4.5	32
Culture-proven infection	20.8	46
Hyperbilirubinemia	3.2	28

VV access is the predominant mode of support in adults with respiratory failure, accounting for about 70% of initial modes of those reported to the Registry for 2004. The mode of support in adult ECLS was not recorded prior to 1998.

The complications profile for adults is similar to that of pediatrics (Table 7), except for a higher proportion of patients requiring inotropic agents for support (57% for adults vs. 38% for pediatrics). Cannulation site and surgical site bleeding occurred in 12% and 22%, respectively. GI bleeding was infrequent (4%). The infection rate was identical to that of pediatric patients (21%).

Cardiac support

The number of cases of ECLS for cardiac support reported to the ELSO Registry has shown a steady annual increase over the past decade (Figures 7-10). Over 5,500 cases were reported to the ELSO Registry by the end of 2004, with an overall survival of 40%. The majority are neonatal (37%) and pediatric patients (55%), with adults comprising the remainder (8%). The cumulative survival has decreased slightly but consistently over the past several years (44% in 1994). This is most likely because of the increasing complexity of the cases referred and accepted for ECLS.

Congenital defects in the perioperative period constitute the vast majority of cardiac diagnoses, with an overall survival of 39% (Table 8). Cardiomyopathy, myocarditis, cardiogenic shock, and cardiac arrest account for most of the remaining diagnoses. Myocarditis is associated with a better survival than other diagnoses. Cardiac transplant support accounted for 4% of cases, post-operative support 78%, bridge to

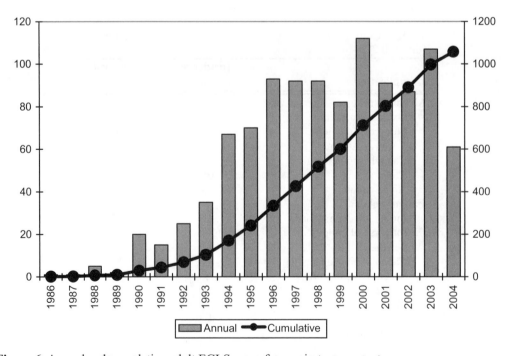

Figure 6. Annual and cumulative adult ECLS cases for respiratory support.

Table 6. Survival and support duration in adult ECLS by diagnosis (through 2004).

Diagnosis	Total cases	Avg. run time (hrs)	Survival (%)
Viral pneumonia	88	259	63
Bacterial pneumonia	191	237	52
Aspiration pneumonia	32	217	56
ARDS, post-op/trauma	136	240	51
ARDS, non-post-op/trauma	200	260	51
ARF, non-ARDS	59	204	63
Other	352	177	49

Table 7. Complications of ECLS in adult respiratory support (through 2004).

Complication	Incidence (% reported)	Survival (%)
Mechanical		
Oxygenator failure	18.0	42
Pump malfunction	4.1	35
Raceway rupture	0.7	29
Cannula problems	10.8	40
Clots	9.5	55
Air in circuit	1.1	58
Patient-related		
Intracranial hemorrhage	2.6	22
Intracranial infarction	1.9	35
Seizures	1.9	45
Cannulation site bleeding	12.2	45
Surgical site bleeding	22.2	35
GI bleeding	4.3	24
Hemolysis	5.2	27
Pulmonary hemorrhage	5.0	26
Culture-proven infection	21.2	41
Hyperbilirubinemia	4.3	13

Table 8. Survival and support duration in cardiac ECLS by diagnosis (through 2004).

Age group	0-30 days			31 days-<1 year			1 year-<16 years		
	Total cases	Avg. run time (hrs)	Survival (%)	Total cases	Avg. run time (hrs)	Survival (%)	Total cases	Avg. run time (hrs)	Survival (%)
Congenital defect	2,119	141	36	1,366	143	42	769	133	40
Cardiac arrest	27	104	26	27	142	26	52	118	40
Cardiogenic shock	24	163	50	12	76	33	34	107	32
Cardiomyopathy	73	203	66	65	227	46	204	201	53
Myocarditis	29	256	41	35	230	57	99	188	61
Other	185	178	44	168	155	42	276	146	43

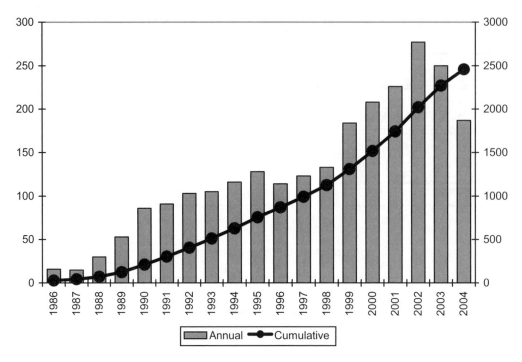

Figure 7. Annual and cumulative ECLS cases for cardiac support in the 0-30 day age group.

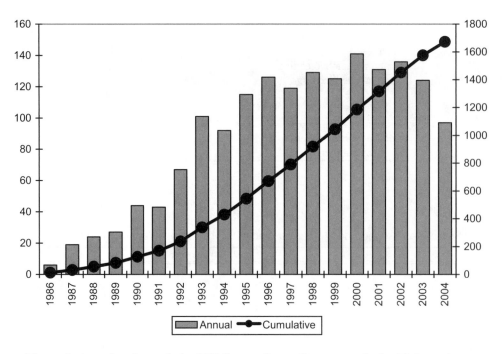

Figure 8. Annual and cumulative ECLS cases for cardiac support in the 30 day to 1-year age group.

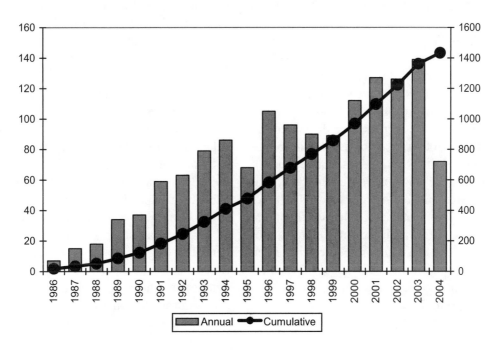

Figure 9. Annual and cumulative ECLS cases for cardiac support in the 1 year to 16-year age group.

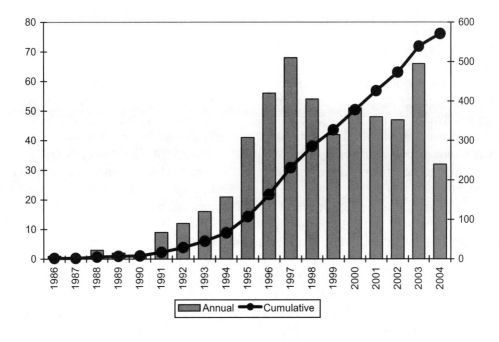

Figure 10. Annual and cumulative ECLS cases for cardiac support in the >16-year age group.

transplant 5%, and the remaining 13% were for non-post-operative cardiac support.

The Registry contains data for the major groups of cardiac operations performed for the correction of left-to-right shunts, left-sided obstructive lesions, hypoplastic left heart syndrome, right-sided obstructive lesions, cyanotic heart disease with increased or decreased pulmonary blood flow, and unclassified lesions.

Surgical site bleeding was reported in 29% of patients. The most common complication was the requirement for inotropes, which was reported in 52% of patients. Cardiac dysrhythmias occurred in 20% and infectious complications in 11%. Renal dysfunction requiring intervention was reported in about 30%. Mechanical complications, including cannula problems, were not common.

Summary

The ELSO Registry remains an important and comprehensive database on the application and outcomes of ECLS for respiratory and cardiac failure in all age groups. It is a significant source of information for the clinical practice of ECLS and for support of academic research.

The ELSO Registry is a source for data upon which an individual institution can benchmark its performance against the international experience. The re-design of the database allows for improved data retrieval and generation of ad hoc reports on short notice. Improved data entry has reduced delays and errors in data management.

The Registry has weaknesses in addition to its strengths. It can capture summary information, but cannot provide the in-depth information which may be needed to support clinical practice. It is a voluntary registry, and therefore does not capture the full domestic, and especially the international experience. Even with well-defined data submission forms and instructions, the misinterpretation of fields, especially for complications, can lead to errors in reporting and analysis. Outcome data are very limited, as the Registry only captures basic outcome information.

The re-designed Registry is more readily capable of growth and expansion because of the additional reporting of new pre-ECLS support treatments, devices and other technological changes, and the listing of mechanical and clinical complications. Growth can now take place without changes in the underlying structure of the database, and, thus, can be implemented in a timely fashion. Data entry and retrieval via the World Wide Web has improved timely reporting of data and assists in capturing international data. The Registry now allows for the integration of specialized data collection projects without modifications to the database structure, such as an addendum to enhance cardiac support data or the inclusion of an expanded outcomes database.

References

1. Conrad SA, Rycus PT, Dalton HJ. Extracorporeal Life Support Registry Report 2004. *ASAIO J* 2005; 51:4-10.

2. Roy BJ, Rycus P, Conrad SA, Clark RH. The changing demographics of neonatal extracorporeal membrane oxygenation patients reported to the Extracorporeal Life Support Organization (ELSO) Registry. *Pediatrics* 2000; 106:1334-1338.

3. Zapol WM, Snider MT, Hill JD, et al. Extracorporeal membrane oxygenation in severe acute respiratory failure. A randomized prospective study. *JAMA* 1979; 242:2193-2196.

4. Morris AH, Wallace CJ, Menlove RL, et al. Randomized clinical trial of pressure-controlled inverse ratio ventilation and extracorporeal CO_2 removal for adult respiratory distress syndrome. *Am J Respir Crit Care Med* 1994; 149:295-305.

11

Legal Considerations During ECLS

Edward B. Goldman, J.D.

Introduction

This chapter will discuss the legal process and legal aspects of the doctor-patient relationship, malpractice and defenses, and the probability of risk in this area. Discussion will then turn to informed consent, followed by the rules of research. The chapter will then conclude with a discussion of the treatment process.

The legal process

Law is a system of social control. The symbol of justice holding a scale is appropriate for the legal system since the system is always trying to strike a balance of rights and responsibilities. For example, the First Amendment to the United States Constitution grants all citizens the right of free speech but does not allow one to yell "fire!" in a crowded theater.

Law is based on the notion that, in an adversary system, conflicts can be resolved in a way that is just and fair for both society and litigants. Because law is based on an adversary system, its rules differ substantially from health care. For example, an expert witness in the legal system is hired to advance the point of view of one side to a dispute, not to render an impartial opinion.

The legal system establishes guidelines for conduct within this adversary system. Inevita-bly, if guidelines are to be clear and predictable, they will by nature have an element of arbitrariness. For example, the rule in law called the statute of limitations states that a claim brought past a certain point of time is stale and cannot be heard in the courts. The period of time is set by the state legislatures and can vary from state to state. Thus, in one state an injured party may have two years to bring a lawsuit for malpractice, while in an adjacent state, an injured party may have three years.

When other routes fail, the legal system searches for truth and conflict resolution through litigation. Litigation occurs after the facts being disputed, and this provides opportunities to recount facts after the incident in question has occurred. Of course, this recreation of fact can create a "reality" far different from what really occurred. Decisions that are made in split seconds in the operating room can be examined two years after the fact over a matter of hours or days in the courtroom.

Indeed, the whole notion of "facts" is viewed differently by health care professionals and lawyers. Physicians are generally inductive, going from physical observation to conclusion, while lawyers are deductive, moving from general principles to conclusions. A general principle for lawyers may not be seen as fair in every case, but one that best balances the needs of society and individuals. A physician may conclude that a neonatal patient needs ECMO and would benefit from transfer to an ECMO center. After the fact, an attorney deducing from the general principle of "first do no harm" may, with the assistance of expert witnesses, conclude that the patient would have been better served by intensive care in the facility rather than risking deterioration during transfer.

The adversarial nature of the legal system, the "recreation of reality" problem, and the difference in definition of fact, are compounded by the problem of retroactivity. The legal system in civil law cases (disputes about property or injury) decides whether to award compensation only after the injury occurs. This allows the litigants to hire expert witnesses who reason backward and determine whether care was appropriate. Of course, hindsight is always 20/20 and, when reasoning backward, experts may often express an opinion that care should have been rendered in a different manner.

The system has specific rules of evidence and proof. The party claiming the right to compensation (the plaintiff) has the burden of proof and must present sufficient evidence to sustain a case before a trier of fact. In a civil case, the burden of proof is called "the preponderance of the evidence". The party with the burden of proof must prove a case by 51% certainty or better. This "preponderance" standard is used in civil law when compensation is what is at stake. In a criminal case, where life and liberty are at stake, the standard is "beyond a reasonable doubt", a much higher standard of proof. Therefore, in a civil case, the plaintiff can win by showing their case is slightly more likely than the defendant's, whereas in a criminal case, the state must prove beyond a reasonable doubt that the defendant is guilty.

Health care professionals are often not comfortable with the legal system's approach to reimbursement for injury. Typically, health care professionals seek certainty and want a system more akin to a mortality and morbidity conference. This creates tension between health care professionals and the legal system.

Individuals involved in the legal system should never lose sight of the fact that law is a process, and the procedural rules must be observed. Cases proceed in a specified fashion, and the parties engage in a sort of ritualized warfare out of which conflicts are resolved by a trier of fact. The aim of the system is both to resolve a conflict and to do so in a way that produces a just outcome.

With this background, the chapter will proceed to a specific discussion of malpractice issues.

Civil liability

The doctor-patient relationship

Health care professionals are responsible only for the care of their patients. The creation of the doctor-patient relationship is a contractual matter, although few health care professionals think of it in this way. Legally, what occurs is that a prospective patient asks whether a physician will provide care. The physician decides whether or not they wish to undertake this responsibility. The physician agrees to provide care so long as the patient agrees to pay for the care and be a participant in the process. Either side can terminate the contract at any time except that the health care professional cannot terminate in a way which would cause injury to the patient. Termination that would cause injury is called "abandonment" and is defined as a physician discontinuing a relationship when it is reasonably likely that harm would occur. An extreme example of abandonment would be if a patient was placed on ECMO and the physician then said, "I have decided that I am going to take a long weekend, and therefore, I am discontinuing ECMO." A physician may terminate doctor-patient relationship only in a way that does not harm the patient. The patient, however, can terminate the relationship at any time even if termination would cause injury to the patient. A typical example of termination by a patient is leaving a hospital against medical advice. Here, the patient is warned that leaving the hospital would be dangerous to his or her health, but the patient may decide to leave anyway. With competent adult patients, the physician need only document that the patient has refused medical advice. For minors, where the parents want to refuse care, the physician can use the child abuse and neglect laws to treat the patient while the legal system resolves whether care should continue.

In an emergency, the doctor-patient relationship is created when the patient arrives at (or near) the emergency room. Any facility with an emergency room is legally bound to create a relationship with any patient needing emergency care. Equally, when an ECMO unit accepts a patient in transfer, the unit and its staff have agreed to create a relationship.

Federal law via the Emergency Medical Treatment and Active Labor Act (EMTALA) requires a screening exam and subsequent stabilization for emergency patients seen at an emergency facility.[1] This means that any patient seen at an emergency department must receive an exam to determine if they need treatment and if so, the nature and extent of the condition. Then, the patient must receive care designed to stabilize their condition regardless of their ability to pay for the care prior to transfer to another medical facility.

Once the doctor-patient relationship has been created, it is the obligation of the patient to provide the facts necessary for the doctor's diagnosis and treatment and to comply with the medical regimen. It is the responsibility of the physician to treat the patient in the same way that other similarly situated, reasonably prudent practitioners would. This is referred to in the legal system as the "standard of care" rule.

Malpractice

Malpractice simply means a claim by a patient that a medical professional has breached the standard of care, resulting in harm to the patient. It is no different than any other civil lawsuit for injury except that, in medical cases, it generally requires testimony from expert witnesses. A malpractice case could be brought against an architect for improper design of a structure resulting in injury, a lawyer for inappropriate legal advice resulting in injury, or a physician for inappropriate diagnosis or treatment resulting in injury. The elements of malpractice are the existence of a doctor-patient relationship, duty, breach of duty, causation ("proximate cause"), and damages.

Duty means the obligation of the health care professional to provide treatment in the same manner as any other similarly situated, reasonably prudent practitioner. This means that treatment must be rendered according to commonly accepted norms in the profession. In areas involving advanced treatment such as ECMO, the physician's duty is to exhaust standard methods of treatment before proceeding to new approaches until the new approaches have been demonstrated to be as good or better than existing modalities of treatment.

Breach of duty is a circumstance where the practitioner does not act in a reasonably prudent fashion. Together, duty and breach of duty are commonly referred to as "the standard of care". The standard of care can arise from general education and experience in the field (i.e., doing things the way that you were taught to do them), or it can arise from standards created by a governing body. For example, the American College of Obstetrics and Gynecology provides guidelines which describe standard ways to provide care.[2] Standards can also come from consensus development conferences and from state or federal law. For example, in some states, state legislators mandate how informed consent must be obtained for certain procedures. For example, the laws in Maine and Texas specify the elements of consent for specific procedures.[3,4]

Even if a standard of care may have been violated, this, in and of itself, will not necessarily allow a plaintiff to win a lawsuit. The plaintiff must also demonstrate that the violation resulted in an injury. These are the elements of "proximate cause" and "damages". To take an extreme example, air introduced into an IV system would constitute a violation of a standard of care. However, if the air was removed before damage occurred to the patient, there would be no viable malpractice case. If, however, air was introduced, and hypoxic brain injury resulted, all elements (relationship, duty, breach, proximate cause, and damage) of a claim would be present. The breach must be a cause of the injury.

Damages in a malpractice suit consist of economic damages and non-economic damages. Economic damages include hospital costs, lost wages, need for future health care, and costs of adaptive equipment. Non-economic damages are pain and suffering. Many states have, through tort reform, limited the amount of damages available to a plaintiff. For example, in many states, if a patient receives compensation for post-injury hospital care from an insurance company, the plaintiff cannot claim the cost of that care as damages. Similarly, in states with caps on non-economic damages, plaintiffs are limited to a specific dollar amount of recovery. For example, California, Michigan, and other states have a specific dollar cap on non-economic damages.[5]

Product liability

In product liability cases, claims can be brought not just against individuals, but also against equipment manufacturers. For example, if a catheter tip shears off in a patient, a claim may be brought against the physician for improper technique or against the company for improper design of the catheter. Product liability cases are brought against manufacturers on the theory that the manufacturer failed to take reasonably appropriate steps to make the product safe for its intended use. With ECMO, there may be claims against manufacturers for improper design of equipment. A claim might be made, for

example, that setup of a system allowed lines to be damaged by friction, that fluids were not appropriately warmed, or that safeguards were not in place to prevent a flow of oxygen into the system, causing air embolism. In these cases, the claim would be made against the manufacturer. The manufacturer could argue that the material was manufactured properly and was being used improperly by the end user. A manufacturer may argue that a piece of equipment was inappropriately modified by a hospital, or that it was used without following the appropriate maintenance standards. Typically, cases against manufacturers are brought for design and manufacturing defects.

Defenses

Once a plaintiff brings a suit, a defendant has an opportunity to raise both factual and legal defenses. Factual defenses might include claims that care was delivered appropriately; that a patient was non-compliant; that a third party, such as a manufacturer or subsequent treating physician, was responsible; or that the plaintiff's claim is factually inaccurate. Legal defenses include the statute of limitations or other defenses provided by state or federal law. The statute of limitations sets a time within which a plaintiff must bring a suit or lose the right to bring that claim. These statutes are state specific. Generally, the statutes for adults require a claim to be brought within two or three years from the date of injury; however, statutes for children vary widely. In some states, children do not have to sue until after they become legal adults. In other states, children must sue by a specified time. For example, in Michigan a newborn has until age 10 to bring a claim.[6] In other states, if the injury results in damage so that the patient can never regain competency, claims can be brought at any time. If a suit is not brought within the relevant statute of limitations for the particular state where the injury occurred, then the claim cannot go forward regardless of how meritorious it is on its facts.

Another common defense is "comparative negligence". This means that the patient's negligence caused or contributed to the injury. The patient's negligence is then factored into the equation to determine how much compensation, if any, the patient can receive. For example, a physician may warn a patient not to operate heavy equipment for 48 hours post-surgery. If, during the 48 hours, the patient operates heavy equipment and is injured, the physician would be seen to have no negligence, while the patient would be seen to have full responsibility for his or her actions. This would result in a verdict of no cause of action for the plaintiff.

Application to ECMO

A claim could be brought in ECMO cases for improper diagnosis or treatment. An improper diagnosis claim could argue that the physician should have been aware of the existence of ECMO and its utility in a particular patient's case. An improper treatment claim could argue that a patient was placed on ECMO when there were contraindications such as intracranial hemorrhage. Cases could also be based on claims of improper maintenance of equipment, improper monitoring, improper follow-up, improper transfer, or any other deviation from the standard of care.

Probability of risk

Although there have been a few malpractice cases involving ECMO use in the U.S., the likelihood of a claim is not high so long as the equipment is well maintained, the staff is appropriately trained, ECMO equipment is used correctly, and patients are monitored appropriately. Currently, treatment, at least of neonates, is well established with generally accepted inclusion and exclusion criteria and generally accepted approaches for treatment.

Informed consent

The rule of informed consent states that health care professionals cannot conduct invasive procedures without prior consent of the patient. The patient must be competent to give or withhold consent. Patients may be unable to consent because of age or medical status. Patients under the legal age of majority cannot consent unless they are emancipated pursuant to state law. Typically, minors can be emancipated when they are married, in the armed services, or because a court has held that they can be responsible for their own actions. Adults are competent so long as they understand the nature and consequences of their actions. Adults may be incompetent if they are unconscious, developmentally disabled, psychotic, or unable to express an opinion about their care. If a patient is not competent, then a guardian needs to be appointed for the patient. The guardian then makes decisions on behalf of the patient. In ECMO cases involving children, parent(s) or a court appointed guardian would consent to treatment.

The rule of informed consent says that the nature of the proposed procedure, its significant risks, its possible benefits, and treatment alternatives need to be explained to the competent patient or guardian for the incompetent patient. A choice then needs to be made by the patient or guardian. It is the responsibility of the provider to explain options to the patient or guardian. The provider can, and should, indicate a professional opinion, but it is up to the patient to make the choice. If the patient makes a choice that the provider does not feel is appropriate, then the provider can look at options for ending the doctor-patient relationship without abandonment or attempt to demonstrate that the patient is not competent and suggest that a guardian be appointed.

In the event of a true life- or limb-threatening emergency, care can be provided without obtaining informed consent. However, this is a rare circumstance, and typically, there is sufficient time to have a discussion with a patient or guardian before therapy is initiated.

Competent adults can make choices which cannot be contested. However, in certain limited cases, if parents are making choices for their children that are felt by the health care providers to be inappropriate, cases can proceed to court for resolution. The most typical case is where a parent, for religious reasons, refuses a blood transfusion for the child. In this case, courts reason that since the child has not made a free election for the religion, the parents cannot put the child at risk. Accordingly, the courts appoint a guardian for the child and the guardian then can consent to a blood transfusion.[7]

Paying attention to informed consent is important for two reasons. First, it is necessary to avoid legal liability. Treatment in a non-emergency situation without consent constitutes an assault and battery for which the professional rendering the treatment can be held liable. Second, discussion of the procedure and its risks, benefits, and alternatives helps to create rapport between the treatment provider and patient. This rapport is important in establishing a good therapeutic relationship.

Informed consent is a process of information exchange. The results of the process should be charted in the medical record or on an informed consent document, but the critical part of the exercise is the exchange of information. The document is merely a memorial that the discussion took place and was understood by the patient. The document also shows the choice made by the patient.

The rules of research

Research occurs when health care professionals are interested in expanding the boundaries of knowledge. Research is a careful approach to proving or disproving a hypothesis through data obtained pursuant to a protocol. Rules for research funded by the U.S. government are set forth in Federal regulations written pursuant to the National Research Act of 1974 and the Federal Privacy Regulations.[8] The Federal Government rules are a reaction to past abuses where researchers conducted studies without consent from patients, or against the best interest of the patients.[9] While this chapter cannot discuss the Health and Human Services and the Food and Drug Administration rules or the privacy and security regulations in any detail, they are well explained in governmental websites.[10,11]

The rules for research require submission of protocols to institutional review boards for a review of the appropriateness of the research before it can be carried out on human subjects. There are very specific rules for research involving minors. For example, the regulations require that researchers respect infants and children by protecting them from all but "minimal risk". Minimal risk is defined as the risks involved in provision of health care. Any research carrying more than minimal risk for children is allowed only if there is an expectation of direct health-related benefit for the subject child, or if there is "a minor increase over minimal risk" with the possibility of generalized knowledge about the child's specific disease.[12] Creation of a database specifically for research purposes is also governed by the Federal rules of research and privacy regulations.

ECMO was initiated in the 1970s and 1980s and its role in improving the survival for neonatal respiratory failure was described by Bartlett et al.[13,14] Three randomized, controlled trials have been performed in this patient population and all have shown that ECMO significantly improves survival.[15-17] ECMO for neonatal respiratory failure became a commonly accepted modality; it is no longer subject to research rules, but rather is considered the standard of care for patients who meet the relevant eligibility criteria.

Legal implications as ECMO develops

As indications for ECMO develop, there is a question of how ECMO should be provided. National organizations such as the ELSO Registry publish documents serving as references for physicians. These documents suggest considerations for treatment. As data develop, the considerations for treatment become more concrete. However, there are always new modalities of treatment. Just as ECMO for neonates was originally experimental, new proposed treatments could be evaluated against ECMO for specific neonatal indications.

Data can be aggregated to allow for epidemiologic studies of the long-term results of ECMO. Of course, if the ELSO Registry data is used for research, it must be created in accordance with the HIPAA privacy regulations and the federal research rules and must be IRB approved. ELSO Registry data collection provides sufficient data allowing ECMO to be reviewed longitudinally. This demonstrates the efficiency of ECMO as well as its complications.

The standard of care is the level at which a competent physician is expected to practice. In newly developing areas of medicine such as ECMO there is no clearly defined standard of care until there is common agreement on how practice should occur. In the early phases of any new innovation in medicine the first approaches are seen by the legal system as research or "innovative care" and they do not establish a uniform standard of care by which practitioners may be judged. It is only after the medical profession agrees on how the procedure is to be performed that a standard of care by which practitioners can be measured emerges. In other words, having a group like ELSO suggest guidelines in this developing field does not mandate that all practitioners must strictly follow those guidelines. Instead, practitioners are in a continual quality improvement process designed to improve the field.

Conclusion

ECMO is a rapidly developing field so the standard of care is, in a real sense, a moving target. Patients are by definition critically ill,

so intervention, assuming consent, is generally seen as preferable to non-intervention. Collection of data to show the efficacy of ECMO is important. Rapport with patients and families enhances trust and avoids claims of malpractice. Although this is a field dominated by critically ill patients and rapid advances in technology, the risk of lawsuit is low. Careful, prudent practice will minimize the risk of lawsuit while providing appropriate treatment for critically ill patients.

References

1. Federal Emergency Medical Treatment and Active Labor Act (EMTALA), 42 CFR, Parts 413, 482, and 489. Available at: www.emtala. com. Accessed May 27, 2005.
2. American College of Obstetrics and Gynecology. Available at: www.acog.org. Accessed May 27, 2005.
3. Texas law, Article 4590, the Medical Liability and Insurance Improvement Act.
4. Maine law, Title 24, Insurance Chapter 21, Maine Health Security Act Section 2905, Informed Consent to Health Care Treatment.
5. Pace NM, Zakaras L, Golinelli D. *Capping Non-economic Awards in Medical Malpractice Trials.* Santa Monica, California: Rand Corp.; 2004.
6. Michigan Compiled Laws, Annotated Section 600.5851(7).
7. Goldman EB, Oberman HA. Legal aspects of transfusion of Jehovah's Witnesses. *Transfus Med Rev* 1991; 5:263-270.
8. United States Department of Health and Human Services. Health Insurance Portability and Accountability Act of 1996 (HIPAA). HIPAA Privacy and Security Regulations, 45 CFR Section 164.512.
9. Levine R. *Ethics and Regulation of Clinical Research.* New Haven, Connecticut; Yale University Press; 1988.
10. United States Department of Health and Human Services. Health Insurance Portability and Accountability Act of 1996 (HIPAA).

Available at: www.hhs.gov/ocr/hipaa. Accessed May 27, 2005.

11. United States Department of Health and Human Services. Office for Human Research Protections. Available at: www.hhs.gov/ohrp/. Accessed May 27, 2005.

12. Additional Protections for Children Involved as Subjects in Research; 45 CFR 46 Subpart D Section 46.406.

13. Bartlett RH, Andrews AF, Toomasian JM, Haiduc NJ, Gazzaniga AB. Extracorporeal membrane oxygenation for neonatal respiratory failure: forty-five cases. *Surgery* 1982; 92:425-433.

14. Kanto WP, Jr. A decade of experience with neonatal extracorporeal membrane oxygenation. *J Pediatr* 1994; 124:335-347.

15. Bartlett RH, Roloff DW, Cornell RG, Andrews AF, Dillon PW, Zwischenberger JB. Extracorporeal circulation in neonatal respiratory failure: a prospective randomized study. *Pediatrics* 1985; 76:479-487.

16. O'Rourke PP, Crone RK, Vacanti JP, et al. Extracorporeal membrane oxygenation and conventional medical therapy in neonates with persistent pulmonary hypertension of the newborn: a prospective randomized study. *Pediatrics* 1989; 84:957-963.

17. UK Collaborative ECMO Trial Group. UK collaborative randomised trial of neonatal extracorporeal membrane oxygenation. *Lancet* 1996; 348:75-82.

12

ECMO Ethics in the Twenty-first Century

Tracy K. Koogler, M.D. and John Lantos, M.D.

Introduction

Today's use of ECMO exists in a state of limbo. On one hand, it is standard therapy for many conditions, and on the other hand, it is considered experimental for some diagnoses. In busy ICUs across the country, doctors have fairly well-defined indications for initiating ECMO in cardiac, pediatric, and neonatal cases. Surgeons will routinely request that ECMO teams "be prepared" before the surgeons undertake difficult cardiac operations or repair of congenital diaphragmatic hernia (CDH). However, there are many clinical situations in which ECMO has not been well studied, and debates about the appropriateness of ECMO use in these circumstances continue.

The underlying clinical dilemma is similar to that with any innovative therapy. We may not know with absolute certainty when ECMO is clinically indicated or whether it will be successful, but we use it in situations where it seems to offer the best hope of survival. The decision is based on a clinical judgment about whether the potential benefits of ECMO outweigh the risks. ECMO holds the possibility of cure but may also give families false hope, increase the patient's suffering, and prolong the dying process.

ECMO was developed as a temporary therapy in order to allow recovery of pulmonary function in neonates with single organ dysfunction. Children with chronic diseases and co-morbidities were excluded.[1,2] This initial use evolved into physicians utilizing ECMO for numerous causes of respiratory and cardiac failure in all age groups.[3] Recently, advances in medical management of respiratory failure, such as high frequency oscillators and inhaled nitric oxide, have decreased the need to use ECMO for isolated respiratory failure.[4,5] At the same time, the customary clinical indications for ECMO have shifted. Many institutions now report success with ECMO in treating children with malignancies,[6,7] asthma,[8] trauma,[9,10] and rejection following heart and lung transplant.[11-14] ECMO is also used as a bridge to heart and lung transplant,[15,16] as post-operative support following complex heart surgery,[17,18] and perioperatively for repair of CDH.[19] Randomized trials have not been completed for any of these conditions in pediatric patients or in adults. For some, there are only case reports of success with no comprehensive reporting of failures.

The lack of evidence may be inevitable. Unlike the situation with neonates, the evaluation of ECMO for older children is complicated by the sheer diversity of clinical indications and the small number of patients with each disease process who will require heroic measures such as ECMO. In this situation, it is often impractical to do randomized trials. Decisions concerning the necessity or potential benefits of ECMO will be individual decisions for physicians, patients, and families to make.

Because there is little evidence from clinical trials to guide decisions, clinical judgment becomes more important. Doctors who consider ECMO must first determine whether to offer it at all, and then how long to continue ECMO while waiting for a failing organ to recover or for a transplant to become available. They must carefully consider issues of communication with patients and decide how to explain the current uncertainties about the utility of ECMO. Such situations raise a number of interesting and unique ethical dilemmas. We will discuss the process of informed consent and the ethical techniques that have been commonly used in other situations where an innovative treatment is proposed for a patient who lacks decision-making capacity.

Informed consent

One "typical" scenario for ECMO use in the pediatric ICU involves a patient who is emergently transferred from an outside hospital with severe respiratory distress refractory to conventional medical therapies. The patient arrives at the tertiary care institution with unstable vital signs. The ECMO team prepares to cannulate the patient as the intensivist attempts to achieve adequate oxygenation and ventilation with various therapeutic interventions.

The intensivist or surgeon meets with the parents of a child or the family/surrogate of an adult patient and quickly explains the critical situation the patient is facing. Previously, the family has been told by doctors at the referring hospital that their loved one could die. Now they are told, "We must place the patient on ECMO immediately; it is the only way we can try to save his/her life."

This is not the ideal situation in which to obtain informed consent for innovative therapy; nevertheless, certain standard tenets of informed consent should guide the discussion. It is im-

portant for the surrogate decision-makers to understand the most serious ECMO complications, particularly death, intracranial bleeding, and life threatening circuit complications. It is crucial to state that there are no guarantees that ECMO will be successful. The family should be told that use of ECMO involves a time-limited trial. They should be given an estimate of when efficacy will be reevaluated. This information can be put in a standard written format. This allows the family an opportunity to read it again at a later time when they are not hurried and emotionally distraught.

A second typical scenario for ECMO is one in which non-emergency ECMO use is considered part of a larger treatment plan. This situation may arise before a complex congenital heart surgery or during the evaluation of a patient with heart failure who is being placed on a transplant list. The patient with respiratory or circulatory failure whose response is not optimal to medical therapy may also be a candidate for early discussion. In many instances, these patient's condition progresses rapidly and are often only hours from admission to placement on ECMO. Ideally, if a surgeon or intensivist believes there is a reasonable chance the patient may need ECMO in the future, then early discussion, when the parties involved are calm and time is not constrained, is ideal to present a realistic view of ECMO.

These two situations are similar in that both require careful consideration of the type of information given to patients or surrogates, and the type of cautions that should be included. Given the recurrent nature of these dilemmas, one good solution would be to develop a standardized informed consent form which could serve as a template for discussion about the risks and benefits of ECMO.

In most cases of ECMO, informed consent will come from a parent or a surrogate, because the patients are critically ill and unable to make decisions for themselves. The substituted judgment standards for children and adults differ, with the best interest standard being utilized for children or individuals who have never had decision-making capacity, while substituted judgment is used in the case of formerly competent adults.

Best interest standard

Parents and legal surrogates of children (up to 18 years of age) make decisions based on the best interest standard. This standard means that based on background, values, ethnicity, and family make-up, decisions are made which they believe are in the child's best interest. Parents have been given this right and responsibility, because it is inherent to child-rearing. Parents choose in what manner they raise their children (e.g., schools, religious practice, and home environment). A child's best interest is determined by a view of the child's situation in its entirety. The physician's role is to recommend therapies in the child's medical interest and allow the family to determine if the medical goals are compatible with the child's overall best interest.

Traditionally, physicians do not override the parental decisions unless not doing so will directly harm the child, or the parental decision will result in neglect. In such cases, court intervention is sought. One example of such an override based on the best interest standard, would be a child who is being raised as a Jehovah's Witness and requires a blood transfusion.

In the past, doctors have been reticent to seek court orders to override parental refusals of ECMO. There have been three reasons for this. First, survival after ECMO, though high, was far from certain. Second, the burdens of treatment imposed by ECMO were seen as extraordinary. Finally, the long-term sequelae of ECMO were not well quantified. Taken together, these led doctors to be cautious in their insistence upon ECMO if parents refused, and the need for ECMO seemed to be a reliable threshold at which the child's best interest could be deemed unclear, the indications for treatment ambiguous, and the long-term outcomes uncertain. There may be some situations in which that is no longer the case. For example, the cumulative survival in the ELSO Registry for babies with meconium aspiration who receive ECMO is 94%. Such a survival rate may, in itself, create a moral obligation for doctors to seek court approval to override parental refusals.

Substituted judgment

Although children below a certain age cannot make medical decisions for themselves, they usually have parents that are their recognized legal guardians. The situation regarding incompetent adults presents a case that can be more complicated as one must identify the appropriate surrogate.

The simplest case is one in which a formerly competent adult designated a proxy decision maker using a durable power of attorney for healthcare (DPAH). The DPAH is a legal document allowing a competent adult to authorize another person to make medical decisions on his or her behalf.

If a DPAH does not exist — as is the case for most patients— then, ideally, the patient is asked prior to becoming incapacitated who should make medical decisions for him. When authorizing a surrogate, it is best if only one person is named; if more than one is given, then the patient must indicate which decision-maker should be asked first. This information should be recorded in the patient's medical record after confirmation that the designated person accepts this role should it be needed. If the physician has not had the opportunity to discuss this with the patient, then state law is consulted to determine whether surrogacy issues are legislated. Most states have such laws which typically list types of individuals suitable to make medical decisions for a person who lacks decision-making ability. The lists are compiled in a hierarchical fashion, with spouse typically being first, adult children second, parents third, and friends or acquaintances designated last. The individual designated is expected to make decisions based on what the patient would do. Thus, this is referred to as "substituted judgment" rather than a "best interest" decision.

While a DPAH has the authority in most states to allow any decision the person could have made, the surrogate has some limitations on options when choosing life-prolonging therapies such as ECMO. A few states require proof of knowledge of prior patient wishes concerning withdrawal or withholding of life-prolonging therapies. If the physician believes that the surrogate in this situation is going against what the patient had previously requested for medical care, then the physician can challenge the decision. However, because of the high risk of ECMO, a physician should have very good cause to question the surrogate decision maker.

Emotions

Unlike other discussions physicians may have with families and surrogates, discussions surrounding ECMO are usually charged with emotion because of the critical nature of the situation. Therefore, despite realizing the risks and benefits of the procedure, many families will instruct the physician to do anything that might increase the risk for survival no matter how slight. The crisis situation often clouds rationality, and many never really hear or understand the potential long-term sequelae or potential for death despite ECMO. Therefore, one must reiterate to families the potential complications during subsequent conversations including daily updates about bleeding and infection risks, and the likelihood of a favorable outcome.

ECMO and futility

One of the most difficult issues surrounding ECMO involves considerations of medical futility which arise in three different ways:

situations in which doctors think ECMO will not work, situations in which doctors think ECMO is inappropriate because of the patient's underlying condition, and situations in which ECMO has been started but appears to be ineffective.

The first scenario, where doctors think ECMO will not work, rarely raises ethical dilemmas. Most families do not know to request or demand ECMO in the way they might know to request CPR. Instead, when doctors think ECMO is not indicated, they simply do not offer it. To the extent that dilemmas arise in this situation, they are usually intraprofessional dilemmas, that is, disagreements among doctors about whether or not ECMO should be offered. These may be situations where ECMO use is most experimental or innovative. When ECMO is offered in these situations, it is crucial that parents understand that its use is non-standard.

In some situations, doctors deem ECMO inappropriate because of the patient's underlying condition. One example is the use of ECMO in patients with Trisomy 13 or 18. In these cases, the decision to not offer ECMO is based upon a combination of two factors: the patient's poor prognosis for survival and the patient's poor prognosis for quality-of-life in the event of survival. Decisions to not offer ECMO based on poor prognosis for survival are more easily defensible than those based on the doctors' assessment of quality-of-life.

Finally, there are situations in which ECMO is initiated but is not producing the expected outcome. In a sense, these situations are similar to those in which there is poor prognosis for survival. However, because they involve withdrawal, rather than the withholding of ECMO, they are viewed differently. While lawyers and philosophers agree that withholding and withdrawing are legally and morally equivalent, doctors and families understand that emotionally they are not. In order to anticipate and address the special issues that arise with the withdrawal of ECMO, doctors should always include the idea of a "time-limited trial" as part of the initial consent process.

Time-limited trial

ECMO therapy should be offered as a time-limited trial and be described as such to all involved parties from the beginning. The medical team should determine a best estimate of how long the patient will need to receive ECMO therapy to adequately recover function and be weaned from ECMO. This time period will be based on the type of injury and the anticipated time course to healing. Data show that ECMO for cardiac failure after heart surgery continued beyond 3-5 days results in poor outcomes,[18,20] and ECMO beyond 2 weeks may not improve respiratory failure.[6] In the early days of ECMO, there was a marked decline in survival after 2 weeks. More recent data suggests that, although the longer a patient is on ECMO, the lower the survival rate, many patients have been supported more than 2 weeks and have survived.[21,22] Thus, today, there is no easily definable time period after which ECMO should be considered futile. Nevertheless, families should be told that the likelihood of success will be periodically reevaluated, so that ECMO does not become simply an extraordinary and artificial prolongation of the dying process. Each program should describe a time period after which ECMO might be considered futile and be withdrawn at the time of consent and discussed daily so that the family recognizes that, if there is no improvement within a certain period of time, goals will need to be changed and ECMO removed, potentially resulting in the death of the patient. To families, the patient may appear the same on day 1 of ECMO as on day 14, and they will not understand the need to remove the life-prolonging therapy. They may question why ECMO cannot continue indefinitely to give the patient every chance to get better.

Paris et al. discuss a case in which parents request that ECMO be continued after the physicians believe the therapy is no longer beneficial. The patient had a pulmonary contusion and hemorrhage secondary to trauma.[23] The article discusses how physicians have no obligation to continue a therapy that will not improve the outcome for the patient. If the time-limited trial has passed and there is no evidence of improvement, then the therapy has unfortunately been a failure and should be discontinued unless the physicians believe additional therapy, such as listing for transplant, may be beneficial. Further, if the patient develops complications that indicate ECMO is not improving the patient's health, but is causing harm or merely prolonging the dying process, it is justified to discuss these complications with the family and withdraw ECMO before the time trial is completed.

Palliative care

Palliative care is essential when the patient is going to die despite having received ECMO. Preparation of the family for discontinuation of ECMO and discussions concerning what the family would like to do in preparation for removal of the circuit is crucial. Does the patient require religious ceremony such as baptism, last rites, or other religious blessings? Does the family want to be present during discontinuation of the circuit? Did the patient wish to be an organ or tissue donor? Do the parents wish to hold the child during removal from ECMO? Who should be in the room with the family? These questions must be considered, and reasonable requests should be granted, since, for most of these families, these may be the only decisions they truly make, while other decisions have been made by the physicians with family agreement.

Most infants can be placed in the parent's arms prior to clamping the circuit. It should be explained to the parents that the circuit may alarm after the child is lowered into their arms. Allowing the parents to hold their baby prior to death which for some, may be the first time they have held their child, is critically important. Older children and adults can have their hands held during discontinuation of ECMO. A palliative care team can also help the family in the coming months to deal with their loss and provide support.

Families whose children receive ECMO and survive are also likely to benefit from palliative care services. Palliative care services will provide the emotional support to deal with a critically ill child as well as the potential transition to chronic illness which may result from the original insult. Chronic illnesses may include lung disease or neurological sequelae. The patient may require immunosuppressive medications for a transplant. The parents of an ECMO survivor are unlikely to take a completely healthy child home from the hospital. It is likely that the child will require some therapy, such as rehabilitation, supplemental oxygen, mechanical ventilation, or a feeding tube. They may also have seizures, developmental delay, cerebral palsy, or learning disabilities. Support from chaplains, social workers, and other specialists will minimize the trauma of this ICU experience. Unfortunately, most adult palliative care services are unable to provide these services; however, other support services for the inevitable transitions for the adult patient and family are beneficial.

Summary

ECMO has proven effective in treating acute respiratory and cardiac decompensation. Failures as well as successes should be reported so that more information is available to physicians when determining which patients may or may not benefit from this therapy and which conditions may lead to certain failure.

ECMO must be considered a time-limited trial, and physicians should administer it with the anticipation of a maximal length of trial. The time period should be relayed to the family and the medical team. The patient should be assessed daily to determine if the time period should be altered or other treatments considered such as transplant. If the time period expires and improvement is not seen, then it is the physician's ethical obligation to make the critical decision to remove ECMO, since it has failed to fulfill its goal.

Family support during this time of critical illness is crucial to help with the transition to caring for a family member with chronic medical issues or losing a family member. Palliative care teams, chaplains, and social workers may all be instrumental in achieving these goals.

If ECMO is unsuccessful, allowing the family some choices about the method of withdrawal of ECMO and the presence of family is imperative. As we continue to provide extraordinary therapies to save lives, we must also remember to provide extraordinary care when technological therapies fail and death is inevitable.

References

1. Bartlett RH, Gazzaniga AB, Toomasian J, Coran AG, Roloff D, Rucker R. Extracorporeal membrane oxygenation (ECMO) in neonatal respiratory failure. 100 cases. *Ann Surg* 1986; 204:236-245.

2. Toomasian JM, Snedecor SM, Cornell RG, Cilley RE, Bartlett RH. National experience with extracorporeal membrane oxygenation for newborn respiratory failure. Data from 715 cases. *ASAIO Trans* 1988; 34:140-147.

3. Conrad SA, Rycus PT, Dalton H. Extracorporeal life support registry report. *ASAIO Journal* 2005; 51:4-10.

4. Hintz SR, Suttner DM, Sheehan AM, Rhine WD, Van Meurs KP. Decreased use of neonatal extracorporeal membrane oxygenation (ECMO): how new treatment modalities have affected ECMO utilization. *Pediatrics* 2000; 106:1339-1343.

5. Hui TT, Danielson PD, Anderson KD, Stein JE. The impact of changing neonatal respiratory management on extracorporeal membrane oxygenation utilization. *J Pediatr Surg* 2002; 37:703-705.

6. Masiakos PT, Islam S, Doody DP, Schnitzer JJ, Ryan DP. Extracorporeal membrane oxygenation for nonneonatal acute respiratory failure. *Arch Surg* 1999; 134:375-379.

7. Linden V, Karlen J, Olsson M, et al. Successful extracorporeal membrane oxygenation in four children with malignant disease and severe Pneumocystis carinii pneumonia. *Med Pediatr Oncol* 1999; 32:25-31.

8. MacDonnell KF, Moon HS, Sekar TS, Ahluwalia MP. Extracorporeal membrane oxygenator support in a case of severe status asthmaticus. *Ann Thorac Surg* 1981; 31:171-175.

9. Steiner RB, Adolph VR, Heaton JF, Bonis SL, Falterman KW, Arensman RM. Pediatric extracorporeal membrane oxygenation in posttraumatic respiratory failure. *J Pediatr Surg* 1991; 26:1011-1014.

10. Fortenberry JD, Meier AH, Pettignano R, Heard M, Chambliss CR, Wulkan M. Extracorporeal life support for post-traumatic acute respiratory distress syndrome at a children's medical center. *J Pediatr Surg* 2003; 38:1221-1226.

11. Hoffman TM, Spray TL, Gaynor JW, Clark BJ 3rd, Bridges ND. Survival after acute graft failure in pediatric thoracic organ transplant recipients. *Pediatr Transplant* 2000; 4:112-117.

12. Mitchell MB, Campbell DN, Bielefeld MR, Doremus T. Utility of extracorporeal membrane oxygenation for early graft failure following heart transplantation in infancy. *J Heart Lung Transplant* 2000; 19:834-839.

13. Dahlberg PS, Prekker ME, Herrington CS, Hertz MI, Park SJ. Medium-term results of extracorporeal membrane oxygenation for severe acute lung injury after lung transplantation. *J Heart Lung Transplant* 2004; 23:979-984.

14. Oto T, Rosenfeldt F, Rowland M, et al. Extracorporeal membrane oxygenation after lung transplantation: evolving technique improves outcomes. *Ann Thorac Surg* 2004; 78:1230-1235.

15. Levi D, Marelli D, Plunkett M, et al. Use of assist devices and ECMO to bridge pediatric patients with cardiomyopathy to transplantation. *J Heart Lung Transplant* 2002; 21:760-770.

16. Hopper AO, Pageau J, Job L, Heart J, Deming DD, Peverini RL. Extracorporeal membrane oxygenation for perioperative support in neonatal and pediatric cardiac transplantation. *Artif Organs* 1999; 23:1006-1009.

17. Kulik TJ, Moler FW, Palmisano JM, et al. Outcome-associated factors in pediatric patients treated with extracorporeal membrane oxygenator after cardiac surgery. *Circulation.* 1996; 94:II63-68.

18. Aharon AS, Drinkwater DC, Churchwell KB, et al. Extracorporeal membrane oxygenation in children after repair of congenital cardiac lesions. *Ann Thorac Surg* 2001; 72:2095-2101.

19. Heiss K, Manning P, Oldham KT, et al. Reversal of mortality for congenital diaphragmatic hernia with ECMO. *Ann Surg* 1989; 209:225-230.

20. Mehta U, Laks H, Sadeghi A, et al. Extracorporeal membrane oxygenation for cardiac support in pediatric patients. *Am Surg* 2000; 66:879-886.

21. Linden V, Palmer K, Reinhard J, et al. High survival in adult patients with acute respiratory distress syndrome treated by extracorporeal membrane oxygenation, minimal sedation, and pressure supported ventilation. *Int Care Med* 2000; 26:1630-1637.

22. Frenckner B, Palmer P, Linden V. Extracorporeal respiratory support and minimally invasive ventilation in severe ARDS. *Minerva Anestesiol* 2002; 68:381-386.

23. Paris JJ, Schreiber MD, Statter M, Arensman R, Siegler M. Beyond autonomy-physicians' refusal to use life-prolonging extracorporeal membrane oxygenation. *N Engl J Med* 1993; 329:354-335.

13

Economics of ECLS

Robert H. Bartlett, M.D. and Robin A. Chapman, R.N.

Introduction

Anyone walking into a modern ICU in any country is first impressed with the intense, professional, and highly technological atmosphere, and second with what must be an enormous expense. Any health care professional who spends a month in any modern ICU perceives that most patients recover, but some suffer expensively only to die or to be discharged to permanently non-productive lives. Daily, the question arises: Is it worth it? ECLS is an obvious example of the dilemma: how much time, effort, and money can we afford to spend on a single individual? ECLS is not very costly when as compared with other high-tech therapies. It is less expensive than organ transplant, cancer chemotherapy, or the cost of maintenance hemodialysis for 1 year. The cost accrues over a short time in very accountable categories; however, the patient is often a small child, and the outcome is uncertain. Recently in a study by Angus et al., the high cost of nitric oxide (NO) was examined and they concluded that although the initial costs were high with NO treatment, the cost effectiveness profile was favorable.[1] This demonstrates that therapies with high initial costs can become cost effective if the therapy is successful and leads to many productive years of life. This aspect of ECMO was recently studied in a 4-year follow up to the UK collaborative ECMO trial.[2] The study concluded that ECMO was cost effective when compared to conventional treatment at 4 years.

As the indications for ECMO broaden, patient selection becomes a factor in ECMO's cost effectiveness, as was recently highlighted in a study by Van Litsenberg et al.[3] Therefore, the question, "Is this worth it?" is epitomized at the ECMO bedside. The answer to this question requires various facts which we will enumerate in this chapter. It also includes some intangible variables which must be addressed. The implications of the costs and benefits to a single patient, workers, payers, and to society have been addressed in several retrospective and prospective studies which we will examine, all in an effort to address this challenging question.

Formal reports regarding the costs and benefits of ECLS are based on neonatal patients. Walsh-Sukys[4] compared resource utilization and outcome at 20 months of age in 43 neonates treated with ECLS to 26 infants with respiratory failure who did not receive ECLS. The hospital charges were similar (about $60,000). Schumacher et al.[5] conducted a prospective, randomized study comparing the costs and outcome in neonates treated with ECLS at 50% mortality risk to neonates treated with ECLS at 80% mortality risk. The hospital charges were similar (about $51,000). However, the ICU stay was shorter and the neurological complications less in the early ECLS group.

ECLS for cardiac support has led to a dramatic improvement in the survival of children with congenital heart defects. The survival rate for cardiac ECMO is ~40%, leading some to question the utility of an expensive therapy such as ECLS in this patient population. Mahle et al. utilized an accepted cost-efficacy of <$50,000 per quality-adjusted life-year saved; the authors concluded that salvage ECMO in the cardiac population resulted in a $24,386 per quality-adjusted life-year saved and that ECMO was an economically viable treatment option in this high risk population. [6]

Using statewide databases, the number of neonatal cases considered for ECLS can be estimated, and the impact on neonatal mortality per dollar can be calculated.[7,8] The cost effectiveness of ECLS compared to other treatment can be analyzed using information from the ELSO Registry and some assumptions. Schumacher et al.[9] used this approach to estimate the number and costs of additional survivors with ECLS and included the added costs of caring for survivors with chronic pulmonary or neurological conditions.

The cost of ECLS is moderate compared to the cost of treating other serious diseases. However, the percentage of healthy survivors is much higher than that seen with stroke, cancer, or heart attack, for example. Moreover, the survivors of cardiac or respiratory failure treated with ECLS are younger, so the number of quality life years per treatment is high as compared to other expensive treatments which are often justified by quality life years.[10] By this measure, ECLS is economically sound.

The financial and intangible costs of maintaining an ECLS program are similar worldwide. The reimbursement system varies considerably between countries, as do the budgets for health care. In the U.S., any care which extends a healthy productive life is considered legitimate regardless of cost. In life-threatening situations such as those requiring ECLS, care is given by doctors and hospitals regardless of the individual's ability to pay. An elaborate system of identifying costs and charges exists in the U.S., and the insurance carriers and tax-supported agencies pay enough to cover the "bad debt" incurred by doctors and hospitals. In other countries, the reimbursement system ranges from a fee-for-service approach resembling that of the U.S. to a fixed annual rate for physicians and hospitals regardless of the amount or type of care rendered. Obviously, any decision by an individual physician, a hospital, a health care payor, or a society will depend on the variables of the reimbursement system for that group or individual. Therefore, the answer to the value question for any technology will be different for each person involved and for each societal group. In this chapter we will focus on the U.S. system for costs, charges, and reimbursement. Those existing within other systems can then modify this information to apply to their own health care finance systems. This chapter was prepared with the recognition that ECLS is only conducted in major medical centers, typically academic medical centers.

Costs

The costs of maintaining ECLS capability are fairly easily enumerated: equipment, supplies, personnel, and some additional costs. In this section we will identify the specific costs associated with a hypothetical ECMO program with the capability for treating one patient at a time and a history of treating 20 patients per year: 10 newborn, 5 pediatric, and 5 adult respiratory failure patients. Low and high cost estimates are derived. Finally, the costs are analyzed per day of ECLS and per case. The personnel needed for a full-time team are identified for active centers anticipating this need.

The equipment required for a single case is shown in Table 1. This list assumes that a fully stocked and equipped ICU is the venue for the procedure. It is not necessary to have a separate room or location identified for ECLS, it is not necessary to use the OR for cannulation (although a scrub team from the OR is helpful), and it is not necessary to use additional space or nursing personnel than that usually allotted to a critically ill patient with respiratory failure. In fact, the need for ICU nursing time is usually decreased when patients are on ECLS, assuming that there is a separate specialist managing the pump and the patient. The essential equipment is the blood pump, a servo-regulation system for the pump, a flow meter (usually integral to the pump), a method to monitor pressures and saturation in the extracorporeal circuit, a device for measuring whole-blood activated clotting time (ACT), an oxygen flow regulator and pressure pop-off valve, a circulating water bath to maintain the temperature in the heat exchanger, an emergency battery, and a small cart to carry this equipment. All of this equipment can be purchased pre-packaged at a cost of ~$48,000; assembled from individual components which costs about $21,000; or made up from used equipment (which any hospital accustomed to

doing cardiac surgery has in its research lab) which has a parts cost of ~$1,000. The only piece of equipment which is unique to the ECLS system is the servo-regulation system to control inlet or suction pressure generated by the pump. Most ECMO centers buy the commercially available servo-regulation system for ~1,500 from OriGen Biomedical (Austin, TX).

Any roller pump which will accommodate ¼-, 3/8-, and ½-inch tubing is acceptable. Any pressure and online venous saturation monitoring system can be adapted for use by the ECLS system. There are commercially available online blood gas sensors which are convenient, but not necessary. It is necessary, however, to measure inlet and outlet pressure on the membrane lung. This can be done with a dedicated system, which is quite inexpensive, or with the pressure transducers available in any ICU. The battery should be of sufficient size to operate the pump alone (not the water bath) for 1 hour. Batteries used for a computer power system's back-up are the most economical. Circulating water baths intended to maintain normothermia over long periods and specifically designed for

Table 1. Equipment for ECLS.

	Used components	New components	Integrated system
Pump	OR equipment	$10,000	$45,000
Pump servo-regulation	Make on-site	$3,000	
Bladder box	$100		
Pressure sensors	ICU equipment	$1,000	
Saturation monitor	ICU equipment	ICU equipment	
Water bath	Blanket warmer	$3,000	
Battery	$500	$1,000	
Cart	ICU equipment	$1,500	
Gas flow meter	ICU equipment	ICU equipment	
Gas valve	RT equipment	$50	
Other (e.g., clamps, cords)	$50	$50	
ACT machine	Borrow from Dialysis	$2,500	$2,500
Total	**$650**	**$22,100**	**$47,500**
Back-up			
List of components	0	0	0
Used components	–	$650	–
Complete system	–	$22,100	$47,500
Total with back-up	**$650**	**$44,200**	**$95,000**

ECLS are commercially available. Any continuous source of 38°C water can be used (such as systems designed for heating blankets), with the knowledge that these systems are not intended for weeks of continuous use and are not capable of rapid cooling or heating.

Although servo-regulated roller pumps are the least expensive and the most reliable for prolonged extracorporeal circulation, other types of pumps described in this book are useful for prolonged support. Centrifugal pumps are commonly used, although without some type of servo-regulation they can cause high negative pressures resulting in hemolysis. Some of the newer centrifugal pumps (e.g., Jostra Magnetically Suspended Rotor Pump, Jostra AG, Hirrlingen, Germany) are better suited to prolonged ECLS. As long as the inlet pressure does not exceed –300 mm Hg during inlet clamping at a specific rpm, the pump can be used at that rpm without major risk of hemolysis. Heat generation and thrombosis in the pump head are still potential problems with centrifugal pumps. The ideal pump for prolonged extracorporeal support is a peristaltic pump; however, no such pump is currently commercially available.

In addition to the equipment necessary to manage a single patient, at least one back-up component should be available for each part of the system. This may require having a duplicate, unused, complete system available at all times, or may be simply a list of equipment which can be located in the OR, laboratory, or ICU storage area when needed. However, the back-up equipment may be needed emergently on any night or weekend, so the back-up equipment must be truly immediately available. With all these considerations, the cost of equipment for an ECMO program might range from $3-95,000 (Table 1). A safe and reasonable approach is to buy a new equipment component system and use old, recently-serviced equipment as a back-up, all of which will cost ~$28,000.

Disposable supplies

Disposable supplies must be provided for each case, and must be custom designed for patient size and the type of vascular access. Enough supplies must be kept on hand to respond to any type of patient and to replace disposable components as necessary. The supplies needed for the hypothetical ECMO center are listed in Table 2. The annual supply costs for a typical ECMO center are $68,300. We have estimated conservatively, for safety, that 2 oxygenators and 2 circuits will be needed for each patient, but this is an overestimate and will result in some surplus stock. The supplies needed specifically for the ECMO system are oxygenators, various sizes of conduit tubing, connectors, Luer locks, pigtail adapters and stop cocks, a small venous bladder for servo-regulation, disposable components needed for pressure monitoring and venous saturation monitoring, a heat exchanger, and tubes and syringes for blood sampling and ACT measurements. The entire extracorporeal circuit, with the exception of the oxygenator and access catheters, can be purchased as custom-made tubing packs that include all the supplies, plus extra ones, necessary for priming and cannulation. Although commercially assembled tubing packs are convenient and safe, it is certainly possible to assemble the circuit components ahead of time, sterilize the entire system with gas sterilization, and achieve considerable cost savings. If an institution assembles its own tubing packs on-site, it is important to allow appropriate time for sterilization and full degassing. It is particularly important to have connectors and tubing in all appropriate sizes, and other components individually wrapped and sterilized in order to deal with any circuit emergency. The only ECMO-specific drug requirement is heparin, although there will be increased requests to the pharmacy for antibiotics, sedatives, and narcotics, as well as extra demands on the blood bank.

Personnel costs relate to non-physician hospital-based personnel only. Resident and staff physicians do not receive any specific salary for the care of ECLS patients, although in most U.S. hospitals the physician costs and charges are accounted for separately from the hospital-based personnel costs and charges. The hospital should provide appropriate reimbursement for the time that the ECMO physicians spend administering the program although, at present, most hospitals do not. The personnel costs unique to the ECLS program begin with a full-time coordinator and include part-time or full-time ECMO specialists to comprise the entire ECMO team. The team may include individuals whose backgrounds are in nursing, respiratory therapy, perfusion, or medicine. Team members may be assigned: full-time to the ECLS program, full-time to the ECLS program, rotating to other hospital duties when there are no ECLS patients, or assigned to other hospital programs such as nursing, respiratory therapy, or perfusion and rotating to ECLS patients as needed. A variation of the latter approach is to train most or all of the nurses and respiratory

therapists in the ICU to manage ECLS. This is the most economical approach, but is difficult to maintain because of turnover and training costs. Considering vacation time, sick time, and unforeseen events, 6 full-time positions are necessary to provide 24-hour, 7-day coverage for ECMO. For our hypothetical center to hire a coordinator and 6 full-time specialists to treat 20 patients a year seems unreasonable ($15,000 per patient in personnel costs alone). However, a part-time team is less reliable and requires more training and more on-call time. An individual hospital may require paying overtime for the specialists' time carried out by employees who have other full-time or part-time jobs in the hospital. Our hypothetical center hired a coordinator and 2 full-time specialists. In addition, they have 15 part-time specialists drawn from the nursing and respiratory therapy personnel of the ECMO ICU so that ICU personnel can cover for breaks, meals, and unexpected absences. The coordinator and the full-time specialists provide 80% of the bedside ECMO care. They may work 50-60 hours a week when a patient is on ECLS, but their hospital allows paid days

Table 2. Supplies needed for 20 ECLS cases over one year.

Supplies			
Oxygenators			
Medtronic	0.8	20 @ $515	$10,300
	1.5	10 @ $515	$5,150
	4.5	10 @ $500	$5,000
Tubing Packs (tubing, venous bladder, heat exchanger, connectors)*			
	Infant	20 @ $500	$10,000
	Pediatric	10 @ $600	$6,000
	Adult	10 @ $600	$6,000
Back-up supplies			
Tubing, connectors, pigtails, stopcocks			$1,000
Access catheters			
Infant: 8F, 10F, double lumen VV			
Pediatric: 17F, 21F			
Adult: 23F, 25F			$11,350
ACT tubes			$1,500
Office supplies, telephone			$1,000
Total			**$57,300**

*Tubing packs can be constructed at 30% the cost of purchasing pre-made.

off in compensation when there is no ECLS patient. If the team worked in a hospital that did not allow such paid days off, the cost would be considerably more because of the increased costs of overtime pay.

The major cost incurred for any individual ECLS patient is the personnel cost for ECLS specialists. This cost is directly proportional to the time a patient is on bypass. Adults and pediatric patients will incur more cost than neonatal patients. A reasonable estimate of the hourly cost of the ECMO specialist is $50/hour, assuming this includes salary, benefits and indirect costs, on-call pay, training time, and time spent on other ECLS-related duties, including the cost of a full-time coordinator. Therefore, the estimated personnel specialists' cost is $1,200/day, so the personnel cost for a typical 4-day neonatal run is $4,800, a typical 10-day pediatric run is $12,000, and a typical 15-day adult run is $18,000.

A full-time coordinator is essential, regardless of whether the program treats 12 patients or 100 patients per year. In addition to day-to-day care of patients, the coordinator is responsible for maintaining equipment and supplies, managing schedules, training and education, triaging patients, maintaining policies and procedures, managing the hospital budget, and coordinating follow-up care. The coordinator can come from a background of perfusion, respiratory therapy, or nursing. However, because the ICU management of patients on ECLS will eventually become a routine part of bedside nursing management, in most circumstances it is desirable that the coordinator be a nurse. When a program exceeds 20 patients per year, the coordinator is too busy to spend significant time at the bedside. When a program approaches 50 patients per year, an administrative secretary and an equipment manager should be added.

The most critical personnel decisions relate to the number of patients that can be treated simultaneously. To have the capability to treat 2 or 3 patients simultaneously usually requires a full-time team of 6-10 specialists or a very large and well-trained part-time team.

Other costs

Other costs associated with an ECLS program include the cost of training team members (physicians, ICU nurses, and respiratory therapists); the expenses of laboratory animal training; administrative costs (including quality assurance, record maintenance, office and equipment storage space, computers, telephones, parking); and the cost of patient follow-up. The cost of quality assurance and Joint Commission on Accreditation of Healthcare Organization (JCAHO) requirements are met in most centers by membership in ELSO, which provides detailed data comparing ECMO center performance. The ECMO program will place additional requirements on other hospital departments, particularly nursing, respiratory therapy, pharmacy, radiology, blood bank, laboratory pathology, and rehabilitation. Whatever transport system the hospital uses for critically ill patients will be required to transport patients referred for ECMO and may become involved with on-ECMO transports, depending on the nature of the referral base. With all these considerations, the actual cost of our hypothetical ECMO center is $298,000 per year (Table 3). This could range from $174,600 to $425,900 per year (for an integrated system with 4 full-time specialists). Assuming that the total cost for providing ECLS for 20 patients is $300,000 per year, the cost per case is $15,000. The cost related to specific types of patients is provided in Table 4.

A hospital or HMO administrator looking at an annual cost of $300,000 for a 20-patient ECMO program might consider the expense excessive. ECLS is a complex technology that has a definite economy of scale and usage. Like organ transplantation, it is a good example of an activity that should be limited to a few regionally-based centers. Although it may not always be convenient for patients' families, and may be dissatisfying to the medical and nursing staff, most hospitals would be better off financially to refer all patients who require complicated intensive care to regional referral centers. However, there is another side to the ledger, discussed below.

Charges and reimbursement

In the U.S., charges to patients and insurance carriers are itemized in detail based on current procedural terminology (CPT) codes for physicians. These codes identify only the names of specific charge items for hospitals (e.g., 24

Table 3. Annual direct costs for ECLS program.

	Actual	Lowest cost	Highest cost
Equipment	$25,000	$1,000	$98,000
Supplies	$57,300	$50,000	$57,300
Personnel			
Coordinator @ $60/hr.	$60,000	$60,000	$60,000
Full time team @ $50/hr.	$100,000	0	$200,000
Part time team @ $3/hr.	$45,000	$60,000	0
Other			
Training	$3,000	$3,000	$3,000
Lab	$3,000	borrowed	$3,000
ELSO membership	$980	$980	$980
Travel, education	$3,000	0	$3,000
Miscellaneous	$1,000	0	$1,000
Total	**$298,280**	**$174,980**	**$426,280**

Table 4. Costs for specific types of ECLS patients.

Estimated costs	
Total program cost	$300,000
Cost per patient (20 patients)	$15,000
ECLS days	
Newborn @ 4 days	40 days
Pediatric @ 10 days	50 days
Adult @ 15 days	75 days
Total	165 days
Cost per patient day	$1,818
Cost per patient	
Newborn	$7,272
Pediatric	$18,180
Adult	$27,270
Estimated total hospital cost	
Newborn	$20,000
Pediatric	$45,000
Adult	$90,000

hours in an ICU, use of a ventilator, supplying a bronchoscope) or physicians (e.g., hourly care in an ICU, management of a ventilator, performing a bronchoscopy). The charges for each item are based on direct and indirect costs, plus a charge for anticipated bad debt, and a small profit margin. On average, the total charge is roughly 3 times the actual cost. The charges rendered by hospitals account for 80% of total cost, and 20% are rendered by physicians. The bills for these services are usually separate; in fact, there may be several hospital bills and additional invoices from several doctors for a single case. If all of the patient care is conducted in an insurance-owned system (e.g., the Kaiser system or the British National Health Service), a single theoretical "bill" for all the patient care goes to the account holding the assets. All of this reimbursement is done in retrospect; that is, at the end of the case or the end of the year, the total expenses are tallied up, the amount of reimbursement is added up, and the balance is determined. In the U.S. system, it is possible to determine the total cost, the total charges, and the total reimbursement, along with the profit or loss, for each individual hospitalization although this is rarely done. More commonly, individual patient costs are estimated based on a series of assumptions and averages. Individual patient charges are accurately identified, but hospital accounting of reimbursement is usually based on some global income amount divided by some number of patients, or more commonly by identifying the classification of insurance carriers for a group of patients, calculating a payment-per-charge ratio, and multiplying the result by the number of patients. This common approach to the accounting of hospital finances seems bewildering and misleading to physicians who are responsible for administrating ECLS or other hospital programs. This type of approach to hospital accounting can identify whether the entire hospital made or lost money in a year, but is not useful when it comes to administrating a small program like an ECLS program. Hospital

accountants can study the ECLS program, but without specific questions and help from the program administrator, the financial results may be deceptive.

To determine hospital and professional income for managing an ECMO program 6 simple questions must be answered: 1) what was the total number of patients referred for or because of ECLS; 2) How many referred patients were turned away and why; 3) how many referred patients were admitted to the hospital; 4) how many of these patients were treated with ECLS; 5) for the patients admitted to the hospital, what was the total hospital bill for each patient; 6) what was the reimbursement for each patient. With the answer to these questions, the financial status of the ECMO program can be described.

Documentation of the number of referrals, turn-aways, transports, and actual admissions must be kept by the ECLS program. It is important to keep specific records on each of these categories, particularly turn-aways. If the overall analysis indicates that each case is profitable for the hospital, then the decision to increase the size of the program will depend on the number of referrals declined because of lack of ECMO facilities or lack of ICU beds. It is important to record the number of patients transferred for ECLS because all of these patients are counted as patients in the ECLS referral base. In a typical program, less than half of these patients will actually require ECLS, but the bills are paid for all patients, so the financial analysis of the ECMO program must include both the cost and the income related to patients who are not treated with ECLS. Hospital charges associated with ECLS are shown in Table 5. To determine the actual hospital bill and true reimbursement for each individual patient, it is necessary to go to the hospital cashier's office with a list of patients, registration numbers, and specific hospital dates. Reimbursement takes 5-10 months, so the reimbursement side of this accounting must be updated a year or more after each patient is discharged. The hospital financial office will need the same list of names and dates to estimate reimbursement, but they will probably do it based on the mix of insurance carriers rather than the actual reimbursement figures. Typical hospital charges for ECLS patients related to other diagnoses and procedures are shown in Table 6.

Hospitals

In the U.S., the Federal and state governments use tax dollars to support health care for the elderly (Medicare), and the indigent (Medicaid and others). The federal government has developed a separate reimbursement system that applies to federally-supported health care. In this system, hospitals are paid a fixed fee for each patient admission based on diagnosis, not care provided. There are approximately 500 diagnosis-related groups (DRGs) codes ranging from acute respiratory failure to hysterectomy. The hospital is paid the same amount (with some modifiers) whether the patient is hospitalized for one day or one month. The payment per DRG is arbitrary and not based on actual data. For example, the highest paying DRG is tracheostomy, and one of the lowest is neonatal intensive care. It has been proposed that the DRG code for ECLS be the same as the one for tracheostomy, (i.e., DRG 541) because of the complexity and expense involved. The DRG system relates only to federally-supported Medicare and Medicaid payment programs, but many private insurance

carriers are using the federal DRG system for reimbursement as well.

Physicians

Physicians are paid for procedures according to a system called CPT. There are thousands of CPT codes, ranging from a simple history and physical to ligation of patent ductus arteriosus. Physicians decide how much they charge for each CPT, and insurance carriers decide how much they will pay per CPT. Medicare and Medicaid assign a payment value to each CPT based on a relative value scale, which attempts to assign payment according to complexity. If a new procedure does not have a CPT (e.g., extracorporeal liver support), there is a long, cumbersome method to establish a CPT. CPT codes related to ECLS are shown in Table 7.

ECLS is a good example of the principle that it costs money to make money. Although an ECLS program is very expensive for a relatively small number of patients, with a prudent approach to costs, and accounting done by the physician director or coordinator, almost all ECMO programs can generate a profit for the hospital and the individual physicians.

Table 5. Typical hospital charges related to ECLS.

Charges	
ICU/day	$1,000
Ventilator/day	$750
ECMO set-up	$4,500
ECMO/day	$3,000
Oxygenator	$2,500
OR team/hour	$286
Hemofiltration/day	$225

Table 6. Typical annual charges for diagnoses and procedures.

Diagnoses/procedures	
Cataract	$6,000
Myocardial infarction	$25,000
Coronary bypass	$40,000
Hemodialysis	$40,000
Respiratory failure	
Newborn	$50,000
Pediatric	$100,000
Adult	$150,000
Respiratory failure plus ECLS	
Newborn	$50,000
Pediatric	$100,000
Adult	$150,000
Breast cancer	$100,000
Major trauma	$150,000
Liver transplant	$250,000

Intangible costs and benefits of ECLS

Although an ECLS program may be very profitable for a hospital, the intangible costs and benefits far outweigh the actual dollars. Depending on the individuals involved, the balance of intangible assets may be strongly positive or strongly negative. Needless to say, any institution considering instituting an ECLS program should consider the bottom line in the intangible category before proceeding to any direct financial analysis.

For the hospital or HMO, the primary intangible benefit is the level of sophistication and education of the hospital and resident staff in the ICUs involved with the ECLS program. Because of the complexity of the physiology, the difficulties with patient care, and the understanding of laboratory tests and interpretations required, the ICU staff achieves a high level of technical expertise. Although immeasurable, every ECLS center finds that the general care of ICU patients, particularly ventilator patients, improves dramatically: ICU stays decrease; the need for blood gases, x-rays, and laboratory tests usually decreases; and there is improvement in the overall approach to anticoagulation, ventilator care, fluids, electrolyte management, and sedative and paralytic drugs. As care improves, the incidence of adverse events and lawsuits decreases, and the type of patients that can be accepted for care increases,

thus increasing the overall referral population. Some programs such as neonatology, pediatrics, pediatric cardiology, and diagnostic radiology have measurable increases in patient activity. As the reputation of the hospital is enhanced, the best available resident applicants, nursing applicants, and other staff seek out these institutions. Valuable physicians remain, providing stability and leadership. Patient and family contacts from follow-up visits allow successful relationships to be established with referring physicians and hospitals, resulting in an increased number of referred patients. Assuming the institution is managed well, more patients are always a benefit rather than a cost.

Intangible costs to the institution inevitably come with increased numbers of more complex patients. Ancillary services such as laboratory, radiology, anesthesia, pharmacy, nutrition support, critical care nursing, and respiratory therapy will have to be increased. Blood bank, OR, housekeeping, ER, and transport will have new and unique challenges. Each patient represents a potential lawsuit. If the administrator views increased numbers and complexity of patients as a cost rather than a benefit, the ECLS program will bring added expense.

For the staff and resident physicians, the intangible benefits are inherently obvious. The opportunity to save lives does not come along often in medical practice. ECLS offers that opportunity on a regular basis, and even if it

Table 7. Typical professional fees related to ECLS.

CPT		
36822, 36810	ECLS cannulation	$2,500
33960	ECLS care, first 24 hours	$2,500
33961	ECLS care, subsequent 24 hours	$1,500
99291	Critical care/first hour	$250
99292	Critical care, subsequent care/hour	$200
99295	NICU care/initial hour	$250
99296	NICU care/subsequent/hour	$200
90996	Hemofiltration management/day	$300
99193	Institution and first hour cardiopulmonary bypass	$600
99190	Pump oxygenator management/hour	$300

only occurs 50% of the time it is intensely satisfying. ECLS is currently the state-of-the-art in high technology intensive care. Knowledge and understanding of the bioengineering and physiology involved brings all other aspects of critical care management to a higher level. Involvement with ECLS automatically brings online monitoring, oxygen kinetic physiologic monitoring, calorimetry and protein balance monitoring, hemofiltration, chronic neuromuscular blockade monitoring, advanced ventilator management techniques, and a variety of other intensive care procedures into focus. For academic physicians, the benefit of studying cardiac and pulmonary disease and the opportunity to work on the forefront of clinical life support research usually means a career in which laboratory research is in an adjuvant rather than a primary priority. This association with advanced technology in patient care that has a measurable and favorable endpoint leads to overall physician satisfaction and results in recruitment and retention of the best doctors who have an interest in critical care. Financial income related to ECLS-referred patients is a minor benefit.

The costs to physicians are high, and should be considered carefully before establishing an ECLS program. ECLS patients are always acute emergencies and consume days to weeks at the bedside, without regard for the hour of the day, holidays, vacations, or family plans. Although physicians are accustomed to being on call, ECLS requires being available and often physically in the hospital every day and every week for extended periods. This applies, in some degree, to every physician involved with the program. Before beginning an ECLS program, an enthusiastic pediatric or adult intensivist must ascertain the commitment of surgeons, radiologists, cardiologists, and other physicians who might be needed on a moment's notice for an ECLS patient. For academic physicians, time spent at the bedside means time not spent at the laboratory bench.

Is it worth it?

Several years ago, a prominent physician responsible for health care in a small African country visited the University of Michigan ECMO program. After seeing a few patients, he commented that the cost of an ICU with an ECMO program designed for 20-30 patients was more than the entire public health budget for his country. If the worth of money spent for health care means the most good for the most people, then an ECLS program would not be prudent in this example. Health care funds might be better spent on education, birth control, water purification, or malaria prevention.

The answer to the value question of whether or not ECMO is worth the expense depends on the responder. To the patient or family, the opportunity for a return from acute, lethal illness to prolonged productive life is worth it regardless of the cost. If the survival rate were only 10%, or if the severe disability rate were 30%, efforts expended on an individual patient would not be worth the agony and expense imparted to the majority of dead or disabled patients and families. But with survival ranging from 50-90% and disability ranging from 5-15% to the individual patient the effort is definitely worth it if the chance of survival with conventional therapy is <50%.

For the physicians, the opportunity to salvage the dying patient is always worth the effort when the outcome is good. The question of value, however, must be individually answered by each physician involved, weighing hours at the bedside against hours not spent in other activities (e.g., office, laboratory, OR, time off).

For hospital staff, the value comes in the satisfaction of returning sick patients to a healthy and prolonged life. The demands on time and lifestyle imposed on the physicians by ECLS are not felt by most hospital staff, who generally work on an hourly, salaried basis and work the same number of hours regardless of the activity. Although some hospital staff see ECLS as merely extra intensive work, most of the staff, from the housekeepers to the ICU nurses, consider the balance to be positive. For the ECLS specialist team and coordinator, ECLS offers a new and usually exciting career opportunity, which brings new knowledge, extra satisfaction, and usually supplemental income.

For hospital administrators, the value of an ECLS program is measured in dollars, no matter how humanitarian the outlook of the administrator. As discussed in some detail above, a hospital administrator who regards an increase in patients as an asset will consider that the ECLS program is worth it while an administrator who considers additional patients a liability will not.

The same reasoning applies to managers of insurance companies and HMOs. Prepaid insurance programs cater to younger working individuals. They avoid the liability of diseases of the elderly, but accept the liability of diseases of the young (trauma, obstetrical complications, newborn emergencies, and acute, lethal diseases such as severe respiratory failure). Although an acute lethal disease is unusual, it is always expensive, particularly when it is followed by chronic disability. Trauma care is much more of a problem for managed care companies than acute respiratory failure. Nonetheless, because each hospitalization is a liability relatively unrelated to income, any managed care or HMO administrator may view an ECLS program as a liability. An HMO administrator who reads current literature may come to realize that the cost of ECMO-treated newborn patients is the same or less than similar patients treated with conventional ventilation; therefore, a newborn ECMO program might be considered an asset. Eventually, the same studies will be conducted on pediatric and adult cases, although the resulting analysis might not be as favorable.

Finally, the value to society depends on the characteristics of that society. For the small African nation with a very limited health care budget, it would not be financially sound to have an ECLS program, and for that matter an intensive care program for infants or adults. For a society like that of the U.K., decisions about programs like transplantation and ECLS are based on financial analysis. The National Health Service sponsored a prospective, randomized study of ECLS compared to conventional ventilator management in newborn infants, with the final endpoint being neurological and developmental status at age one. There were more than twice as many healthy survivors in the ECLS group; therefore, ECLS produced many more quality life years than conventional treatment.[2] In France, Italy, Sweden, Japan, and other similar countries, the financial ability exists to devote a higher per capita amount of funds to be spent on health care. Whenever there is a good chance that a patient will return to a normal, healthy, productive life, almost any cost is justified, and the societal arguments become more scientific than financial.

References

1. Angus DC, Clermont G, Watson S, Linde-Zwirble WT, Clark RH, Roberts MS. Cost-effectiveness of inhaled nitric oxide in the treatment of neonatal respiratory failure in the United States. *Pediatrics* 2003; 124:1351-1360

2. Petrou S, Edwards L. Cost effectiveness analysis of neonatal extracorporeal membrane oxygenation based on four years results from the UK Collaborative ECMO trial. *Arch Dis Child Fetal Neonatal Ed* 2004; 89:F263-68

3. Van Litsenburg R, De Mos N, Edell D, Grivenwald C, Bohn DJ, Parshuram CS. Resource and health outcomes of paediatric extracorporeal membrane oxygenation. *Arch Dis Child Fetal Neonatal Ed* 2005; 90: F176-7

4. Walsh-Sukys MC, Bauer RE, Cornell DJ, Friedman HG, Stork EK, Hack M. Severe respiratory failure in neonates: Mortality

and morbidity rates and neurodevelopmental outcome. *J Pediatr* 1994; 125:104-110.

5. Schumacher RE, Roloff DW, Chapman R, Snedecor S, Bartlett RH. Extracorporeal membrane oxygenation in term newborns. A prospective cost-benefit analysis. *ASAIO J* 1993; 39:873-879.

6. Mahle W, Forbess J, Kirshbom P, et al. Cost-utility analysis of salvage cardiac extracorporeal membrane oxygenation in children. *J Thorac Cardiovasc Surg* 2004; 129:1084-90

7. Schumacher, RE. Effect of Extracorporeal membrane oxygenation on the infant mortality rate. *Pediatr Res* 1991; 29:265A.

8. Wegman ME. Annual summary of vital statistics. *Pediatrics* 1991; 88:1081-1092.

9. Schumacher RE. ECMO: Will this therapy be as efficacious in the future? *Ped Clin N Amer* 1993; 40:1005-1022.

10. Backhouse ME, Mauskopf JA, Jones D, et al. Economic outcomes of colfosceril palmitate rescue therapy in infants weighing 1250g or more with respiratory distress syndrome: Results from a randomised trial. *Pharmacoeconomics* 1994; 6:358-369.

14

Safety Issues of ECLS

Matthew C. Scanlon, M.D.

Introduction

The issue of patient safety is not new to medicine; however, there has been increasing awareness of the scope and complexity of the problem over the last decade. At its core, the patient safety problem is not a "people" problem; instead, it is a problem with systems within health care. ECMO is an example of a complex system within health care. This chapter will explore essential concepts of patient safety and how to apply these concepts to the delivery of ECMO. Additionally, tools available for improving safety of these systems will be discussed.

The lexicon of patient safety

Precision in the use of language has never been a requirement for the provision of health care. Keeping with this spirit, the patient safety field is prone to confusing jargon. The following definitions are offered in an attempt to minimize confusion. Patient safety is simply the freedom from preventable injury.[1] A widely accepted definition of error draws from the work of James Reason,[2] who has defined error as consisting of two possible types of failure. First is an error of execution where a correct plan of action is not carried out correctly. An example of this would be administering an incorrect heparin dose to a patient going on ECMO as a result of using the wrong patient weight. Second are errors of planning where the incorrect plan is applied to a situation. Errors in planning may be executed flawlessly but are wrong, because the plan itself is wrong. An illustration of a planning error is initiation of treatment for persistent pulmonary hypertension of the newborn when, in fact, the patient has a cyanotic congenital heart lesion.

The vast majority of errors in health care do not reach patients, and a subset of those that reach patients cause no harm. These events are called near-miss and no-harm events, respectively. Similarly, not all events that cause harm to patients are preventable. This distinction is central to the difference between adverse drug events (ADEs) and adverse drug reactions (ADRs). ADEs are injuries to patients that result from an error, and are thus preventable. ADRs are injuries to patients that occur in the course of normal, correct medical care. An example of the latter is an idiosyncratic, anaphylactic reaction resulting from the administration of a medication to a patient for the first time. In the absence of a history of reactions to that drug or similar drugs, the ability to anticipate and prevent the injury is not possible.

Systems thinking

To understand patient safety, one must first recognize the importance of systems in the way care is delivered. The Institute of Medicine, drawing from James Reason's studies of error, defines a system as "a set of interdependent elements interacting to achieve a common aim".[3] The interdependent elements represent both people and technology or equipment. This definition fits with prevailing concepts of systems in the human factors literature.[4] For any given process (for example, the transfer of a patient from a referring hospital for ECMO cannulation), there is a sequence of parts (including people) and actions that must occur to accomplish the desired goal. An understanding of the role of systems is a necessary prerequisite to improving safety.

While not necessarily intuitive, the concept of interdependent elements interacting with one another is not foreign to those caring for critically ill patients. Care providers are taught about individual organ systems (e.g., pulmonary or circulatory); however, not all health care providers understand the interaction among these individual systems in the context of the system as a whole. Cardiopulmonary interactions are witnessed daily in an ICU with interventions to one system often leading to predictable (and sometimes unpredictable) changes in the next. The interconnectedness of elements in a system, be it physiologic or process related, is recurrent in health care and central to patient safety efforts.

An understanding of the individual systems in health care is necessary but not sufficient. Before efforts can effectively be made to improve safety, there is a need to appreciate the importance of interactions and feedback both within and between systems. Numerous systems and subsystems exist in health care. A group of physicians, nurses, and respiratory therapists working to cannulate a child for ECMO in an ICU can be viewed as one system. This system may interact with other systems (e.g., lab, radiology) as well as impact other systems (e.g., patient care units asked to take emergent transfers to create bed spaces). The patient care room in which the cannulation is occurring

resides in the larger system of the ICU itself. Specific issues, including staffing, location of resuscitation carts and medications, and other patient's conditions, all influence the care in the room. Finally, hospital issues, as a larger system, interact with both the system of the ICU, and the care provided within. In the same way, ECMO can be viewed as a system, within larger systems. Only by recognizing how almost everything required to provide ECMO can be viewed as part of a system or process can one begin to think about safety.

The systems that both involve and affect ECMO can often be described as complex adaptive systems. This concept has significant leadership implications that are beyond the scope of this chapter. Interested readers are directed to other works comparing complex adaptive systems with the mechanistic systems that are less common in health care.[5]

As an appreciation of the ubiquitous presence of systems in health care develops, an understanding of the inherent complexity of many systems should follow. Health care has been compared to other systems such as nuclear energy and aviation, both of which have been described as tightly coupled.[6] A system that is tightly coupled has a series of steps where each must occur correctly for the subsequent step to occur. By virtue of being tightly coupled, the system has neither tolerance nor slack for failure at a preceding step. There is no room for error between the steps in the process, either in sequence or, as is often the case, in timing. In contrast, a loosely coupled system is one in which failure at a step can occur and the remaining steps in the process may still occur correctly, or there is ability to compensate easily for the failed step. A simplistic example of a tightly coupled system in health care is the preparation for ECMO. An ECMO pump must be prepared and primed before cannulation can safely begin. Cannulation is necessary prior to providing bypass support. In this simplified example, failures at any step will lead to delay; the steps allow for little variation in process; and, the majority of steps must occur sequentially. These features of complex, tightly coupled systems are endemic in health care settings.

The importance of recognizing the systems-based nature of health care lies in the fact that most events causing patient harm are the result of poorly designed systems of care. To illustrate this concept, one need only consider the phenomena of inadvertent potassium chloride administration, resulting in cardiac arrest. While a simplistic perspective focuses on the fact that ultimately a nurse administered an unintended dose of potassium, this ignores the complex systems which make this type of event inevitable and recurrent in many health care settings. That is, the potassium administration resulted from numerous contributing factors: hospital policies that allow the storage of potassium on patient care units, the common problem of look-a-like medication vials and labels, the practice of taking vials of medication to bedsides, and punitive hospital cultures coupled with a tort environment that prevents hospitals from sharing the lessons they have learned with other hospitals. The final step to assure safety is "a person must do the right thing without mistake." In light of the data on human performance, a system designed to depend on flawless human performance is destined for failure.

One approach to identifying an event that has occured as the result of flawed systems is to apply the "substitution test".[7] Applying this test, one asks, "All things being equal, is it possible that, if another person were in this situation, the same event could have happened?" If the answer is "yes", then focusing on the human performance without addressing systems problems will simply result in changing the persons involved. The system is not fundamentally safer.

The concept of shifting from blaming individuals to focusing on redesigning systems faces several barriers. First, historically, health care has had a punitive approach to events that lead to harm. It is much easier to punish or re-educate someone then to deal with the underlying system problems. Second, the shift from blaming individuals to focusing on systems is often mistaken for advocating for a system that does not hold people accountable for individual actions. To the contrary, a health care organization that focuses on learning from errors and improving systems without punishing those involved, while also holding individuals accountable for reckless violations, has been argued to be a more just culture.[8]

With a foundation in the language of safety and the concepts of systems, the next sections will explore specific vulnerabilities in the safe application of ECMO.

Specific safety issues related to ECMO

The challenge of maintaining expertise

Central to the safe use of any technology is the development and maintenance of expertise. Whether it is an IV infusion pump or an ECMO circuit, safe use is predicated on the end users being skilled at both the use and troubleshooting of the technology. Practice makes perfect; however, familiarity and skill with a technology is influenced by several factors. For instance, a technology that is used infrequently is more likely to rely on memory or recall for safe use. There is a greater risk for error in human performance when dependent on recall.[9]

Compounding the problem of infrequent use is the issue of having a large number of providers that may be required to maintain the necessary skill set. For example, a large ICU may easily have more than 100 nurses who are expected to assure the safe operation of the pump. The greater the number of nurses, the more extensive nursing training will be required. At the same time, it is less likely that any given nurse will be interacting with the pump during use with a given patient. One adaptation to this is limiting the pool of ECMO providers to a smaller set. However, this creates risk by having a smaller pool of individuals with the necessary skills for providing ECMO care. There is an increased risk that one of the nurses with critical skills will be unavailable at the time needed.

As a way of balancing the need to maintain expertise with an infrequently used technology, simulation is being used in an increasing number of health care settings to maintain or develop competencies.[10-13] While creating a full simulation laboratory for the sole use of ECMO is impractical, it is reasonable to recommend regular competency renewal through the use of the ECMO circuit drills. In particular, specific crises such as tubing rupture or pump failure can then be safely simulated with an opportunity for staff to develop appropriate responses.

ECMO, patient safety, and the use of technology

Another challenge to the use of technologies, particularly those that are life-sustaining, is the need for usability. Usability has been described as the degree to which people can quickly and easily use technology to perform a specific task.[14] Technology that is truly usable has a common set of attributes[15] including:

- ease of learning
- optimization of efficiency
- ease of remembering how to use (if memory is required at all)
- difficulty in committing errors
- ease of satisfying the needs of the end user

Additionally, usable technology features consistency in appearance and function, timely and obvious feedback with interactions, minimal modes of use which fit prevalent mental models, minimal reliance on memory, clear and unambiguous labeling, and the avoidance of clumsy automation.

The concept of usability can be understood by thinking about common, household devices such as videocassette recorders or clock radios. Despite the widespread use of such technologies, they remain difficult to use. The lack of relative usability of VCRs and clock radios has resulted in institutionalized workarounds. Specifically, VCR Plus technology and hotel "wake up calls" are patches to poorly designed technology. Unfortunately, end users seldom recognize that the problem is with the design of the technology.[16] Instead, if a person has difficulty using a device, the failure is usually attributed to the user's inadequate training, a lack of competency, or a personal failing when using technology.

A small, but growing, number of publications explore the link between the poor usability of health care technology and errors or harm to patients.[17-19] While there are no published reports of specific usability problems linked to ECMO, the nature of the technology would suggest that "user error" may be more related to the complexity of the technology. For example, safe and error free interaction relies heavily on memory, as interactions with the pump are not intuitive, especially in the face of pump failure. The process of manually cranking the pump in the face of pump failure, or the act of "flashing the bridge", both represent clumsy automation that may result in devastating harm to patients if done improperly. The network of tubing interspersed througout the multiple components (e.g., filters, oxygenators) usually does not have clear and unambiguous labeling. Instead, the two sides of the circuit may be distinguished only by a red or blue colored label, or by tracing the tubing back to the patient or pump. Unfortunately, it is likely that errors that have occurred to date have been blamed on the people using the devices rather than flawed design. At a minimum, the question of the usability of ECMO technology suggests opportunities for further study.

There are practical solutions to assist with the issue of technology with poor usability. One simple technique is the use of direct observation of end users interacting with the technology. Direct observation may lead to the discovery of workarounds and other practices that staff have developed to compensate for poorly designed technology. Workarounds are shortcuts in processes that staff use to compensate for poorly usable technology, lack of necessary resources (other people, information, or supplies), or policies that don't reflect the actual work that needs to be performed. In turn, steps can be taken to try to mitigate the risk associated with workarounds, and the information can be shared with other providers. Barriers associated with this technique include the time required to perform observations, the potential of resistance by staff to being observed, and the limitation that potentially beneficial or problematic practices need to be both observed and recognized for what they are.

The use of checklists is a second method that can decrease the risks associated with complex technology. For example, the ECMO pump requires a reliance on memory by virtue of its design. Checklists can be used to avoid undesired events that occur because of memory lapses or missed steps. Research on "the human factor" has found that the rate of forgetting something in the absence of reminders occurs at 1 per 100 opportunities. With the addition of reminders, this rate drops to 3 omissions per 1000 opportunities.[20] Considering that the preparation of an ECMO pump may occur in an urgent or emergent setting, there is a greater risk of missing key steps. Research has shown that the chance of failure increases 11-fold with a time shortage.[21] Short of fundamental redesign of ECMO pumps from an end-user perspective, the introduction of standard checklists may minimize the risk of forgetting essential steps either in pump/circuit preparation, or in the sequence of required events leading up to cannulation.

Team training and ECMO

Whether or not it is explicitly recognized as such, the safe provision of ECMO support is a team activity. Team work is necessary for each step, including pre-cannulation resuscitation, stabilization and evaluation of the patient, preparation of the circuit, medications and blood administration, and maintenance of both the patient- and ECMO-related technology. Each of these steps may involve a unique mix of individuals who may have limited experience working together.

The relevance of teamwork to patient safety has grown out of research in aviation safety. Studies of black box recordings after airline disasters have revealed a recurrent theme of impaired communication and an absence of teamwork. In response, formal training of teams, often called crew resource management (CRM), has become a standard component of all airlines' training programs. Studies of team interactions of health care, particularly in the OR setting, have revealed dysfunctional interactions similar to those found in the cockpit.[22] As a result, there is a growing push for providing formal team training to groups that interact in analogous health care situations. Team training has and is being studied among surgical teams, obstetrical teams, and teams that provide resuscitation.[23-26] In light of the complexity of safely initiating, maintaining, and coming off ECMO, as well as the grave consequences of a failure in these processes, there is significant potential for applying team training concepts to ECMO. This observation is consistent with prior ECMO-related publications.[27]

One means of improving communication is through the use of the "SBAR" technique. This technique applies a standard framework to effectively convey concerns to team members, especially in the face of hierarchical team composition. There is a known barrier to communication that results from having team members of different levels of authority working together.

This barrier, coupled with inconsistency in the content and method of delivery of information and experience with negative feedback results in poor communication and preventable risk to patient care. A nurse may feel challenged in communicating concerns about a patient effectively to a resident or attending physician. SBAR involves four steps to facilitate communication: situation, background, assessment, and recommendations (Table 1). The application of this technique is believed to improve both the effectiveness of communication as well as critical thinking skills among those initiating a conversation.[28] While there is no published data about the relation between ineffective communication and poor outcome on ECMO, it is reasonable to suggest that timely communication of concerns may have implications for their outcome.

A second strategy of benefit, particularly at the time of cannulation and decannulation, is the use of pre-procedural briefings and debriefings. Modeled on pre-flight briefings used in aviation, these briefings are designed to create a shared understanding of factors that may influence the outcome of the procedure. Considerations include patient condition, equipment, surgical tools, medications and blood products, potential complications, and other resources which may be needed. A model of this communication tool used at Orange County Kaiser provides specific opportunity for the surgeon, OR coordinator, scrub nurse, and anesthesiologist to share their concerns in a concise and timely manner. Upon completion of the procedure, the same team members are given a chance to share observa-

tions of what worked well and what could be improved. Use of this methodology at Kaiser has been associated with fewer adverse events, decreased nurse turnover, improved perceptions of a safe work environment, and improved perceptions of communication.[28] In light of the complexity of successful ECMO cannulation and decannulation, there may be a role for implementing briefings and debriefings in the context of ECMO care. In turn, key findings could then be shared with all the participants who are involved in the ECMO cannulation and decannulation processes, thus avoiding each team from having to "find" problems on their own.

ECMO and infections

Secondary infection is a known complication of ECMO therapy. Potential risk factors include underlying illness, prior cardiac surgery, disruption of skin barriers by cannula placement, relative immunosuppression, frequent accessing of the ECMO circuit during medication, blood administration, laboratory draws, and the use of antibiotics. Traditionally, hospital-acquired infections in health care have been viewed as an unavoidable risk associated with receiving care. However, there is growing opposition to the view that "infections happen" and that the risk is acceptable. In patient safety circles, hospital-acquired infections are instead viewed as a process failure that may be preventable, and, thus thought of as an error.[29] Based on this belief that hospital-acquired infections are preventable and should not be tolerated, in 2005 the Joint Commission on the Accreditation of Healthcare Organizations (JCAHO) implemented a National Patient Safety Goal requiring hospitals to review all hospital-acquired infection related deaths as sentinel events.[30]

Published rates of hospital-acquired infection associated with patients on ECMO range from 5-26%.[31,32] The retrospective review at one center with 26% incidence of hospital-acquired

Table 1. SBAR methodology.

Step	Key communications
Situation	What is happening now with the patient, including acute changes?
Background	What are the factors or events leading up to the situation or change?
Assessment	What does the person initiating communication believe is happening?
Recommendation	What the person initiating communication proposes/seeks in the way of action?

infection found that 78% were in the cardiac population. In the same series, 3 of 24 (12.5%) ECMO patients with hospital-acquired infections died secondary to the infection. In light of changes in the patient safety community, as well as the opinion of regulatory and accreditation bodies towards hospital-acquired infections, it would be advisable to perform a systematic review of steps that could be implemented to minimize infection risks on ECMO. At a minimum, steps associated with the reduction of central line infection rates may provide a starting point for risk reduction. Admittedly, it is unlikely that the infection risk will ever be zero. However, by reframing hospital-acquired infections as a potentially preventable complication rather than a "fact of life", there is potential for improvement.

Di(2-ethylhexyl) phthalate and ECMO

Di(2-ethylhexyl) phthalate (DEHP) is a plasticizer used to make polyvinyl chloride (PVC) tubing soft, tougher, and flexible. This is critical to current ECMO design because the circuit is often exposed to hundreds of hours of operation. In addition, DEHP can be found in infusion lines, cardiac bypass circuits, and ventilator circuits. These medical exposures have gained increasing attention because of animal research that has demonstrated that DEHP and other phthalates are both carcinogenic and can cause fetal death, malformations, and future infertility.[33,34] There is divided opinion as to whether the findings from animal models can be extrapolated to humans. A report by the American Council of Science and Health, Inc.[35] stated that the risk from DEHP exposure in medical settings is "unlikely to pose a health risk to even highly exposed humans". This conclusion may be bolstered by a study of 19 adolescents who had been exposed to DEHP during the neonatal period that found no evidence of adverse effects from either a growth or maturational standpoint.[36] While there is no

overwhelming evidence to support the elimination of DEHP and other phthalates from the medical setting, it is foreseeable that there may be increasing pressure to minimize exposure by using alternative materials. It is arguably advisable that the ECMO community continue to monitor this debate and consider alternative strategies in the event that use of DEHP is limited or eliminated.

ECMO in the context of health care

The safety issues described in this chapter have been specific to the performance of ECMO. While a discussion of the large number of risks associated with health care is well beyond the scope of this text, it is critical to appreciate that the performance of ECMO does not occur in a vacuum. Instead, ECMO patients are at risk for all of the known health care process failures that can result in harm. These include misdiagnosis, procedural complications, injuries (including extravasation of intravenous lines and pressure sores), and medication errors. The true rate of these events is largely unknown. However, the estimates of preventable inpatient mortality in U.S. hospitals of between 44,000[37] and 195,000[38] patients per year suggest that there is considerable additional risk beyond that of ECMO. Improving the safety of ECMO care without addressing the more global risks of health care is short-sighted and potentially misguided. In other words, successful rescue of an infant with persistent pulmonary hypertension secondary to diaphragmatic hernia through the use of ECMO support, only to have the child injured or die from a medication error, remains a health care failure. The growing science of investigating medical errors and harm has revealed significant deficits in how health care processes are designed and performed. Improving the safety of ECMO is necessary but not sufficient in the larger context of medical care. Like the larger medical community, providers of ECMO support are faced with difficult decisions whether to proactively address the issues of failed processes and medical harm. However, it is likely that the measures by which health care is evaluated will continue to expand to include measures of safety and quality. Based on this, there is much work remaining in order to provide both safe ECMO support and safe medical care.

References

1. Kohn LT, Corrigan JM, Donaldson MS. Executive Summary. In: Kohn LT, Corrigan JM, Donaldson MS, eds. *To Err Is Human: Building a Safer Health System.* Washington, DC: National Academy Press; 1999: p. 4.

2. Reason JT. *Human Error.* New York, NY: Cambridge University Press; 1990.

3. Kohn LT, Corrigan JM, Donaldson MS. Why do errors happen? In: Kohn LT, Corrigan JM, Donaldson MS, eds. *To Err Is Human: Building a Safer Health System.* Washington, DC: National Academy Press; 1999: pp. 49-69.

4. Czaja SJ. Systems design and evaluation. In: Salvendy G, ed. *Handbook of human factors and ergonomics.* 2nd ed. New York, NY: John Wiley and Sons, Inc.; 1997: pp.17-41.

5. Zimmerman B, Lindberg C, Plsek P. *Edgeware: insights from complexity science for health care leaders.* Irving, TX: VHA Inc.; 1998.

6. Perrow C. *Normal Accidents: living with high-risk technologies.* 2nd ed. New York, NY: Basic Books; 1994.

7. Johnston, N. Do blame and punishment have a role in organizational risk? *Flight Deck,* Spring 1995; pp. 33-36.

8. Marx D. Patient safety and the "just culture": a primer for health care executives. New York, NY: Columbia University; 2001. Available at: http://www.mers-tm.net/support/Marx_Primer.pdf, accessed 3/20/2003. Columbia University under a grant provided by the National Heart, Lung, and Blood Institute developed a medical event reporting system for transfusion medicine.

9. Park KS. Human Error. In: Salvendy G, ed. *Handbook of human factors and ergonomics.* 2nd ed. New York, NY: John Wiley and Sons, Inc.; 1997; pp. 150-174.

10. Gaba DM. Future vision of simulation in health care. *Qual Safety Health Care* 2004; 13 (Suppl 1):i2-i10.

11. Byrne AJ, Greaves JD. Assessment instruments used during anaesthetic simulation: review of published studies. *Br J Anaesth* 2001; 86:445-450.

12. Schwid HA, Rooke GA, Carline J, et al. Evaluation of anesthesia residents using mannequin-based simulation: a multiinstitutional study. *Anesthesiol* 2002; 97:1434-1444.

13. Small SD, Wuerz RC, Simon R, Shapiro N, Conn A, Setnik G. Demonstration of high-fidelity simulation team training for emergency medicine. *Acad Emerg Med* 1999; 6:312-323.

14. Dumas JS, Redish JC. *A Practical Guide to Usability Testing.* Rev. ed. Exeter, UK: Intellect Press; 1999.

15. Neilsen J. *Usability Engineering.* Amsterdam, Netherlands: Morgan Kaufmann; 1993.

16. Norman D. *The Design of Everyday Things.* New York, NY: Currency Doubleday; 1988.

17. Scanlon M, Gosbee J. Computer physician order entry and the real world: we're only humans. *Jt Comm J Qual Safety* 2004; 6:342-346.

18. Murff HJ, Gosbee JW, Bates DW. Human factors and medical devices. In: Wachter RM, ed. *Making Health Care Safer: A Critical Analysis of Patient Safety Practices.* 2001. AHRQ Publication No. 01-E058. Available at: http://www.ahrq.gov/clinic/ptsafety/chap41a.htm. Accessed March 12, 2004.

19. Fairbanks RJ, Caplan S. Poor interface design and lack of usability testing facilitate medical error. *Jt Comm J Qual Safety* 2004; 30:579-584.

20. Park KS. Human Error. In: Salvendy G, ed. *Handbook of human factors and ergonomics.* 2nd ed. New York, NY: John Wiley and Sons, Inc.; 1997:150-174.

21. Reason JT. Understanding the adverse events: the human factor. In: Vincent C, ed. *Clinical Risk Management.* London, UK: BMJ Books; 2001:9-30.

22. Helmreich H, Merritt AC. *Culture at Work in Aviation and Medicine: National, Organizational and Professional Influences.* Aldershot, UK: Ashgate; 1998.

23. Miller LA. Safety promotion and error reduction in perinatal care: lessons from industry. J Perinat Neonat Nurs 2003; 17:128-138.

24. Knox GE, Simpson KR, Garite TJ. High reliability perinatal units: an approach to the prevention of patient injury and medical malpractice claims. J Healthc Risk Manag 1999; 19:24-32.

25. Small SD, Wuerz RC, Simon R, Shapiro N, Conn A, Setnik G. Demonstration of high-fidelity simulation team training for emergency medicine. Acad Emerg Med 1999; 6:312-323.

26. Joint Commission on Accreditation of Healthcare Organizations. Preventing infant death and injury during delivery. Sentinel Event Alert [series online]. Jul 2004; 30:1-2. Available at: http://www.jcaho.com/.

27. Klein MD, Whittlesey GC. ECMO in the Hospital Setting. In: Zwischenerger JB, Bartlett RH, eds. *ECMO: Extracorporeal Cardiopulmonary Support in Critical Care.* Extracorporeal Life Support Organization: Ann Arbor, MI; 1998: pp. 191-205.

28. Leonard M, Graham S, Bonacum D. The human factor: the critical importance of effective teamwork and communication in providing safe care. *Qual Saf Health Care* 2004; 13(Suppl 1):i85-90.

29. Kohn LT, Corrigan JM, Donaldson MS. Safety activities in health care organizations. In: Kohn LT, Corrigan JM, Donaldson MS, eds. *To Err Is Human: Building a Safer Health System.* Washington, DC: National Academy Press; 1999:267-268.

30. Joint Commission on the Accreditation of Healthcare Organizations. *Facts about the 2005 National Patient Safety Goals.* Available at: http://jcaho.com/accredited+organizations/patient+safety/05+ npsg/npsg_facts.htm. Accessed February 2, 2005.

31. Zwischenerger JB, Upp JR. Emergencies during Extracorporeal Membrane Oxygenation and their Management. In: Zwischenerger JB, Bartlett RH, ed. *ECMO: Extracorporeal Cardiopulmonary Support in Critical Care.* Extracorporeal Life Support Organization: Ann Arbor, MI; 1998:221-251.

32. O'Neill J, Schutze G, Heulitt M, et al. Nosocomial infections during extracorporeal membrane oxygenation. *Intens Care Med* 2001; 27:1247-1253.

33. Lovekamp-Swan T, Davis BJ. Mechanisms of phthalate ester toxicity in the female reproductive system. *Env Health Persp* 2003; 111:139-145.

34. Shea KM, Academy of Pediatrics Committee on Environmental Health. Pediatric exposure and potential toxicity of phthalate plasticizers. *Pediatrics* 2003; 111:1467-1474.

35. Koop CE, Juberg DR, Benedek EP, et al. A scientific evaluation of health effects of two plasticizers used in medical devices and toys: a report form the American Council on Science and Health. *MedGenMed* 1999; 22:E14.

36. Rais-Bahrami K, Nunez S, Revenis ME, et al. Follow up study of adolescents exposed to di(2-ethylhexyl) phthalate (DEHP) as neonates on extracorporeal membrane oxygenation (ECMO) support. *Env Health Persp* 2004; 112:1339-1340.

37. Kohn LT, Corrigan JM, Donaldson MS. Executive Summary. In: Kohn LT, Corrigan JM, Donaldson MS, eds. *To Err Is*

Human: Building a Safer Health System.
Washington, DC: National Academy Press;
1999:1-17.

38. Healthgrades, Inc. In-hospital deaths
from medical errors at 195,000 per year,
Healthgrades Study finds. July 27, 2004.
Available at: http://www.healthgrades.com/
PressRoom/index.cfm?fuseaction =Press-
Releases. Accessed December 13, 2004.

15

Regulatory Issues Related to ECLS

Ronald B. Hirschl, M.S., M.D.

Introduction

ECLS is a technique employing medical devices intended to provide prolonged cardiopulmonary support to patients with heart or lung failure.[1-3] The U.S. Food and Drug Administration (FDA) does not review or approve medical procedures and cannot approve ECLS, but does regulate the medical devices used. These devices are regulated under authority first established by the U.S. Congress in 1938. In 1976, following several amendments to the Act of 1938 that authorized this empowerment, the FDA's authority was extended to regulate and ensure the safety and effectiveness of all medical devices sold in the U.S.

Subsequently, devices have been classified on the basis of the risk of illness or injury that could occur should the device fail and regulatory controls have been established to assure device safety and effectiveness. The classifications and controls have been implemented through an approval process that is founded on regulations pertaining to the 1976 Amendments to the Food, Drug and Cosmetics Act (FD&C) and the Safe Medical Devices Act (SMDA) of 1990.

The application and implications of the SMDA are diverse and complex. These include marketing, labeling, medical reporting, and off-label use. The applicable controls and regulations that have been put in place for the SMDA, or are in the process of being developed, are intended to result in the provision of safe and effective ECLS devices for medical use and the enhancement of patients' health status.

Summary of the statutory authority of the FDA for medical devices

In 1906, the U.S. Congress passed a Food and Drugs Act to prohibit interstate commerce in misbranded and adulterated foods, drinks, and drugs.[4] Devices were not included in this legislation. In 1938, Congress enacted the Federal FD&C Act that placed some therapeutic medical devices within FDA jurisdiction. Over the years, the FD&C Act was amended several times. Based on findings of device-related patient injuries in the Cooper Report of 1970, U.S. Congress passed the Medical Device Amendments of 1976 and extended the FDA's authority to ensure the safety and effectiveness of all medical devices sold in the U.S. Under the 1976 Amendments, the FDA was required to classify all devices into three classes; Class I, II, or III. In 1990, the FD&C Act was again amended to enhance the FDA's enforcement capability.[5] The current FDA Modernization Act (FDAMA) was passed in 1997 (Table 1).[6] This Act ordered the most wide-ranging reforms in FDA practices since 1938. It included measures to accelerate the review of devices and to regulate advertising of unapproved uses of approved devices. Finally, the Medical Device User Fee and Modernization Act (MDUFMA) of 2002 established medical device review fees to support the process for review of device applications. More importantly, the Act established performance goals for FDA device review, the ability for companies to use FDA–accredited persons to inspect qualified manufacturers, rules for the reprocessing of single-use devices, additional funds for post-market surveillance, and a means for using online labeling for devices. Finally, it dictated that panels reviewing devices for pre-market approval would include one or more pediatric experts, where appropriate, in order to develop safe and effective pediatric devices.[7]

Device classification

All devices are assigned to one of three regulatory classes (Table 2). The classes are based on the level of control necessary to assure the safety and effectiveness of the device.

Class I devices

Class I devices require general controls. These are the baseline requirements of the FD&C Act that apply to all medical devices. Unless specifically exempted by regulation, Class I devices consist of those for which general regulatory controls are sufficient to provide reasonable assurance of safety and effectiveness. These devices are subject to the least regulatory control. They are not considered to present an unreasonable risk of illness or injury. General controls consist of device listing, registration of manufacturers, manufacturing devices in accordance with the Good Manufacturing Practices (GMP) regulation, labeling, and submission of a Premarket Notification [510(k)] prior to marketing a device (Table 3). Approximately

---

Table 1. The content of the FDA Modernization Act of 1997.

Title II. Improving regulation of devices

Sec. 201. Investigational device exemptions

Sec. 202. Special review for certain devices

Sec. 203. Expanding humanitarian use of devices

Sec. 204. Device standards

Sec. 205. Scope of review; collaborative determinations of device data requirements

Sec. 206. Pre-market notification

Sec. 207. Evaluation of automatic class III designation

Sec. 208. Classification panels

Sec. 209. Certainty of review timeframes; collaborative review process

Sec. 210. Accreditation of persons for review of pre-market notification reports

Sec. 211. Device tracking

Sec. 212. Post-market surveillance

Sec. 213. Reports

Sec. 214. Practice of medicine

Sec. 215. Noninvasive blood glucose meter

Sec. 216. Use of data relating to pre-market approval; product development protocol

Sec. 217. Clarification of the number of required clinical investigations for approval

The entire act may be found at http://www.fda.gov/cder/guidance/105-115.htm.

Table 2. The regulations from the amended FD&C Act which describe device classification.

SEC. 513. [360c] (a)(1) There are established the following classes of devices intended for human use:

(A) Class I, general controls—

(i) A device for which the controls authorized by or under section 501, 502, 510, 516, 518, 519, or 520 or any combination of such sections are sufficient to provide reasonable assurance of the safety and effectiveness of the device.

(ii) A device for which insufficient information exists to determine that the controls referred to in clause (i) are sufficient to provide reasonable assurance of the safety and effectiveness of the device or to establish special controls to provide such assurance, but because it—

(I) is not purported or represented to be for a use in supporting or sustaining human life or for a use which is of substantial importance in preventing impairment of human health, and

(II) does not present a potential unreasonable risk of illness or injury, is to be regulated by the controls referred to in clause (i).

(B) Class II, special controls—A device which cannot be classified as a class I device because the general controls by themselves are insufficient to provide reasonable assurance of the safety and effectiveness of the device, and for which there is sufficient information to establish special controls to provide such assurance, including the promulgation of performance standards, post-market surveillance, patient registries, development and dissemination of guidelines (including guidelines for the submission of clinical data in pre-market notification submissions in accordance with section 510(k)), recommendations, and other appropriate actions as the Secretary deems necessary to provide such assurance. For a device that is purported or represented to be for a use in supporting or sustaining human life, the Secretary shall examine and identify the special controls, if any, that are necessary to provide adequate assurance of safety and effectiveness and describe how such controls provide such assurance.

(C) Class III, pre-market approval—A device which because—

(i) it

(I) cannot be classified as a Class I device because insufficient information exists to determine that the application of general controls are sufficient to provide reasonable assurance of the safety and effectiveness of the device, and

(II) cannot be classified as a Class II device because insufficient information exists to determine that the special controls described in subparagraph (B) would provide reasonable assurance of its safety and effectiveness, and

(ii)

(I) is purported or represented to be for a use in supporting or sustaining human life or for a use which is of substantial importance in preventing impairment of human health, or

(II) presents a potential unreasonable risk of illness or injury, is to be subject, in accordance with section 515, to pre-market approval to provide reasonable assurance of its safety and effectiveness.

The entire FD&C act may be seen at http://www.fda.gov/opacom/laws/fdcact/fdctoc.htm.

93% of all Class I devices are exempt from the premarket notification process. A listing of exempt cardiopulmonary bypass (CPB) devices and their classification is provided on the FDA Web Site (www.fda.gov/).[8] Examples of Class I devices are accessory equipment such as a mounting bracket for an oxygenator or system priming equipment.[7] These devices have no contact with blood and are used in the bypass circuit to "support, adjoin, or connect components, or aid in the set-up of the extracorporeal line."

Class II devices

Class II devices are those that cannot be classified as Class I devices because the general controls by themselves are insufficient to provide reasonable assurance safety and effectiveness. Reasonable assurance for Class II devices can be obtained by applying special controls. Special controls may include mandatory performance standards, special labeling requirements, post-market surveillance, patient

registries, or guidance documents. Examples of Class II devices include heat exchangers, blood tubing, pressure gauges, and monitors. Examples of FDA-cleared, ECLS Class II devices are provided in Table 4.

Class III devices

Class III devices usually support or sustain human life, are of substantial importance in preventing the impairment of human health, or present a potential, unreasonable risk of illness or injury. Class III devices require an in-depth assessment of safety and effectiveness and cannot be classified as Class I or II devices as the controls therein alone are insufficient to provide a reasonable assurance of safety and effectiveness. In general, the Class III devices are either new devices that are "not substantially equivalent" to any previously marketed device, or are devices in which failure would be catastrophic to patient health. They may undergo a pre-market approval (PMA) process in which in vitro, animal study, and/or clinical trial data

Table 3. Regulations related to pre-market notification or 510(k) which is the most frequent method of device "clearance" and is specifically applied to those devices which are substantially equivalent to predicate devices and which are not of Class III.

510 (k) Each person who is required to register under this section and who proposes to begin the introduction or delivery for introduction into interstate commerce for commercial distribution of a device intended for human use shall, at least ninety days before making such introduction or delivery, report to the Secretary (in such form and manner as the Secretary shall by regulation prescribe)—

> (1) the class in which the device is classified under section 513 or if such person determines that the device is not classified under such section, a statement of that determination and the basis for such person's determination that the device is or is not so classified, and
> (2) action taken by such person to comply with requirements under section 514 or 515 which are applicable to the device.

SEC. 520. [360j] (a) Any requirement authorized by or under section 501, 502, 510, or 519 applicable to a device intended for human use shall apply to such device until the applicability of the requirement to the device has been changed by action taken under section 513, 514, or 515 or under subsection (g) of this section, and any requirement established by or under section 501, 502, 510, or 519 which is inconsistent with a requirement imposed on such device under section 514 or 515 or under subsection (g) of this section shall not apply to such device.

are used to evaluate the device. This is in addition to the general and special controls that are applied to Class I and Class II devices. The only exceptions to the PMA requirement are devices that were on the market in 1976 and were originally classified as Class III. To date, some of those devices, such as oxygenators, have been re-classified. These exceptions are reviewed under the 510(k) process. Examples of Class III devices include centrifugal pumps. Examples of devices approved by the FDA for ECLS are provided in Table 4.

As previously stated, pre-market notifications are also known as 510(k) applications. At least 90 days prior to first-time marketing of a device in the U.S., a pre-market notification must be submitted to the FDA. These applications provide enough information to demonstrate that the device is "substantially equivalent" to a predicate device. That is, one that is currently, legally marketed in the U.S. Unless a device is exempt, a pre-market notification is required when marketing the device for the first time or when there has been a substantial modification to the device. A change to the intended use, or population, or a significant design change may affect the safety and effectiveness and would require a 510(k). These 510(k) applications are "cleared" by the FDA if the device is found to be substantially equivalent to the predicate device. If a device is determined to be "not substantially equivalent" it is considered a Class III device and a pre-market approval must be obtained.

Regulatory approval process

One question that quickly arises is how manufacturers can distribute Class II and Class III devices for evaluation before they are approved for marketing since some devices may require clinical data for clearance or approval. Authorization to allow investigational devices to be tested on human subjects is required and may be obtained in the form of an Investigational Device Exemption (IDE). The IDE allows manufacturers to distribute devices to clinical investigators for use on human subjects. The FD&C Act authorizes the FDA to exempt these devices from certain requirements of the Act that would apply to devices in commercial distribution. FDA approval of the IDE is not required for "non-significant" risk devices,

Table 4. Frequently used ECLS devices and the device classification and whether clearance or approval for ECLS has been granted.

Device	Class	FDA approved for ECLS
Roller pump	II	none
Centrifugal pump	III	none
Blood tubing/cannula	II	Kendall infant VV catheter Origen cannula
Heat exchanger	II	Medtronic ECMOTHERM II Gish heat exchanger – HE-1
Oxygenator	II	Medtronic 600,800,1500
Bladder box	I	Zimmer
Reservoir	II	Gish ECMO bladder
S_vO_2 monitor	II	none
ACT monitor	II	none
Stopcock	II	none
Bubble detector	II	none

although Institutional Review Board (IRB) approval and adherence to IDE regulations is still necessary.

The process for FDA approval of a device is based on its classification. Class I devices follow the general controls described unless the devices were exempted from particular requirements before their intended marketing. Class II devices also follow a 510(k) clearance path, but require special controls. These may include performance standards, data based on in vitro, animal, and/or clinical studies, guidelines for 510(k) submissions, advisory panel evaluation, device labeling, post-market evaluation, and device tracking. Class III devices follow a PMA process that involves an in-depth review of the safety and effectiveness of the device, along with the general (Class I) and applicable special controls (Class II). Often, an advisory committee consisting of persons with expertise related to the device under consideration is convened to provide independent review and to advise the FDA.

Regulatory processes for marketing ECLS devices

When the U.S. Congress passed the Medical Devices Amendments of 1976, numerous potential ECLS devices were already in use for cardiopulmonary bypass (CPB). Such devices were "grandfathered" in without formal clearance. This was done to establish baseline information for a cohort of CPB devices that could serve as predicate devices upon which subsequent CPB equipment could be evaluated. These devices are known as pre-amendment devices, and include those in commercial distribution prior to May 28, 1976. All devices introduced since that date must be approved prior to marketing by the FDA. Based on the SMDA, even those pre-amendment devices that are considered Class III must now be either reclassified or requested.

Issues with ECLS devices

Labeling of a device is based on the data provided from the manufacturer to the FDA. It includes details on the intended use, methods of use, contraindications, warnings, precautions, patient selection information, and a summary of clinical data. Especially pertinent to the use of CPB devices for ECLS is the duration of use labeling, which typically limits the use of CPB equipment to 6 hours. Generally, CPB devices are not, therefore, labeled for ECLS use.

Once 510(k) or PMA is obtained, device manufacturers may market the device. However, Medical Device Reporting regulations (21 CFR, Part 803) require that manufacturers report to the FDA all instances where marketed devices may have caused or contributed to a death or serious injury. This requirement also applies if a device has malfunctioned and death or serious injury would be likely to occur if the malfunction were to recur. All device users must provide to the manufacturer or the FDA information which suggests that a device has or may have contributed to serious injury or death. This information must be reported within 10 working days of a patient's injury or death. Such information is also summarized for the FDA by each device user on an annual basis. Finally, the FDA may require manufacturers to track a Class II or III device as part of routine post-market surveillance.

Implications of using an ECLS device off-label

The goal of the FD&C Act regulations is to oversee manufacturing, marketing, and sales of devices for specific uses. The focus of such regulations is not intended to, "limit or interfere with the authority of the health care practitioner to prescribe or administer any legally marketed device to a patient for any condition or disease within the legitimate health care practitioner-patient relationship." It is not illegal, therefore, to use devices in an "off-label" manner. It is, however, illegal for a manufacturer to promote an unapproved use of a legally marketed device. For example, a manufacturer may not label their device for ECLS use until the device has been approved for ECLS use. Physicians may also obtain devices that are not legally marketed for use in their practice by prescription via the custom device exclusion of the FD&C Act (Table 5). It is specified in the regulations, however, that such devices should not be generally available to, or generally used by, other physicians. This exclusion legally allows use of custom devices in a very limited fashion, and would generally not apply to devices used for ECLS.

The intent of the FDA is altruistic and worthy: provide patients and physicians with safe and effective devices. Clearly, a balance must be maintained between provision of needed devices to patient populations and appropriate regulation of such devices. The FDA has encouraged regulations that strike a healthy balance between these competing forces.

References

1. Hirschl RB. Extracorporeal Life Support. In: O'Neill JA, ed. *Pediatric Surgery* Chicago, IL: Year Book Medical Publishers, Inc.; 1998: page 89-102.

2. Bartlett R, Roloff DW, Custer J, Younger JG, Hirschl R. Extracorporeal life support: The University of Michigan experience. *JAMA* 2000; 283:904-908.

3. ELSO Registry. Ann Arbor, Michigan: Extracorporeal Life Organization; 2004.

4. Food and Drug Administration. Federal Food and Drugs Act of 1906 (The "Wiley" Act). Available at http://www.fda.gov/opacom/laws/wileyact.htm. Accessed July 24, 2005.

5. Food and Drug Administration. Federal Food, Drug, and Cosmetic Act. Available at http://www.access.gpo.gov/uscode/title21/chapter9_.html. Accessed July 24, 2005.

Table 5. The Custom Device Exclusion in the FD&C Act that details the capability of any physician to prescribe a device which is not commercially distributed for use by a manufacturer, is not generally used by other practitioners, and is to be used for a specific patient or in the practice of that physician/dentist.

Federal Food, Drug, and Cosmetic Act, as Amended, Chapter V; Subchapter A§520(b)(A)(I)(ii)(B)
Sections 514 and 515 do not apply to any device which, in order to comply with the order of an individual physician or dentist (or any other specially qualified person designated under regulations promulgated by the Secretary after an opportunity for an oral hearing) necessarily deviates from an otherwise applicable performance standard or requirement prescribed by or under section 515 if

(1) the device is not generally available in finished form for purchase or for dispensing upon prescription and is not offered through labeling or advertising by the manufacturer, importer, or distributor thereof for commercial distribution, and
(2) such device—
(A) (i) is intended for use by an individual patient named in such order of such physician or dentist (or other specially qualified person so designated) and is to be made in a specific form for such patient, or
(ii) is intended to meet the special needs of such physician or dentist (or other specially qualified person so designated) in the course of the professional practice of such physician or dentist (or other specially qualified person so designated), and
(B) is not generally available to or generally used by other physicians or dentists (or other specially qualified persons so designated).

6. Food and Drug Administration Modernization Act of 1997. Available at http://www.fda.gov/cder/guidance/105-115.htm. Accessed July 24, 2005.

7. Food and Drug Administration. Medical Device User Fee and Modernization Act of 2002. Available at http://www.fda.gov/oc/mdufma. Accessed July 24, 2005.

8. Food and Drug Administration. Title 21—Food and Drugs, Subchapter H-Medical Devices, Part 870 Cardiovascular Devices, Subpart E—Cardiovascular Surgical Devices [21CFR, Subpart E §870.4200(a)(b)]. Available at http://www.accessdata.fda.gov/scripts/cdrh/cfdocs/cfcfr/CFRSearch.cfm?CFRPart=870&showFR=1&subpartNode=21:8.0.1.1.21.5. Accessed July 24, 2005.

16

ECLS Administrative and Training Issues

Jeanne E. Braby, R.N., M.S.N., C.C.R.N., Barbara M. Haney, R.N.C., M.S.N., C.P.N.P., and Patricia A. English, M.S., R.R.T.

Introduction

ECLS procedures are complex, high risk, utilize many health care resources, and are unpredictable in terms of volume and timing. Certain institutional requirements are essential for safe, economical, and effective use of ECLS. A hospital administrator would want to ensure that all appropriate systems were in place to support the program. The areas to scrutinize include essential support systems, physical facilities and equipment, "team" or personnel issues, and quality assurance. Each area impacts and interacts with the other.

The Extracorporeal Life Support Organization (ELSO) has developed "ELSO Guidelines for ECMO Centers"[1] which outlines the institutional requirements for effective use of ECMO. ELSO recognizes that differences in regional and institutional regulations may result in variations from these guidelines. Nevertheless, it is an important reference for both current and future ECLS centers. All ELSO guidelines are reviewed and revised every three years, and are available on the ELSO website (www.elso. med.umich.edu).

ECLS Centers should be located in tertiary care centers with a tertiary level NICU, pediatric ICU, and/or adult ICU. In order to achieve and maintain clinical expertise and operate cost effectively, ECLS centers should be located in geographic areas that can support a minimum of 6 ECLS patients/center/year. These centers providing ECLS services should be actively involved in ELSO, including participation in the ELSO Registry.

Essential support systems

Certain institutional support systems are essential for the safe provision of comprehensive ECLS services. Centers providing ECLS services must have the ability to provide additional clinical support from biomedical engineers and consultants in pediatric and/or adult neurology, nephrology, and occupational and physical therapy, along with developmental and rehabilitation specialists. In addition, it is essential that physicians and other medical personnel who routinely provide care for pediatric/adult cardiology, cardiovascular surgery, general surgery, cardiovascular perfusion, anesthesiology, neurosurgery, radiology, and genetics be on-call 24 hours/day. Support facilities with staff such as a laboratory for blood gas, blood chemistry, and hematological testing; blood bank; and radiology, including cranial ultrasound and CT scan, must also be available around the clock. Furthermore, cardiovascular OR facilities with cardiopulmonary bypass (CBP) capabilities should be located within the hospital and, once again, be available 24 hours/day.

Facilities and equipment

ECLS may be provided in a centralized intensive care location or in multiple ICUs. It is not necessary to have a special ECLS unit.[2] If the space allotted for ECLS is located outside the ICU, it should be in close proximity to and have appropriate communication with the ICU to assure additional staff support for any emergency. As cannulation, decannulation, and other surgical procedures are often performed at bedside, adequate lighting and surgical instruments are required.

To be prepared for potential emergencies, back-up components of the ECLS system and the circuit must be available, as well as appropriate training of the staff in managing ECLS emergencies. Other chapters in this book are devoted to the specifics involved in ECLS equipment and anticoagulation (Chapters 6 and 3, respectively). Each center should establish an effective system for inventory and ordering to ensure adequate supplies are available at all times. Equipment maintenance and cleaning is essential. A process must be in place to ensure that the manufacturer's suggested periodic maintenance is performed. This process will be unique to the individual center and may involve the biomedical engineering department, cardiopulmonary perfusion services, ECLS team members, or designated ECLS equipment technicians.

Often, situations arise which necessitate transport of the ECMO patient – to another ICU, the OR, cardiac catheterization, or another ECLS center. Each center is responsible for developing procedures and equipment for safe in-hospital transport to prevent interruption of ECLS. This requires policies, procedures, and training on the considerations for safely transporting ECLS patients. Insuring uninterrupted power supply (UPS) during transport is essential. Transport of the ECLS patient to another ECLS center is uncommon, extremely complex, and involves many issues, regulations and circuit modifications. It also may require different equipment than that normally used at a given institution. For these reasons, most centers do not provide inter-hospital ECLS transport. Each center must develop guidelines and identify resources, such as contacting other regional centers that provide inter-hospital transport for transporting the patient on ECLS outside their institution (See Chapter 9).

Team and training issues

The overall operation of each ECLS program should be the responsibility of a physician designated as the medical director. The medical director should be either board-certified or eligible for certification and can be a neonatologist, a critical care specialist, or a pediatric, cardiovascular, or thoracic surgeon.

ECLS physicians provide 24-hour coverage for the ECLS patient, and may include neonatologists, pediatric, or adult critical care specialists; neonatal or critical care fellows, or other physicians who have completed at least three years of post-graduate pediatric, surgical, or adult medical training and have specific ECLS training. All ECLS physicians should meet the requirements of their subspecialty training as set forth by their specific governing board (e.g., the American Board of Surgery or American Board of Pediatrics) in addition to having received institution-specific ECLS training.

Each center should have an ECLS coordinator(s) responsible for the non-physician management of ECLS. The ECLS coordinator should be an experienced neonatal, pediatric, or adult intensive care registered nurse, registered respiratory therapist, or certified clinical perfusionist with ECLS experience. The responsibilities of coordinators vary among centers, but typically include supervision and training of all team members, continuing education, maintenance of equipment, quality assurance monitoring, policy and procedure development, and collection of patient data. In addition, the

ECLS coordinator acts as a clinical resource for all team members.

The ECLS director and coordinator should work collaboratively to develop standard medical and nursing order sets as well as formal policies and procedures regarding all aspects of ECLS. This enhances the effectiveness of the ECLS program. Procedures involved with the equipment and circuit as well as institutional criteria for ECLS should be developed. Each center develops specific indications and contraindications for ECLS appropriate for the practices at that center. Adherence to guidelines can avoid cannulation when contraindicated and minimize costs. Guidelines for the transport of the patient on ECLS should also be included. These policies and procedures should be readily available to all team members and regularly reviewed.

The ECLS specialist is the clinician trained to manage ECLS under the direction of an ECLS-trained physician. ECLS specialists are registered nurses, registered respiratory therapists, certified perfusionists, or physicians who have strong neonatal, pediatric, or adult intensive care backgrounds. Specialists provide care to the patient on ECLS with primary responsibility for maintaining appropriate extracorporeal support, troubleshooting equipment, and assessing the circuit. In addition to the ECLS specialist, a bedside neonatal, pediatric, or adult intensive care nurse provides direct patient care throughout the ECLS course. In some centers, both the bedside nurse and the specialist managing the ECLS system are trained ECLS specialists. This allows the roles to be fluid and provides an immediate resource for troubleshooting, problem-solving, emergencies, and scheduling of breaks.

Because of the diversity of ECLS programs, each center must develop its own training program based on their patient population, equipment, and responsibilities of team members. Since the educational backgrounds of ECLS specialists differ, each center will need to adjust its training program based on their staff's specific needs. For example, respiratory therapists will need more time to learn about transfusion procedures, IV pumps, and medications, whereas nurses may need more education in gas physics and perfusionists will need to learn more about the effects of long-term bypass and patient care assessment. In addition, the bedside nursing staff will need additional training on caring for an ECLS patient along with a basic understanding of ECLS.

It is helpful to include representatives from other patient care services who are involved with the ECLS program in some portions of the training. This may include representatives from transfusion, radiology, OR staff, laboratory medicine, and biomedical engineering. This will help improve communication among hospital services and will allow other services to understand and anticipate the needs of the ECLS patient. Whatever the team composition, the training process should include team-building activities.

Good team communication is probably the most important skill for the ECMO team to maintain. Optimal care of ECLS patients requires that specialized knowledge from multiple disciplines be integrated. Integration is best accomplished through frequent, respectful interaction, and skilled communication. In today's healthcare system, working collaboratively with others is as important to successful ECLS care as expert clinical skills are to the individual practitioners. According to data from the Joint Commission of Accreditation of Healthcare Organizations (JCAHO), a breakdown in team communication is a top contributor to sentinel events.[3] The chapter on safety includes more information on this topic (See Chapter 14).

Selecting clinicians to train as ECLS specialists

The strength of an ECLS team is largely dependent on the ECLS specialists and the communication between them. Functioning in the role of an ECLS specialist is not a job suited for everyone. It is essential that clinicians are aware of all job expectations including training requirements, continuing education, alternate shift work, and on-call hours. In most ECLS programs, specialists are given a fair amount of responsibility and are required to work under stressful conditions. Characteristics of ECLS specialists are found in Table 1. When recruiting personnel, individuals with these qualities should be sought.

Gaining ECLS competency

The ECLS coordinator is responsible for the training of ECLS specialists and assuring their ongoing competency. JCAHO standard HR 1.20 states, "The hospital has a process to ensure that a person's qualifications are consistent with his or her job responsibilities."[4] It further states that health care leaders need to define the required competence and qualifications of staff in all programs. The ECLS coordinator's role in competency assessment is to determine staff qualifications and job responsibilities, determine the competencies required for each job, implement a competency system for verification, identify staff development needs, and develop a plan should a case arise where an employee does not meet standards.

Competency can be defined as an individual's performance of a procedure, skill, or

Table 1. Characteristics valued in ECLS specialists.

Characteristic
• Technically adept
• Able to work in stressful situations
• Good communication skills
• Good critical thinking skills
• Team player
• Flexible with patient assignments
• Flexible with scheduling

job function in a particular setting, according to established guidelines and standards. Established guidelines and standards for ECLS should be found in each institution's policies and procedures. ELSO has developed "ELSO Guidelines for Training and Continuing Education of ECMO Specialists"[5] and "Guidelines for ECMO Centers" which can be used as a reference for both current and future ECLS centers. The most current versions of the guidelines can be found on the ELSO Web site (www.elso.med. umich.edu).

In the early years of ECLS, many institutions created their own training manual, or used manuals from other centers.[6] There are resources available from ELSO to support ECLS centers with their training. The ECMO Redbook is one example; ELSO also has a Specialist Training Manual[7] and both are available for purchase. Each chapter of the training manual includes review questions that can be used to assure that the learning objectives are met.

Didactic course

Training outlines and objectives designed for the specific needs of each center are key to developing a successful didactic course. It may help to consider the principles of adult learning prior to developing a course. All ECLS centers should begin their training preparation by reviewing the "ELSO Guidelines for Training and Continuing Education of ECMO Specialist", which recommends that a new ECMO program offer a didactic course lasting 24-36 hours, followed by water drills and animal sessions. The recommendations for an experienced center are the same, except that animal labs are not required. Instead, a new specialist should be precepted by an experienced specialist at the bedside.

There are many topics to include in a didactic course. A sample outline is provided in Table 2. A good place to start an ECLS training course is with an "Introduction to ECLS." This

Table 2. ECLS didactic topics.

Subject	Topics
Introduction to ECLS	• History • Current status of ECLS in neonates, pediatrics, adults, and eCPR • Overview of ELSO • Review of ELSO Registry data • Indications and contraindications in neonates, pediatrics, and adults • ECLS vs. CPB • Pre-ECLS evaluation - Therapies - Blood sampling - Echocardiogram - Head ultrasound
Physiology of common diseases treated with ECLS	• Persistent pulmonary hypertension of the newborn • Meconium aspiration syndrome • Sepsis • Neonatal pneumonia • Congenital diaphragmatic hernia • Adult respiratory distress syndrome • Post-op cardiac
Gas exchange	• Oxygen content, delivery, consumption • Normal gas exchange • Membrane gas exchange • Effecting gas exchange with pump, sweep flow, carbogen, CO_2
Ventilator/airway management during ECLS	• Resting ventilator settings • FiO_2 challenge • Suctioning • Nitric oxide
Methods of providing ECLS support	• Venoarterial (VA) • VV with double lumen cannula (DLC) • VV • Cephalad cannula • Conversion from VV to VA
Physiology of ECLS support	• VA • VV • VV-DLC
Blood products	• Whole blood • PRBC • Platelets • Cryoprecipitate • FFP • 25% Albumin • 5% Albumin

Subject	Topics
Coagulation	• Normal coagulation • Anticoagulation • Monitoring anticoagulation - Activated clotting times - Anti-thrombin III levels - D-dimers - Fibrinogen levels - PT/PTT • Heparin management
ECLS equipment	• ECLS pump • Membrane oxygenators • Heat exchangers • ECLS equipment supply box • UPS • Water bath • Bladder controller • Membrane pressure monitors • Blood flow monitor • ACT machine • Additional circuit components • Cannulas • CVVH interface with ECLS circuit
Calculations	• Oxygen content • Sweep flows • Drug dosages • Urine output • Total fluids/hourly fluids • Heparin requirement
ECLS orders and documentation	• ECLS flow sheet • ECLS report • Standing orders/target values
Circuit priming	• Circuit assembly - Use of pre-primed circuits ▪ CO_2 prime ▪ Negative pressure application ▪ Crystalloid prime ▪ Albumin prime ▪ Blood prime ▪ Additional circuit medications - Heparin - 25% albumin - Calcium gluconate - Tham/sodium bicarbonate

Subject	Topics

Cannulation and ECLS initiation	• Preparing the patient
	• Setting alarms
	• ACT instrument quality control
	• Analyzing circuit anticoagulation
	• Initiating bypass
	  - Beginning and advancement of blood flow
	  - Monitoring circuit pressures
	  - Monitoring patient heart rate, blood pressure, saturation levels
	  - Sweep gas changes
	  - Assessing cannula position
	  - Cannula security
	  - Documentation at start-up
	  - Back-up equipment
	  - Specialist, bedside nurse, ECLS physician roles

Medications	• Therapeutic category
	• Medication use during ECLS
	• Mechanism of actions
	• Usual dosages
	• Potential side effects
	• Drugs commonly given during ECLS:
	  - Anticoagulants
	  - Antibiotics
	  - Analgesics, narcotics, sedatives
	  - Anticonvulsants
	  - Antifibrinolytics
	  - Antihypertensive agents
	  - Cardiovascular agents
	  - Diuretics
	  - Electrolyte solutions
	  - Gastrointestinal agents
	  - Paralytics

ECLS lab schedule	• Frequently monitored lab values • ECLS effect on lab values
Patient complications during ECLS	• Bleeding • Clotting • Air embolization • Hypovolemia • Hypervolemia • Arrhythmias associated with ECLS • Cardiac stun • Blood pressure instability • Electrolyte imbalance • Cardiac arrest on ECLS • Renal failure • Inadvertent decannulation

Subject	Topics
Mechanical complications	• Oxygenator • Pump • Blood warming unit • Pressure monitors • Bladder controller/servo-regulation monitoring system • Bladder box • Heat exchanger • Circuit disruption-connectors, pigtails, raceway • Flow sensor failure
Weaning from ECLS	• VA vs. VV (differences and similarities) • How and why • Monitoring during weaning process • Trial off ECLS
Decannulation	• Preparing the patient • Preparing the circuit • Specialist, bedside nurse, ECLS physician roles • Management of the patient post-decannulation • Disposing of the ECLS circuit
ECLS transport	• Preparing for transport • Personnel needed • Roles during transport • Patient management in OR • Expectation of UPS • Back-up equipment
Stocking	• Stocking the ECLS cart
Special considerations	• Managing two ECLS patients • Unit-specific considerations • ECLS parents/families • Dealing with multiple medical/surgical teams

course should include discussion of the history of ECLS. An understanding of past successes and failures will lead to a better understanding of the basis for current practice. The history of ECLS should include information from clinical research trials as well as advances in equipment development. This session may also include discussion related to the general indications for ECLS as well as the risks and benefits. Center-specific indications and contraindications for ECLS should be discussed.

Specialists should be aware of pre-ECLS therapies that may have been used in potential ECLS patients including inhaled nitric oxide (iNO), high frequency oscillation, surfactant administration, permissive hypercapnia, and prone positioning. They should also be aware of the pre-ECLS orders that need to be completed. These orders include informed consent for ECLS and consent for blood transfusions. Pre-ECLS laboratory sampling tests need to be completed along with blood product type and crossmatch for all patient populations. Echocardiograms and head ultrasounds are routinely performed on neonatal patients. Room set-up and ECLS initiation should be discussed, and all documentation tools should be reviewed.

Institutions that provide ECLS to neonatal patients should discuss normal neonatal physiology. Included therein would be fetal circulation, transitional circulation, and normal newborn circulation. It is important that each student have a clear understanding of the physiology and pathophysiology of the diseases commonly treated with ECLS. This would include, at a minimum, persistent pulmonary hypertension of the newborn, meconium aspiration syndrome, congenital diaphragmatic hernia, and neonatal sepsis or pneumonia.

Those programs providing ECLS to pediatric and adult patients would include discussion on diseases specific to those populations; similarly, centers using ECLS for cardiac support would educate their specialists on the anatomy and circulation of both pre-operative and post-operative congenital heart disease, cardiomyopathy, myocarditis, and cardiac transplantion.

It is imperative that each ECLS specialist gains a complete understanding of blood gas interpretation and gas exchange. This includes understanding the concepts of oxygen content, oxygen delivery and consumption, CO_2 production and elimination, and how each interacts under normal conditions and with extracorporeal support. All team members should be able to explain how changes in the ECMO pump and sweep flow will affect gas exchange. Ventilator and airway management may be included in this session.

Although each center should focus the majority of teaching on the ECLS technique that is site-specific, it is also important to discuss the different types of support in use at other centers. Blood product administration, coagulation management, and medications commonly used in the blood prime and during ECLS should be reviewed. Each trainee should know how to run

an activated clotting test (ACT) and be aware of factors affecting the result. ECLS weaning and decannulation procedures should be discussed. In addition, a basic understanding of intra-hospital ECLS transport should be reviewed.

It is critical that all specialists gain a thorough understanding of ECLS equipment used in their institution. Every specialist should know how to set alarm parameters, be aware of the factors that would cause alarm conditions, and demonstrate the appropriate response to the alarm. Many alarm conditions can be simulated in water drill sessions where the response of the specialist can be observed. Finally, time should be spent discussing mechanical complications and preventative measures. During this session, a review of the most recent ECLS Registry report may be helpful. The Registry report highlights the common problems reported by participating centers and their incidence. For comparison, the report also indicates the rate of occurrence of each problem at the individual center. Information on patient follow-up could be included here. It is important for specialists to be familiar with patient outcomes in order to appreciate the risks and benefits associated with ECLS.

Priming

Priming an ECLS circuit refers to the method used to prepare the circuit for patient use. Additional training and practice for ECMO primers is required in order to prepare the ECLS circuit in a safe and timely fashion. Depending on individual experience, a review of sterile technique may be needed prior to teaching individuals to prime.

Training individuals to prime an ECLS circuit has two primary aspects. The first is teaching the steps in a logical order that accomplishes the goal of the prime. This becomes the prime "recipe". Secondly, the focus turns to the speed of the process. Because ECLS is often needed urgently with little, if any, advance notice, those responsible for priming the circuit need to perform the procedure rapidly. In addition, it is essential that the primer understand the purpose of each step in the priming process.

Prior to allowing individuals to prime alone, a priming trainee should demonstrate the procedure accurately and within a pre-established time frame. Repeated "practice" of the technique is necessary to maintain the accuracy and speed. For centers with few cases, some maximum interval between performing either a practice or actual prime will help to maintain their skill level.

Priming practices vary among institutions and depend on the type of oxygenator or membrane in the system. In general, there are common components to priming a circuit with a silicone membrane: circuit assembly, air displacement with CO_2, application of negative force to the circuit, fluid filling of all components followed by circulating albumin to reduce blood circuit interactions, and replacement of the fluid with blood and medications.

The medications typically used in the prime are a buffering agent to create a normal pH, heparin for anticoagulation, and calcium to counter the citrate effect. Once the circuit is primed, the sweep flow is initiated to add oxygen and remove CO_2. A sample priming procedure is outlined in Table 3.

Each center must identify a team of personnel who prime the ECLS circuit and provide assistance for troubleshooting and component replacement. The composition of the priming team varies from center to center. In some centers all of the specialists are primers; whereas in other centers, only perfusionists or a small group of specialists prime. Regardless of the team make-up, a system must be in place to insure that an ECLS primer is always readily available. Some centers have ECLS primers in-house at all times, while others have established an on-call system.

All ECLS specialists should be familiar with what is involved in the priming process. All specialists should know what blood products are used and the dosage of all medications used in the process of priming. This will allow a more thorough understanding of potential patient problems after the circuit is connected to the patient.

Water drills

ECLS circuits can be assembled, fluid filled, and run in non-clinical settings. This allows for opportunities to mimic many of the situations that occur during an actual ECLS run and is commonly referred to as a water drill. Water drills should be small enough to allow for hands-on experience by each individual. Table 4 shows a sample water drill session. The basic session should include a discussion and demonstration of all equipment including an explanation of the circuit configuration and function, alarm functions, and how to do a routine circuit assessment. Infusion and sampling ports should be identified, along with basic troubleshooting. At the end of the session, all trainees should be able to describe each piece of equipment, know what each alarm represents (including identification of the high and low pressure points within the circuit), and perform all basic procedures.

Table 3. Priming outline.

Task
• Obtain all appropriate equipment
• Assemble ECLS circuit using sterile technique
• Infuse CO_2 to displace air
• Apply a negative pressure to the silicone membrane
• Fluid fill the circuit with a crystalloid solution
• Coat circuit with albumin
• Displace fluid with blood and medications
• Circulate blood prime
• Warm circuit
• Obtain labs
• Add sweep gas prior to initiating support

Additional preparation for responding to emergencies can be practiced during water drills. Table 5 suggests topics to cover during an emergency session. In these sessions, the trainee will practice performing emergency functions such as repairing a raceway rupture and removing air from the circuit. Depending on the specialist's role, replacing a heat exchanger, bladder, and oxygenator should also be practiced. At the end of this session, each specialist should be able to promptly identify and correct any mechanical circuit problem. Specialists should also know how to respond appropriately to power failures, should practice clamping off ECLS, and know how to manually power the pump (hand cranking). The instructor will need to assess each trainee and determine by observation if they are competent in performing the technical skills necessary to manage simulated ECLS emergencies.

Animal lab sessions

Animal labs are performed in accordance with institutional animal care guidelines. New ECLS centers should conduct animal labs for a 24-72 hour period. This will decrease the number of animals needed and will simulate the around-the-clock management requirements of the ECLS patient. Each trainee should participate in a 4-8 hour session. The sessions should be small enough to allow for hands-on practice and allow the trainee to practice such tasks as blood product administration, IV solution and medication administration, blood gas, ACT, and other laboratory sampling. Each trainee should be able to make changes on the pump and assess how the changes affect the animal. The student can gain an understanding of heparin management by assessing ACT results and adjusting the heparin rate. Physician orders and appropriate

Table 4. Basic water drills.

Subject	Topics

Equipment	• Review of disposable circuit
	  - Sampling ports
	  - Oxygenator
	  - Heat exchanger
	• Pump controls, alarms
	• Pressure monitoring
	• Sweep gas monitoring
	• Oxygen analyzer
	• Water heater
	• Air bubble detector
	• Flow meter

Basic procedures	• Circuit assessment • Pump head occlusion checks • Drawing blood samples • Running ACTs • Drawing pre- and post-membrane blood gases • Changing stopcocks • Administering platelets and other blood products • Administering medications • Setting up hemofiltration/dialysis

documentation tools such as the ECLS flow sheet should be used. It is vitally important for new centers to repeat these sessions until all team members are competent in managing ECLS systems.

Verifying ECLS competency

ECLS competency can be verified by observation in actual clinical settings or in simulated settings. There are three skills to consider when assessing competency - technical, critical thinking, and interpersonal. Verification is the objective process of assuring that a staff member can perform the competency based on specific performance criteria used to ensure accurate and safe practice. Performance criteria must be outlined in a policy, procedure, standard, guideline, or reference. A sample ACT competency form is located in Table 6.

Technical skills include psychomotor activities that are part of every job. ECLS technical skills are easy to verify in a simulated water lab session. The instructor can observe the specialist performing the procedure. One example might be observing the specialist repairing a tubing rupture. True competency can only be verified by observation in actual patient situations. It is only under real-life, stressful situations that the specialist's ability level can be most accurately determined. For this reason, it is important to practice infrequently used skills on a regular

Table 5. Emergency procedures.

Procedure
• Clamping off ECMO
• Hand cranking pump
• Repairing tubing ruptures
• Replacing raceway tubing
• Removing venous air
• Removing arterial air
• Power failure
• Changing out an oxygenator
• Changing out other components

basis. Each center should determine their own timeline for competency evaluation based on their specific needs.

Critical thinking skills include decision-making, prioritizing, troubleshooting, and responding to actual or potential events. A written test can be used to assess for knowledge, in fact, the ELSO guidelines recommend that all specialists take an annual oral and/or written exam. Specific ECLS problems and the knowledge of how to handle them can be simulated in an animal or water lab session. The verifier can then observe if the ECLS specialist responds appropriately. Since ECLS is a high risk/low volume procedure, these skills should be evaluated on a regular basis. Again, each center needs to determine its own timeline for evaluation based on its specific needs.

Interpersonal skills reflect the ability to communicate effectively with individuals and groups. Professional communication skills include written, spoken, and non-verbal skills. Co-workers can identify ECLS specialists who lack the appropriate interpersonal skills. The difficulty lies in objectively identifying those skills. Some of the communication behavioral indicators include demonstrating courtesy, being respectful, and practicing good listening and feedback skills.

Developing new ECMO competencies

Initial ECLS competencies may be completed in a set time frame and will need to be verified on a regular basis. Each specialist should demonstrate acceptable performance in skills and decision-making ability in the ECLS setting. In general, ongoing or new competencies need to be developed after answering the following questions:

1. Are there new procedures, polices, equipment, or initiatives? An example would be a new in-line gas monitoring system or new ECLS pump.

Table 6. Competency checklist.

| COMPETENCY CHECKLIST | Employee Name: _____ |

Title: ACT (Activated Clotting Test)

OBJECTIVE STATEMENT (following this competency, the participant should be able to...):
To demonstrate competence in performing an ACT.

KNOWLEDGE OR TECHNICAL RESOURCES:
- ECMO Training Manual
- Electronic Hemochron QC and Patient Log

VALIDATION OF COMPETENCY:

A.   Knowledge (cognitive) Criteria

Circle the correct answer:

1. Electronic QC's must be performed:
    a. Every 8 hour shift when patients are tested
    b. Every 12 hour shift when patients are tested
    c. Once a day
2. ACTs may decrease:
    a. After an increase in urine output
    b. After platelets are given
    c. Both of the above
    d. None of the above
3. The P214 test tubes should be used when patients have received Aprotinin:
    a. True
    b. False
4. The first response to an ACT of 40 would be to:
    a. Notify the physician
    b. Give a heparin bolus and increase the drip
    c. Repeat the test

B.   Technical (psychomotor) Skills
    ____   Tap tube to bring powder to the bottom.
    ____   Clear the pigtail and stopcock of stagnant blood.
    ____   Withdraw 0.4 cc blood.
    ____   Simultaneously inject blood into tube and start ACT machine by depressing start button.
    ____   Close the cap on tube and flick gently 5-7 times to assure mixture of clotting substances.
    ____   Insert the tube into test well and rotate clockwise one turn after the green detector light comes on.

    Documentation:
        Record results on the patient's flow sheet.
        Repeat any questionable results.

C.   Department-specific Requirements (if applicable)

D.   Comments

Competency	Validated by	Date
Initial		
Annual		

Competency Review Requirements:
New employees: Competency must be validated initially and annually thereafter.
Employees (ongoing): Competency must be validated annually

2. Are there changes or revisions in procedures, policies, equipment, or initiatives? An example would be a change in ACT quality analysis mandated by CLIA regulations.
3. What are the non-routine practices, procedures, equipment, or skills needed? An example would be the occasional use of hemofiltration.
4. What are the problem-prone aspects of ECLS? These can be identified through quality improvement data, incident reports, staff surveys, and other forms of evaluation.
5. What are the high-risk aspects of this job? High risk is anything that would lead to harm, death, or legal action. Unfortunately, this about covers everything to do with ECLS.

Maintaining ECMO competency

ECLS centers need to ensure that all team members obtain the appropriate education and experience to remain competent. The ELSO guidelines recommend that water drills be held at a minimum of every 6 months. It is also suggested that an annual examination be used to verify the knowledge and skills of all specialists. Team members should be required to have a minimum number of pump hours in an established time period. If the number of hours is not met, then retraining should be undertaken.

ECLS specialist team meetings should be held on a regular basis to identify any pertinent issues and to provide continuing education. Frequencies of these meetings should be based on the size of the team and the volume of ECLS patients treated. Attendance records should be monitored and team members should be required to attend a certain number of meetings.

It can be a struggle to provide educational offerings that remain interesting and challenging, especially for experienced team members who have been doing ECLS for a long time. Many

ECLS centers have come up with ideas to assist others such as developing an ECLS crossword puzzle with clues hinting at the intended ECLS answer. Another idea is to have ECMO trivia such as ECMO jeopardy or ECMO trivial pursuit. Initiating an "ECLS question of the week" via email or on a bulletin board can stimulate discussion and be another tool to promote ECLS education. Sample test questions may soon be available on the ELSO Web site, and in the future there may be an ELSO sponsored, web-based "self-assessment tool."

ECLS-net

Another avenue for continued education is via the ECLS-net–an Internet-based list-serve comprised of health care professionals involved in the development and implementation of ECLS. It is overseen by moderators to ensure that postings are of appropriate content and are available only from authorized participants. Directions on how to subscribe to ECLS-net can be found on the website www.ecls-net.net. The ECLS-net provides a medium for ECLS centers throughout the U.S. and abroad to share ideas regarding such topics as technique, equipment, and procedures. It is an important tool for identifying practice variations and for collaboration. It can be used for rapid clinical patient consultations as well as for requesting information concerning clinical practices or program organization. Specialists can learn from other specialists who have experience in managing ECLS patients and problems. All clinical situations are presented without any patient identifiers. Ideas from the ECLS-net can be useful for another center's situation. As with all Internet chatter, the information needs to be dealt with cautiously.

Evaluation and institutional certification of the ECMO specialist

At this time there is not a national certification for ECLS specialists. Each institution is responsible for evaluating and certifying its own team members. A written evaluation of each specialist's training should be maintained. This evaluation should include documentation of course attendance, successful performance at water drills and/or animal sessions, and completion of all required skills lists and/or competencies. In addition, each specialist should obtain a passing grade on a written and/or oral exam. Institutional certification can be granted after successfully completing the training course requirements and passing the exam. Sample certification requirements are shown in Table 7.

Periodic review of the ECLS specialist's knowledge and skill level is essential. The frequency and the skills to be assessed are center-specific. Each center should develop specific requirements for recertification. All training expectations need to be established as well as criteria indicating success (e.g., a passing score on a test and a minimum number of pump hours). In addition, requirements for attendance and participation in team meetings should be specified. Sample recertification requirements are listed in Table 8.

Ensuring quality

Promoting and maintaining quality in an ECLS program is essential. Continuous qual-ity improvement is required by accrediting agencies; moreover, ECMO programs have a responsibility to their patients to monitor outcomes and continually seek opportunities for improvement. Membership in ELSO is of paramount importance. ELSO supports many quality improvement tools for centers to utilize such as national meetings that facilitate important collaboration, publications, research studies, and the Registry.

Each institution needs to comply with the various governing agencies that monitor care. For example, ACT testing is considered a moderately complex point of care test (POCT). Several POCT regulations for quality control apply to ACT testing. Strict adherence to these requirements is essential and all specialists should be aware of the regulations and procedures for following electronic and liquid quality controls.

National meetings

An essential component of any quality ECLS program is ongoing active participation at national ECLS meetings. There are several national meetings every year offering opportunities for benchmarking and collaboration as well as promotion of scientific advancement

Table 7. Requirements for ECLS certification.

Certification requirement
• Minimum of 1 year critical care experience prior to training
• Attendance at all didactic sessions
• Attendance at all laboratory sessions
• Participation in ECLS water/emergency drills
• Completion of percepted pump time
• Completion of technical skills list and/or competencies
• Successful completion of written/oral exam with passing score

Table 8. Requirements for ECLS re-certification.

Re-certification requirement
• Attendance at all ECLS update sessions
• Verification of ECLS competency
• Participation in bi-annual ECLS disaster/water drills
• Passing score on annual written or oral examination
• Attendance at required team meetings
• Performance of required number of pump hours per quarter

and basic education. These include the ELSO annual meeting that is usually held in the fall, and the Children's National Medical Center's Annual Symposium for ECMO and Advanced Therapies for Respiratory Failure held in the spring. Another conference that is designed for ECLS specialists is the Specialist Education ECMO (SEECMO) meeting. SEECMO is sponsored by rotating ELSO member institutions.

ELSO Registry

One of the main activities of the ELSO organization is maintenance of a central data registry. Formal reporting of the data occurs twice annually. Each member institution receives collective International Summary reports as well as Center-specific reports. More details about the Registry are included in chapter 10.

The International and Center-specific ELSO Registry reports provide the foundation for a quality ECLS program. ECLS programs should regularly and routinely review their outcomes and compare these with the international results. The Registry reports provide one mechanism for this comparison, with an opportunity for an institution to benchmark itself against the rest of the international ECLS community. However, in comparing some outcome statistics, it is important to realize there are potential limitations to the use of these reports. When interpreting and comparing outcomes, it is essential to interpret the data with the understanding that there is a lack of consensus among programs regarding many diagnostic and monitoring parameters during the course of a patient on ECLS. For instance, centers using the Center-specific report to compare their rate of hemolysis, as determined by plasma hemoglobin measurements, with the International Summary must recognize that not all centers measure plasma hemoglobin.

The Registry also cannot provide in-depth information regarding clinical practice, as the reports are limited to the data that are reported. Regular review of all recent ECLS-related literature is essential, in addition to participation in ECLS-net and national meetings.

Formal ECLS committee program evaluation

It is the responsibility of each center to ensure that ongoing quality improvement occurs. A multi-disciplinary ECLS team should be developed including all key ECLS team members. ELSO guidelines recommend that formal team meetings be held on a regular basis. These formal multi-disciplinary meetings, with written minutes, should review clinical cases, equipment, administrative and educational needs, and other pertinent issues. Minutes to these meetings should be available to all ECLS team members. The multi-disciplinary ECLS team should have quality assurance review procedures in place for annual internal ECLS evaluation. It should be expected that all team members have the responsibility to promote and maintain a quality program.

A prompt review of any major complication or death should be held both with ECLS team members and with the responsible morbidity and mortality committee in the hospital. These reviews should be conducted under the relevant quality assurance laws for the state where the center is located. Formal clinical-pathological case reviews with a multi-disciplinary approach should be regularly conducted.

Summary

Although providing ECLS to critically ill patients is complex and uses many health care resources, it can be very rewarding to the institution, staff, and, especially, the infants, children, adults, and families served. Meticulous attention to the areas of essential support systems, physical facilities and equipment, team and personnel issues, and quality assurance are the foundations of a successful ECLS program.

References

1. ELSO guidelines for ECMO centers. Available at: http://www.elso.med.umich. edu/guide.htm. Accessed May 25, 2005.

2. Klein MD, Stockmann PT. ECMO in the hospital setting. In: Zwischenberger JB, Steinhorn RH, Bartlett RH, eds. *ECMO Extracorporeal Cardiopulmonary Support in Critical Care*. 2nd ed. Extracorporeal Life Support Organization; 2000: 237-252.

3. Joint commission on accreditation of healthcare organizations. Root causes of sentinel events 1995-2003. Available at: http://www.jcaho.com/accredited+organizations/ambulatory+care/sentinel+events/root+causes+of+sentinel+event.htm. Accessed May 25, 2005.

4. Comprehensive accreditation manual for hospitals: the official handbook. Available at: http://intranet.chw.org/display/displayFile.asp?docid=6840&filename=/Groups/JCAHO/2005_CAMH_Update_1.pdf. Accessed May 25, 2005.

5. ELSO guidelines for training and continuing education of ECMO specialists. Available at: http://www.elso.med.umich.edu/guide.htm. Accessed May 25, 2005.

6. Rosenberg EM. ECLS technical manuals. In: Zwischenberger JB, Steinhorn RH, Bartlett RH, eds. *ECMO Extracorporeal Cardiopulmonary Support in Critical Care*. 2nd ed. Extracorporeal Life Support Organization; 2000: 193-198.

7. Van Meurs K. *ECMO Specialist Training Manual*. 2 ed. Ann Arbor, Michigan: ELSO; 1999.

17

Neonatal Respiratory Failure: Pathophysiology and Management

Kathryn N. Farrow, M.D. and Robin H. Steinhorn, M.D.

Introduction

Survival of the newborn is dependent upon the adaptation of the fetal cardiopulmonary system to the sudden demands of extrauterine life. Some infants fail to achieve or sustain the normal decrease in pulmonary vascular resistance (PVR) at birth, leading to severe respiratory distress and hypoxemia, which is referred to as hypoxemic respiratory failure or persistent pulmonary hypertension of the newborn (PPHN).

Hypoxemic respiratory failure, often associated with PPHN, is a major clinical problem in the neonatal ICU and can contribute significantly to morbidity and mortality in full-term and premature neonates. Neonatal respiratory failure affects nearly 80,000 newborns per year and is responsible for up to half of all neonatal mortality.[1] Nearly one-third of all infants with respiratory failure are term or near-term and are potential candidates for neonatal extracorporeal support. Newborns with hypoxemic respiratory failure and/or PPHN are at risk for severe asphyxia and its complications, including death, neurologic injury, and other problems. These infants typically present shortly after birth with respiratory distress and cyanosis, but a structurally normal heart. The incidence of severe PPHN is estimated at 0.2% of live-born term infants.[2]

Respiratory failure and hypoxemia in the term newborn results from a heterogeneous group of disorders, and the therapeutic approach and response often depends on the underlying disease. Appropriate and timely interventions are essential to prevent progression to circulatory failure and death.

The fetal pulmonary vasculature

During fetal life, the pulmonary circulation undergoes striking developmental changes in vascular growth and structure. These are accompanied by maturational changes in function. Because the placenta, not the lung, serves as the organ of gas exchange, less than 10% of the combined ventricular output is circulated through the pulmonary vascular bed, and most of the right ventricular output crosses the ductus arteriosus to the aorta. Despite increases in vascular surface area, PVR increases with gestational age when corrected for lung or body weight, suggesting that vascular tone actually increases during late gestation and is high prior to birth. Therefore, in utero, pulmonary pressures are equivalent to systemic pressures due to elevated PVR.

There are multiple pathways involved in maintaining high pulmonary vascular tone in utero. Some of the known pulmonary vasoconstrictors in the normal fetus include low oxygen tension, endothelin-1 (ET-1), and leukotrienes. In addition, there is relatively low basal production of vasodilator products such as prostacyclin (PgI_2) and nitric oxide (NO).

Normal pulmonary vascular transition

Pulmonary endothelial cells play a central role in the pulmonary vascular transition through the production and release of numerous mediators that act on smooth muscle cells. The main endothelial products which are currently believed to be responsible for the pulmonary vasodilatation at transition include arachidonic acid metabolites and nitric oxide (NO).

As gestation progresses, these mediators of the vasodilatory pathways become more dominant. In particular, NO production increases at the time of birth.[3] Pulmonary expression of endothelial nitric oxide synthase (eNOS) and its downstream target, soluble guanylate cyclase (sGC), increases during late gestation.[4,5] Ultimately, increased NO production and sGC activity lead to increased cyclic guanosine monophosphate (cGMP) concentrations in vascular smooth muscle cells, which then leads to vasorelaxation by decreasing intracellular calcium. Acute or chronic inhibition of NOS in fetal lambs produces pulmonary hypertension following delivery, indicating its importance in the normal pulmonary vascular transition.[3,6]

The prostacyclin pathway is another potentially important vasodilatory pathway in the normal transition to extrauterine life. Cyclooxygenase (COX) is the rate-limiting enzyme that generates prostacyclin from arachadonic acid. Both COX-1 and COX-2 are found in the lung, but COX-1 is upregulated during late gestation.[7] This upregulation leads to an increase in prostacyclin production in late gestation and early postnatal life.[8,9] Prostacyclin interacts with adenylate cyclase to increase intracellular cyclic adenosine monophosphate (cAMP) levels, which then lead to vasorelaxation.

At the time of birth, multiple factors intervene to regulate these pathways. As a result, pulmonary artery pressure decreases to approximately 50% of systemic pressure and pulmonary blood flow increases by 10-fold.[10-12] The most critical signals for these transitional changes are mechanical distension of the lung, a decrease in CO_2 tension, and an increase in oxygen tension in the lungs. When near-term fetal lambs are ventilated without changing the tensions of CO_2 or oxygen, pulmonary blood flow increases to approximately two-thirds of levels normally observed following birth.[13,14] Similarly, near-term fetal lambs can be exposed to oxygenation without ventilation through hyperbaric oxygenation of the ewe. Under these conditions, fetal PVR decreases and pulmonary blood flow increases to levels comparable to those seen after birth.[15,16]

Oxygen stimulates the activity of both eNOS and COX-1 immediately after birth, leading to increased levels of NO and prostacyclin.[17-19] Likewise, oxygen stimulates the release of adenosine triphosphate (ATP) from oxygenated red blood cells (RBCs), which also increases the activity of both eNOS and COX-1.[20-23] Finally, shear stress regulates the synthesis of NO in the fetal circulation. During transition, an initial increase in pulmonary blood flow in response to ventilation or oxygenation leads to increased shear stress in the vasculature, which in turn further increases NO production.[19,24,25] Thus, events in utero and at the time of birth that impair these critical transition steps will ultimately lead to elevated pulmonary pressures and the symptomatic infant with PPHN.

Pathophysiology of PPHN

PPHN can be thought of as one of three types: 1) the abnormally constricted pulmonary vasculature due to parenchymal diseases such as meconium aspiration syndrome (MAS), respiratory distress syndrome (RDS), and sepsis; 2) the structurally abnormal vasculature, also known as idiopathic PPHN; or 3) the hypoplastic vasculature as seen in congenital diaphragmatic hernia (CDH). The pathophysiology of each type is dependent on the point in gestation when the normal transition to extrauterine life fails.

Parenchymal lung disease: meconium aspiration syndrome

The most common cause of PPHN is meconium aspiration syndrome (MAS), which affects 25–30,000 infants with 1,000 deaths annually in the U.S.[26] Approximately 13% of all live births are complicated by meconium-stained fluid, but only 5% of these infants subsequently develop MAS.[27] In these cases, the infant passes meconium while still in utero, usually in response to stressful stimuli. The affected infant then aspirates the meconium into its airways, where it impedes ventilation immediately after birth. While the traditional belief is that aspiration occurs with the first breath after birth, more recent data suggest that for the more severely affected infants, it most likely occurs in utero.[26,27] In either case, meconium aspiration injures the lung through multiple mechanisms including mechanical obstruction of the airways, chemical pneumonitis due to inflammation, activation of complement, inactivation of surfactant, and vasoconstriction of pulmonary vessels. Meconium acts as an airway obstruction with a "ball-valve" effect, preventing adequate ventilation in the immediate postnatal period. The subsequent air trapping makes the risk of pneumothorax in the infant approximately 15-33%.[26]

Meconium also appears to also have toxic effects in the lungs that are mediated by inflammation.[26,27] Within hours of the meconium aspiration event, neutrophils and macrophages are found in the alveoli and lung parenchyma.[28] The release of cytokines such as tumor necrosis factor alpha (TNFα), interleukin 1-ß (IL-1ß), and interleukin-8 (IL-8) may directly injure the lung parenchyma and lead to vascular leakage, causing a pneumonitis with pulmonary edema, which in turn continues to interfere with the ventilation required to trigger postnatal pulmonary vasodilation.[29,30] Meconium also activates the alternative complement pathway, but not the classical and lectin pathways.[31] In a piglet model of MAS, the meconium-induced complement activation precedes cytokine release, and the increase in complement activation correlates with worsening lung dysfunction. In fact, the subgroup of piglets that died from MAS had substantially higher levels of complement activation.[32] There is also evidence that meconium injury may also directly trigger postnatal release of vasoconstrictors such as ET-1, thromboxane A2 (TXA2), and prostaglandin E2 (PGE2), which also play a role in the development of PPHN.[33,34]

In the early 1990s, it was recognized that in addition to its obstructive and pro-inflammatory effects, meconium inactivates surfactant.[35] Meconium displaces surfactant from the alveolar surface and inhibits its ability to lower the alveolar surface tension. Lung lavage fluid from infants with MAS has been shown to contain known surfactant inhibitors such as albumin and phosphatidylserine.[36] Additionally, meconium has been shown to contain increased levels of phospholipase A2, which appears to be, in part, responsible for the surfactant inactivation.[37] The resulting functional surfactant deficiency in infants with MAS leads to alveolar atelectasis, decreased lung compliance, and poor oxygenation.[26]

Idiopathic PPHN

Idiopathic (or "black-lung") PPHN is the second most common etiology of PPHN and is most common in term and near-term (>34 weeks gestation) newborns. Evaluation of these infants at autopsy shows significant remodeling of their pulmonary vasculature with vessel wall thickening and smooth muscle hyperplasia. Further, the smooth muscle extends to the level of the intra-acinar arteries (Figure 1), which does not normally occur until much later in the postnatal period.[38,39] As a result, these infants do not appropriately vasodilate their pulmonary vasculature in response to birth-related stimuli, and they present with profound hypoxemia and clear, hyperlucent lung fields on chest radiograph, thus the term "black-lung" PPHN (Figure 2).

The pathophysiology of this abnormally remodeled pulmonary vasculature is the subject of intense investigation. One cause of idiopathic PPHN is constriction of the fetal ductus arteriosus in utero from exposure to non-steroidal anti-inflammatory drugs (NSAIDs) during the third trimester.[40] From studies utilizing a fetal lamb model, ductal constriction in utero is known to cause an increase in fetal pulmonary artery pressure, pulmonary vascular remodeling, and a subsequent failure to transition to extrauterine life.[41-43] Recent studies have demonstrated the presence of ibuprofen and naproxen in the meconium of the infant, which implies in utero exposure. Further, the concentration of these drugs in the meconium correlates with the incidence and severity of idiopathic PPHN. However, not all infants with NSAID exposure had PPHN, suggesting biologic or genetic susceptibility in those infants who develop severe disease.[44]

There is growing evidence that infants with idiopathic PPHN suffer from disruptions of the NO-cGMP, prostacyclin-cAMP, and the endothelin signaling pathways (Figure 3). Decreased levels of both expression and activity of eNOS have been documented in infants with PPHN, as well as in the ductal-ligation lamb model of PPHN.[45-47] In addition to eNOS disruption, PPHN lamb models also demonstrate an uncoupling of eNOS from the chaperone protein, heat shock protein 90 (hsp 90). Decreased hsp90:eNOS interactions lead to decreased NO synthesis and increased superoxide production by eNOS.[22] Nicotinamide adenine dinucleo-

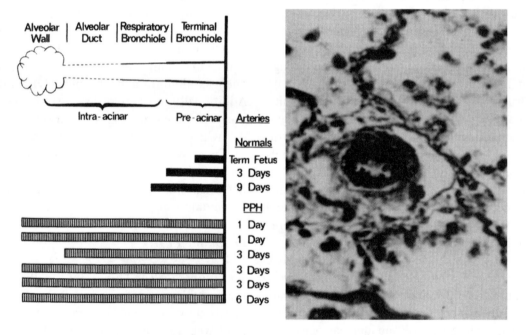

Figure 1: Vascular maldevelopment is a hallmark of PPHN. The pulmonary vessels show thickened walls with smooth muscle hyperplasia. Further, the smooth muscle extends to the level of the intra-acinar arteries which does not normally occur until much later in the postnatal period. (Murphy JD, Rabinovitch M, Goldstein JD, Reid LM. *J Pediatr* 1981; 98:962).

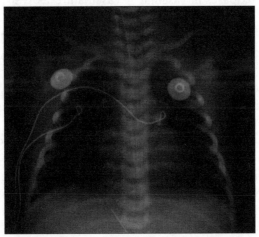

Figure 2: Chest radiograph of an infant with idiopathic PPHN. Note the clear lung fields with decreased vascularity. These findings are sometimes called "black-lung" PPHN.

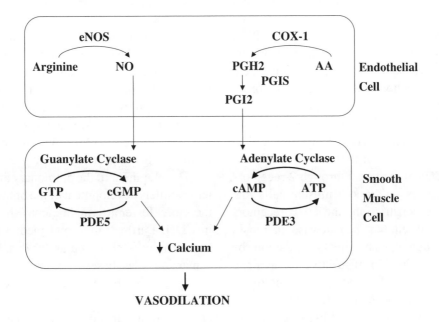

Figure 3. NO and prostacyclin signaling pathways in regulation of vascular tone. NO is synthesized by NOS from the terminal nitrogen group of L-arginine. NO stimulates sGC to increase intracellular cGMP. PGI2 is an arachidonic acid metabolite formed by COX-1 and prostacyclin synthase (PGIS) in the vascular endothelium. PGI2 stimulates adenylate cyclase in vascular smooth muscle cells, which increases intracellular cAMP. Both cGMP and cAMP indirectly decrease free cytosolic calcium resulting in smooth muscle relaxation, which leads to vascular dilation. Specific phosphodiesterases hydrolyze cGMP and cAMP, thus regulating the intensity and duration of their vascular effects.

tide phosphate (NADPH) oxidases in vascular smooth muscle may also serve as a source of superoxide, which leads to vasoconstriction and smooth muscle hypertrophy.[48] Additionally, not only is there less NO production and more production of reactive oxygen species, but vessel studies from PPHN lamb models also suggest that soluble guanylate cyclase is less sensitive to the NO that is present, leading to less cGMP in the vascular smooth muscle.[49] Finally, in addition to decreased cyclic guanyl monophosphate (cGMP) production, increased activity of phosphodiesterase (PDE5) has been reported in PPHN lamb models, which may lead to increased cGMP destruction.[50] Thus, PPHN following ductal constriction leads to failed transition by decreasing available cGMP, which is important for vasodilation, and increasing superoxide, which stimulates vasoconstriction.

While prostacyclin appears to be important in the normal pulmonary vascular transition, less is known about the potential dysregulation of the prostacyclin-cAMP pathway in PPHN. However, new evidence suggests that production of the vasoconstrictor arachadonic acid metabolite thromboxane increases in pulmonary hypertension resulting from hypoxia.[51]

Circulating levels of the potent vasoconstrictor endothelin-1 (ET-1) are elevated in lambs and newborn infants with PPHN.[52,53] ET-1 effects are mediated through 2 receptors, ET-A receptors on smooth muscle cells that mediate vasoconstriction, and ET-B receptors on endothelial cells that mediate vasodilation. In addition, endothelin may affect vascular tone by increasing production of reactive oxygen species such as superoxide and hydrogen peroxide, which also act as vasoconstrictors.[54-56] Thus, the elevated endothelin levels in PPHN may lead to increased vasoconstriction through preferential stimulation of ET-A receptors and through increased production of superoxide.

These data indicate that idiopathic PPHN is the result of a complex pathological process that includes structural remodeling of the pulmonary vasculature as well as disruption of multiple signaling pathways, most notably endothelin and NO. Since multiple pathways are involved, effective treatment will likely require multiple therapeutic agents.

Congenital diaphragmatic hernia

CDH occurs in 1 of every 2-4,000 live births and accounts for 8% of all major congenital anomalies. CDH is an abnormality in diaphragm development resulting in a defect that allows abdominal viscera to enter the chest and compress the lung. Herniation occurs most often in the posterolateral segments of the diaphragm, and 80% of the defects occur on the left side. While compression of the lung in utero is believed to produce lung hypoplasia, there is some evidence that the lung hypoplasia may be a primary event that occurs independently of the diaphragmatic defect.[57] Because severe CDH develops early in the course of lung development, airway divisions are limited in both the affected and contralateral lungs. Therefore, CDH is characterized by a variable degree of pulmonary hypoplasia associated with a decrease in cross-sectional area of the pulmonary vasculature and possible dysfunction of the surfactant system. Because airspace development follows airway development, alveolarization is similarly reduced.

Development of the pulmonary arterial system parallels development of the bronchial tree; therefore, fewer arterial branches are observed in CDH. Further, abnormal medial muscular hypertrophy is observed as far distally as the acinar arterioles. In severe cases, left ventricular hypoplasia is observed. Pulmonary capillary blood flow is decreased because of the small cross-sectional area of the pulmonary vascular bed, and flow may be further decreased by abnormal pulmonary vasoconstriction.

The reported survival rate for CDH varies widely, depending on whether the disease is diagnosed before or after birth. Tertiary referral centers with ECMO capability report that up to 75% of infants with CDH survive.[57] In contrast, antenatal diagnosis has been associated with lower survival at 42%.[58] CDH is no longer thought to require immediate surgery, since the primary problem after birth is not herniation of abdominal viscera into the chest, but severe pulmonary hypoplasia and associated pulmonary hypertension. However, the medical management of CDH remains a major challenge for the clinician.

Treatment of PPHN

The initial treatment of the newborn with PPHN includes correction of underlying conditions including polycythemia, hypothermia, and hypoventilation, as well as correction of hypoglycemia, hypocalcemia, anemia, and hypovolemia. While the use of alkalinizing agents remains controversial, correction of metabolic acidosis is routine. Cardiac output and systemic oxygen transport must be optimized through the support of cardiac function, and perfusion with volume and inotropic agents (dobutamine, dopamine, and milrinone). Increasing systemic arterial pressure may improve oxygenation in some cases by reducing right-to-left extrapulmonary shunting.

The goal of mechanical ventilation is to achieve "optimal" lung volume to allow for lung recruitment while minimizing the risk for lung injury. Failure to achieve adequate lung volumes at or above functional residual capacity contributes to hypoxemia and high PVR in newborns with PPHN. For instance, some newborns with parenchymal lung disease associated with PPHN will improve oxygenation and decrease right-to-left extrapulmonary shunting in response to lung recruitment during high frequency oscillatory ventilation (HFOV). A favorable response to HFOV is most likely to occur in infants with homogenous lung disease due to respiratory distress syndrome or pneumonia.[59] However, mechanical ventilation using excessive pressures can produce acute lung injury, pulmonary edema, decreased lung compliance, and lung inflammation due to increased cytokine production and lung neutrophil accumulation. The development of ventilator-induced lung injury is an important determinant of clinical course and eventual outcome of newborns with hypoxemic respiratory failure, and postnatal lung injury exacerbates the degree of pulmonary hypertension. Infants that have received prolonged mechanical ventilation and exposure to high oxygen concentrations (>10-14 days) have higher mortality following extracorporeal support and may be excluded from consideration for ECMO due to concerns about irreversible lung injury. Furthermore, overexpansion of the lung beyond 9-10 ribs may paradoxically worsen pulmonary hypertension because overdistended alveoli may compress capillaries and small arterioles.

The use of forced alkalosis to produce pulmonary vasodilation remains controversial. Hyperventilation has been shown in 2 small case series to decrease mean pulmonary artery pressure and improve PaO_2. Animal studies have shown that this effect is dependent on the increase in pH rather than changes in $PaCO_2$.[60] The benefits of these short-term physiologic changes have not been systematically studied in clinical trials. In addition, extreme alkalosis may decrease cerebral perfusion, cause systemic vasodilation, and decrease oxygen unloading from hemoglobin at the tissue level. Some adverse outcomes, such as hearing loss, appear to be related to the extent and duration of hyperventilation.[61,62]

Parenchymal lung disease of the term and near-term infant is often associated with surfactant deficiency and/or inactivation. As noted above, surfactant dysfunction has been demonstrated in MAS, with a concentration-dependent inhibition of pulmonary surfactant activity occurring at meconium concentrations much lower than those required for inhibition by plasma protein and blood cell components.[35]

Single-center trials have shown that surfactant improves oxygenation in infants with MAS,[63] and a large multi-center trial demonstrated that surfactant treatment decreased the need for ECMO.[64] The reduction in the need for ECMO was most apparent in infants treated early (oxygenation index [OI] of 15-22) and in infants with primary diagnoses of MAS or sepsis.[64] In contrast, a recent report indicates that surfactant therapy does not reduce death, need for ECMO, or other morbidities in infants with CDH.[65] Thus, surfactant may be an important tool in optimizing lung inflation in infants with parenchymal lung disease, except for those with CDH.

Inhaled nitric oxide

Before the availability of inhaled NO (iNO), selective pulmonary vasodilatation was not clinically possible. iNO has many of the characteristics of an ideal selective pulmonary vasodilator. It has a rapid and potent vasodilator effect. Because it is a small gas molecule, NO can be delivered through a ventilator directly to airspaces approximating the pulmonary vascular bed. Once in the blood stream, NO binds avidly to hemoglobin, preventing systemic vasodilator effects.

Early animal studies and human case reports rapidly led to multi-center randomized, placebo-controlled, blinded trials to test the effectiveness of iNO in term and near-term infants with PPHN. These trials demonstrated that iNO significantly decreases the need for ECMO in newborns with PPHN,[66,67] although it has not been shown to reduce mortality or length of hospitalization. In addition, follow-up studies at 12-24 months have shown that iNO does not significantly increase the incidence of chronic lung disease (CLD), or adverse neurodevelopmental sequelae.[68,69] This is an interesting observation that may indicate that the underlying disease is associated with early neurological injury.

Several of the randomized trials had sufficient patient entry to assess response as a function of the underlying lung disease. The most consistent finding is that iNO does not reduce the need for ECMO in infants with unrepaired CDH.[66,70] The infants with CDH enrolled in these 2 studies had relatively severe illness at the time of enrollment, as indicated by a high OI. While it is possible that iNO may be beneficial for the infant with CDH if delivered prior to the onset of severe respiratory failure, this has not yet been demonstrated.

Initiation of iNO

An initial echocardiographic evaluation is needed to exclude structural heart lesions and establish the presence of pulmonary hypertension. The use of iNO is contraindicated in congenital heart diseases that is dependent on right-to-left shunting across the ductus arteriosus. This would include infants with critical aortic stenosis, interrupted aortic arch, and hypoplastic left heart syndrome. In addition, iNO may worsen pulmonary edema in infants with obstructed total anomalous pulmonary venous return due to the fixed venous obstruction. The use of iNO should be reserved for post-operative care in these patients after the obstruction has been surgically corrected.

In general, iNO should be initiated when the OI exceeds 25, the entry criteria for the multi-center randomized studies noted above. A recent study demonstrated that beginning iNO earlier in the disease course with an OI of >15 did not change the incidence of ECMO and/or death, or improve other patient outcomes.[71]

Dose of iNO

The recommended initial dose of iNO is 20 ppm. Early studies in animals and infants used iNO doses as high as 80-100 ppm.[72] However, in large clinical trials, inhalation of these higher dosages produced no better outcomes than lower doses of 20 ppm. For instance, in the Neonatal Inhaled Nitric Oxide Study (NINOS) trial, 47% of infants failed to respond to 20 ppm iNO (defined by an increase in PaO_2 of >20 torr). When the iNO dose was increased to 80 ppm, only 15% of these infants responded with an increase in PaO_2 of >10 torr.[67]

The role of initiating therapy with doses <20 ppm is not clear. Cornfield et al. randomized infants with PPHN to an initial iNO dose of 2 or 20 ppm,[73] and found that infants randomized to 2 ppm NO did not have any improvement in oxygenation and did not improve even after iNO was increased to 20 ppm. Tworetsky et al. directly measured pulmonary arterial pressure in 7 neonates with PPHN during inhalation of NO.[74] iNO improved oxygenation at 5 ppm, but peak improvement in the pulmonary-to-systemic arterial pressure ratio was observed at an NO dose of 20 ppm. Together, these data suggest improved oxygenation does not always reflect an optimal decrease in PVR and that an initial dose of 20 ppm may be the most appropriate for the initial treatment of PPHN. However, a recent study enrolled infants with an OI of <25, and found that iNO at 1-2 ppm was as effective as higher concentrations.[75] The authors also noted that low doses did not attenuate responses to higher doses of iNO. While interesting, these results need to be confirmed before concluding that lower doses of iNO are safe and effective in infants with moderate respiratory disease.

Toxicity of iNO

It is important to monitor for potential toxicities associated with the use of iNO. Higher iNO doses (80 ppm) may be associated with toxicity. The reaction of NO with oxygen produces nitrogen dioxide (NO_2), which is highly toxic to pulmonary epithelial cells. Current delivery devices measure NO_2 continuously at the bedside using electrochemical cells to avoid toxic levels.

NO binding to hemoglobin produces methemoglobin. Activity of methemoglobin reductase is often reduced in the neonatal period, and high levels of methemoglobin could aggravate hypoxia. Methemoglobin levels should be measured several times in the first 24 hours of therapy, and subsequently at 24-hour intervals. Fortunately, NO_2 levels >2 ppm and methemoglobin levels >5% have generally been reported only in infants receiving high doses of iNO (i.e., 80 ppm).[76]

An additional concern is that NO increases platelet cGMP, which inhibits platelet aggregation and could increase bleeding complications. While iNO increases bleeding time in healthy adults,[77] bleeding complications such as intracranial hemorrhage have not increased in infants treated with iNO. However, if unexpected bleeding occurs in the clinical setting, discontinuation of iNO should be considered.

Extremely hypoxic infants who are candidates for iNO therapy are typically treated with high fractions of inspired oxygen, which could lead to oxidative stress in the lung. Increased production of the potent oxidant peroxynitrite may occur through reaction of NO with superoxide ion produced in inflamed lungs, leading to further oxidative damage to all pulmonary cells and nitration of proteins. Damaged cells and inactivated proteins and enzymes can lead to further hypoxia and failed vasodilatation. Continued requirement for aggressive respiratory support can lead to chronic lung injury, which can eventually become irreversible. Therefore, the duration of exposure to hyperoxia is an important consideration when bearing in mind the reversibility of lung disease prior to cannulation for ECMO.

Weaning and rebound pulmonary hypertension

Once a pulmonary vascular response to 20 ppm is established and stable, efforts to wean both iNO and FiO_2 should be made, knowing that the combination of these two gasses can generate several toxic products. During weaning of iNO, the goal should be adequate oxygen delivery rather than sustained hyperoxia. A PaO_2 of 60-80 mm Hg is generally adequate to accomplish sufficient oxygen saturation of hemoglobin. Once oxygenation is established, iNO can usually be weaned to 5 ppm within 24 hours Subsequently, most infants will tolerate continued weaning of iNO over several days. It should be noted that recommendations for weaning iNO are varied, and various large trials have used different protocols effectively.

Although weaning is usually well tolerated, stopping iNO can sometimes be difficult due to rebound pulmonary hypertension. Clinically, acute withdrawal of iNO can be associated with a dramatic worsening of hypoxia. Rebound pulmonary hypertension is more likely to be observed in those infants exposed to higher iNO doses for several days. It can usually be avoided by stepwise weaning to 1 ppm, with discontinuation of iNO from that dose. Mild decreases in PaO_2 necessitating a transient increase in inspired oxygen may still be seen. This can often be tolerated, although some infants only respond to reinstitution of iNO. Often, subsequent attempts at withdrawing iNO are successful after slow gradual reduction in the dose. The iNO delivery device allows weaning to 0.5 ppm prior to final discontinuation.

Other considerations

Severe parenchymal lung disease may be associated with poor responsiveness to iNO in newborns with PPHN. In the NINOS trial, iNO did not reduce need for ECMO in infants with respiratory distress syndrome (RDS) and MAS.[67] In a subsequent trial where lung expansion was first optimized using surfactant and/or high frequency ventilation (HFV), iNO significantly reduced the need for ECMO in infants with RDS and MAS.[66] An additional, randomized, multi-center trial demonstrated

that for infants with PPHN associated with severe parenchymal disease, response rates for HFOV and iNO together were better than HFOV alone or iNO with conventional ventilation.[78] These results have led to the recommendation that lung inflation should be optimized using HFOV prior to the use of iNO.

When there is a poor response to iNO, the clinician should carefully consider whether ventricular function is adequate. For instance, left ventricular dysfunction is often associated with high left atrial and pulmonary venous pressures. iNO may not produce a sustained improvement in oxygenation if there is pulmonary venous hypertension and pulmonary edema.

Use of iNO in the non-ECMO center

Because of the relative ease of delivery of iNO, this therapy is used at non-ECMO centers. Although iNO produces a marked improvement in oxygenation in many infants with PPHN, this improvement does not always occur and is not always sustained. The ideal clinical use of iNO should never delay transfer to an ECMO center.

Abrupt discontinuation of iNO can destabilize an infant due to rebound pulmonary hypertension. This is especially likely in those infants exposed to higher doses for several days and can occur even if there was no initial response to iNO. Therefore, continuing iNO during transport is essential and provisions must be in place to accomplish transport to the ECMO center without interruption of iNO treatment. The referring center should work in close collaboration with the receiving ECMO center to prospectively establish appropriate iNO failure criteria and mechanisms for the safe and timely transfer of infants to the collaborating ECMO center.

Finally, because the use of iNO has not been demonstrated to reduce the need for ECMO in infants with CDH, iNO should be used in non-ECMO centers only for acute stabilization of these infants when necessary, followed by immediate transfer to an ECMO center.

Interactions between ECMO and new therapies

Following the introduction of HFV, surfactant, and iNO therapies in the early 1990s, recent reports have shown that patient demographics of neonatal ECLS has changed.[79] ELSO Registry data indicate that use of these therapies has increased steadily over the last 10 years in neonates with respiratory failure secondary to PPHN, MAS, CDH, RDS, sepsis, and other disorders (Figure 4).[80] From 1992-2001, the number of neonates cannulated for ECLS has decreased by >40%. These new therapies have played a major role in the decreased utilization of ECMO observed over the last 10 years.

In addition, the type of patient cannulated for ECMO appears to be changing. The number of infants with MAS cannulated for ECMO has steadily decreased over the last 10 years, and in 2003, MAS was no longer the most common indication for ECMO. In contrast, the number of infants with CDH has stayed constant. There-fore, the population appears to have shifted to infants that require more prolonged ECMO support.

Some physicians have speculated that these new treatment modalities may delay ECLS cannulation and as a result, negatively impact those infants that continue to require ECMO. Gill et al. studied neonates with MAS cannulated for ECMO from 1989-1998.[81] They found that NO and HFV use resulted in a delay of ECLS cannulation and concluded that this delay in cannulation was associated with an increase in mortality and a prolonged hospital stay. We recently examined data from the ELSO Registry between 1996-2001.[82] We found that NO, HFV, and surfactant use were not associated with any adverse outcomes during ECMO, including increased hours on ECMO or increased time to extubation. Further, NO use was associated with a small but significant decrease in ECMO mortality (P=0.04) even when controlled for diagnosis, age of cannulation, use of HFV and surfactant use. As ECMO is proven therapy for severe respiratory failure, it is reassuring to learn that these new therapies have not had a negative impact on the most severely affected infants.

Alternate pulmonary vasodilators

While iNO is often effective in reversing PPHN, alternative therapies may be useful in cases in which the response to NO is inadequate or unsustained. The best-known alternative agent may be tolazoline, which is a potent endothelium-independent vasodilator. Unfortunately, the efficacy of tolazoline was limited by systemic hypotension, and it is no longer manufactured in the U.S.

Other vasodilators have been investigated as adjunct therapies in the management of infants with severe PPHN. Magnesium sulfate ($MgSO_4$) has vasodilator effects through antagonism of calcium entry into vascular smooth muscle cells. Case reports indicate that IV

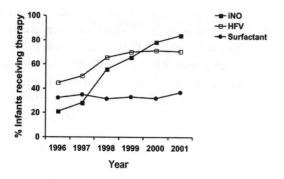

Figure 4. Data from the ELSO Registry on the use of NO, HFV, and surfactant prior to cannulation for ECMO. The percent of infants treated with NO increased 4-fold and the percent of infants treated with HFV almost doubled from 1996-2001. The use of surfactant did not significantly change.

MgSO$_4$ infusion may improve oxygenation in infants with PPHN,[83] but these have not been confirmed by clinical trials, and the potential for systemic vasodilatation and hypotension will likely limit clinical use. Adenosine and ATP cause NO-dependent pulmonary vasodilatation in fetal lambs,[84] and pilot studies indicate a potential benefit in infants.[85] Moya et al. have recently suggested that treatment with the unique gas O-nitrosoethanol (ENO) may increase the endogenous pool of S-nitrosothiols in the airway and circulation, thereby providing a new treatment strategy for PPHN.[86] They recently found that ENO produced sustained improvements in postductal arterial oxygenation and systemic hemodynamics in 7 neonates.[87]

Since the response to iNO is believed to be mediated primarily by activation of soluble guanylate cyclase and activation of cGMP-dependent protein kinase, it is logical to pursue other mechanisms that might enhance cGMP accumulation. Inhibition of cGMP-metabolizing PDE5 activity may increase cGMP concentrations and may result in pulmonary vasodilation and/or increase the efficacy of iNO. Dipyridamole, which has been used for many years to inhibit platelet aggregation, inhibits cGMP metabolism. While there have been anecdotal reports of its use in human infants,[88,89] dipyridamole may be associated with systemic hypotension in the newborn period[90] and needs to be used with caution in this age group. More potent and specific experimental inhibitors of PDE5 have been tested with encouraging results, indicating the feasibility of this therapeutic strategy.

Sildenafil is a potent and highly specific PDE5 inhibitor recently approved by the FDA for the treatment of male erectile dysfunction. In experimental lambs with pulmonary hypertension induced by a thromboxane analog, both enteric and aerosolized sildenafil dilated the pulmonary vasculature and augmented the pulmonary vascular response to iNO.[91,92] IV sildenafil was found to be a selective pulmonary vasodilator with efficacy equivalent to iNO in

a piglet model of meconium aspiration,[93] although hypotension resulted when it was used in combination with iNO.[94] Reports of the use of enteric and IV sildenafil in adults and pediatric patients with pulmonary hypertension are appearing,[95,96] and a randomized trial was recently completed examining the benefit of enteric sildenafil for adult pulmonary arterial hypertension. Sildenafil may attenuate rebound pulmonary hypertension after withdrawal of iNO.[97,98] However, studies to date have been limited in newborn infants because sildenafil is available only in enteric form. An IV preparation is currently under investigation in newborns with PPHN.

Similar to cGMP, cAMP also stimulates vasodilatation, and therapies aimed at increasing cAMP have been used for pulmonary hypertension. One potential approach is to use milrinone to inhibit PDE3, the phosphodiesterase that metabolizes cAMP (Figure 3). Milrinone has been shown in animal studies to decrease pulmonary artery pressure and resistance and to act additively with iNO.[99] A recent report indicates it may decrease rebound PPHN after discontinuation of iNO.[100] Systemic hypotension may limit the usefulness of milrinone.

Prostacyclin (PGI$_2$) stimulates membrane-bound adenylate cyclase, increases cAMP, and inhibits pulmonary artery smooth muscle cell proliferation in vitro.[101] Although the use of systemic infusions of PGI$_2$ may be limited by the development of systemic hypotension, inhaled PGI$_2$ has been shown to have vasodilator effects limited to the pulmonary circulation.[102] Reports in children have been encouraging, but to date there have been few reports of inhaled PGI$_2$ use in neonates with PPHN. The actions of inhaled PGI$_2$ and iNO appear to be additive in humans[103] and even synergistic in animal studies.[104] Rebound PPHN following withdrawal of iNO has been mitigated by IV PGI$_2$ in children with PPHN following CDH.[105] Kelly et al. recently reported the use of inhaled PGI$_2$ to treat 4 infants with severe PPHN who were unresponsive to iNO, and observed rapid improvements in oxygenation in all infants.[106] A recent report indicates that brief inhalations of another prostaglandin mediator, PGE_1, may also improve oxygenation in newborns with severe hypoxemic respiratory failure.[107]

New studies indicate that scavengers of reactive oxygen species such as superoxide dismutase (SOD) may augment responsiveness to iNO. Since iNO is usually delivered with high concentrations of oxygen, as described above, there is the potential for enhanced production of free radicals such as superoxide and peroxynitrite. Further, experimental models of PPHN have been shown to be associated with increased production of superoxide.[22,48] SOD scavenges and converts superoxide radical to hydrogen peroxide, which is subsequently converted to water by the enzyme catalase. Administration of recombinant human superoxide dismutase (rhSOD) has been accomplished in preterm infants without adverse effects and with strong trends toward decreased pulmonary morbidity.[108] In lambs with pulmonary hypertension, a single dose of intratracheal rhSOD dilated the pulmonary circulation and enhanced the pulmonary vascular effects of iNO.[109] This therapeutic approach may have multiple beneficial effects. Scavenging superoxide may make iNO more available to stimulate vasodilatation and may also reduce oxidative stress and limit lung injury. Human trials are anticipated.

Summary

New therapies such as iNO, HFV, and surfactant have significantly decreased the use of ECMO in term infants with hypoxic respiratory failure. Awareness of the scientific basis for and human experience with the use of these therapies is imperative in order to use them in the most safe and effective manner. Meanwhile, ongoing investigation adding to our understanding of the etiology of respiratory failure and PPHN is essential to bring additional effective therapies to the bedside. The ultimate goal is to not simply to decrease the need for ECMO, but to decrease mortality and morbidity, and improve the overall outcome for this high-risk population of infants.

References

1. Angus DC, Linde-Swirble WT, Clermont G, Griffin MF, Clark RH. Epidemiology of neonatal respiratory failure in the United States. *Am J Resp Crit Care Med* 2001; 164:1154-1160.

2. Walsh-Sukys MC, Tyson JE, Wright LL, et al. Persistent pulmonary hypertension of the newborn in the era before nitric oxide: practice variation and outcomes. *Pediatrics* 2000; 105:14-20.

3. Abman SH, Chatfield BA, Hall SL, McMurtry IF. Role of endothelium-derived relaxing factor during transition of pulmonary circulation at birth. *Am J Physiol* 1990; 259:H1921-H1927.

4. Halbower AC, Tuder RM, Franklin WA, Pollock JS, Forstermann U, Abman SH. Maturation-related changes in endothelial nitric oxide synthase immunolocalization in developing ovine lung. *Am J Physiol* 1994; 267:L585-L591.

5. Bloch KD, Filippov G, Sanchez LS, Nakane M, de la Monte SM. Pulmonary soluble guanylate cyclase, a nitric oxide receptor, is increased during the perinatal period. *Am J Physiol* 1997; 272:L400-L406.

6. Fineman JR, Wong J, Morin III FC, Wild LM, Soifer SJ. Chronic nitric oxide inhibition in utero produces persistent pulmonary hypertension in newborn lambs. *J Clin Invest* 1994; 93:2675-2683.

7. Brannon TS, MacRitchie AN, Jaramillo MA, et al. Ontogeny of cyclooxygenase-1 and cyclooxygenase-2 gene expression in ovine lung. *Am J Physiol* 1998; 274:L66-L71.

8. Brannon TS, North AJ, Wells LB, Shaul PW. Prostacyclin synthesis in ovine pulmonary artery is developmentally regulated by changes in cyclooxygenase-1 gene expression. *J Clin Invest* 1994; 93:2230-2235.

9. Leffler CW, Hessler JR, Green RS. The onset of breathing at birth stimulates pulmonary vascular prostacyclin synthesis. *Pediatr Res* 1984; 18:938-942.

10. Dukarm RC, Steinhorn RH, Morin FC, 3rd. The normal pulmonary vascular transition at birth. *Clin Perinatol* 1996; 23:711-726.

11. Konduri GG. New approaches for persistent pulmonary hypertension of newborn. *Clin Perinatol* 2004; 31:591-611.

12. Cassin S, Dawes GS, Mott JC, Ross BB, Strang LB. The vascular resistance of the foetal and newly ventilated lung of the lamb. *J Physiol* 1964; 171:61-79.

13. Reid D, Thornburg K. Pulmonary pressure-flow relationships in the fetal lamb during in utero ventilation. *J Appl Physiol* 1990; 69:1630-1636.

14. Teitel D, Iwamoto H, Rudolph A. Changes in the pulmonary circulation during birth-related events. *Pediatr Res* 1990; 27:372-378.

15. Morin FC, 3rd, Egan EA. Pulmonary hemodynamics in fetal lambs during development at normal and increased oxygen tension. *J Appl Physiol* 1992; 73:213-218.

16. Morin FC, 3rd, Egan EA, Ferguson W, Lundgren CE. Development of pulmonary vascular response to oxygen. *Am J Physiol* 1988; 254:H542-H546.

17. Shaul PW, Wells LB. Oxygen modulates nitric oxide production selectively in fetal pulmonary endothelial cells. *Am J Respir Crit Care Med* 1994; 11:432-438.

18. Shaul PW, Campbell WB, Farrar MA, Magness RR. Oxygen modulates prostacyclin synthesis in ovine fetal pulmonary arteries by an effect on cyclooxygenase. *J Clin Invest* 1992; 90:2147-2155.

19. Black SM, Johengen MJ, Ma ZD, Bristow J, Soifer SJ. Ventilation and oxygenation induce endothelial nitric oxide synthase gene expression in the lungs of fetal lambs. *J Clin Invest* 1997; 100:1448-1458.

20. Konduri GG, Theodorou AA, Mukhopadhyay A, Deshmukh DR. Adenosine triphosphate and adenosine increase the pulmonary blood flow to postnatal levels in fetal lambs. Pediatr Res 1992;31:451-457.

21. Steinhorn RH, Morin FC, 3rd, Van Wylen DG, Gugino SF, Giese EC, Russell JA. Endothelium-dependent relaxations to adenosine in juvenile rabbit pulmonary arteries and veins. *Am J Physiol* 1994; 266:H2001-H2006.

22. Konduri GG, Ou J, Shi Y, Pritchard KA. Decreased association of hsp90 impairs endothelial nitric oxide synthase in fetal lambs with persistent pulmonary hypertension. *Am J Physiol Heart Circ Physiol* 2003; 285:H204-H211.

23. Pearson JD, Slakey LL, Gordon JL. Stimulation of prostaglandin production through purinoceptors on cultured porcine endothelial cells. *Biochem J* 1983; 214:273-276.

24. Uematsu M, Ohara Y, Navas JP, et al. Regulation of endothelial cell nitric oxide synthase mRNA expression by shear stress. *Am J Physiol* 1995; 269:C1371-C1378.

25. Ayajiki K, Kinderman M, Hecker M, Fleming I, Busse R. Intracellular pH and tyrosine phosphorylation but not calcium determine shear stress-induced nitric oxide production in native endothelial cells. *Circ Res* 1996; 78:750-758.

26. Gelfand SL, Fanaroff JM, Walsh MC. Controversies in the treatment of meconium aspiration syndrome. *Clin Perinatol* 2004; 31:445-452.

27. Wiswell TE. Advances in the treatment of the meconium aspiration syndrome. *Acta Paediatr Suppl* 2001; 436:28-30.

28. Davey AM, Becker JD, Davis JM. Meconium aspiration syndrome: physiological

and inflammatory changes in a newborn piglet model. *Pediatr Pulmonol* 1993; 16:101-108.

29. de Beaufort AJ, Bakker AC, van Tol MJD, Poorthuis BJ, Schrama AJ, Berger HM. Meconium is a source of pro-inflammatory substances and can induce cytokine production in cultured A549 epithelial cells. *Pediatr Res* 2003; 54:491-495.

30. Zagariya A, Bhat R, Uhal B, Navale S, Freidine M, Vidyasagar D. Cell death and lung cell histology in meconium aspirated newborn rabbit lung. *Eur J Pediatr* 2000; 159:819-826.

31. Castellheim A, Lindenskov PHH, Pharo A, Fung M, Saugstad OD, Mollnes TE. Meconium is a potent activator of complement in human serum and in piglets. *Pediatr Res* 2004; 55:310-318.

32. Lindenskov PHH, Castellheim A, Aamodt G, Saugstad OD, Mollnes TE. Complement activation reflects severity of meconium aspiration syndrome in newborn pigs. *Pediatr Res* 2004; 56:810-817.

33. Soukka H, Jalonen J, Kero P, Kaapa P. Endothelin-1, atrial natriuretic peptide and pathophysiology of pulmonary hypertension in porcine meconium aspiration. *Acta Paediatr* 1998; 87:424-428.

34. Soukka H, Viinikka L, Kaapa P. Involvement of thromboxane A2 and prostacyclin in the early pulmonary hypertension after porcine meconium aspiration. *Pediatr Res* 1998; 44:838-842.

35. Moses D, Holm BA, Spitale P, Liu MY, Enhorning G. Inhibition of pulmonary surfactant function by meconium. *Am J Obstet Gynecol* 1991; 164:477-481.

36. Dargaville PA, South M, McDougall PN. Surfactant and surfactant inhibitors in meconium aspiration syndrome. *J Pediatr* 2001; 138:113-115.

37. Schrama AJ, de Beaufort AJ, Sukul YRM, Jansen SM, Poorthuis BJ, Berger HM. Phospholipase A2 is present in meconium and inhibits the activity of pulmonary surfactant: an in vitro study. *Acta Paediatr* 2001; 90:412-416.

38. Murphy JD, Rabinovitch M, Goldstein JD, Reid LM. The structural basis of persistent pulmonary hypertension of the newborn infant. *J Pediatr* 1981; 98:962-967.

39. Haworth SG. Pulmonary vascular remodeling in neonatal pulmonary hypertension. *Chest* 1988; 93:133S-138S.

40. Manchester D, Margolis HS, Sheldon RE. Possible association between maternal indomethacin therapy and primary pulmonary hypertension of the newborn. *Am J Obstet Gynecol* 1976; 126:467-469.

41. Abman SH, Shanley PF, Accurso FJ. Failure of postnatal adaptation of the pulmonary circulation after chronic intrauterine pulmonary hypertension in fetal lambs. *J Clin Invest* 1989; 83:1849-1858.

42. Morin FC, 3rd. Ligating the ductus arteriosus before birth causes persistent pulmonary hypertension in the newborn lamb. *Pediatr Res* 1989; 25:245-250.

43. Wild LM, Nickerson PA, Morin FC, 3rd. Ligating the ductus arteriosus before birth remodels the pulmonary vasculature of the lamb. *Pediatr Res* 1989; 25:251-257.

44. Alano MA, Ngougmna E, Ostrea EM, Konduri GG. Analysis of nonsteroidal antiinflammatory drugs in meconium and its relation to persistent pulmonary hypertension of the newborn. *Pediatrics* 2001; 107:519-523.

45. Villanueva ME, Zaher FM, Svinarich DM, Konduri GG. Decreased gene expression of endothelial nitric oxide synthase in newborns with persistent pulmonary hypertension. *Pediatr Res* 1998; 44:338-343.

46. Pearson DL, Dawling S, Walsh W, et al. Neonatal pulmonary hypertension: urea-cycle intermediates, nitric oxide production and carbamoylphosphate synthetase function. *New Eng J Med* 2001; 344:1832-1838.

47. Shaul PW, Yuhanna IS, German Z, Chen Z, Steinhorn RH, Morin FC, 3rd. Pulmonary endothelial NO synthase gene expression is decreased in fetal lambs with pulmonary hypertension. *Am J Physiol Lung Cell Mol Physiol* 1997; 272:L1005-L1012.

48. Brennan LA, Steinhorn RH, Wedgwood S, et al. Increased superoxide generation is associated with pulmonary hypertension in fetal lambs: a role for NADPH oxidase. *Circ Res* 2003; 92:683-691.

49. Steinhorn RH, Russell JA, Morin FC, 3rd. Disruption of cGMP production in pulmonary arteries isolated from fetal lambs with pulmonary hypertension. *Am J Physiol Heart Circ Physiol* 1995; 268:H1483-H1489.

50. Hanson KA, Ziegler JW, Rybalkin SD, Miller JW, Abman SH, Clarke WR. Chronic pulmonary hypertension increases fetal lung cGMP phosphodiesterase activity. *Am J Physiol* 1998; 275:L931-941.

51. Fike CD, Zhang Y, Kaplowitz MR. Thromboxane inhibition reduces an early stage of chronic hypoxia-induced pulmonary hypertension in piglets. *J Appl Physiol* 2005; 31:31.

52. Kumar P, Kazzi NJ, Shankaran S. Plasma immunoreactive endothelin-1 concentrations in infants with persistent pulmonary hypertension of the newborn. *Am J Perinatol* 1996; 13:335-341.

53. Rosenberg AA, Kennaugh J, Koppenhafer SL, Loomis M, Chatfield BA, Abman SH. Elevated immunoreactive endothelin-1 levels in newborn infants with persistent pulmonary hypertension. *J Pediatr* 1993; 123:109-114.

54. Wedgwood S, McMullan M, Bekker JM, Fineman JR, Black SM. Role for endothelin-1-induced superoxide and peroxynitrite production in rebound pulmonary hypertension associated with inhaled nitric oxide therapy. *Circ Res* 2001; 89:357-364.

55. Wedgwood S, Dettman RW, Black SM. ET-1 stimulates pulmonary arterial smooth muscle cell proliferation via induction of reactive oxygen species. *Am J Physiol Lung Cell Mol Physiol* 2001; 281:L1058-L1067.

56. Wedgwood S, Black SM. Endothelin-1 decreases endothelial NOS expression and activity through ETA receptor-mediated generation of hydrogen peroxide. *Am J Physiol Lung Cell Mol Physiol* 2005; 288: L480-487.

57. Doyle NM, Lally KP. The CDH Study Group and advances in the clinical care of the patient with congenital diaphragmatic hernia. *Semin Perinatol* 2004; 23:174-184.

58. Harrison DG, Adzick NS, Estes JM, Howell LJ. A prospective study of the outcome for fetuses with diaphragmatic hernia. *JAMA* 1994; 271:382-384.

59. Paranka MS, Clark RH, Yoder BA, Null DMJ. Predictors of failure of high-frequency oscillatory ventilation in term infants with severe respiratory failure. *Pediatrics* 1995; 95:400-404.

60. Schreiber MD, Heymann MA, Soifer SJ. Increased arterial pH, not decreased PaCO2 attenuates hypoxia-induced pulmonary vasoconstriction in newborn lambs. *Pediatr Res* 1986; 20:113-117.

61. Bifano E, Pfannensteil A. Duration of hyperventilation and outcome in infants with persistent pulmonary hypertension. *Pediatrics* 1988; 81:657-661.

62. Ferrara B, Johnson DE, Chang PN, Thompson TR. Efficacy and neurologic outcome of profound hypocapneic alkalosis for the treatment of persistent pulmonary hypertension in infancy. *J Pediatr* 1984; 105:457-461.

63. Findlay RD, Taeusch W, Walther FJ. Surfactant replacement therapy for meconium aspiration syndrome. *Pediatrics* 1996; 97:48-52.

64. Lotze A, Mitchell BR, Bulas DI, Zola EM, Shalwitz RA, Gunkel JH. Multicenter study of surfactant (beractant) use in the treatment of term infants with severe respiratory failure. Survanta in Term Infants Study Group. *J Pediatr* 1998; 132:40-47.

65. Van Meurs K and the CDH Study Group. Is surfactant therapy beneficial in the treatment of the term newborn infant with congenital diaphragmatic hernia? *J Pediatr* 2004; 145:312-316.

66. Clark RH, Kueser TJ, Walker MW, Southgate WM, Huckaby JL, Perez JA, et al. Low dose nitric oxide therapy for persistent pulmonary hypertension of the newborn. *N Engl J Med* 2000; 342:469-474.

67. Neonatal Inhaled Nitric Oxide Study Group. Inhaled nitric oxide in full-term and nearly full-term infants with hypoxic respiratory failure. *New Engl J Med* 1997; 336:597-604.

68. Neonatal Inhaled Nitric Oxide Study Group. Inhaled nitric oxide in term and near-term infants: neurodevelopmental follow-up of the neonatal inhaled nitric oxide study group (NINOS). *J Pediatr* 2000; 136:611-617.

69. Clark RH, Huckaby JL, Kueser TJ, et al. Low-dose nitric oxide therapy for persistent pulmonary hypertension: 1-year follow-up. *J Perinatol* 2003; 23:300-303.

70. Neonatal Inhaled Nitric Oxide Study Group. Inhaled nitric oxide and hypoxic respiratory failure in infants with congenital diaphragmatic hernia. *Pediatrics* 1997; 99:838-845.

71. Konduri GG, Soliman A, Sokol GM, et al. A randomized trial of early versus standard inhaled nitric oxide therapy in term and near-term newborn infants with hypoxic respiratory failure. *Pediatrics* 2004; 113:559-564.

72. Roberts JD, Fineman JR, Morin FC, 3rd, et al. Inhaled nitric oxide and persistent pulmonary hypertension of the newborn. *New Eng J Med* 1997; 336:605-610.

73. Cornfield DN, Maynard RC, deRegnier RO, Guiang III SF, Barbato JE, Milla CE. Randomized, controlled trial of low-dose inhaled nitric oxide in the treatment of term and near-term infants with respiratory failure and pulmonary hypertension. *Pediatrics* 1999; 104:1089-1094.

74. Tworetzky W, Bristow J, Moore P, et al. Inhaled nitric oxide in neonates with persistent pulmonary hypertension. *Lancet* 2001; 357:118-120.

75. Finer NN, Sun JW, Rich W, Knodel E, Barrington KJ. Randomized, prospective study of low-dose versus high-dose inhaled nitric oxide in the neonate with hypoxic respiratory failure. *Pediatrics* 2001; 108:949-955.

76. Davidson D, Barefield ES, Kattwinkel J, Dudell G, Damask M, Straube R, et al. Inhaled nitric oxide for the early treatment of persistent pulmonary hypertension of the term newborn: A randomized, double-masked, placebo-controlled, dose-response, multicenter study. *Pediatrics* 1998; 101:325-334.

77. Hogman M, Frostell C, Arnberg H, Hedenstierna G. Bleeding time prolongation and NO inhalation. *Lancet* 1993; 341:1664-1665.

78. Kinsella JP, Truog WE, Walsh WF, et al. Randomized, multicenter trial of inhaled nitric oxide and high-frequency oscillatory ventilation in severe, persistent pulmonary hypertension of the newborn. *J Pediatr* 1997; 131:55-62.

79. Hui TT, Danielson PD, Anderson KD, Stein JE. The impact of changing neonatal respiratory management on extracorporeal membrane oxygenation utilization. *J Pediatr Surg* 2002; 37:703-705.

80. Extracorporeal Life Support Organization. Neonatal ECMO Registry: Extracorporeal Life Support Organization (ELSO); 2004 July 2004.

81. Gill BS, Neville HL, Khan AM, Cox Jr. CS, Lally K. Delayed institution of ex-

tracorporeal membrane oxygenation is associated with increased mortality rate and prolonged hospital stay. *J Pediatr Surg* 2002; 37:7-10.

82. Fliman P, deRegnier RO, Rankin L, Kinsella J, Reynolds M, Steinhorn R. Neonatal Extracorporeal Life Support in the Modern Era. *Pediatr Res* 2004; 55:479A.

83. Wu T, Teng R, Yau KT. Persistent pulmonary hypertension of the newborn treated with magnesium sulfate in premature neonates. *Pediatrics* 1995; 96:472-474.

84. Konduri GG, Mital S. Adenosine and ATP cause nitric oxide-dependent pulmonary vasodilation in fetal lambs. *Biol Neonate* 2000; 78:220-229.

85. Konduri GG, Garcia DC, Kazzi NJ, Shankaran S. Adenosine infusion improves oxygenation in term infants with respiratory failure. *Pediatrics* 1996; 97:295-300.

86. Moya MP, Gow AJ, McMahon TJ, et al. S-nitrosothiol repletion by an inhaled gas regulates pulmonary function. *Proc Natl Acad Sci U S A* 2001; 98:5792-5797. Epub 2001 Apr 24.

87. Moya MP, Gow AJ, Califf RM, Goldberg RN, Stamler JS. Inhaled ethyl nitrite gas for persistent pulmonary hypertension of the newborn. *Lancet* 2002; 360:141-143.

88. Thebaud B, Saizou C, Farnoux C, Hartman JF, Mercier JC. Dypiridamole, a cGMP phosphodiesterase inhibitor, transiently improves the response to inhaled nitric oxide in two newborns with congenital diaphragmatic hernia. *Intensive Care Med* 1999; 25:300-303.

89. Kinsella JP, Torielli F, Ziegler JW, Ivy DD, Abman SH. Dipyridamole augmentation of response to nitric oxide. *Lancet* 1995; 346:647-648.

90. Dukarm RC, Morin FCI, Russell JA, Steinhorn RH. Pulmonary and systemic effects of the phosphodiesterase inhibitor dipyridamole in newborn lambs with persistent

pulmonary hypertension. *Pediatr Res* 1998; 44:831-837.

91. Weimann J, Ullrich R, Hromi J, Fujino Y, Clark MWH, Bs C, et al. Sildenafil is a pulmonary vasodilator in awake lambs with acute pulmonary hypertension. *Anesthesiology* 2000; 92:1702-1712.

92. Ichinose F, Erana-Garcia J, Hromi J, et al. Nebulized sildenafil is a selective pulmonary vasodilator in lambs with acute pulmonary hypertension. *Crit Care Med* 2001; 29:1000-1005.

93. Shekerdemian LS, Ravn HB, Penny DJ. Intravenous sildenafil lowers pulmonary vascular resistance in a model of neonatal pulmonary hypertension. *Am J Respir Crit Care Med* 2002; 165:1098-1102.

94. Shekerdemian LS, Ravn HB, Penny DJ. Interaction between inhaled nitric oxide and intravenous sildenafil in a porcine model of meconium aspiration syndrome. *Pediatr Res* 2004; 55:413-418. Epub 2004 Jan 7.

95. Ghofrani HA, Wiedemann R, Rose F, Schermuly RT, Olschewski H, Weissmann N, et al. Sildenafil for treatment of lung fibrosis and pulmonary hypertension: a randomised controlled trial. *Lancet* 2002; 360:895-900.

96. Schulze-Neick I, Hartenstein P, Li J, et al. Intravenous sildenafil is a potent pulmonary vasodilator in children with congenital heart disease. *Circulation* 2003; 108: II167-173.

97. Keller RL, Hamrick SE, Kitterman JA, Fineman JR, Hawgood S. Treatment of rebound and chronic pulmonary hypertension with oral sildenafil in an infant with congenital diaphragmatic hernia. *Pediatr Crit Care Med* 2004; 5:184-187.

98. Atz AM, Wessel DL. Sildenafil ameliorates effects of inhaled nitric oxide withdrawal. *Anesthesiology* 1999; 91:307-310.

99. Deb B, Bradford K, Pearl RG. Additive effects of inhaled nitric oxide and intravenous milrinone in experimental pulmonary

hypertension. *Crit Care Med* 2000; 28:795-799.

100. Thelitz S, Oishi P, Sanchez LS, et al. Phosphodiesterase-3 inhibition prevents the increase in pulmonary vascular resistance following inhaled nitric oxide withdrawal in lambs. *Pediatr Crit Care Med* 2004; 5:234-239.

101. Wharton J, Davie N, Upton PD, Yacoub MH, Polak JM, Morrell NW. Prostacyclin analogues differentially inhibit growth of distal and proximal human pulmonary artery smooth muscle cells. *Circulation* 2000; 102:3130-3136.

102. Zobel G, Dacar D, Rodl S, Friehs I. Inhaled nitric oxide versus inhaled prostacyclin and intravenous versus inhaled prostacyclin in acute respiratory failure with pulmonary hypertension in piglets. Pediatr Res 1995; 38:198-204.

103. Rocca GD, Coccia C, Pompei L, et al. Hemodynamic and oxygenation changes of combined therapy with inhaled nitric oxide and inhaled aerosolized prostacyclin. *J Cardiothorac Vasc Anesth* 2001; 15:224-227.

104. Hill LL, Pearl RG. Combined inhaled nitric oxide and inhaled prostacyclin during experimental chronic pulmonary hypertension. *J Appl Physiol* 1999; 86:1160-1164.

105. Hermon M, Golej J, Burda G, Marx M, Trittenwein G, Pollak A. Intravenous prostacyclin mitigates inhaled nitric oxide rebound effect: A case control study. *Artif Organs* 1999; 23:975-978.

106. Kelly LK, Porta NF, Goodman DM, Carroll CL, Steinhorn RH. Inhaled prostacyclin for term infants with persistent pulmonary hypertension refractory to inhaled nitric oxide. *J Pediatr* 2002; 141:830-832.

107. Sood BG, Delaney-Black V, Aranda JV, Shankaran S. Aerosolized PGE1: a selective pulmonary vasodilator in neonatal hypoxemic respiratory failure results of a Phase I/II open label clinical trial. *Pediatr Res* 2004; 56:579-585. Epub 2004 Aug 4.

108. Davis JM, Parad RB, Michele T, et al. Pulmonary outcome at 1 year corrected age in premature infants treated at birth with recombinant human CuZn superoxide dismutase. *Pediatrics* 2003; 111:469-476.

109. Steinhorn RH, Albert G, Swartz DD, Russell JA, Levine CR, Davis JM. Recombinant human superoxide dismutase enhances the effect of inhaled nitric oxide in persistent pulmonary hypertension. *Am J Respir Crit Care Med* 2001; 164:834-839.

18

ECMO for Neonatal Respiratory Failure

Krisa P. Van Meurs, M.D., Susan R. Hintz, M.D., and Arlene M. Sheehan R.N., N.N.P., M.S.

Introduction

The first successful use of ECMO in a full-term newborn was in 1976.[1] Data that accumulated afterward suggested that ECMO was successful when compared to historical controls.[2,3] Ultimately, several randomized trials were performed, the first at the University of Michigan by Dr. R.H. Bartlett, published in 1985.[4] This trial used a "randomized play-the-winner" statistical method where the chance of randomly assigning an infant to one treatment or the other is influenced by the treatment outcome of previously enrolled study patients. The trial concluded with only one patient assigned to the conventional arm who died and 11 that received ECMO and survived. The second trial was performed by Dr. P. O'Rourke at Boston Children's Hospital and published in 1989.[5] This trial also used a study design intended to limit the number of deaths in the group receiving the inferior therapy. Randomization continued until 4 deaths occurred in either group. The trial concluded after 4 of 10 babies died in the conventional medical therapy arm. All 9 infants in the ECMO group survived. Neither of these trials was deemed to be conclusive as they were small and used adaptive designs known to introduce bias. In the U.S., further trials were not performed as accumulating data documented survival of approximately 80% for patients with neonatal respiratory failure.[1,3] In the U.K. a randomized controlled trial published in 1996 determined that ECMO improved survival to 1 year when compared with conventional management (32% versus 59%, respectively, relative risk 0.55, 95% confidence interval 0.39-0.77, P=0.0005).[6]

Indications

All infants considered for ECMO should receive a complete history, physical examination, chest and abdominal radiographs, complete blood count and differential, coagulation studies, serum electrolytes with BUN and creatinine, cranial ultrasound, and echocardiogram.

Gestational age

The requirement for systemic anticoagulation places significant limitations on the population treated. Currently, most ECMO centers exclude infants <34 weeks. Gestational age has been found to be the most powerful predictor of intracranial hemorrhage (ICH).[8] Infants <34 weeks were found to have a near 50% incidence of ICH, while infants 34 to <36 and 36 to <38 weeks gestation had odds ratios for ICH of 4.1 and 2.1, respectively. Hirschl et al. reported that infants ≤34 weeks had lower survival (63% vs. 84%, P<0.001) and a higher prevalence of ICH (37% vs. 14%, P<.001) when compared to term infants.[9] Review of ELSO Registry data (1995–2002) demonstrated that advancing gestational age was associated with a progressive increase in survival (57% at 34 weeks to 79% at 40 weeks) and decreasing rate of ICH (20% at 34 weeks to 5% at 40 weeks).[10] The survival for infants at 33 weeks gestation dropped to 39% with a 26% incidence of ICH. In a recent analysis of ELSO Registry data, Hardart concluded that post-conceptual age was better than either gestational or postnatal age as a predictor of ICH.[11]

Birth weight

Although 2 kg is generally considered to be the lower limit, infants small for gestational age but ≥34 weeks should not be excluded. A higher rate of ICH and mortality has been documented in this low birth weight group.[12] Revenis et al. examined survival and the rate of ICH in infants 2.0 to 2.5 kg and found a higher mortality when compared to infants >2.5 kg (34% vs. 11%, P<0.0005). Major ICH was highly correlated with death. In infants with a birth weight <2 kg, catheter size may be a limiting factor. However, new, thin-walled catheters have improved flow characteristics making this less of an issue.

Reversible lung disease

More than 10-14 days of mechanical ventilation is considered to be a relative contraindication. Chronic lung injury induced by prolonged mechanical ventilation and exposure to high oxygen concentrations may not improve within the time period that ECMO can be used safely. Early ECMO consultation allows time to judge the disease progression and intervene before irreversible injury occurs.

Infants with irreversible lung disease due to conditions such as surfactant B deficiency, alveolar capillary dysplasia, or pulmonary hypoplasia may be placed on ECMO prior to definitive diagnosis of these conditions. Placement on ECMO allows time for the diagnosis to be confirmed.

Uncontrolled bleeding or coagulopathy

The requirement for systemic heparinization places ECMO patients with pre-existing coagulopathy or bleeding at high risk for continued, uncontrollable hemorrhage. Attempts should be made to correct coagulation abnormalities prior to placement on ECMO. Severe, uncorrected coagulopathy or bleeding, such as pulmonary hemorrhage, are relative contraindications. Arnold et al. documented the presence of coagulation abnormalities prior to ECMO as well as the reduction in coagulation factors and activation of the coagulation cascade on bypass.[13] The authors postulate that these abnormalities contribute to bleeding complications on ECMO, and an aggressive approach to replacement may be prudent. Nevertheless, neonates with significant coagulopathy or pulmonary hemorrhage have been successfully managed on ECMO.[14] An exchange transfusion for infants with severe disseminated intravascular coagulation (DIC) has been used to rapidly normalize coagulation prior to ECMO.

Intracranial hemorrhage

The need for heparinization also precludes the treatment of infants with significant ICH. Most ECMO centers exclude infants with grade 2 or greater hemorrhage. Some centers will consider individual cases for ECMO in a patient with a grade 2 hemorrhage.

Congenital heart disease

Congenital heart disease should be ruled out with an echocardiogram prior to ECMO. Some diagnoses such as total anomalous pulmonary venous return may be missed. ECMO may be needed in some cases to stabilize infants with congenital heart disease considered too ill for immediate cardiac surgery or to allow for diagnostic procedures such as cardiac catheterization. ECMO has been used with increasing frequency to support neonates following heart surgery (see Chapter 28).

Decision to not provide full support

Newborns with lethal anomalies such as Trisomy 13 and 18 are generally not considered to be appropriate ECMO candidates. Infants with severe and irreversible brain injury should be excluded, but it is inherently difficult to make this diagnosis in a precise manner. Most physicians opt to err on the side of caution, offering ECMO. Stabilization on ECMO may allow for performance of studies such as head computed tomography (CT) or electroencephalography (EEG) to clarify the prognosis.

Respiratory entry criteria

Various criteria have been used to select a population with a predicted mortality of 80% or greater. The various criteria used by ECMO centers are listed in Table 1.[15,16] Each of these criterion is limited by institutional specificity, retrospective data collection, and changes in intensive care over time. The oxygenation index (OI) is the most commonly utilized criteria. The use of an OI >40 for 3 hours in the U.K. trial selected a control group with a 61% mortality, slightly lower than the 80% as originally suggested.[7] Some have advocated that ECMO be used in infants with a lower OI. Schumacher et al. documented that infants randomized to receive ECMO at an OI >25 but <40 had a shorter length of hospitalization and lower hospital charges than those infants who received ECMO using an OI >40.[17] There was also a trend toward improved outcomes at 1 year of age.

Diseases treated

The diagnoses treated with ECMO include meconium aspiration syndrome (MAS), congenital diaphragmatic hernia (CDH), idiopathic pulmonary hypertension, sepsis/pneumonia, respiratory distress syndrome (RDS), air leak

Table 1. Neonatal ECMO criteria.

General inclusion and exclusion criteria
Gestational age ≥34 weeks or birth weight ≥2000g
No significant coagulopathy or uncontrolled bleeding
No major intracranial hemorrhage (ICH)
Reversible lung disease with length of mechanical ventilation <10-14 days
No uncorrectable congenital heart disease
No lethal congenital anomalies
No evidence of irreversible brain damage

Respiratory entry critera*	
$A_aDO_2^\dagger$	>605-620 mm Hg‡ for 4-12 hr.
Oxygenation index (OI)§	>35-60 for 0.5-6 hr.
PaO_2	<35 to <60 mm Hg for 2-12 hr.
Acidosis and shock	pH <7.25 for 2 hr. or with hypotension
Acute deterioration	PaO_2 <30 to <40 mm Hg

*   50% of ECMO centers use more than one respiratory entry criteria.

†   At sea level.

‡ $\dfrac{P_{atm} - 47 - PaCO_2 - PaO_2}{FiO_2}$

§ $\dfrac{MAP \times FiO_2 \times 100}{PaO_2}$

syndrome, and others. Recently, novel uses of ECMO have been reported in the neonatal population including bridge to transplantation, hydrops fetalis, viral pneumonia (herpes simplex virus and adenovirus), and cardiomyopathy. It has also been used as support for other procedures such as complex tracheal reconstruction or as part of the ex-utero intrapartum treatment (EXIT) to ECMO procedure.[18] With the EXIT procedure, the fetus with in utero diagnosis of severe airway anomaly, obstructive neck mass, complicated CDH, or cystic adenomatoid malformation (CCAM) undergoes surgical correction while receiving placental support. The fetal head and neck only are delivered via cesarean section and uteroplacental circulation is maintained to support the fetus during the surgical procedure. Ideally the infant is intubated prior to delivery of the torso and umbilical cord. In the event the intubation is not possible, or the pulmonary status of the fetus is compromised, the neck is cannulated and the fetus is placed on ECMO support prior to delivery. The indications for EXIT to ECMO are controversial.

The ECMO team

Neonatal ECMO requires a highly specialized multidisciplinary team. The team is composed of surgical personnel including a senior surgeon (pediatric, cardiovascular, or thoracic), a surgical assistant, a surgical scrub nurse, and a circulating OR nurse; medical personnel consisting of a physician (neonatologist, pediatric intensivist, or pediatric surgeon) trained in management of ECMO patients and cannulation techniques and responsible for medical management of the infant during the procedure; a bedside intensive care nurse (neonatal or pediatric ICU) who will monitor vital signs, record events, and administer the required medications; a respiratory therapist who will change ventilator settings; a circuit specialist (cardiovascular perfusionist, RN, or RT) specially trained in this procedure who will prime the pump; and a bedside ECMO specialist (RN, RT, or CV perfusionist with special training in ECMO management) who will manage the ECMO system after the patient has been placed on ECMO. Ongoing involvement of other appropriate sub-specialties such as cardiologists, pediatric and cardiovascular surgeons, pediatric radiologist, neurodevelopmental psychologist, and biomedical engineers are essential to ensure high-quality, tertiary care and state-of-the-art practice in the field.

Cannulation

Preparation

The decision to proceed to ECMO may be a difficult one, but the ECMO team should be prepared to cannulate without delay once the decision is made. The procedure is usually performed at the bedside in the critical care unit while strictly observing the infection control and sterility practices consistent with an OR environment. In addition to the equipment, monitoring devices, and medications standard to any critical care unit, electrocautery, surgical head lamps, and other light sources should be readily available.

A radiograph cassette should be in place under the patient before initiating the procedure so that the catheter(s) position can be quickly confirmed. Preparation and correct positioning of the patient is crucial to the success of the cannulation. The infant is placed supine with a roll under the right neck and shoulders, and the head is turned to the left to facilitate right cervical cannulation. The cannulation site is prepped and draped in sterile fashion. Positioning may be particularly challenging if a rigid high-frequency oscillatory ventilator is in use. Nonetheless, it is essential for respiratory therapists to be able to access ventilatory equipment to ensure relative patient stability during the procedure, as well as to make rapid ventilator changes after initiation of bypass to avoid hypocarbia.

Anesthesia for the cannulation should include a narcotic (e.g., morphine, fentanyl) for pain control, and a muscle relaxant for paralysis. A local anesthetic such as lidocaine is also frequently used. As with any surgical or interventional procedure, meticulous and constant attention to vital signs, pulse oximetry, and medication and fluid administration is essential. To that end, it is important to prepare and drape the patient assuring easy access to infusion pumps, deep venous lines, and arterial ports throughout the procedure so that medications can be given and blood sampling can be performed.

Modes of neonatal ECMO

There are two general forms of ECMO used for the neonatal population: venoarterial (VA) and venovenous (VV). For neonatal VA ECMO, the right carotid artery and internal jugular vein are cannulated, whereas for VV ECMO a single double-lumen catheter is inserted in the internal jugular vein.[19,20] In VV ECMO, the single catheter is used to both drain and return blood to the right atrium. Although VV ECMO is currently considered to be the preferred ECMO mode for neonatal respiratory failure, it is not possible in every situation. The principle advantage to VV ECMO is the fact that carotid artery ligation is unnecessary. In addition, normal pulsatility can be maintained, and left ventricular stun can be avoided. A significant challenge to the use of VV ECMO is the absence of direct cardiovascular support. However, no specific level of inotropic or ventilatory support has been identified which definitively precludes VV ECMO for neonatal respiratory failure.[21] In fact, cardiac performance has been shown to improve after initiation of VV ECMO, and inotropic support can frequently be weaned.[21,22] Renal function may also be transiently more compromised in VV vs. VA ECMO.[21] Also, in infants <2.5 kg or those with extremely small jugular vessels, it may not be technically feasible to place a double-lumen VV cannula.

Procedure

VA cannulation: A transverse incision is made and the right carotid artery and internal jugular vein are exposed and dissected, and proximal and distal ligatures are placed. The largest cannulas that can safely be inserted should be chosen to ensure adequate drainage and return. Heparin (50-100 units/kg) is given to the patient prior to insertion of the cannulas. The carotid artery is usually cannulated with an 8-10F arterial catheter, and the vein with a 12-14F venous catheter. The proximal ligature around the carotid is tied, and the cannulas are secured with distal ligatures. Correct cannula position should be verified immediately by radiograph. The arterial cannula should be at the junction of the right common carotid artery and the aortic arch, and the tip of the venous cannula should in the right atrium. If questions arise regarding placement, echocardiography can be helpful in determining the exact position of the cannula tip.

VV cannulation: Traditionally, VV cannulation has been performed using an open surgical technique.[23] The procedure is the same as for VA cannulation, except the carotid artery is not cannulated. The tip of the double-lumen venous catheter should be in the mid-right atrium, with the arterial port positioned flat against the infant's neck and behind the ear while the head is midline in order to direct oxygenated blood returning from the circuit toward the tricuspid valve. Other methods of cannulation for neonatal VV ECMO have been described, including the modified or semi-Seldinger technique.[24] This procedure involves exposure of the vein as previously described, but does not require ligation of the internal jugular vein. A puncture is made above the incision site, a guidewire is passed, and successive dilations are performed before the cannula is placed. The modified Seldinger method may allow for improved hemostasis and a potentially less complex cannulation. If conversion to VA ECMO is required, only dissection and exposure of the carotid artery is required. Percutaneous access for VV ECMO in the neonatal population has also been described,[25] but is not routinely performed.

Ligation of the internal jugular has been implicated as a potential factor in ECMO-associated neurologic injury through a mechanism of cerebral congestion and hypertension.[26] In addition to cannulation techniques that avoid internal jugular ligation such as the modified Seldinger, routine placement of a cephalad jugular drainage catheter has been used. This method also has the potential benefit of augmenting venous return and decreasing recirculation and cerebral venous decompression.[27] A recent review of ELSO Registry data did not demonstrate significant differences in neonatal outcome or complication rates in those infants receiving double-lumen VV ECMO, with or without a cephalad catheter.[28]

Initiation of bypass

Once the cannulas are placed, bypass is initiated by connecting the cannulas to the ECMO circuit in a sterile fashion, taking care to connect the arterial cannula to the arterial side of the circuit. Meticulous attention must be given to preventing introduction of air at the site of connection, thus avoiding air embolus upon initiation of bypass. The circuit flow is reduced to 20 ml/kg/min, and the clamps are removed. Circuit flow is gradually increased over the next 15-30 minutes to reach the desired flow rate, which is typically 100-120 ml/kg/min.

Vital signs must be observed rigorously during the initiation of bypass. Hypocalcemia is a frequent cause of cardiovascular instability, particularly in VV ECMO cases.[29] Hypotension is common, but usually transient. Hypovolemia frequently occurs at the initiation of bypass due to circuit distensibility and is readily treated with volume infusion. Unpacked platelets are given routinely after the initiation of bypass. Depending on the clinical scenario, packed red blood cells (RBCs), fresh frozen plasma (FFP), or cryoprecipitate may also be required. Other causes of hypotension should be investigated during this critical period. Complications such as pneumothorax, hemothorax, cardiac tamponade, or hemorrhage should be considered. Mechanical causes for inadequate venous drainage include inappropriate cannula placement, catheter kinking, inadequate patient bed height, inadequate venous cannula diameter, and bladder malfunction.

As bypass flow is increased, ventilatory support should be decreased to rest settings quickly. The goal of these settings is to maintain adequate oxygenation and lung distension while limiting barotrauma. FiO_2 can usually be rapidly decreased to 0.21-0.30 in response to rising pulse oximetry values. It is essential to avoid hypocarbia, which has been linked with neurologic sequelae such as hearing loss and cerebral palsy.[30] Similarly, care should be taken not to correct hypercarbia too quickly. Given the efficiency of the membrane in removing CO_2, peak inspiratory pressure (PIP) and rate can be quickly decreased to rest settings once ECMO flow is established. Higher peak end expiratory pressures (PEEP) are used in some centers to prevent complete atelectasis and to shorten the length of the ECMO run. Post-oxygenator, mixed venous, and patient blood gases should be performed shortly after the initiation of bypass.

Despite adequate pain control prior to and during cannulation, initiation of ECMO can lead to sequestration of fentanyl and morphine in the circuit and membrane.[31] Physicians and nurses should be alert to signs and symptoms of pain during this early period and administer additional narcotics as needed.

Activated clotting time (ACT) is checked soon after the initiation of ECMO and every 15 minutes until the ACT reaches approximately 300 seconds. At that point, a continuous heparin infusion is started, and the ACT is checked every 15 minutes until stable. Typical ACT range is

180-200 seconds depending on the instrument used. ACT target goals may be altered depending on the clinical scenario.

Management of neonates on ECMO

Fluids and nutrition

In addition to the usual fluid requirements, an infant on ECMO will experience water loss through the oxygenator of 2 ml/m²/hr. Nevertheless, many, if not most, infants are edematous at the time of cannulation or become edematous while on ECMO. Initial daily fluid intake is limited to 60-100 ml/kg/day. In specific clinical situations, such as substantial fluid overload prior to ECMO initiation, a diuretic regimen may be initiated early in the ECMO course. Sepsis or hypoxic-ischemic injury may also be associated with significant capillary leak during this early period, and aggressive diuresis can lead to intravascular depletion. A natural diuresis phase is usually evident as cardiac output improves, capillary leak resolves, and fluid mobilization occurs. Some practitioners choose to begin diuretics at this later phase in the ECMO course. If renal failure is persistent despite adequate fluid resuscitation, hemofiltration may be initiated.

Neonates on ECMO are usually not fed enterally. Caloric intake is optimized through the use of total parenteral nutrition (TPN). Protein in the form of amino acids is added, although renal protein preparations such as Aminosyn RF may be necessary if the blood urea nitrogen (BUN) is elevated.[32] Many centers use lipid emulsions as part of the TPN regimen, although some centers limit lipid infusions during the early days of treatment due to concern about their use in the context of severe respiratory disease.[33,34] Ranitidine is added prophylactically to TPN at a dose of 2 mg/kg/day to attempt to limit the significant complication of gastritis-associated gastric bleeding exacerbated by anticoagulation.[35]

Serum electrolytes are monitored at least daily, and glucose is checked every 4-6 hours. Serum sodium levels may be high due to the high sodium content of blood products. However, both sodium and potassium requirements may be increased among patients receiving routine diuretics. Calcium and magnesium requirements may be higher than usual. Metabolic alkalosis may become evident due to exposure to large amounts of blood products containing the anticoagulant citrate-phosphate-dextran (CPD).

Respiratory

Routine oral and endotracheal suctioning is performed every 4-6 hours. Changes in secretions, particularly if blood-tinged, should be noted. Treatment of pulmonary hemorrhage varies with the severity of the event, and includes limitation of suctioning, increasing PEEP, decreasing ACT target range, and instillation of dilute epinephrine. Exogenous surfactant administration in the setting of severe neonatal respiratory failure should be continued during the ECMO course.[36,37]

Patient arterial blood gases, along with circuit pre- and post-oxygenator blood gases, are obtained every 6-8 hours. Daily chest radiographs are obtained to confirm line, catheter, and tube position; assess lung volume changes and areas of significant atelectasis or collapse; and to evaluate free air. A large or tension pneumothorax requires placement of a chest tube using electrocautery if necessary, particularly when obstructing venous return. Radiograph findings combined with frequent or continuous tidal volume measurements provide the practitioner with the data needed to formulate a weaning plan.

Cardiovascular

Neonates with severe respiratory failure are frequently managed prior to ECMO with inotropic agents. Once VA ECMO is initiated, all inotropes can usually be rapidly weaned. Some centers continue low-dose dopamine during VA ECMO to improve renal perfusion. It was previously suggested that infants undergoing VV ECMO would require continued, higher dose inotropic support during the ECMO run. However, it is now clear that VV and VA ECMO patients maintain similar mean arterial pressures (MAPs) and may be weaned from inotropes with equal success. Knight et al. found no significant differences in inotrope index after VA and VV ECMO initiation and found that MAP was higher among VA than VV ECMO patients only during the first two hours of the ECMO run.[38]

Hematologic

Routine hematologic laboratory studies are obtained while on ECMO bypass; hemoglobin and hematocrit are obtained every 8-12 hours and platelet count every 6-8 hours. Packed RBCs are given to keep the hematocrit >40% in order to maximize oxygen carrying capacity. In specific cases, a higher hematocrit may be targeted; this maneuver can be especially pertinent for VV ECMO patients who may have marginal oxygenation. Platelet counts are usually kept >80,000/mm³, although clinical issues such as active bleeding, prematurity, or need for surgical intervention may require a higher threshold. Platelet transfusion results in decreased ACT; thus, routine heparin boluses in conjunction with platelet transfusion are used. ACTs should be monitored before and after platelet transfusion. Fibrinogen level is maintained at >150 mg/dl through the use of cryoprecipitate or FFP. Prothrombin time (PT) is monitored at least daily or more often, particularly in the setting of sepsis-associated coagulopathy. FFP should be given to correct prolonged PT; ACT should be monitored before and after plasma administration. Persistent or worsening coagulopathy, which is minimally responsive to blood product administration, may be related to circuit-associated DIC. Further evidence of this phenomenon might be obtained by visual inspection of the circuit for clots, increasing serial D-dimer levels, and rising pre-oxygenator pressures. Antithrombin III, protein C, and protein S deficiencies should be considered in patients for whom circuit clotting is a persistent problem.[39,40]

ACT is checked every 1-2 hours, more frequently if: ACT is unstable; if platelets, FFP, or cryoprecipitate have been administered; or if heparin infusion has been changed. The targeted ACT range is 180-200 seconds (depending on the instrument used); however, this may be decreased if active bleeding or other clinical issues are present. In general, heparin infusion should not be completely discontinued. Many centers maintain a minimal heparin infusion rate of 10-15 units/kg/hour. If ACT levels are persistently above or below range, the underlying cause should be investigated.

Neurologic

Infants with severe respiratory failure are frequently heavily sedated, narcotized, and paralyzed prior to the initiation of ECMO. However, after ECMO is established, paralysis is generally not required for the neonatal patient and should be discontinued. Similarly, the use of sedatives and narcotics should be curtailed in order to facilitate frequent and reliable neurologic examination. Of course, routine pain level scoring should be implemented and appropriate response evaluated throughout the ECMO course.

Intracranial hemorrhage (ICH) is one of the most significant complications of neonatal ECMO. Head ultrasound (HUS) should be performed prior to the initiation of ECMO, with serial daily HUS commencing 12-24 hours after cannulation. Khan et al. have reported that over 90% of ICH cases occur in the first 5 days of ECMO therapy.[41] Abnormalities in serial EEGs during ECMO have also been shown to be valuable in predicting mortality and neurologic morbidity.[42,43] Conversely, the combination of normal serial HUS and EEG without significant abnormalities on ECMO appears to be highly predictive of normal post-ECMO neuroimaging (MRI or CT).[44]

Weaning from ECMO

Numerous issues must be considered when making the decision to wean from ECMO. No absolute weaning criteria can apply to every clinical situation. Adequate pulmonary and cardiac recovery, with weaning to minimal ventilator and inotrope support, is clearly the optimal goal. The risk of continuing ECMO must be carefully considered when compared to the potential benefit. In some cases, an echocardiogram on low pump flow may provide additional useful information.

Weaning is the gradual decrease in ECMO support over a period of time until idling flow (~20 ml/kg/min) is achieved. As flow is decreased, ACT target range is increased slightly to reduce clot formation, and ACT is, therefore, more frequently monitored. The minimum flow rate for a 1/4-inch circuit is generally considered to be 80-100 ml/min. During the period of weaning, ventilator support is increased above rest settings as needed, vital signs and pulse oximetry are carefully observed, and frequent patient blood gases are monitored. Idle flow is maintained for several hours to ensure the infant is tolerating minimal ECMO support.

At this point, some centers advocate a period of trial off ECMO. For VA ECMO, this involves temporarily removing the patient from ECMO support by clamping the venous limb, unclamping the bridge, and clamping the arterial limb. Pump flow is increased to 150-200 ml/min to mitigate circuit clot formation, and sweep gas is disconnected. All infused medications and fluids are removed from the circuit and infused directly to the patient. The

heparin infusion continues into the circuit unless the trial off period is to last >15 minutes, in which case, it too, is infused directly into the patient. Vital signs and pulse oximetry are monitored carefully. Patient blood gas and ACT from the patient and circuit should be obtained every 15 minutes. The cannulas should also be unclamped (flashed) every 10-15 minutes. The length of the trial off varies, but in general does not last more than 1-3 hours. If the trial off is successful, decannulation is planned. If decannulation cannot be performed immediately, the patient should be returned to low-flow ECMO. Many centers do not perform a trial off, particularly if the indication for ECMO was neonatal respiratory failure and pulmonary recovery on ECMO was rapid, and discontinue ECMO after idle flow is tolerated for several hours.

For VV ECMO, pump flow is gradually weaned as outlined above. The oxygenator is then "capped off" by disconnecting the sweep gas line and running a piece of tubing from the oxygentator gas inlet to the oxygenator gas outlet. Because no direct circulatory support is provided by VV ECMO, this maneuver essentially provides a trial off ECMO. Careful monitoring of vital signs, pulse oximetry and serial patient blood gases should be undertaken as described for the VA ECMO weaning process, and adjustments in ventilator setting made as necessary. In-line pre-oxygenator saturations reflect the patient's true mixed venous saturations once the oxygenator is capped off.

Decannulation

Preparation

If the patient has tolerated weaning and/or trial off procedures, surgical decannulation is performed. Full medical and surgical teams and appropriate equipment should be available as previously described for cannulation. A roll is placed under the right shoulder and neck, and the site is prepped and draped in a sterile fashion. The patient is given analgesia (morphine or fentanyl), sedation if necessary, and is paralyzed. Prior to paralysis, ventilator settings are increased. As noted previously, the security of the endotracheal tube and access to lines and ports are crucial during the procedure. After surgeons drape the patient, bypass is discontinued by clamping the venous line, unclamping the bridge, and clamping the arterial line. All infused medications and fluids, except for the heparin, are moved from the circuit to the patient.

Decannulation

VA decannulation: Exploration and thorough inspection of the cannulation site should be performed. The arterial cannula is usually removed first. Each vessel is controlled, the cannula clamped and withdrawn, and the vessel ligated. Reconstruction of the carotid artery is performed in some institutions. Short term results have been favorable;[45,46] however, relatively little are known about long-term vessel patency and neurologic outcome after reconstruction. Levy et al. demonstrated patent carotid arteries by ultrasound among 27 patients followed to up to 29 months.[47] In a small group of neonatal ECMO survivors, Cheung and colleagues reported decreasing frequency of normal ultrasound studies from 92% at 6 months and 46% at 4 years.[48] Hemodynamically significant stenosis was present in only two children, and none of the children were clinically symptomatic. Others have reported an association of transmural necrosis and increased length of the ECMO run, suggesting that length of time on ECMO should be considered in the decision to reconstruct the carotid artery.[49] Upon inspection, if infection at the site is suspected, reconstruction is contraindicated. In addition, a risk of recurrent embolic phenomenon has been suggested with carotid artery reconstruction. Further long-term data will be useful in determining whether, and in what circumstances, carotid artery reconstruction should be undertaken.

VV decannulation: If the open technique cannulation has been used, the site should be explored carefully, the vessel controlled, and cannula removed with vessel ligation. If the modified Seldinger cannulation technique has been used, clearly no exploration is required. A mattress suture is placed around the cannula, the cannula is withdrawn, and the suture is tied.

Complications

Given the complexity of the ECMO circuit and the critical nature of the ECMO patient's illness, the potential for complications when using this therapy is high. For good reason, the acronym ECMO is sometimes used to mean "Extra Complex Medical Operation." In the discussion which follows, complications related to ECMO therapy will be discussed with regard to diagnosis, prevention, treatment, and effect on patient outcome.

Bleeding and thrombosis

Both in terms of morbidity and mortality, bleeding and thrombosis are the most significant of all ECMO complications (Tables 2 and 3).[10] Maintaining adequate levels of anticoagulation to prevent clotting, while avoiding overheparinization and bleeding, is one of the greatest challenges of the ECMO clinician. The causes of bleeding on ECMO are related to pre-existing coagulopathy, circuit related platelet and factor consumption, and use of heparin.[50]

Bleeding

Bleeding complications can be relatively inconsequential, such as cannula site oozing, or catastrophic, such as uncontrollable surgical site hemorrhage. Minor bleeding is common and occurs at sites of invasive lines or incision. This includes nasal bleeding from nasogastric (NG) tubes, tracheal bleeding from ETT suctioning, and urethral bleeding from urinary catheters.

Persistent oozing can also occur at entry sites of peripheral and central lines, chest tubes, and the ECMO cannulation site. Removal or replacement of the line is generally not indicated and may in fact worsen the problem. Minor bleeding is generally managed by correcting coagulopathy and thrombocytopenia and lowering the target ACT range. Topical hemostatic agents such as thrombin glue may also be helpful. At times, persistent, even brisk bleeding cannot be stopped and is tolerated throughout the run. In this event, the patient is transfused with appropriate blood products as needed to maintain blood volume and avoid coagulopathy. Because gastritis may occur, all ECMO patients receive H_2 blocker or antacid.[35]

Catastrophic bleeding is much less common, but if uncontrolled may lead to a premature end to the ECMO run. The most common location of significant bleeding is the cannulation site. Massive bleeding is more likely when the cannulation is thoracic. Hemorrhage can occur at any surgical incision and is a potentially major complication whenever surgery is performed while on ECMO, as in the case of CDH repair. Control of massive bleeding usually involves surgical re-exploration and intervention. It may also be necessary to limit or even stop heparinization, keeping a primed circuit available in the event of sudden circuit clotting. Aminocaproic acid (Amicar), aprotinin, and recombinant activated Factor VII are drugs that

Table 2: Cumulative incidence of patient and circuit bleeding complications and associated survival of neonatal ECMO respiratory patients.[10]

Site of bleeding	Reported to Registry (%)	Survival to discharge* (%)
Surgical site	6.1	46
Cannulation site	6.3	67
CNS hemorrhage	5.9	45
Cardiovascular tamponade	0.4	38
Pulmonary hemorrhage	4.4	45
Raceway rupture	0.3	62
Other tubing rupture	0.7	74

*Overall cumulative neonatal ECMO survival rate to transfer or discharge in 2005: 77%.

Table 3: Cumulative incidence of clotting and associated survival of neonatal respiratory patients.[10]

Site of clot	Reported to Registry (%)	Survival to discharge* (%)
Oxygenator	18.4	67
Bridge	11	68
Bladder	16.3	70
Hemofilter	2.5	44
Other circuit site	5.1	59
DIC	1.5	38
CNS infarct	8.5	55

*Overall cumulative neonatal ECMO survival rate to transfer or discharge in 2005: 77%.

have been used to control bleeding in patients undergoing surgery and to prevent ICH (see Chapter 38). Results with these interventions have been mixed. Wilson et al demonstrated reduction in overall incidence of bleeding with the use of Amicar.[51] Horwitz et al. studied the use of Amicar to prevent ICH in 29 neonates on ECMO excluding CDH patients. There was no significant difference in the incidence of ICH or thrombotic complications in the Amicar vs. control groups (23% vs. 12.5%).[52] Downard et al. in 2003 reviewed Boston Children's experience with Amicar over a 10-year period and concluded that Amicar significantly reduced surgical site bleeding, but not ICH.[53] The authors did not recommend Amicar use for the infant at risk for ICH. An increased number of circuit changes were required in the Amicar-treated group, but other thrombotic complications were not increased.

Pulmonary hemorrhage occurs in 4% of ECMO patients and can be difficult to control. Increased PEEP and correction of coagulopathy with lowering of ACT target ranges is usually successful in stopping hemorrhage. On occasion, uncontrollable bleeding from the endotracheal tube or chest tube will lead to discontinuation of bypass support.

ICH is the most devastating of the bleeding complications associated with ECMO. According to the July 2005 ELSO Registry report, 5.9% of neonatal patients experience intracranial hemorrhage with an associated survival rate of 45%.[10] Development of intracranial bleed or extension of pre-existing bleed usually leads to termination of ECMO. Hardart et al. utilized the ELSO Registry to explore the etiology of ICH in neonates on ECMO.[8] They found that gestational age was the strongest predictor of ICH. Other pre-ECMO factors with high correlation were acidosis, primary diagnosis of sepsis, coagulopathy, and treatment with epinephrine. Rates of ICH were not different between patients treated with VV vs. VA ECMO or those treated with or without cephalic jugular drainage.

Circuit disruption is an additional potentially catastrophic bleeding complication. Inadvertent decannulation, raceway rupture and tubing disconnection can all lead to fatal blood loss. Prevention of circuit disruption is of critical importance. A primary task of the ECMO specialist is careful and frequent inspection of the cannula and circuit lines. The cannula position with relation to the incision should be continuously observed by both the bedside nurse and circuit specialist. Patient sedation must be adequate to avoid catheter displacement. Any cannula site bleeding must be evaluated promptly.

Roller pump raceway rupture is uncommon when super-tygon raceway tubing is used.[54] Nevertheless, hourly inspection of the raceway by the specialist should be performed. For long runs, walking of the raceway is also recommended. Tubing disconnection is prevented by use of connector ties and avoidance of high circuit pressure. The arterial side of the circuit is more likely to experience high pressure generated by the roller pump. Care must be taken to avoid leaving clamps on the circuit tubing when ECMO is initiated. Clotting within the membrane oxygenator will obstruct blood flow and lead to even higher pressure within the circuit tubing. If unnoticed or untreated, it can lead to rupture of the tubing at the oxygenator inlet. Use of servo-regulated pressure systems that slow or stop the pump for high pressure will alert the specialist to circuit obstruction.[55]

Thrombosis

Clotting and thrombotic complications can be as catastrophic as hemorrhage. Circuit clotting is one of the most common mechanical complications seen in ECMO patients and is associated with a lower survival rate (see Table 3).[10] Although clot formation within the circuit is unavoidable, it can be limited by maintaining adequate heparinization and circuit flow rates. Circuit clots may embolize, leading to obstruction of blood flow in the circuit. A second concern is the potential for clots to embolize to the patient. Visible clots within the circuit are more common on the venous, low flow side of the circuit, particularly at connection sites and the bottom of the bladder. Change-out of these components is usually not performed unless the clots are obstructing flow, in which case total circuit change-out may be preferable. Visible clots on the arterial side of the circuit, (e.g., at the top of the oxygenator or in the heat exchanger) should lead to a complete circuit change because of the embolic potential. Clotting is often not apparent on visual inspection and must be monitored by lab analysis, which should include daily coagulation studies with D-dimer determination. Circuit DIC, as evidenced by visible clots, rising D-dimer values, fibrinogenemia, and platelet consumption is managed by complete change-out of the ECMO circuit.

Patient embolic complications are difficult to diagnose, and the incidence is not known. Microemboli cannot be imaged, and the effect of microemboli on organ function has not been studied. Cerebral infarct is seen in 8.5% of neonatal respiratory ECMO patients.[11] VV ECMO is felt to be safer than VA with regard to thrombi due to the potential for the pulmonary bed to act as a filter.

Circuit air

Air emboli can have similar consequences to embolized clots, but occur less commonly. Air on the venous side of the circuit is generally easier to manage than arterial air, as the circuit is designed to trap air at multiple sites. Air on the arterial side of the circuit constitutes an ECMO emergency requiring temporary cessation of bypass support while the air is contained and removed.

Air can enter the ECMO circuit from multiple sites. The most common way is by introduction through IV lines, with medication administration, and during transfusions and blood draws. Certainly, prevention of air entry should be stressed through meticulous performance of routine nursing tasks. Administration of fluids and medications post-pump should be avoided when possible. Due to negative pressure on the venous line, air can be entrained from a malpositioned ECMO cannula side port or by way of a faulty connection. It is also possible to entrain venous air via loose cannula ties, especially with trans-thoracic cannulation.

Cavitation is another means by which air may enter the circuit. The functional bladder box or venous pressure monitor prevents this complication by servo-regulating pump flow when venous drainage is inadequate. The area of tubing between the venous reservoir and the pump is susceptible to cavitation. Kinking or clamping of this tubing will result in rapid air entry pre-oxygenator. This section of tubing should be protected by careful positioning and stabilization to prevent kinking.

At the level of the membrane oxygenator, air entry can occur in two ways. A tear in the membrane allows communication between the air and blood phases. If pressure on the air side of the membrane exceeds pressure in the blood compartment, air will cross over to the blood phase and enter the patient. This complication is prevented by use of a pop-off manometer on the gas line to prevent pressurization of the gas phase. Air can also be introduced by "supersaturation", where partial pressure of oxygen increases to a point where gas bubbles out of solution. Avoidance of supersaturation can be assured by monitoring of post-oxgenator blood gases with a goal of keeping the PaO_2 less than 500 mm Hg.

Once air is identified, it should be removed promptly if on the venous side of the circuit, and emergently if on the arterial side. Air post-oxygenator should be managed by coming off bypass and supporting the patient by conventional means until the air has been removed.

Hemolysis

Hemolysis can be caused by excessive shearing force on the RBC membrane. This may occur when circuit pressure is high, especially where blood is being forced through narrow channels. A pre-oxygenator circuit pressure which exceeds 400 mm Hg may increase hemolysis. The transmembrane pressure, or the difference between pre- and post-membrane pressures, should also be noted. Transmembrane pressure in excess of 150 mm Hg can indicate clotting within the membrane and a need for oxygenator change-out. Hemolysis can also occur when negative forces are high, as with a dysfunctional pump servoregulator, or with pumping via centrifugal pump. Finally, over-occluded roller pumps will cause hemolysis. RBC lysis with hemolysis may also be related to circuit-disseminated intravascular coagulation (DIC) or high circuit temperature. Hemolysis is suspected when a patient develops otherwise unexplained hyperbilirubinemia and is diagnosed by laboratory evaluation of the plasma-free hemoglobin. Treatment involves identification and correction of the cause and may require circuit change.

Inadequate ECMO support

At times, pump flow on VA or VV bypass may be inadequate to support patient need as indicated by acidosis, hypoxia, or hypotension. Inadequate support can be due to flow limitation from decreased venous drainage or myocardial dysfunction.

Inadequate venous drainage can have multiple causes, the most common of which is hypovolemia. This can be readily corrected with colloid infusion in most cases. At times though, it is complicated by capillary leak, which may require massive volume infusion until the capillary leak resolves. Other causes of decreased venous return to the circuit include venous catheter malposition; clotting, kinking or clamping of the catheter or venous line; or patient tension pneumothorax or cardiac tamponade. Treatment depends on the underlying etiology.

In the patient on VV bypass, cardiac function may be suboptimal, necessitating inotropic

and volume boluses. If the patient is hypoxic or acidotic, it may be necessary to convert to VA bypass.

Equipment failure

Failure of a critical ECMO circuit component will by definition cause patient decompensation. Oxygenator failure occurs in about 6% of neonatal ECMO runs with an associated survival rate of 55%.[10] The cause may be fluid accumulation in the membrane, clotting, or membrane leak. A wet or clotted membrane will exhibit a loss in ability to exchange gas. Increasing gas sweep flow will dry out a wet membrane. Excessive clotting can only be treated by membrane change-out. A leaking membrane is usually carefully observed, with change-out only if blood loss is excessive. With a membrane blood leak it is important to monitor the gas phase carefully, as a blood clot in the gas outlet can cause pressurization of the gas phase, leading to air embolus. Use of a pop-off manometer on the gas line will audibly alert the specialist to development of this complication and prevent over-pressurization of the gas phase.

Heat exchangers rarely fail, but a leak could potentially lead to contamination of the patient blood stream with non-sterile water. Complications could include hemodilution, hemolysis, and infection.

Malfunction of gas flow equipment can lead to hypoxia or hypercarbia. The membrane oxygenator efficiently exchanges carbon dioxide (CO_2), and some ECMO centers blend CO_2 or carbogen into the sweep gas to prevent hypocarbia. This practice can potentially lead to inadvertent delivery of excessive CO_2. Use of an in-line blood gas monitoring device can help monitor for this complication. Alternatively, many centers adjust sweep flow gases to a very low level and thus eliminate the need for CO_2 blending.

Failure of the pump necessitates emergency response with rapid change-out of equipment. In this case, the patient is clamped off bypass and supported using conventional means while the problem is diagnosed and corrected. If the patient condition has improved to the point that ECMO can safely be terminated, conventional support is continued and plans are made to decannulate.

Cardiac complications

Cardiac stun is a term used to describe decreased cardiac contractility not uncommonly seen in VA ECMO patients in the first hours and days on bypass.[56] The etiology of "stun" is controversial but is likely caused by myocardial ischemia with decreased coronary blood flow. Stun can be exacerbated by malposition of the arterial catheter with flow directed towards the aortic valve. Stun is rarely seen on VV bypass, possibly because coronary blood is well oxygenated and supplied by normal flow patterns. Patients with stun demonstrate narrowed pulse pressure and a very high patient arterial PO_2. The sweep FiO_2 is lowered to prevent hyperoxia. A echocardiogram should be obtained to check arterial catheter position. Stun nearly always resolves spontaneously.

Hypertension is frequently seen in neonates on VA support and is significant enough in about 13% of neonatal ECMO cases to require vasodilator therapy.[10] The cause of hypertension is likely related to peripheral vasoconstriction and increased afterload. The non-pulsatility of the ECMO pump flow on VA bypass may trigger the renin-angiotension system with subsequent rise in blood pressure. Treatment includes weaning of pump flow, while maintaining adequate perfusion, and use of vasodilators.

Arrhythmia on ECMO in neonatal patients with respiratory failure occurs infrequently. It can be caused by metabolic disturbance such as hypocalcemia[57] or by venous catheter malposition. Cardiac ultrasound can be used to evaluate catheter position. Arrhythmia is generally well tolerated on VA bypass but can constitute an emergency if the patient is on VV support.

Persistence of a patent ductus arteriosus has been described in neonates on ECMO. Treatment with indomethacin is contraindicated due to platelet dysfunction and thrombocytopenia. Most patients respond to diuretic therapy and fluid restriction. Ductal ligation on ECMO has been performed successfully, but is generally unnecessary.[58]

Renal complications

Renal dysfunction in neonates on ECMO is often linked to pre-ECMO hypoxia and hypotension. Also contributing to decreased renal function may be the kidney's response to non-pulsatile VA pump flow. Many neonates exhibit decreased urinary output in the first 24-48 hours on bypass, with spontaneous resolution over time. Low-dose dopamine infusion may be used to increase renal perfusion.

Volume overload pre-ECMO is common, and the need for volume support on ECMO may continue due to capillary leak. Diuresis is usually promoted with aggressive use of diuretics once capillary leak has resolved. If the patient's urinary output remains insufficient, use of ultrafiltration to treat volume overload can be instituted.

A small number of ECMO patients will develop acute renal failure with anuria and will require hemofiltration with dialysis. This involves addition of dialysate or renal replacement fluid to the ECMO ultrafiltration circuit. This system will remove solutes as well as fluid.

Infection

Considering the ECMO patient exposure to instrumentation and blood exposure to artificial surface, infection is a surprisingly rare complication on ECMO. Between the years 2000 and 2004, the rate of culture proven infection reported to the ELSO Registry was, on average, 6%.[10] ECMO patients who develop sepsis on bypass have higher complication rates and decreased survival. Lung recovery is delayed, prolonging the ECMO run. Septic infants have a higher incidence of bleeding, thrombosis, seizures, and metabolic derangement.[59] Broad spectrum antibiotic coverage is used by most ECMO centers throughout the run, and many also run routine surveillance cultures.

Neurologic complications

As a group, patients who are placed on ECMO have experienced significant pre-ECMO physiologic instability. Patients are potentially exposed to hypotension, acidosis, alkalosis, hypercarbia, and profound hypoxia, putting them at risk for neurologic sequelae. In addition, the ECMO run exposes the patient to carotid and jugular ligation, heparinization, coagulopathy, and hypertension, all of which predispose to neurologic complication.[55,60] ICH and infarct remain significant causes of ECMO mortality and morbidity. The combined incidence as reported to ELSO in 2004 was 14.4% with an overall survival of 28%.[10] One promising neuroprotective strategy is the use of mild hypothermia (see Chapter 35). The safety of this therapy when used in conjunction with ECMO was studied in a pilot investigation in 2003 by Horan et al.[61] They found no evidence of clinical or circuit complication related to cooling or rewarming.

Graft-versus-host-disease

Transfusion associated graft vs host disease (TA-GVD) is a rare but nearly always fatal complication of ECMO. Several case studies of neonates contracting this disease after ECMO therapy have been reported.[62] TA-GVD is caused by host response to donor T-lymphocytes, with subsequent organ involvement of skin, liver, spleen, bone marrow, and thymus. It is entirely prevented by adequate irradiation of blood products (>1500 rads).

DEHP exposure

Di(2-ethylhexyl)phthalate (DEHP) is a chemical added to vinyl to make it pliable. The polyvinyl chloride tubing of the ECMO circuit is manufactured with the addition of DEHP. It is recognized that this chemical leaches out of the plastic when it is in contact with blood. Animal studies have linked DEHP to teratogenic and carcinogenic effects on the liver, lungs, and reproductive organs.[63] One study in neonates treated with ECMO revealed detectable levels of DEHP in serum, liver, heart, and testicular tissues, and traces in the brain.[64] Given the prolonged exposure to DEHP from the ECMO circuit, the potential for toxicity is high. Further studies of ECMO and DEHP are in progress

Survival and outcome

To date 19,939 neonates with respiratory failure have been treated with ECMO; 85% were successfully decannulated and 77% survived to discharge.[10] The cumulative survival statistics are highest for meconium aspiration syndrome at 94% and lowest for CDH at 52% (Table 4). Changes in intensive care and the introduction of new therapies such as surfactant, selective antibiotic prophylaxis for mothers and babies, high frequency ventilation, and iNO have reduced the numbers of infants who require ECMO. The current survival statistics for specific diagnoses have remained relatively stable except for CDH. The number of CDH infants treated with ECMO has remained unchanged, but survival rates have decreased from 60% in 1990 to 42% in 2004.

Medical and neurodevelopmental outcome of the ECMO patient is encouraging, considering the severity of illness in the newborn period. Analysis of outcome studies performed in persistent pulmonary hypertension of the newborn (PPHN) survivors treated with conventional medical therapy, iNO, and ECMO yield grossly equivalent morbidities and outcomes.[65] This suggests that neurodevelopmental outcome is more related to the underlying illness than to the therapeutic intervention utilized.

Chronic lung disease (defined as oxygen use at 28 days) is seen in 15% of ECMO survivors, but long-term oxygen use is uncommon except in infants with CDH. Hospitalization for respiratory problems in the first year of life is needed in approximately 25%.[66] Normal somatic growth is seen in ECMO-treated children except those with CDH.

Progressive high-frequency sensorineural hearing loss is seen in 3-21% of ECMO-treated infants.[67] An important aspect is the delayed onset, making diagnosis problematic. The position statement by the Joint Committee on Infant Hearing in 2000 added PPHN and ECMO as risk indicators for hearing loss and recommended audiologic evaluation every 6 months until 3 years of age.[68]

Numerous investigators have reported on the neurodevelopmental outcome of the ECMO patient and consistently report Bayley scores in the normal range in the first 2 years of life.[69-71] Fewer studies of ECMO survivors at older ages have been performed.[72] Glass et al. reported that by 5 years of age, mean IQ scores remain in the normal range, but are lower than controls (96 vs. 115, P<0.001).[73] Approximately 15% of ECMO

survivors at age 5 had a major handicap, most commonly mental retardation, while <5% had severe or profound impairment. Nevertheless, 50% of ECMO survivors have an increased risk of learning and behavioral problems when compared to normal controls. As a result of these deficits, ECMO survivors are vulnerable to academic and psychosocial difficulties.

Changing demographics of ECMO

As previously mentioned, a number of new treatments have been used for neonatal respiratory failure, including high frequency-ventilation, surfactant replacement, and iNO over the last decade.[74-81] The use of some of these pre-ECMO therapies has been observed to decrease the need for ECMO.[75-80]

Roy et al. used the ELSO Registry to study the changes in health care practices for infants with neonatal respiratory failure from 1988-1998.[74] Although there was no change in gestational age, gender, chronologic age, or pre-ECMO blood gases, there were significant differences in pre-ECMO therapies used, ventilator practices, and the diagnostic categories treated. The use of high-frequency ventilation, surfactant, and iNO increased dramatically over the study period. The pre-ECMO PIP decreased

Table 4. Changes in ECMO survival by diagnosis.[10]

Diagnoses	Cumulative patients (N)	Cumulative survival* (%)	2004 patients (n)	2004 Survival* (%)
MAS	6805	94	117	91
CDH	4770	52	166	42
Sepsis	2699	74	25	76
PPHN	3077	78	90	67
RDS	1398	84	6	50
Other	1436	64	97	57
All	19,939	77	665	64

*Survival to discharge or transfer.
MAS: meconium aspiration syndrome
CDH: congenital diaphragmatic hernia
PPHN: persistent pulmonary hypertension of the newborn
RDS: respiratory distress syndrome

from 47 ±10 to 39 ±12. The percent of ECMO patients with respiratory distress syndrome decreased from 15-4% while the percent with CDH increased from 18-26%. The number of infants treated annually with ECMO has steadily declined from 1500 patients in 1991 to approximately 1000 patients in 1997. The number of ECMO centers has been relatively stable since 1993, so the average number of patients treated at an ECMO center has decreased from 18 to 9 while the average length of an ECMO run for the non-CDH population increased from 124 ±67 to 141 ±104 hours. The use of VV ECMO has increased to 32%. The rate of ICH has remained stable. Mortality for all neonatal respiratory failure increased from 18-22%, but this increase is due both to the relative increase in the percentage of ECMO patients with CDH and the downward trend for survival in these patients.

Review of the neonatal ELSO Registry data for July 2005 demonstrates ongoing demographic changes (Figure 1). ECMO use continues to decline with 665 cases reported to the Registry for 2004.[10] Dramatic decreases in the use of ECMO for respiratory distress syndrome and sepsis/pneumonia are also noted with only 33 and 8 patients treated in 2004, respectively. There has also been a steady downward trend in the use of ECMO for MAS; it is no longer the most common indication for ECMO. The number of CDH infants placed on ECMO continues to be stable at ~250 per year, but the survival rate continues to decline.

Summary

It has been nearly 30 years since ECMO was first successfully used to treat a newborn with respiratory failure. This experience as

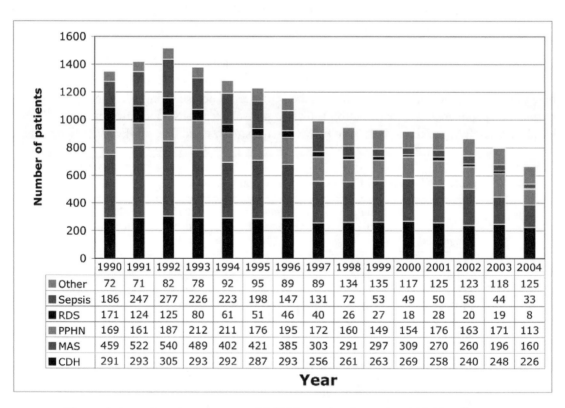

Figure 1. Annual respiratory neonatal ECMO runs by diagnosis, 1990-2004.[10]

documented by the ELSO Registry, as well as randomized control trials, have demonstrated the successful use of ECMO in this patient population, especially when compared to other age and diagnostic groups. Therapies such as iNO, surfactant, and high frequency ventilation have led to a decrease in the utilization of ECMO for certain neonatal disease states. This trend has resulted in fewer patients receiving ECMO treatment, and those that do receive treatment have longer, more complicated runs. Bleeding and clotting and their sequelae remain significant sources of morbidity and mortality. The future challenge for neonatal ECMO centers will lie in developing techniques to limit complications and improve survival, while treating fewer and more complex patients.

References

1. Bartlett RH, Gazzaniga AB, Jefferies MR, Huxtable RF, Haiduc NJ, Fong SW. Extracorporeal membrane oxygenation (ECMO) cardiopulmonary support in infancy. *Trans Am Soc Artif Intern Organs* 1976; 22:80-93.
2. Bartlett RH, Andrews AF, Toomasian JM, Haiduc NJ, Gazzaniga AB. Extracorporeal membrane oxygenation for newborn respiratory failure: forty-five cases. *Surgery* 1982; 92:425-433.
3. Short BL, Miller MK, Anderson KD. Extracorporeal membrane oxygenation in the management of respiratory failure in the newborn. *Clin Perinatol* 1987; 14:737-748.
4. Bartlett RH, Roloff DW, Cornell RG, Andrews AF, Dillon PW, Zwischenberger JB. Extracorporeal circulation in neonatal respiratory failure: a prospective randomized study. *Pediatrics* 1985; 76:479-487.
5. O'Rourke PP, Crone RK, Vacanti JP et al. Extracorporeal membrane oxygenation and conventional medical therapy in neonates with persistent pulmonary hypertension of the newborn: a prospective randomized study. *Pediatrics* 1989; 84:957-963.
6. UK collaborative randomised trial of neonatal extracorporeal membrane oxygenation. UK Collaborative ECMO Trial Group. *Lancet* 1996; 348:75-82.
7. Elbourne D, Field D, Mugford M. Extracorporeal membrane oxygenation for severe respiratory failure in newborn infants. *Cochrane Database Syst Rev* 2002; (1): CD001340.
8. Hardart GE, Fackler JC. Predictors of intracranial hemorrhage during neonatal extracorporeal membrane oxygenation. *J Pediatr* 1999; 134:156-159.
9. Hirschl RB, Schumacher RE, Snedecor SN, Bui KC, Bartlett RH. The efficacy of extracorporeal life support in premature and low birth weight newborns. *J Pediatr Surg* 28 1993; 1336-1340; discussion 1341.
10. Neonatal ECMO Registry of the Extracorporeal Life Support Organization (ELSO). Ann Arbor, Michigan, July 2005.
11. Hardart GE, Hardart MK, Arnold JH. Intracranial hemorrhage in premature neonates treated with extracorporeal membrane oxygenation correlates with conceptional age. *J Pediatr* 2005; 145:184-189.
12. Revenis ME, Glass P, Short BL. Mortality and morbidity rates among lower birth weight infants (2000 to 2500 grams) treated with extracorporeal membrane oxygenation. *J Pediatr* 1992; 121:452-458.
13. Arnold P, Jackson S, Wallis J, Smith J, Bolton D, Haynes S. Coagulation factor activity during neonatal extra-corporeal membrane oxygenation. *Int Care Med* 2001; 27:1395-1400.
14. Kolovos NS, Schuerer DJ, Moler FW et al: Extracorporeal life support for pulmonary hemorrhage in children: a case series. *Crit Care Med* 2002; 30:577-580.
15. Beck R, Anderson KD, Pearson GD, Cronin J, Miller MK, Short BL. Criteria for extracorporeal membrane oxygenation

in a population of infants with persistent pulmonary hypertension of the newborn. *J Pediatr Surg* 1986; 21:297-302.

16. Ortiz RM, Cilley RE, Bartlett RH. Extracorporeal membrane oxygenation in pediatric respiratory failure. *Pediatr Clin North Am* 1987; 34:39-46.

17. Schumacher RE, Roloff DW, Chapman R, Snedecor S, Bartlett RH. Extracorporeal membrane oxygenation in term newborns. A prospective cost-benefit analysis. *ASAIO J* 1993; 39:873-879.

18. Hedrick HL. Ex utero intrapartum therapy. *Semin Pediatr Surg* 2003; 12:190-195.

19. Anderson HL, Otsu T, Chapman RA, Bartlett RH. Veno-venous extracorporeal membrane oxygenation (ECMO) using a double-lumen cannula. *Trans ASAIO* 1989; 35:650-653.

20. Rais-Bahrami K, Rivera O, Mikesell GT. Improved oxygenation with reduced recirculation during venovenous extracorporeal membrane oxygenation: Evaluation of a test catheter. *Crit Care Med* 1995; 23:1722-1725.

21. Cornish JD, Clark RH, Ricketts RR, Dykes RD, Wright JA, Kesser K. Efficacy of veno-venous extracorporeal membrane oxygenation for neonates with respiratory and circulatory compromise. *J Pediatr* 1993; 122:105-109.

22. Strieper MJ, Sharma S, Dooley KJ, Cornish JD, Clark RH. Effects of veno-venous extracorporeal membrane oxygenation on cardiac performance as determined by echocardiographic measurements. *J Pediatr* 1993; 122:950-955.

23. Anderson HL, Snedecor SM, Otsu T, Bartlett RH. Multicenter comparison of conventional venoarterial access versus venovenous double-lumen catheter access in newborn infants undergoing extracorporeal membrane oxygenation. *J Pediatr Surg* 1993; 28:530-534.

24. Peek GJ, Firmin RK, Moore HM, Sosnowski AW. Cannulation of infants for venonenous extracorporeal life support. *Ann Thorac Surg* 1996; 61:1851-1852.

25. Reickert CA, Schreiner RJ, Bartlett RH, Hirschl RB. Percutaneous access for venovenous extracorporeal life support in neonates. *J Pediatr Surg* 1998; 33:365-369.

26. Walker LK, Short BL, Traystman RJ. Impairment of cerebral autoregulation during venovenous extracorporeal membrane oxygenation in the newborn lamb. *Crit Care Med* 1996; 24:2001-2006.

27. Pettignano R, Labuz M, Gauthier TW, Huckaby J, Clarki RH. The use of cephalad cannulae to monitor jugular venous oxygen content during extracorporeal membrane oxygenation. *Crit Care* 1997; 3:95-99.

28. Skarsgard ED, Salt DR, Lee SK, ELSO Registry. Venovenous extracorporeal membrane oxygenation in neonatal respiratory failure: does routine, cephalad jugular drainage improve outcome? *J Ped Surg* 2004; 39:672-676.

29. Meliones JN, Moler FW, Custer RJ, et al. Hemodynamic instability after the initiation of extracorporeal membrane oxygenation: role of ionized calcium. *Crit Care Med* 1991; 19:1247-1251.

30. Graziani LJ, Ginglas M, Baumgart S. Cerebrovascular complications and sequelae of neonatal ECMO. *Clin Perinatol* 1997; 24:655-675.

31. Buck ML. Pharmacokinetic changes during extracorporeal membrane oxygenation: implications for drug therapy of neonates. *Clin Pharmacokinet* 2003; 42:403-417.

32. Mascarenhas MR, Kerner JA, Stallings VA. Chapter 78: Parenteral and Enteral Nutrition. In Walker WA, Durie PR, Hamilton JR et al, eds. *Pediatric Gastrointestinal Disease, Third edition.* New York: B.C. Decker Inc. 2000; 1730-1740.

33. Hammerman C, Aramburo MJ. Decreased lipid intake reduces morbidity in sick premature neonates. *J Pediatr* 1988; 113:1083-1088.

34. Helbock HJ, Motchnik PA, Ames BN. Toxic hydroperoxides in intravenous lipid emulsions used in preterm infants. *Pediatrics* 1993; 91:83-87.

35. Kuusela AL, Ruuska T, Karikoski R, et al. A randomized, controlled study of prophylactic ranitidine in preventing stress-induced gastric mucosal lesions in neonatal intensive care unit patients. *Crit Care Med* 1997; 25:346-351.

36. Lotze A, Knight GR, Martin GR. Improved pulmonary outcome after exogenous surfactant therapy for respiratory failure in term infants requiring extracorporeal membrane oxygenation. *J Pediatr* 1993; 122:261-268.

37. Stillerman LR, Gunn SB, Hart JC, Engle WA. Effects of exogenous surfactant on neonates supported by extracorporeal membrane oxygenation. *J Perinatol* 1997; 17:262-265.

38. Knight GR, Dudell GG, Evans ML, Grimm PS. A comparison of venovenous and venoarterial extracorporeal membrane oxygenation in the treatment of neonatal respiratory failure. *Crit Care Med* 1996; 24:1678-1683.

39. Bucur SZ, Levy JH, Despotis GJ, Spiess BD, Hillyer CD. Uses of antithrombin III concentrate in congenital and acquired deficiency states. *Transfusion* 1998; 38:481-498.

40. Edstrom CS, Christensen RD. Evaluation and treatment of thrombosis in the neonatal intensive care unit. *Clin Perinatol* 2000; 27:623-641.

41. Khan AM, Shabarek FM, Zwishenberger JB, et al. Utility of daily head ultrasonography for infants on extracorporeal membrane oxygenation. *J Pediatr Surg* 1998; 33:1229-1232.

42. Korinthenberg R, Kachel W, Koelfen W, Schultze C, Varnholt V. Neurologic findings in newborn infants after extracorporeal membrane oxygenation, with special reference to the EEG. *Dev Med Child Neurol* 1993; 35:249-257.

43. Graziani LJ, Streletz LJ, Baumgart S, Cullen J, McKee LM. Predictive value of neonatal electroencephalograms before and during extracorporeal membrane oxygenation. *J Pediatr* 1994; 125:969-975.

44. Gannon CM, Kornhauser MS, Gross GW, et al. When combined, early bedside head ultrasound and electroencephalography predict abnormal computerized tomography or magnetic resonance brain images obtained after ECMO treatment. *J Perinatol* 2001; 21:451-455.

45. Baumgart S, Streletz LJ, Needleman L, et al. Right common carotid artery reconstruction after extracorporeal membrane oxygenation: vascular imaging, cerebral circulation, electroencephalographic, and neurodevelopmental correlates to recovery. *J Pediatr* 1994; 125:295-304.

46. Taylor BJ, Seibert JJ, Glasier CM, VanDevanter SH, Harrell JE, Fasules JW. Evaluation of the reconstructed carotid artery following extracorporeal membrane oxygenation. *Pediatrics* 1992; 90:568-572.

47. Levy MS, Share JC, Fauza DO, Wilson JM. Fate of the reconstructed carotid artery after extracorporeal membrane oxygenation. *J Pediatr Surg* 1995; 30:1046-1049.

48. Cheung PY, Vickar DB, Hallgren RA, Finer NN, Robertson CMT, Western Canadian ECMO Follow-up Group. Carotid artery reconstruction in neonates receiving extracorporeal membrane oxygenation: a 4-year follow-up study. *J Pediatr Surg* 1997; 32:560-564.

49. Moulton SL, Lynch FP, Cornish JD, Bejar RF, Simko AJ, Krous HF. Carotid artery reconstruction following neonatal extracor-

poreal membrane oxygenation. *J Pediatr Surg* 1991; 26:764-769.

51. Muntean W. Coagulation and anticoagulation in extracorporeal membrane oxygenation. *Artif Organs* 1999; 23:979-983.

52. Wilson JM, Bower LK, Fackler JC, Beals PA, Bergus BO, Kevy SV. Aminocaproic acid decreases the incidence of intracranial hemorrhage and other hemorrhagic complications of ECMO. *J Pediatr Surg* 1993; 28:536-540.

53. Horowitz JR, Cofer BR, Warner BW, Cheu HW, Lally KP, A multicenter trial of 6-aminocaproic acid (Amicar) in the prevention of bleeding in infants on ECMO. *J Pediatr Surg* 1995; 30:1490-1492.

54. Downard CD, Betit P, Chang RW, Garza JJ, Arnold JH, Wilson JM. Impact of Amicar on hemorrhagic complications of ECMO in a ten year review. *J Pediatr Surg* 2003; 38:1212-1216.

55. Toomasian JM, Kerby KA, Chapman RA, Heiss KF, Hirschl RB, Bartlett RH, Performance of rupture resistant polyvinyl chloride tubing. *Proc Am Acad Cardiovasc Perf* 1987; 8:56-59.

56. Zwischenberger JB, Nguyen TT, Upp JR, Jr, et al. Complications of neonatal extracorporeal membrane oxygenation. Collective experience from the Extracorporeal Life Support Organization. *J Thorac Cardiovasc Surg* 1994; 107:838-849.

57. Martin GR, Short BL, Abbott C, O'Brien AM. Cardiac stun in infants undergoing extracorporeal membrane oxygenation. *J Thorac Cardiovasc Surg* 1991; 101:607-611.

58. Meliones JN, Moler FW, Custer JR, et al. Hemodynamic instability after the initiation of extracorporeal membrane oxygenation: role of ionized calcium. *Crit Care Med* 1991; 19:1247-1251.

59. Becker JA, Short BL, Martin GR. Cardiovascular complications adversely affect survival during extracorporeal membrane oxygenation. *Crit Care Med* 1998; 26:1484-1486.

60. Meyer DM, Jessen ME, Eberhart RC, and the Extracorporeal Life Support Organization. Neonatal extracorporeal membrane oxygenation complicated by sepsis. *Ann Thorac Surg* 1995; 59:975-980.

61. Short BM. The effect of extracorporeal life support on the brain: a focus on ECMO. *Semin Perinatol* 2005; 29(1):45-50.

62. Horan M, Ichiba S, Firmin RK, et al. A pilot investigation of mild hypothermia in neonates receiving ECMO. *J Pediatr* 2003; 144:301-308

63. Hatley RM, Reynolds M, Paller AS, Chou P. Graft vs. host disease following ECMO. *J Pediatr Surg* 1991; 26:317-319

64. Rubin RJ, Mess PM. What price progress? An update on vinyl plastic bags. *Transfusion* 1990; 29:358-361.

65. Shneider B, Schena J, Truog R, Jacobson M, Kevy S. Exposure to di(2-ethylhexyl) phthalate in infants receiving extracorporeal membrane oxygenation. *New Engl J Med* 1989; 320:1563.

66. Benitz WE, Rhine WD, Van Meurs KP. Persistent pulmonary hypertension of the newborn. In Sunshine P, Stevenson DK, eds. *Fetal and neonatal brain injury: mechanisms, management, and the risks of practice.* New York: Cambridge University Press 2003; 636-662.

67. Hofkosh D, Thompson AE, Nozza RJ, et al. Ten years of extracorporeal membrane oxygenation: neurodevelopmental outcome. *Pediatrics* 1991; 87:549-555

68. Cheung PY, Robertson CM. Sensorineural hearing loss in survivors of neonatal extracorporeal membrane oxygenation. *Pediatr Rehabil* 1997; 1:127-130.

69. Joint Committee on Infant Hearing, American Academy of Audiology, American Academy of Pediatrics, American Speech-Language-Hearing Association, Directors of Speech and Hearing Programs in State

Health and Welfare Agencies. Year 2000 position statement: Principles and guidelines for early hearing detection and intervention programs. *Pediatrics* 2000; 106:798-817.

70. Glass P, Miller MK, Short BL. Morbidity for survivors of extracorporeal membrane oxygenation. Neurodevelopmental outcome at 1 year of age. *Pediatrics* 1989; 83:72-78.

71. Schumacher RE, Palmer TW, Roloff DW, LaClaire PA, Bartlett RH. Follow-up of infants treated with extracorporeal membrane oxygenation for newborn respiratory failure. *Pediatrics* 1991; 87:451-457.

72. Bennett CC, Johnson A, Field DJ, Elbourne D, UK Collaborative ECMO Trial Group. UK collaborative randomised trial of neonatal extracorporeal membrane oxygenation: Follow-up to age 4 years. *Lancet* 2001; 357:1094-1096.

73. Nield, TA, Langenbacher D, Poulsen MK, Platzker AC. Neurodevelopmental outcome at 3.5 years of age in children treated with extracorporeal life support: Relationship to primary diagnosis. *J Pediatr* 2000; 136:338-344.

74. Glass P, Wagner AE, Papero PH, et al. Neurodevelopmental status at age five years of neonates treated with extracorporeal membrane oxygenation. *J Pediatr* 1995; 127:447-457.

75. Roy BJ, Rycus P, Conrad SA, Clark RH, for the Extracorporeal Life Support Organization (ELSO) Registry. The changing demographics of neonatal extracorporeal membrane oxygenation patients reported to the Extracorporeal Life Support Organization (ELSO) Registry. *Pediatrics* 2000; 106:1334-1338.

76. Wilson JM, Bower LK, Thompson JE, Fauza DO, Fackler JC. ECMO in evolution: The impact of changing patient demographics and alternative therapies on ECMO. *J Pediatr Surg* 1996; 31:1116-1123; discussion 1122-1123.

77. Hintz SR, Suttner DM, Sheehan AM, Rhine WD, Van Meurs KP. Decreased use of neonatal extracorporeal membrane oxygenation (ECMO): How new treatment modalities have affected ECMO utilization. *Pediatrics* 2000; 106:1339-1343.

78. The neonatal inhaled nitric oxide study group (NINOS). Inhaled nitric oxide in full term and nearly full term infants with hypoxic respiratory failure. *N Engl J Med* 1997; 336:597-604.

79. Roberts JD Jr., Fineman JR, Morin FC III, et al. Inhaled nitric oxide and persistent pulmonary hypertension of the newborn. *N Engl J Med* 1997; 336:605-610.

80. Clark RH, Kueser TJ, Walker MW, et al. Low-dose nitric oxide therapy for persistent pulmonary hypertension in the newborn. Clinical inhaled nitric oxide research group. *N Engl J Med* 2000; 342:469-474.

81. Lotze A, Mitchell BR, Bulas DI, et al. Multicenter study of surfactant (beractant) use in the treatment of term infants with severe respiratory failure. Survanta in Term Infants Study Group. *J Pediatr* 1998; 132:40-47.

82. Clark RH, Yoder BA, Sell MS. Prospective, randomized comparison of high-frequency oscillation and conventional ventilation in candidates for extracorporeal membrane oxygenation. *J Pediatr* 1994; 124:447-454.

19

Congenital Diaphragmatic Hernia and ECMO

Amir M. Khan, M.D. and Kevin P. Lally, M.D.

Introduction

Congenital diaphragmatic hernia (CDH) is an abnormality of diaphragm development which permits abdominal viscera to herniate into the thoracic cavity. CDH was first described in 1679 by Lazarus Riverius, who incidentally noted a CDH on a post-mortem exam in a 24-year-old. In 1701, the classical clinical and post-mortem findings of an infant with CDH were noted by Sir Charles Holt in the philosophical transactions of the Royal Society of London. Giovanni Battista Morgagni, in 1761, described the anterior diaphragmatic hernia which today bears his name. Finally, in 1848, Victor Bochdalek described patients with both right and left posterolateral diaphragmatic hernias, commonly known today as a Bochdalek hernia.

CDH occurs in approximately 1 in 2,000-4,000 births. Males are more commonly affected, with a 1.5:1 male:female ratio. The recurrence risk for future pregnancies is ~2%. Worldwide, the frequency is the same as that in the U.S.[1,2] While the mechanisms involved remain largely unclear, the result is a defect in the diaphragm that allows abdominal viscera to herniate into the chest cavity. Approximately 95% occur in the posterolateral portion of the diaphragm and of these, 80% occur on the left side.[3] The presence of abdominal contents in the chest cavity can compress the lung and is thought to impair lung development, resulting in pulmonary hypoplasia. However, some animal models have suggested that lung hypoplasia may also occur independently.[4] In addition to the small lungs, abnormalities of the pulmonary vasculature result in pulmonary hypertension, a significant and severe problem in infants with CDH.

The presence of chromosomal defects and/or cardiac anomalies in infants with CDH has lead to the thinking that the disease involves a spectrum of problems including pulmonary hypoplasia, chromosomal defects, and cardiac anomalies.[2]

Diagnosis

CDH is commonly diagnosed before birth by ultrasound. In some series, over half of CDH patients were diagnosed prenatally.[5] The diagnosis is made antenatally by finding bowel loops in the thoracic cavity with a shift of the heart into the opposite chest cavity. Additionally, the position of the fetal liver in relation to the chest cavity is used to diagnose CDH. However, the clinical usefulness of these diagnostic tools remains controversial.

After delivery, infants with CDH often present with cyanosis and respiratory distress soon after birth although severity of clinical presentation can range from asymptomatic to severely ill. Physical examination shows the abdomen to be flat or scaphoid, and, on auscultation, air entry is reduced on the affected side (Figure 1). A chest radiograph confirms the presence of gastrointestinal loops in the chest (Figure 2). Once air is present in the bowel, multiple loops of air-filled bowel can be identified in the chest. A nasogastric tube may be seen on a chest radiograph in the thorax if the stomach is herniated. There is a shift of the heart and mediastinum away from the side of the hernia.

Management

In infants with CDH, respiratory distress may be progressive with rapidly worsening hypoxemia, hypercarbia, and acidosis. Therefore, post-delivery respiratory support with intubation and ventilation is usually required. A nasogastric tube should be passed. Gas exchange and acid-base status should be assessed. Continuous pre-ductal pulse oximetry is valuable in the management of PPHN. Bag-and-mask ventilation in the delivery room should be avoided because the stomach and intestines can become distended with air, which can further compromise pulmonary function. In addition to respiratory support, infants with CDH may also require cardiovascular support in the form of inotropes. Given the increased incidence of cardiac anomalies and chromosomal defects, an echocardiogram and chromosome analysis is essential in these infants.

Mechanical ventilation

Infants with CDH develop varying degrees of hypoxemic respiratory failure (HRF). The severity of HRF is thought to be related primarily to the degree of pulmonary hypoplasia. Most infants with CDH and resulting HRF require endotracheal intubation and mechanical ventilation. With the advent of neonatal mechanical ventilation in the 1960s, many CDH infants with previously fatal HRF survived to undergo surgical repair. As an understanding of perinatal physiology grew, the presence of pulmonary hypertension and extra-pulmonary shunting was appreciated. Studies found that pulmonary vascular resistance (PVR) could be modulated by changing the pH and pCO_2, leading to the widespread use of hyperventilation to control hypoxemia in these infants.[6] Although this strategy was effective in reducing PVR, the amount of ventilator support required to achieve the desired effect was sometimes high and led to significant ventilator-induced lung injury. Wung et al. showed that some of the mortality in CDH infants was, in fact, due to ventilator-

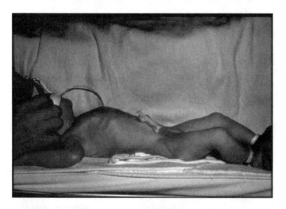

Figure 1. Photograph of an infant with a scaphoid abdomen. Such presentation would be very suggestive of CDH.

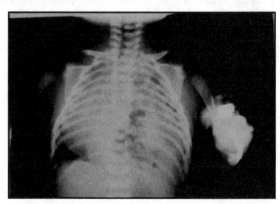

Figure 2. Chest radiograph of an infant with CDH. There are bowel loops visible in the left chest with the heart shifted towards the right chest.

induced lung injury.[7] Studies have suggested that gentle ventilation with permissive hypercapnea reduces the mortality in neonates who meet ECMO criteria.[8] In many ECMO centers, current ventilation strategy focuses on minimizing barotrauma by allowing spontaneous ventilation with minimal set respiratory rates, pressure-limited ventilation, tolerance of high $PaCO_2$, minimal sedation, and avoidance of paralysis. Using this strategy, several authors have reported survival approaching 90%.[9,10]

High frequency oscillatory ventilation (HFOV) has been shown in animal models to cause less lung injury than conventional mechanical ventilation. For this reason, there has been some interest in exploring its use in infants with CDH. However, the benefit of HFOV in CDH remains controversial. Paranka et al. found HFOV to be of little benefit when used in a high-pressure lung recruitment strategy in patients with CDH.[11] Others have shown that when used as the initial mode of therapy, HFOV can be an effective mode of mechanical ventilation in CDH.[12,13]

In summary, while the optimum mode of ventilation in CDH remains controversial, there clinical data suggest that management strategies designed to limit lung distention and barotrauma may result in improved survival.

Inhaled nitric oxide

PPHN remains a significant problem in infants with CDH. Multiple factors, including decreased cross-sectional area of the pulmonary vascular bed due to lung hypoplasia, increased medial thickness of the pulmonary arteries, and blunted oxygen-induced vasodilation, are thought to contribute to the pulmonary hypertension seen with CDH. Inhaled nitric oxide (iNO) is a selective pulmonary vasodilator which improves oxygenation and decreases the need for ECMO in neonates with respiratory failure secondary to PPHN. Unfortunately, results in patients with CDH have been discouraging.

When used as a rescue therapy for post-operative infants with CDH and severe respiratory failure, iNO does not improve overall survival or reduce the need for ECMO.[14,15] However, NO may be useful in patients with CDH, as many infants with CDH have pulmonary hypertension and right heart failure that may last for months or longer.[16]

Other management options

In addition to the above-mentioned common management options, other modalities used in CDH include prenatal steroids, fetal surgical interventions, and postnatal surfactant replacement. Data regarding their effectiveness remain mixed and their use is controversial.[3]

ECMO

The first report of the use of ECMO for infants with CDH was by German et al. in 1977.[17] He reported on 4 infants with severe respiratory failure who were placed on ECMO after repair, resulting in one survivor. ECMO was initially used to treat infants with severe hypoxemia after surgical repair of CDH. CDH was treated as an emergent surgical condition in the 1970s and 1980s; hence, the infants who were placed on ECMO post-operatively and often had significant ventilator-induced lung injury. In the late 1980s, the role of pulmonary hypertension in CDH was increasingly recognized, and surgical intervention was delayed until the pulmonary hypertension resolved. As a result of these changes, ECMO is now used as a component in a strategy of pre-operative stabilization, and the majority of infants with CDH who receive ECMO are placed on bypass before surgical correction.[18,19]

ECMO Criteria

ECMO is generally reserved for infants that fail maximal medical management. The expanded use of gentle ventilation and permissive hypercapnea has led some centers to institute ECMO in infants with CDH earlier than it had been in the past in order to avoid ventilator-induced lung injury. The criteria used to determine failure of conventional therapy have changed significantly over the past 20 years. A number of different parameters have been used in an attempt to predict those patients with a high risk of death (Table 1). Currently, the most widely used indication for ECMO is the failure to respond to medical therapy. Clearly, this may vary depending on the center and patient, but strict entry criteria that can accurately predict high mortality for the CDH patient prior to ECMO have not been published.[20-24]

Timing of ECMO

Data from the CDH Study group show that most CDH infants placed on ECMO are cannulated prior to repair. By 2002, data for 2,077 patients with CDH were reviewed, showing that 770 patients (37%) were treated with ECMO. Only 15% of the infants were placed on ECMO after CDH repair. Analysis of trends shows that in 1995, ECMO was used after repair in 20% of the patients as opposed to only 5% in 2001.[25] These data clearly show how ECMO has become a component of pre-operative stabilization as opposed to being a post-operative rescue therapy.

Efficacy of ECMO

ECMO provides effective short-term support for respiratory failure and, therefore, reversibility of the underlying disorder is important when considering ECMO therapy. This fundamental selection criterion presents an interesting dilemma when it comes to infants with CDH. The degree of respiratory failure in CDH depends on the severity of pulmonary hypertension and pulmonary hypoplasia. Pulmonary hypertension is potentially reversible but may persist in some infants and lead to progressive right heart failure. The severity of pulmonary hypoplasia, on the other hand, is variable and will not spontaneously improve substantially in a week or two. These underlying problems appear to result in a less favorable outcome for infants treated with ECMO for CDH as opposed to other diagnoses. The overall survival of infants with CDH reported to the ELSO Registry is about 52% and is lowest among all etiologies of neonatal HRF requiring ECMO. Furthermore, analysis of the ELSO Registry data for neonates requiring ECMO for CDH by Stevens et al. shows that survival has decreased from 64% in 1990 to 52% in 2001.[26] Other studies have shown an improvement in mortality with the use of ECMO.[27,28] The usefulness of ECMO in CDH was examined in two studies which showed similar survival rates, but one used ECMO in 50% of the infants with CDH,

Table 1. ECMO criteria.

Author	Criteria for ECMO
Sebald[20]	OI of >40 for 4 hr. or PaO_2 of <40 for 2 hr.
Boloker[10]	Preductal oxygen saturation <80% refractory to ventilator manipulation
Somaschini[21]	OI >40 or PaO_2 <40
Nagaya[22]	Emergent: OI >40 or PaO_2 <40 or $PaCO_2$ >100 for 2 hr. Preventative: FiO_2 >0.9 or MAP >12 for 24 hr.
vd Staak[23]	A-aDO$_2$ >610 for 8 hr. or OI >40 3/5 consecutive blood gases
Howell[24]	A-aDO$_2$ >610 for 8 hr. or OI >40 for 2 hr.

versus 1% in the other, suggesting that interventions other than ECMO may be responsible for improved outcome.[9,29]

Based on the observations previously described, better selection criteria may improve morbidity and mortality among infants with CDH that require ECMO. Among the factors that determine the outcome of CDH, pulmonary hypoplasia is thought to be the most important. However, the degree of pulmonary hypoplasia is difficult to assess prenatally. Attempts have been made to use alveolar arterial oxygen gradient, best pre-ductal hemoglobin saturations, post-ductal arterial PaO_2, and the severity of hypercarbia during the stabilization period. Based on different combinations of the above-mentioned parameters, some centers have developed algorithms for stratifying infants and offer ECMO only to infants who have the best chance of survival (Table 1).

However, because CDH is a disease with a wide spectrum of severity and medical stabilization strategies differ among centers, comparing outcomes remains difficult and controversial. The CDH Study Group has been working since 1995 to develop treatment-independent risk assessment tools to allow accurate comparisons of outcome between centers according to the severity of the disease. Several factors that are available to the clinician in the first 5 minutes such as gender, race, birth weight, Apgar scores, immediate distress, CPR, estimated gestational age (EGA), side of hernia, and prenatal diagnosis have been considered. Of these, birth weight and Apgar scores were found to be the most predictive of outcome. Based on these, a logistic regression equation that estimates the severity of CDH has been published.[1] Applying this equation, a 74% survival in the low-risk group as opposed to 16% in the high-risk group was seen. However, other investigators were unable to confirm these results.[30] Furthermore, the 5-minute Apgar score may not be available as the infant is intubated immediately.

Mode of ECMO in CDH

Traditionally, infants with CDH requiring ECMO have been placed on venoarterial (VA) ECMO. This practice was based largely on the belief that these infants are hemodynamically unstable and do not tolerate venovenous (VV) ECMO. Additionally, concerns about inadequate venous drainage and insufficient oxygen delivery when compared to VA ECMO further reinforced the notion that VA ECMO was the mode of choice in infants with CDH. However, several studies have found VV to be an acceptable initial mode of ECMO for infants with CDH.[31-33] Based on concerns about inadequate venous drainage, there has been a bias to place infants with right-sided CDH on VA ECMO. However, Dimmitt et al. found no difference between right- and left-sided hernias in regard to failure of VV ECMO and the need for conversion to VA.[33] Furthermore, infants who did fail VV and had to be converted to VA ECMO did not have worse outcomes than those who were placed on VA ECMO initially. Based on these studies, it would be prudent to assume that many infants with CDH can be treated with VV ECMO if an adequately sized VV cannula can be placed. Interestingly, Frenckner et al. found that infants with CDH tend to have smaller veins than other infants, which would make cannula placement for VV ECMO more difficult.[34] However, it is not clear if vessel size has played a role in the greater use of VA ECMO in CDH.

CDH surgery on ECMO

The question of optimal timing to repair the defect surfaced when ECMO was used as a part of pre-operative stabilization. Operations on ECMO are high risk because of the potential for anticoagulation-induced bleeding complications. Early reports of surgical repair on ECMO reported significant hemorrhagic complications.[35] Infants who develop significant bleeding while on ECMO have a low survival rate. However, studies have shown that operations can be performed safely and significant bleeding can be avoided as long as the circuit coagulation status is monitored closely. Aminocaproic acid, an inhibitor of fibrinolysis, has been used in ECMO patients that are at high risk for bleeding. In a study by Downard et al., only 5% of infants treated with aminocaproic acid required re-exploration for bleeding on ECMO as opposed to 26% of patients who were not treated.[36] Many centers now use aminocaproic acid in addition to stricter control of circuit coagulation status for infants undergoing surgery for CDH on ECMO. Since aminocaproic acid is an inhibitor of fibrinolysis, the potential complication of its use is increased clot formation and thrombotic complications, including the need for circuit change. However, Downard et al. found that although use of animocaproic acid was associated with an increased need for circuit change, it has no effect on large vessel thrombosis or cerebral infaction.[36]

The optimal time for repair of CDH on ECMO support is unclear. This question has not been critically analyzed, resulting in significant variations among centers. Data from the CDH Study Group shows that of the infants placed on ECMO prior to surgery, 54% were repaired on ECMO as opposed to 30% following ECMO; 16% never underwent repair and all expired.[37] Survival was 83% in infants repaired after ECMO, compared to 49% in those repaired on ECMO. Additionally, the length of hospital stay was shorter (64 vs. 76 days) and need for oxygen lower (56% vs. 64%) among infants repaired after ECMO when compared to those who were repaired on ECMO. In those patients who did undergo repair on ECMO, the timing of operation varied, ranging from repair in the first 24 hours to over 3 weeks. Not surprisingly, infants who were repaired later had lower survival. At the University of Texas Health Science Center at Houston, infants are repaired on ECMO once they have achieved dry weight. If the infants are at or near their dry weights at the time of instituting ECMO, they are repaired within a few days; otherwise, the procedure is delayed until after adequate diuresis.

Long-term outcome of infants with CDH treated with ECMO

Over the past decade, long-term morbidity among survivors of CDH has been increasingly recognized. Infants with CDH placed on ECMO prior to repair appear to have a much higher risk and greater severity of neurological morbidity. Gastroesophageal reflux (GER) is an extremely common finding among CDH survivors and has been reported in 50% of the patients in some series. In one series of patients followed for up to 10 years, a high incidence of nutritional problems was reported, including GER, failure to thrive, and severe oral aversion requiring gastrostomy tube placement.[38,39] Infants with CDH also have greater need for surgical management of GER. In the previous study,[38] 21% of the infants required fundoplication with the highest incidence (68%) among infants that required patch repair of the diaphragmatic defect. Additionally, hernia recurrence has been reported in survivors with increasing frequency and appears to be more prevalent in infants who required a synthetic patch.[39]

An area of major concern for CDH survivors, especially among those that require ECMO for stabilization, is the neurological outcome. There is growing concern that infants with CDH treated with ECMO have a worse neurological outcome when compared to infants that were not treated with ECMO and other non-CDH ECMO-treated patients. Stolar et al. found that 89% of infants treated with ECMO for indications other than CDH were cognitively normal. In contrast, only 60% of infants with CDH treated with ECMO had a normal cognitive outcome.[40] McGahern et al. showed a survival rate of 75% among infants with CDH that were treated with ECMO, of which 67% exhibited signs of neurological compromise.[41] Based on these findings, it has been suggested that the poor neurological outcome may be a function of the severity of the illness, although independent ECMO factors could not be excluded. The U.K. Collaborative ECMO Trial Group reported the 4-year follow-up for infants with CDH in the trial.[42] There were 4 survivors in the ECMO group, but at follow-up, 1 had died and another had severe disability. However, there were no survivors in the control group. Davis et al. reported on the infants with CDH treated with ECMO in the U.K. between 1991- 2000. During this period, 73 infants with CDH were supported with ECMO. Of these, only 46 (63%) were able to wean off ECMO, 42 (56%) survived to hospital discharge and only 27 (37%) survived one year or longer. Of the 27 survivors, only 7 infants were problem-free.[43] These are sobering numbers and add fuel to the growing uncertainty about the utility of ECMO in the CDH infant. Stevens et al. found that over time the length of the ECMO run and the number of complications has increased.[44] The reason for this change is not clear, but the authors suggested that perhaps improvements in ventilator management has led to the sicker infants being placed on ECMO; hence, the longer runs and higher rate of complications. These observations should lead to renewed effort towards redefining the role of ECMO. Specifically, better selection criteria are likely to improve the survival and morbidity rates. Until such time, the role of ECMO will remain controversial for the infant with CDH.

Summary

Infants with CDH may present with severe respiratory that may be unresponsive to medical management and require ECMO for survival. Over the years the role of ECMO in CDH has evolved and is now used as part of lung protective strategy to prevent ventilator-induced lung injury. In spite of greater advances in the management of infants on ECMO, survival rate for infants with CDH treated with ECMO remains the lowest. Additionally, long-term, severe morbidity among survivors remains high. ECMO centers have developed selection criteria to better identify infants with CDH in whom ECMO will be most beneficial. However, selection algorithms that are reliable and reproducible remain elusive.

References

1. The Congenital Diaphragmatic Hernia Study Group. Estimating disease severity of congenital diaphragmatic hernia in the first 5 minutes of life. *J Pediatr Surg* 2001; 36:141-145.

2. Narayan H, De Chazal R, Barrow M, McKeever P, Neale E. Familial congenital diaphragmatic hernia: prenatal diagnosis, management, and outcome. *Prenat Diagn* 1993; 13:893-901.

3. Lally KP. Congenital diaphragmatic hernia. *Curr Opin Pediatr* 2002; 14:486-490.

4. Babiuk RP, Greer JJ. Diaphragm defects occur in a CDH hernia model independently of myogenesis and lung formation. *Am J Physiol Lung Cell Mol Physiol* 2002; 283: L1310-1314.

5. Huddy CL, Boyd PA, Wilkinson AR, Chamberlain P. Congenital diaphragmatic hernia: prenatal diagnosis, outcome and continuing morbidity in survivors. *Br J Obstet Gynaecol* 1999; 106:1192-1196.

6. Drummond WH, Gregory GA, Heymann MA, Phibbs RA. The independent effects of hyperventilation, tolazoline, and dopamine on infants with persistent pulmonary hypertension. *J Pediatr* 1981; 98:603-611.

7. Wung JT, Sahni R, Moffitt ST, Lipsitz E, Stolar CJ. Congenital diaphragmatic hernia: survival treated with very delayed surgery, spontaneous respiration and no chest tube. *J Pediatr Surg* 1995; 30:406-409.

8. Kays DW, Langham MR, Ledbetter DJ, Talbert JL. Detrimental effects of standard

medical therapy in congenital diaphragmatic hernia. *Ann Surg* 1999; 230:340-351.

9. Wilson JM, Lund DP, Lillehei CW, Vacanti JP. Congenital diaphragmatic hernia--a tale of two cities: the Boston experience. *J Pediatr Surg* 1997; 32:401-405.

10. Boloker J, Bateman DA, Wung JT, Stolar CJ. Congenital diaphragmatic hernia in 120 infants treated consecutively with permissive hypercapnea/spontaneous respiration/elective repair. *J Pediatr Surg* 2002; 37:357-366.

11. Paranka MS, Clark RH, Yoder BA, Null DM Jr. Predictors of failure of high-frequency oscillatory ventilation in term infants with severe respiratory failure. *Pediatrics* 1995; 95:400-404.

12. Reyes C, Chang LK, Waffarn F, Mir H, Warden MJ, Sills J. Delayed repair of congenital diaphragmatic hernia with early high-frequency oscillatory ventilation during preoperative stabilization. *J Pediatr Surg* 1998; 33:1010-1014.

13. Cacciari A, Ruggeri G, Mordenti M, et al. High-frequency oscillatory ventilation versus conventional mechanical ventilation in congenital diaphragmatic hernia. *Eur J Pediatr Surg* 2001; 11:3-7.

14. Clark RH, Kueser TJ, Walker MW, et al. Low-dose nitric oxide therapy for persistent pulmonary hypertension of the newborn. Clinical Inhaled Nitric Oxide Research Group. *N Engl J Med* 2000; 342:469-474.

15. Finer NN, Barrington KJ. Nitric oxide for respiratory failure in infants born at or near term. *Cochrane Database Syst Rev* 2001; 4: CD000399.

16. Dillon PW, Cilley RE, Hudome SM, Ozkan EN, Krummel TM. Nitric oxide reversal of recurrent pulmonary hypertension and respiratory failure in an infant with CDH after successful ECMO therapy. *J Pediatr Surg* 1995; 30:743-744.

17. German JC, Gazzaniga AB, Amlie R, Huxtable RF, Bartlett RH. Management of pulmonary insufficiency in diaphragmatic hernia using extracorporeal circulation with a membrane oxygenator (ECMO). *J Pediatr Surg* 1977; 12:905-912.

18. Haugen SE, Linker D, Eik-Nes S, et al. Congenital diaphragmatic hernia: determination of the optimal time for operation by echocardiographic monitoring of the pulmonary arterial pressure. *J Pediatr Surg* 1991; 26:560-562.

19. West KW, Bengston K, Rescorla FJ, Engle WA, Grosfeld JL. Delayed surgical repair and ECMO improves survival in congenital diaphragmatic hernia. *Ann Surg* 1992; 216:454-460.

20. Sebald M, Friedlich P, Burns C, et al. Risk of need for extracorporeal membrane oxygenation support in neonates with congenital diaphragmatic hernia treated with inhaled nitric oxide. *J Perinatol* 2004; 24:143-146.

21. Somaschini M, Locatelli G, Salvoni L, Bellan C, Colombo A. Impact of new treatments for respiratory failure on outcome of infants with congenital diaphragmatic hernia. *Eur J Pediatr* 1999; 158:780-784.

22. Nagaya M, Kato J, Niimi N, Tanaka S, Tanaka T. Analysis of patients with congenital diaphragmatic hernia requiring pre-operative extracorporeal membrane oxygenation (ECMO). *Pediatr Surg Int* 1998; 14:25-29.

23. vd Staak FH, Thiesbrummel A, de Haan AF, Oeseburg B, Geven WB, Festen C. Do we use the right entry criteria for extracorporeal membrane oxygenation in congenital diaphragmatic hernia? *J Pediatr Surg* 1993; 28:1003-1005.

24. Howell CG, Hatley RM, Boedy RF, Rogers DM, Kanto WP, Parrish RA. Recent experience with diaphragmatic hernia and ECMO. *Ann Surg* 1990; 211:793-797.

25. Lally KP, The Congenital Diaphragmatic Hernia Study Group. The use of ECMO for stabilization of infants with Congenital

Diaphragmatic Hernia – A Report of the CDH Study Group (Abstract). In: Surgical Section of the American Academy of Pediatrics; October 19-23, 2002; Boston, MA.

26. ELSO Registry. Ann Arbor, MI: Extracoporeal Life Support Organization; 2004.

27. Finer NN, Tierney AJ, Hallgren R, Hayashi A, Peliowski A, Etches PC. Neonatal congenital diaphragmatic hernia and extracorporeal membrane oxygenation. *CMAJ* 1992; 146:501-508.

28. D'Agostino JA, Bernbaum JC, Gerdes M, et al. Outcome for infants with congenital diaphragmatic hernia requiring extracorporeal membrane oxygenation: the first year. *J Pediatr Surg* 1995; 30:10-15.

29. Azarow K, Messineo A, Pearl R, Filler R, Barker G,. Bohn D. Congenital diaphragmatic hernia--a tale of two cities: the Toronto experience. *J Pediatr Surg* 1997; 32:395-400.

30. Downard CD, Jaksic T, Garza JJ, et al. Analysis of an improved survival rate for congenital diaphragmatic hernia. *J Pediatr Surg* 2003; 38:729-732.

31. Cornish JD, Heiss KF, Clark RH, Strieper MJ, Boecler B, Kesser K. Efficacy of venovenous extracorporeal membrane oxygenation for neonates with respiratory and circulatory compromise. *J Pediatr* 1993; 122:105-109.

32. Heiss KF, Clark RH, Cornish JD, et al. Preferential use of venovenous extracorporeal membrane oxygenation for congenital diaphragmatic hernia. *J Pediatr Surg* 1995; 30:416-419.

33. Dimmitt RA, Moss RL, Rhine WD, Benitz WE, Henry MC, Van Meurs KP. Venoarterial versus venovenous extracorporeal membrane oxygenation in congenital diaphragmatic hernia: the Extracorporeal Life Support Organization Registry, 1990-1999. *J Pediatr Surg* 2001; 36:1199-1204.

34. Frenckner B, Palmer K, Linden V. Neonates with congenital diaphragmatic hernia have smaller neck veins than other neonates-An alternative route for ECMO cannulation. *J Pediatr Surg* 2002; 37:906-908.

35. Lally KP, Paranka MS, Roden J, et al. Congenital diaphragmatic hernia. Stabilization and repair on ECMO. *Ann Surg* 1992; 216:569-573.

36. Downard CD, Betit P, Chang RW, Garza JJ, Arnold JH, Wilson JM. Impact of AMICAR on hemorrhagic complications of ECMO: a ten-year review. *J Pediatr Surg* 2003; 38:1212-1216.

37. Clark RH, Hardin WD Jr, Hirschl RB, et al. Current surgical management of congenital diaphragmatic hernia: a report from the Congenital Diaphragmatic Hernia Study Group. *J Pediatr Surg* 1998; 33:1004-1009.

38. Muratore CS, Utter S, Jaksic T, Lund DP, Wilson JM. Nutritional morbidity in survivors of congenital diaphragmatic hernia. *J Pediatr Surg* 2001; 36:1171-1176.

39. Cortes RA, Keller RL, Townsend T, et al. Survival of severe congenital diaphragmatic hernia has morbid consequences. *J Pediatr Surg* 2005; 40:36-45.

40. Stolar CJ. What do survivors of congenital diaphragmatic hernia look like when they grow up? *Semin Pediatr Surg* 1996; 5:275-279.

41. McGahren ED, Mallik K, Rodgers BM. Neurological outcome is diminished in survivors of congenital diaphragmatic hernia requiring extracorporeal membrane oxygenation. *J Pediatr Surg* 1997; 32:1216-1220.

42. Bennett CC, Johnson A, Field DJ; UK Collaborative ECMO Trial Group. UK collaborative randomised trial of neonatal extracorporeal membrane oxygenation: follow-up to age 4 years. *Lancet* 2001; 357:1094-1096.

43. Davis PJ, Firmin RK, Manktelow B, et al. Long-term outcome following extracorporeal membrane oxygenation for congenital

diaphragmatic hernia: the UK experience. *J Pediatr* 2004; 144:309-315.

44. Stevens TP, Chess PR, McConnochie KM, et al. Survival in early- and late-term infants with congenital diaphragmatic hernia treated with extracorporeal membrane oxygenation. *Pediatrics* 2002; 110:590-596.

20

Neonatal ECMO and the Brain

Billie Lou Short, M.D. and Dorothy Bulas, M.D.

Introduction

ECMO therapy has significantly improved outcome in the newborn with respiratory and cardiac failure. However, morbidity and mortality related to intracranial injury is significant for this population, with the reported frequency of abnormal neuroimaging ranging from 28-52%, depending on techniques and methods of classification.[1-6] This is not unexpected, as most patients are placed on ECMO due to severe hypoxemia from respiratory failure or decreased oxygen delivery from cardiac failure. As ECMO becomes standard clinical practice for infants with respiratory failure, investigations into the outcome of these children must focus not only on survival, but also on the cause of morbidity. A further understanding of factors associated with intracranial injury may allow ECLS techniques to be modified to improve long-term outcome allowing the expansion of these technologies to other populations such as the premature infant.

Pre-ECMO risk factors

Risk factors prior to ECMO associated with cerebral injury include profound hypoxia and acidosis, with many experiencing vasomotor shock and decreased perfusion. Most ECMO infants have experienced some amount of pro-found hypoxia (from hours to days), making it one of the greatest risk factors in the development of cerebral injury. The brain responds to hypoxia by increasing cerebral blood flow (CBF), which maintains cerebral oxygen transport (OT) and cerebral oxygen metabolism ($CMRO_2$).[7] Although mild forms of hypoxia can be tolerated without extensive cerebral injury, prolonged periods of severe hypoxia can result in a loss of cerebral autoregulation leading to a loss of the ability for the brain to maintain OT and $CMRO_2$, and thus, result in brain injury. Several physiologic changes, including asphyxia, hypoxia, and hypercarbia, can all disrupt cerebral autoregulation leaving the cerebral microcirculation vulnerable to alterations in systemic blood pressure.[8-11] In this setting, hypotension can result in ischemic brain injury, whereas hypertension can cause cerebral hyperemia and thus increase the risk for cerebral hemorrhage. Loss of autoregulation in an already injured brain in the presence of systemic heparinization, such as occurs with ECMO, can result in cerebral hemorrhage. Tweed et al. and Short et al. have demonstrated in the newborn lamb that exposure to prolonged hypoxia results in the loss of cerebral autoregulation during the recovery phase from hypoxia.[12,13] In the study by Tweed et al., a 20-minute exposure to a PaO_2 of 30 mm Hg resulted in a loss of cerebral autoregulation for 6 hours following the hypoxic insult. Short et al. exposed newborn lambs to 2 hours of severe hypoxia (SaO_2 = 40%) with carotid artery and jugular vein ligation, simulating the hypoxia seen in patients pre-ECMO. Cerebral autoregulation was evaluated 1 hour after hypoxic insult and was found to be abnormal. When hypoxia recovery was simulated by placing the study animal on ECMO instead of increasing FiO_2 in the ventilator, the effect on cerebral autoregulation was even more profound (Figure 1). At a cerebral perfusion pressure level where CBF decreased, $CMRO_2$ was also decreased, indicating a concerning potential for cerebral injury.

Ashwal et al. has shown in the fetal lamb that the hyperemic post-hypoxia state lasts 4 hours after recovery from hypoxia.[14] These animal studies indicate that the brain may be vulnerable to further insults such as hypotension and/or hypertension during the recovery period from severe hypoxia, and that this high risk period

can be prolonged. The lengths of exposure to hypoxia were relatively short in these studies, causing greater concern for the actual length of vulnerability in the ECMO patient who has been exposed to hours or days of hypoxia.

Respiratory management of these patients, typically involves the two extremes (i.e., hyperventilation or gentle ventilation with hypercapnia) and places these infants at risk for intracranial injury. Although controversial, hyperventilation is still used in some infants with pulmonary hypertension.[15] Several animal studies which evaluated the effect of hyperventilation on the brain, demonstrating an initial decrease of CBF by 20-30%, with normalization of the CBF after 4-6 hours of hyperventilation. Gleason et al. demonstrated this same effect with hyperventilation in the newborn lamb, and extended the study to include the post-hyperventilation period.[16] In this model, after 6 hours of hyperventilation, animals were made acutely normocarbic, simulating what happens when placing an infant on ECMO. At this point, extreme hyperemia occurred, with an increase in CBF of 104%. This hyperemia persisted for the remaining 90 minutes of the study. Since the study did not extend beyond this time period, the exact period needed to normalize the CBF after normalization of $PaCO_2$ is undetermined. As a result of this study, the current clinical practice is to normalize the patient's $PaCO_2$ over a 24 hr. period; the exact period needed to accomplish this safely remains unknown. Hino et al. studied the effect on CBF of acute normalization of $PaCO_2$ after exposure to prolonged hypercapnia in the newborn lamb.[17] It was hypothesized that this might induce a period of cerebral ischemia. Although CBF normally increases dramatically during hypercarbia, normalization of $PaCO_2$ does not result in ischemia. These findings were reassuring, and many centers are now modifying respiratory management to include a "gentle ventilation" or hypercapnic approach to pre-ECMO therapy. However, this study looked only at CBF, and not the effect of prolonged hypercarbia on cerebral autoregulation.

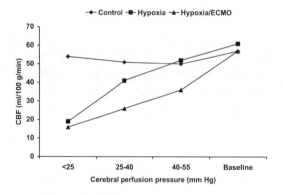

Figure 1. Lower end of an autoregulation curve in newborn lambs after 2 hrs. exposure to hypoxia (SaO_2 40%). Control animals ◆ maintain autoregulation to a cerebral perfusion pressure (CPP) of 25 mm Hg, while animals exposed to hypoxia and then recovered by turning the ventilator FiO_2 to maintain normoxia ■ lost autoregulation at a CPP of 25-39 mm Hg ($P \leq 0.05$). Animals recovered using ECMO to maintain normoxia ▲ lost autoregulation at a CPP of 40-55 mm Hg ($P \leq 0.05$). (Reprinted with permission, Short BL. *Semin Perinatol* 2005; 29:45-50.)

ECMO risk factors

A risk for cerebral injury is introduced by various aspects of the ECMO procedure itself. These include, cannulation and ligation of the carotid artery for venoarterial (VA) ECMO and jugular vein for both VA and venovenous (VV) ECMO, exposure to systemic heparinization, alteration of blood flow dynamics, micro particles including plastics and thrombi dislodging from the circuit, and exposure to high levels of the plasticizer, di-(2-ethylhexyl) phthalate (DEHP).[18] Using near infrared spectrophotometry, Liem et al. demonstrated in patients on ECMO increased cerebral blood volume, loss of autoregulation, reactive hyperperfusion, and hemodilution.[19] Doppler studies of the pericallosal artery in infants on VA ECMO showed a significant change in diastolic flow velocities (Figure 2), representing the effect of the non-pulsatile flow from the ECMO pump. In a study conducted by Taylor et al. in VA ECMO infants, cerebral blood flow changes were compared to left ventricular output data; left ventricular output decreased as the pump flows were increased, resulting in a decrease in the anterior cerebral artery pulsatility index.[20-21] These findings are related to the fact that the cardiac support provided by the pump is non-pulsatile. These changes are not seen in VV ECMO, where cardiac support is not provided.[22] The effect of this altered blood flow pattern on the brain is not fully understood, but it may play a role in the altered cerebral autoregulation seen in VA ECMO patients.

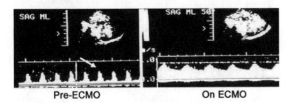

Figure 2. Doppler flow changes seen in the pericallosal artery of a pre-ECMO infant while on ECMO. The increase in diastolic flow is secondary to flow from the non-pulsatile ECMO pump.

Animal studies

Initial findings by Short et al. regarding the acute effects of VA ECMO initiation on the brain did not find altered CBF, $CMRO_2$, cerebral OT, or cerebral oxygen extraction.[23] These studies were conducted at ECMO flows of 150 ml/kg/min. Studies by Rosenberg and Kinsella at ECMO flow rates <100 ml/kg/min showed a drop in CBF.[24] The difference in ECMO flow rate may be responsible for the variance in the findings.

In a study by Hunter et al. the CBF of lambs was measured by laser Doppler flowmetry during VA and VV ECMO. Carotid ligation resulted in a decrease in the CBF to the right cerebral cortex.[25] However, this decrease was transient (60 seconds) and was associated with an elevation of cerebral resistance. With VV ECMO, no change in CBF was observed.[25] Studies by Short et al. using a lamb model did not show ligation of either the carotid artery or jugular vein to have any effect on CBF following exposure to 4 hours of hypoxia.[20]

In the newborn, VA ECMO lamb model, Walker et al. found that the CO_2 reactivity of the brain was preserved while on VA ECMO.[26] Short et al. evaluated the effect on cerebral autoregulation of exposure to VA ECMO in the same lamb model.[27] Exposure to VA ECMO for 1 hour in the healthy newborn lamb resulted in an alteration of cerebral autoregulation. As with hypoxia, right to left blood flow differences were seen in this study when CBF decreased. Although alternations in autoregulation were seen in VV ECMO, they were less severe than those seen in VA ECMO, and no right to left CBF differences were noted.[28] Martinez-Orgado et al. have shown in the newborn piglet that cerebral autoregulation is endothelial-dependent with nitric oxide and calcium-activated potassium channels involved in vasodilation, and endothelial cells and prostanoids involved in vasoconstriction during pressure increase.[29]

Further studies by Short et al. on isolated vessel chamber studies have shown that VA ECMO significantly alters vessel reactivity to acetylcholine (an endothelial-dependent vasodilator), while VV ECMO does not (Figure 3). The vasoconstrictive effect of exposure to N^G-nitro-L-arginine methyl ester (L-NAME), a potent blocker of nitric oxide (NO) production, was markedly blunted in cerebral arteries in study animals exposed to VA ECMO vs. controls with normal pulsatility (Figure 4).[30-31] These findings indicate that the flow and shear stress changes in VA ECMO may alter endothelial reactivity through alterations in the NO pathway. This alteration may be responsible for the changes in autoregulation seen in the VA ECMO animals. This hypothesis has been corroborated by findings that the altered vessel reactivity can be returned to normal after exposure to a NO donor. Other studies have noted endothelial dysfunction in a hypothermic lamb model of cardiopulmonary bypass.[32] Autoregulation changes in a piglet model studied by Martinez-Orgado et al. were shown to be related to endothelial alterations caused by pressure changes.[29] Preckel et al. demonstrated an altered autoregulatory response after NO blockage in their rat model, implicating endothelial dysfunction.[33]

Human studies

There has been concern that ligation of the carotid artery may cause lateralizing cerebrovascular injury. Several early, small studies noted an increase in injuries to the right hemisphere in infants who underwent ligation of the right carotid artery.[34-36] In a larger series by Adolph et al. and Bulas et al. neuroimaging showed no evidence of lateralization.[6,37] In a series of 355 infants using ultrasound, CT, MRI, or clinical evaluation, Graziani et al. also demonstrated no selective or greater injury to the right hemisphere as compared with the left.[38] In a cohort of 31 infants treated with ECMO and evaluated by MRI, there was also no lateralization of major brain lesions.[39] Focal brain lesions were, however, significantly associated with an asymmetric cerebrovascular response to carotid ligation of the right vs. left middle cerebral artery as detected by magnetic resonance angiography (P<0.5).[39] Schumacher et al. has argued that the absence of lateralization of lesions among ECMO-treated neonates is indicative of increased vulnerability of the right hemisphere, since reports of intraventricular hemorrhage and stroke in non-ECMO patients indicate increased vulnerability of the left hemisphere.[5]

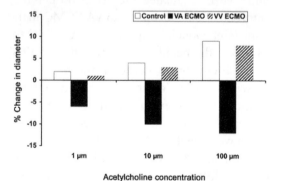

Figure 3. The effect of intraluminal acetylcholine infusion on vascular diameter in control, non-pulsatile (VA) and pulsatile (VV) ECMO. Vasodilation is noted in the vessels from the control and VV ECMO animals with vasoconstriction in vessels exposed to VA or non-pulsatile ECMO indicating altered endothelial reactivity. (Reprinted with permission, Short BL. *Semin Perinatol* 2005; 29:45-50.)

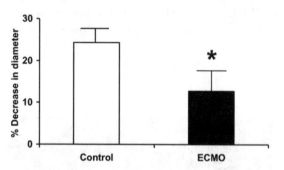

Figure 4. The effect of the intraluminal infusion of L-NAME on vascular diameter in control and non-pulsatile VA ECMO animals. Control animals had a significant vasoconstrictive response compared to animals exposed to VA ECMO (P<0.05) indicating an altered production of NO in the vessels of animals exposed to VA ECMO.[31]

Neuroimaging findings in neonatal ECMO patients

It is believed that premature infants on ECMO are at an increased risk of intracranial hemorrhage due to the presence of a friable germinal matrix with poor supporting stroma.[1,2] Studies have shown that younger infants continue to have a statistically significant increased risk of hemorrhage up to a gestational age of 38 weeks. Notably, only 27% of the hemorrhages originated in the germinal matrix.[6] Although regions of ischemia are at risk for hemorrhage when heparin is used, infarcts in term infants weighing >3 kg typically do not progress into hemorrhages.

Infants with sepsis are also at a high risk for intracranial hemorrhage, possibly due to additional problems with coagulopathy.[40] In a series by Hardart et al. gestational age, sepsis, coagulopathy, and acidosis were all associated with a higher incidence of intracranial hemorrhage.[41,42] Dela Cruz et al. demonstrated that prolonged ACT and low platelet count were also associated with an increase in intracranial hemorrhages.[43] Infants with long ECMO runs, particularly those with CDH, have the highest rate of major non-hemorrhagic lesions. However, with more conservative use of heparin, the risk of partial venous occlusion and microemboli has been shown to increase.[6,44]

Widened interhemispheric fissures have been described in infants on ECMO, with rates as high as 59% (Figure 5).[3,45] Rubin et al. believed this dilatation to be intracranial manifestation of generalized edema.[46] Other authors have suggested that increased sagittal sinus pressure associated with internal jugular vein ligation and cannulation of the superior vena cava is the cause due to decreased cerebrospinal fluid resorption of the arachnoid villi.[47] Widened extra axial space can develop as well, with severe cases noted following superior vena cava thrombosis.[48] VV ECMO tends to result in decreased venous drainage and an increased incidence of dilated interhemispheric fissure and prominent subarach-noid space.[49] Due to the potential risk of venous stasis, cephalic drainage has been used to help prevent neurologic complications by maintaining normal cerebral blood flow and increasing ECMO oxygen delivery.[50]

Ultrasound

Ultrasound is particularly useful in the evaluation of infants on ECMO due to its portability and lack of ionizing radiation. The presence of a large intracranial hemorrhage is a contraindication for ECMO initiation; thus, a screening exam prior to cannulation is critical in the assessment of potential therapeutic options. Ultrasound has been sensitive in the evaluation of large cranial hemorrhages. In a series by Bulas et al. sonography successfully identified 46 of 49 major intracranial hemorrhages, the lesions which have the greatest impact on the infant's acute management.[51] Isolated subependymal hemorrhages have not shown progression and should not prevent the initiation of ECMO therapy.[52]

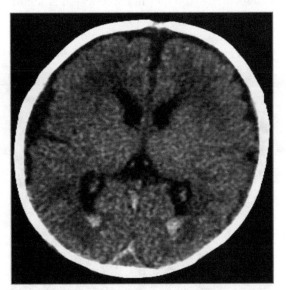

Figure 5. Axial CT image demonstrating mild prominence of the interhemispheric fissure. There is some intraventricular hemorrhage within the occipital lobes bilaterally.

The risk of intracranial hemorrhage is greatest in the first few days on ECMO; therefore, daily cranial sonograms are recommended to rule out evolving intracranial hemorrhage. There is some question as to how long daily sonograms should be performed and this has been reviewed by several centers. In 1996, Biehl found daily sonograms to be cost effective only during the first 3 days on ECMO.[53] In their series, 50% of intracranial hemorrhages occurred in the first 24 hours, 75% by 48 hours, and 85% within 72 hours of initiation of ECMO. Further sonograms were deemed unnecessary unless there was a change in neurological status or multi-organ failure. Khan et al. suggested performing cranial sonograms for the first 5 days on ECMO unless a clinical suspicion was raised.[54]

Large parenchymal hemorrhages are usually identified by ultrasound as focal regions of increased echogenicity (Figure 6).[51] With less than 30% of hemorrhages developing in the germinal matrix, it is crucial to look carefully within the peripheral parenchyma and posterior fossa for unusual regions of increased or decreased echogenicity. If a questionable lesion is identified, close follow-up is needed as these bleeds can increase rapidly in size. Hemorrhages may appear hypoechogenic due to prolonged clotting time and lack of clot formation.

In a series of 117 infants with sonographic or CT evidence of hemorrhage, 64% were parenchymal with 8.5% extraaxial.[30] The most common site for a parenchymal bleed was the cerebellum (27%). Cerebellar hemorrhages can be difficult to identify by ultrasound via the anterior fontanelle. A transmastoid view or imaging via the posterior fontanelle may improve the sonogram's ability to detect these hemorrhages.[55]

Ultrasound is less effective in identifying nonhemorrhagic lesions. Cerebral edema can be difficult to differentiate from the normal state, and Doppler tracings are not useful in the assessment of autoregulation as pulsatility is diminished on VA bypass. Despite these limitations, early screening has been used to identify infants with severe cerebral edema. Von Allmen et al. noted that 63% of infants with evidence of severe edema on pre-ECMO sonograms had a subsequent major intracranial complication (Figure 7).[56] Infarcts, small parenchymal hemorrhages, and extraaxial collections may not be visible on the sonogram. Sonographic

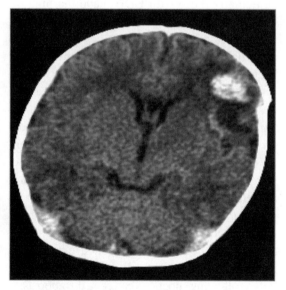

Figure 7. Axial CT demonstrating a moderate sized parenchymal hemorrhagic infarct in the left frontal lobe with some surrounding edema. There is no mass affect.

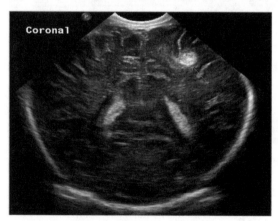

Figure 6. Coronal ultrasound image demonstrating a focal region of increased echogenicity in the left parietal lobe.

distinction between hemorrhagic and ischemic lesions is difficult, as both can be echogenic (Figure 8).

CT and MRI

Numerous studies have demonstrated the superiority of CT and/or MRI in the identification of nonhemorrhagic and small hemorrhagic lesions. CT scans contributed additional information in 73% of neonates with intracranial abnormalities in a series of 286 infants.[51] Of these patients 17 with major lesions went unidentified by ultrasound (Figure 9). Garber et al. noted that in ultrasounds reported as normal, abnormalities were identified by CT in 6.8%.[57]

Follow-up CT/MRI scans provide additional information in 72-93% of ECMO patients initially scanned with ultrasound.[47,51,58,59] In a series of 130 infants with nonhemorrhagic abnormalities, the majority of abnormalities missed by sonography were classified as minor. However, 6 infarcts, 3 diffuse periventricular hypodensities, and 5 moderate atrophies were demonstrated only by CT (Figure 10). Other series have also demonstrated that CT is particularly useful in identifying infarcts, diffuse edema, and atrophy in infants with normal head sonograms.[60]

MRI can provide unique information at follow-up evaluation. Magnetic resonance angiography (MRA) has demonstrated asymmetric cerebrovascular response to carotid ligation of

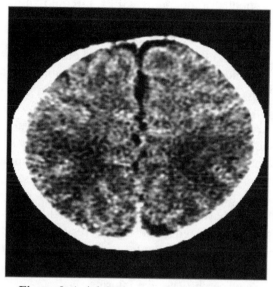

Figure 9. Axial CT image of bilateral parietal edema from ischemia. The ultrasounds were normal.

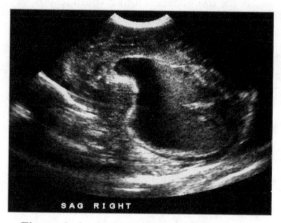

Figure 8. Sagittal ultrasound image demonstrating a large hypoechogenic lesion in the occipital lobe consistent with a large hematoma in a septic infant on ECMO.

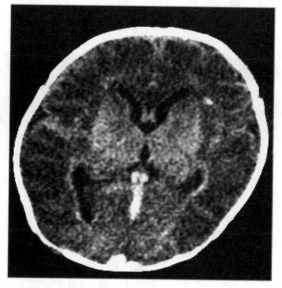

Figure 10. Axial CT image demonstrates diffuse edema with several small, scattered petechial hemorrhages.

the right vs. left middle cerebral artery (MCA).[39] Cerebral proton magnetic resonance spectroscopy has been used to assess potential changes in brain metabolism following carotid ligation.[40] It was hoped that single photon emission computed tomography (SPECT) could show deficits not seen by neuroimaging.[61] However, in a series by Kumar et al. a normal SPECT scan was likely to predict normal outcome but an abnormal SPECT did not predict abnormal outcome.[62] In a recent study using proton magnetic resonance imaging and spectroscopy, 9 neonates were evaluated following ECMO and no difference in right or left basal ganglia was noted, suggesting that ligation of the carotid artery did not produce persistent changes in brain metabolism in the basal ganglia.[40] Larger studies have not yet been reported. As diffusion weighted imaging and higher Tesla scanners become more available, further information may be obtained for the assessment of ECMO-related cerebrovascular injuries.

Conclusion

ECMO is clearly a lifesaving therapy for the newborn infant. The risks for intracranial injury are related both to pre-ECMO events including profound hypoxia and cardiovascular shock and to the ECMO procedure itself, which causes shear-stress changes in blood flow patterns that appear to alter cerebral vascular reactivity and thus, place the patient at risk for cerebral injury. If animal study findings can be extrapolated to the newborn, cerebral circulation may be pressure passive, at least during the initiation of ECMO and treatment of marked blood pressure changes should be undertaken during this period. Concerns have been raised that carotid ligation would result in right-sided cerebral ischemia, but neuroimaging data in this population does not corroborate these concerns. Findings such as widened interhemispheric fissure and posterior fossa hemorrhages do raise concern for a venous obstructive phenomenon

in this population, particularly with VV ECMO. Continued follow-up of the ECMO population with neuroimaging studies in the adolescent population are key to determining the long-term risk of such an event.

References

1. Cilley RE, Zwischenberger JB, Andrews AF, Bowerman RA, Roloff DW, Bartlett RH. Intracranial hemorrhage during extracorporeal membrane oxygenation in neonates. *Pediatrics* 1986; 78:699-704.

2. Sell LL, Cullen ML, Whittlesey GC, et al. Hemorrhagic complications during extracorporeal membrane oxygenation: prevention and treatment. *J Pediatr Surg* 1986; 21:1087-1091.

3. Canady AI, Fessler RD, Klein MD. Ultrasound abnormalities in term infants on ECMO. *Pediatr Neurosurg* 1993; 19:202-205.

4. Luisiri A, Gravis ER, Weber T, et al. Neurosonographic changes in newborns treated with extracorporeal membrane oxygenation. *J Ultrasound Med* 1988; 7:429-438.

5. Schumacher RE, Palmer TW, Roloff DW, LaClaire PA, Bartlett RH. Follow up of infants treated with extracorporeal membrane oxygenation for newborn respiratory failure. *Pediatrics* 1991; 87:451-457.

6. Bulas D, Glass P, O'Donnell RM, Taylor GA, Short BL, Vezina GL. Neonates treated with ECMO: predictive value of early CT and US neuroimaging findings on short-term neurodevelopmental outcome. *Radiology* 1995; 195:407-412.

7. Jones MD, Hudak ML. Regulation of the fetal cerebral circulation. In: Polin RA and Fox WW (eds). *Fetal and Neonatal Physiology.* Philadelphia:W.B. Saunders; 1992: 682-690.

8. Lassen NA. Autoregulation of cerebral blood flow. *Circ Res* 1964; 15(supp):201-204.

9. Paulson OB, Walseman G, Schmidt JF, Strandgaard S. Cerebral circulation under normal and pathologic conditions. *Am J Cardiol* 1989; 63:2C-5C.

10. Strandgaard S, Paulson, OB. Cerebral autoregulation. *Stroke* 1984; 15:413-416.

11. Papile LA, Rudolph AM, Heymann MA. Autoregulation of cerebral blood flow in the preterm fetal lamb. *Pediatr Res* 1985; 19:159-161.

12. Tweed A, Cote J, Lou H, Gregory G, Wade J. Impairment of cerebral blood flow autoregulation in the newborn lamb by hypoxia. *Pediatr Res* 1986; 20:516-519.

13. Short BL, Walker LK, Traystman RJ. Impaired cerebral autoregulation in the newborn lamb during recovery from severe, prolonged hypoxia, combined with carotid artery and jugular vein ligation. *Crit Care Med* 1994; 22:1262-1268.

14. Ashwal S, Majcher JS, Longo L. Patterns of fetal lamb regional cerebral blood flow during and after prolonged hypoxia: Studies during the posthypoxia recovery period. *Am J Obstet Gynecol* 1981; 139:365-372.

15. Walsh-Sukys MC, Cornell DJ, Houston LN, Keszler M, Kanto WP Jr. Treatment of persistent pulmonary hypertension of the newborn without hyperventilation: an assessment of diffusion of innovation. *Pediatrics* 1994; 94:303-306.

16. Gleason CA, Short BL, Jones MD Jr. Cerebral blood flow and metabolism during and after prolonged hypocapnia in newborn lambs. *J Pediatr* 1989; 115:309-314.

17. Hino JK, Short BL, Rais-Bahrami K, Seale WR. Cerebral blood flow and metabolism during and after prolonged hypercapnia in newborn lambs. *Crit Care Med* 2000; 28:3505-3510.

18. Karle VA, Short BL, Martin GR, et al. Extracorporeal membrane oxygenation exposes infants to the plasticizer Di(2-ethylhexyl)phthalate (DEHP). *Crit Care Med* 1997; 25(4):696-703.

19. Liem KD, Hopman JC, Oeseburg B, de Haan AF, Festen C, Kollee LA. Cerebral oxygenation and hemodynamics during induction of ECMO as investigated by near infrared spectrophotometry. *Pediatrics* 1995; 95:555-561.

20. Short BL, Bender K, Walker LK, Traystman RJ. The cerebrovascular response to prolonged hypoxia with carotid artery and jugular vein ligation in the newborn lamb. *J Pediatr Surg* 1994; 29:887-891.

21. Taylor GA, Martin GR, Short BL. Cardiac determinants of cerebral blood flow during extracorporeal membrane oxygenation. *Invest Radiol* 1989; 24:511-516.

22. Holley DG, Short BL, Karr SS, Martin GR. Mechanisms of change in cardiac performance in infants undergoing extracorporeal membrane oxygenation. *Crit Care Med* 1994; 22(11):1865-1870.

23. Short BL, Walker LK, Gleason CA, Jones MD Jr, Traystman RJ. Effect of extracorporeal membrane oxygenation on cerebral blood flow and cerebral oxygen metabolism in newborn sheep. *Pediatr Res* 1990; 28:50-53.

24. Rosenberg AA, Kinsella JP. Effect of extracorporeal membrane oxygenation on cerebral hemodynamics in newborn lambs. *Crit Care Med* 1992; 20:1575-1581.

25. Hunter CJ, Blood AB, Bishai JM, et al, Cerebral blood flow and oxygenation during venoarterial and venovenous extracorporeal membrane oxygenation in the newborn lamb. *Pediatr Crit Care Med* 2004; 5:475-481.

26. Walker LK, Short BL, Gleason CA, Jones MD Jr, Traystman RJ. Cerebrovascular response to carbon dioxide in lambs receiving extracorporeal membrane oxygenation. *Critical Care Med* 1994; 22:291-298.

27. Short BL, Walker LK, Bender KS, Traystman RJ. Impairment of cerebral autoregulation during extracorporeal membrane oxygenation in newborn lambs. *Pediatr Res* 1993; 33:289-294.

28. Walker LK, Short BL, Traystman RJ. Impairment of cerebral autoregulation during venovenous extracorporeal membrane oxygenation in the newborn lamb. *Crit Care Med* 1996; 24:2001-2006.

29. Martinez-Orgado J, Gonzales R, Alonso MJ, Rodriguez-Martinez MA, Sanchez-Ferrer CF, Marin J. Endothelial factors and autoregulation during pressure changes in isolated newborn piglet cerebral arteries. *Pediatr Res* 1998; 44:161-167.

30. Ingyinn M, Lee J, Short BL, Viswanathan M. Venoarterial extracorporeal membrane oxygenation (VA ECMO) impairs basal nitric oxide production in cerebral arteries of newborn lambs. *Pediatr Crit Care Med* 2000; 1(2):161-165.

31. Ingyinn M, Evangelista R, Rais-Bahrami L, et al. Pulsatile ECMO maintains cerebral arterial endothelial function compared to non-pulsatile ECMO in newborn lambs. *Pediatr Res* 2002; 51:48A.

32. Wagerle LC, Russo P, Dahdah NS, Kapadia N, Davis DA. Endothelial dysfunction in cerebral microcirculation during hypothermic cardiopulmonary bypass in newborn lambs. *J Thorac Cardiovasc Surg* 1998; 115:1047-1054.

33. Preckel MP, Leftheriotis G, Ferber C, Degoute CS, Banssillon V, Saumet JL. Effect of nitric oxide blockade on the lower limit of the cortical cerebral autoregulation in pentobarbital-anaesthetized rats. *Int J Microcirc Clin Exp* 1996; 16:277-283.

34. Hofkosh D, Thompson AE, Nozza RJ, Kemp SS, Bowen A, Feldman HM. Ten years of extracorporeal membrane oxygenation: neurodevelopmental outcome. *Pediatrics* 1991; 87:549-555.

35. Mendoza JC, Shearer LL, Cook LN. Lateralization of brain lesions following extracorporeal membrane oxygenation. *Pediatrics* 1991; 88:1004-1009.

36. Hahn JS, Vaucher Y, Bejar R, Coen RW. Electroencephalographic and neuroimaging findings in neonates undergoing extracorporeal membrane oxygenation. *Neuropediatrics* 1993; 24:19-24.

37. Adolph V, Ekelund C, Smith C, Starrett A, Falterman K, Arensman R. Developmental outcome of neonates treated with extracorporeal membrane oxygenation. *J Pediatr Surg* 1990; 25:43-46.

38. Graziani LJ, Gringlas M, Baumgart S. Cerebrovascular complications and neurodevelopmental sequelae of neonatal ECMO. *Clin Perinatal* 1997; 24:655-675.

39. Lago P, Rebsamen S, Clancy RR, et al. MRI, MRA, and neurodevelopmental outcome following neonatal ECMO. *Pediatr Neurol* 1995; 2:294-304.

40. Zimmerman JJ, Deitrich KA. Current perspectives on septic shock. *Pediatr Clin North Am* 1987; 43:131-163.

41. Hardart GE, Hardart MK, Arnold JH. Intracranial hemorrhage in premature neonates treated with ECMO correlates with conceptional age. *J Pediatr* 2004; 145:184-189.

42. Hardart GE, Fackler JC. Predictors of intracranial hemorrhage during neonatal ECMO. *J Pediatr* 1999; 134:156-159.

43. Dela Cruz TV, Stewart DL, Winston SJ, Weatherman KS, Phelps JL, Mendoza JC. Risk factors for intracranial hemorrhage in the extracorporeal membrane oxygenation patient. *J Perinatol* 1997; 17:18-23.

44. Fink SM, Bockman DE, Howell CG, Falls DG, Kanto WP Jr. Bypass circuits as the source of thromboemboli during extracorporeal membrane oxygenation. *J Pediatr* 1989; 115:621-624.

45. Babcock DS, Han BK, Weiss RG, Ryckman FC. Brain abnormalities in infants on extracorporeal membrane oxygenation: sonographic and CT findings. *AJR Am J Roentgenol* 1989; 153:571-576.

46. Rubin DA, Gross GW, Ehrlich SM, Alexander AA. Interhemispheric fissure width in neonates on ECMO. *Pediatr Radiol* 1990; 21:12-15.

47. Matamoros A, Anderson JC, McConnell J, Bolam DL. Neurosonographic findings in infants treated by extracorporeal membrane oxygenation (ECMO). *J Child Neurol* 1989; 4 Suppl:S52-S61.

48. McLaughlin JF, Loeser JD, Roberts TS. Acquired hydrocephalus associated with superior vena cava syndrome in infants. *Childs Nerv Syst* 1997; 13:59-63.

49. Brunberg JA, Kewitz G, Schumacher RE. Venovenous extracorporeal membrane oxygenation: early CT alterations following use in management of severe respiratory failure in neonates. *AJNR Am J Neuroradio* 1993; 14:595-603.

50. Weber TR, Kountzman B. The effects of venous occlusion on cerebral blood flow characteristics during ECMO. *J Pediatr Surg* 1996; 31:1124-1127.

51. Bulas DI, Taylor GA, O'Donnell RM, Short BL, Fitz CR, Vezina G. Intracranial abnormalities in infants treated with extracorporeal membrane oxygenation: update on sonographic and CT findings. *AJNR Am J Neuroradiol* 1996; 17:287-294.

52. Radack DM, Baumgart S, Gross GW. Subependymal (grade 1) intracranial hemorrhage in neonates on extracorporeal membrane oxygenation. Frequency and patterns of evolution. *Clin Pediatr* 1994; 33:583-587.

53. Biehl DA, Stewart DL, Forti NH, Cook LN. Timing of intracranial hemorrhage during extracorporeal life support. *ASAIO J* 1996; 42:938-941.

54. Khan AM, Shabarek FM, Zwischenberger JB, et al. Utility of daily head ultrasonography for infants on extracorporeal membrane oxygenation. *J Pediatr Surg* 1998; 33:1229-1232.

55. Bulas DI, Taylor GA, Fitz CR, Revenis ME, Glass P, Ingram JD. Posterior fossa intracranial hemorrhage in infants treated with extracorporeal membrane oxygenation: sonographic findings. *AJR Am J Roentgenol* 1991; 156:571-575.

56. von Allmen D, Babcock D, Matsumoto J, et al. The predictive value of head ultrasound in the ECMO candidate. *J Pediatr Surg* 1992; 27:36-39.

57. Garber SJ, Sterwart DL, Cook LN, Bond SJ. Evaluation of post ECMO follow-up testing. *ASAIO J* 1998; 44:171-174.

58. Silverboard G, Horder MH, Ahmen PA, Lazzara A, Schwartz JF. Reliability of ultrasound in diagnosis of intracerebral hemorrhage and posthemorrhagic hydrocephalus: comparison with computed tomography. *Pediatrics* 1980; 66:507-514.

59. Amstrong DL, Sauls CD, Goddard-Finegold J. Neuropathologic findings in short-term survivors of intraventricular hemorrhage. *Am J Dis Child* 1987; 141:617-621.

60. Wiznitzer M, Masaryk TJ, Lewin J, Walsh M, Stork EK. Parenchymal and vascular magnetic resonance imaging of the brain after extracorporeal membrane oxygenation. *Am J Dis Child* 1990; 144:1323-1326.

61. Park CH, Spitzer AR, Desai HJ, Zhang JJ, Graziani LJ. Brain SPECT in neonates following extracorporeal membrane oxygenation: evaluation of technique and preliminary results. *J Nucl Med* 1992; 33:1943-1948.

62. Kumar P, Bedard MP, Shankaran S, Delaney-Black V. Post extracorporeal membrane oxygenation single photon emission computed tomography as a predictor of neurodevelopmental outcome. *Pediatrics* 1994; 93:951-955.

21

Outcome and Follow-up of Neonates Treated with ECMO

Penny Glass, Ph.D. and Judith Brown, N.N.P.

Introduction

Given the clinical presentation of critically ill neonates prior to cannulation, the risks inherent to ECMO therapy and the good survival rate, the occurrence of major disability among ECMO survivors is remarkably low. However, ECMO survivors are likely to have medical and developmental issues after discharge from the NICU and tend to be at high risk for learning and/or behavioral problems in childhood. The purpose of this chapter is to summarize the post-ECMO medical issues and the long-term neurodevelopmental outcome status following neonatal ECMO. The chapter concludes with comments about developmental follow-up needs of the ECMO survivor after discharge.

Medical morbidity

After ECMO, major medical concerns include feeding problems, poor somatic growth, chronic lung disease (CLD), and repeated hospitalizations.

Feeding problems

Feeding problems are anticipated following ECMO but need to be differentiated according to whether it is the process of feeding, which may be neurologically based, or whether it is feeding intolerance, which is a gastrointestinal problem. Difficulty with the feeding process would include poor suck/swallow, chronic inability to consume sufficient calories for optimal growth, and/or active food refusal. The majority of ECMO neonates have difficulty initiating a coordinated suck/swallow. This has been variously attributed to interference from tachypnea, generalized central nervous system (CNS) depression, poor hunger drive, soreness in the neck from the surgical procedure or in the throat from intubation, poor oral-motor coordination, and manipulation or compression of the vagus nerve during cannulation/decannulation.[1-3] Difficulty with oral feeding also occurs during withdrawal from narcotic medication. For most ECMO neonates, the problem is usually some combination of these factors. This initial difficulty with oral feeds is usually transient (1-2 weeks); however, appropriate management requires evaluation to determine whether the feeding problem is due to respiratory compromise, lethargic state, or more selective suck/swallow incoordination.

Insufficient caloric consumption is a source of frustration for caregivers. In some circumstances, the standard estimate of caloric need based on the infant's weight may be too high for a relatively lethargic and inactive infant. If the respiratory status is stable and the baby has sufficient suck/swallow, a 3-day trial of on-demand feedings may be in order.

A small but significant proportion of ECMO infants, usually those with significant CLD, develop food refusal which can stem from stressful oral feeding practices begun in the NICU and carried over by the parent after discharge. It can help to initiate feeding as might be offered newborns: stimulation of rooting and sucking reflexes followed by offers of small amounts of food at frequent intervals. The initial feeding goal should focus on a successful feeding process (the baby's well being), rather than volume of intake (the amount consumed from the bottle). Professional sensitivity is necessary to support a delicate balance between attaining a calculated caloric intake for optimal growth and maintaining a nurturing parent-infant relationship.

Feeding intolerance can include vomiting, abdominal distension, gastroesophageal reflux, and esophagitis. These problems reflect abnormal gastrointestinal motility and are not specific to ECMO neonates. Medical and/or surgical intervention may be needed, but many cases resolve within 1-2 weeks.

ECMO infants with a diagnosis of congenital diaphragmatic hernia (CDH) have complex feeding issues that include difficulty establishing oral feeding for the reasons stated above, but feeding intolerance may be anatomical in origin. Feeding is likely to be an ongoing issue for CDH infants. In some centers it is managed aggressively by early insertion of a gastrostomy tube or by fundoplication. More frequently, CDH infants require nasogastric feedings continued after discharge home.[4]

Growth

Normal somatic growth is expected for ECMO treated neonates; therefore, poor growth in post-ECMO infants and children should be evaluated for the underlying cause. Linear growth is affected in the first couple of years in the CDH group. Head circumference below the 5th percentile occurs at a higher than expected rate (10%) and, if occurring in conjunction with a significant brain lesion, is associated with major handicaps at 5 years of age.[5]

Macrocephaly has also been widely reported, which follows a pattern consistent with venous obstruction observed on neonatal neuroimaging. This may resolve without surgical intervention, but needs close monitoring. Macrocephaly may also signify late hydrocephalus following earlier intraventricular hemorrhage.

Chronic Lung Disease

Although ECMO is thought to decrease severe lung disease in survivors, little research has addressed this specific issue. A standard definition of CLD in term infants is oxygen requirement at 28 days. Approximately 15% of neonates treated with ECMO still require oxygen at 28 days. Long-term oxygen requirement (>4 months) is not expected among ECMO survivors, except those with lung hypoplasia.

Significant respiratory sequelae are reported in ECMO survivors during the first 2 years of life, with a high rate of rehospitalization for pulmonary indications, particularly in the first 6 months.[6] Parents of 5-year-old ECMO survivors were twice as likely as parents of normal control children to report the occurrence of at least one episode of pneumonia before the age of 2 (25% vs. 13%). Nearly half of the reported cases of pneumonia in post-ECMO children occurred within the first year, compared to none in control children. More than half of the ECMO rehospitalizations occurred within the first 6 months. Rehospitalization of the ECMO child for respiratory indications does not necessarily reflect a more severe clinical presentation, but may be the pediatrician's response to the child's past medical history or to relieve the parents' anxiety. The rate of respiratory sequelae among ECMO infants in their first year is expected to improve with the routine use of prophylactic treatments such as Synagis.

Reactive airway disease has been defined as recurrent episodes of wheezing which are treated with bronchodilators and/or corticosteroids. By age 2, ECMO-treated neonates are reported to have a lower rate of reactive airway disease than similar infants treated with conventional therapy (18% vs. 35%, respectively).[6] The prevalence of asthma in the normal population of 5- to 11-year-olds is estimated at around 5%.[7] Among the Children's National Medical Center (CNMC) 5-year ECMO cohort, 16% were taking asthma medication at the time of our study, and 10% had been hospitalized at least once for wheezing.

Parents of children treated with ECMO have expressed concern about long-term effects of severe cardiorespiratory problems as a newborn. In a small study of 11-year-old ECMO children and healthy control children, no abnormality on echocardiogram or ECG was evident.[7] The ECMO children, however, had lower exercise tolerance. It is not clear whether this finding is self-limiting or a result of parental anxiety.

Predictors of chronic lung disease

A need for supplemental oxygen beyond 28 days of age is associated with a primary diagnosis of CDH, but is also associated with chronologic age at ECMO cannulation and birthweight.[9] Days from birth to cannulation is a proxy for duration of mechanical ventilation prior to ECMO. Among non-CDH infants, those placed on ECMO earlier had a significantly lower chance of requiring oxygen at 28 days of age.[10] ECMO infants in the lower birthweight range (2.0-2.5 kg) had a greater risk for CLD than those with a higher birthweight (>2.5 kg).[11] From another perspective, the most significant factor in predicting long-term pulmonary outcome in ECMO survivors is the duration of oxygen use following decannulation.[7]

Non-pulmonary rehospitalizations

ECMO children are more likely to be rehospitalized for non-respiratory medical and surgical indications. In the CNMC 5-year ECMO cohort, 11% had been hospitalized for gastroenteritis, flu symptoms, urinary tract infection, or other diagnoses compared to none in the 53 control children.[5] Surgical complications were more frequent and varied among the ECMO children. Rhizotomy, shunt revision, bowel obstruction, urethral valve reconstruction, and diaphragmatic hernia re-repair were each seen in 1 patient, and a ventral hernia, inguinal hernia, and strabismus were seen in 2 patients. None of the control children had major surgery. Both ECMO and control children had similar rates of minor surgeries or fractures (6% and 8%, respectively).

Predictors of medical morbidity

Not surprisingly, CDH infants present the most complex medical outcome seen in ECMO survivors. High rates of hospital readmission, significant gastroesophageal reflux, and associated failure to thrive are commonly seen. However, only a few children with CDH appear to have long-term respiratory complications related to pulmonary hypoplasia. The norm for medical sequelae in non-CDH ECMO children is initial vulnerability to respiratory and non-respiratory sequelae which peaks in the first year. These children become similar to normal children by 5 years of age. The high rate of rehospitalization among the ECMO children for respiratory sequelae still does not address whether the ECMO children were actually sicker or whether the rehospitalization was in response to the neonatal history.

Medical follow-up

Close collaboration with the family's pediatrician is essential, particularly around issues of feeding, reflux medications, pulmonary status, and surgical needs (primarily for CDH). Some ECMO centers prefer to manage the patients' post-ECMO medical needs, but, with the exception of surgical problems, insurance issues are generally encountered when this is performed routinely.

Neurodevelopmental morbidity

As ECMO-treated neonates approach discharge at approximately 1 month of age, virtually all still exhibit signs of general CNS depression, including lethargy, hypotonia (particularly head control), and weak primitive reflexes, consistent with mild to moderate hypoxic-ischemic encephalopathy. By 4 months of age, the typical ECMO infant is functioning in the normal range on standard developmental assessment (e.g., Bayley Scales of Infant Development). Residual hypotonia or mild asymmetry persists in approximately 25% of the infants. Mild motor delay typically accompanies the hypotonia. The prognosis is generally good, by 1-2 years of age, significant developmental delay and/or neurologic abnormality are reported in approximately 10-15%. By 3 years of age, the rate of apparent disability is fairly stable at around 15%, but more subtle problems that may lead to learning disabilities later begin to emerge, particularly in the areas of language or visual/perceptual functioning, and persistent behavioral problems. This general clinical picture persists into school age.

Neurocognitive disability

As a group, in childhood ECMO-treated neonates are expected to function within the normal range with Full Scale IQ around 95 (normal is 85-115), but the IQ scores are significantly lower than children following a normal birth.[5,12-14] Approximately 15% of ECMO children at age 5 have one or more handicapping conditions (Table 1), the most common being mild-moderate mental retardation. The specific handicapping conditions are detailed below in the order of prevalence.

Cognitive impairment is the most common handicapping condition reported in ECMO children. The most severe cases can be identified in the first year, but, for all others, the label of "disability" should be deferred until the child is approaching school age. In the CNMC 5-year cohort, 13% were functioning in the mentally retarded range (Full Scale IQ <70) or had severe learning disability (either Verbal or Performance IQ <70). Profound retardation was rare (1%). Most of the cognitively impaired children tested in the mildly retarded range (Full Scale IQ 50-70). To put these numbers in perspective, an IQ of 50 is the average for a Down syndrome child. Children who are mildly retarded will require continued special education services, but they can learn to read and write sufficient for daily living. They may hold a job, live independently, and marry. Achieving functional independence as an adult removes the label of mental retardation. Children with moderate to severe cognitive impairment (Full Scale IQ <50) have a permanent handicap.

Neuromotor disability

Moderate hypotonia and lethargy are common findings among ECMO infants at the time of hospital discharge and among non-ECMO infants with a clinical history of hypoxic-ischemic encephalopathy. In ECMO infants, symptoms improve dramatically over the next 4 months and sufficiently resolve such that acquisition of motor milestones should be on course by the second half of the first year. Asymmetry in tone

Table 1. Neurosensory disability at age 5 following neonatal ECMO.

Children with disability	Percent
Total	15%
Cognitive impairment	13%
Motor disability	6%
Seizure disorder/epilepsy	2%
Bilateral SNHL*	5%
Cortical visual impairment	2%

*SNHL=sensorineural hearing loss

is frequently reported in early examinations, but this finding is not limited to ECMO children.[5] Persistent functional asymmetry after 4 months of age could represent a lateralizing brain lesion and deserves further evaluation.

Unlike the preterm infant, motor handicap among ECMO children is unlikely to occur alone, but rather as an accompaniment to more severe degrees of mental retardation, reflecting more diffuse brain injury. Estimates across different studies of ECMO-treated neonates place the incidence of severe cerebral palsy (CP) in childhood at less than 5%. The rate of occurrence of mild CP is ~20%, but this incidence is confounded by changes with age as well as different diagnostic criteria. In the CNMC 5-year cohort, a diagnosis of CP was present in 5% and usually concomitant with cognitive impairment. One child was profoundly impaired and another was paraplegic, although cognitively normal. Otherwise, the remaining 150 children in the CNMC 5-year ECMO cohort were ambulatory. None of the 53 control children had an abnormal neurological exam, but equal proportions (25-30%) of the ECMO and control children were found to have "suspect" neurological findings. "Soft neurological signs" are not reliable indicators of neuropathology in young children.

Seizure disorder

Neonatal seizures are traditionally associated with acute neurologic disease and poorer long-term outcome, including cerebral palsy and epilepsy.[15] During the acute NICU course, both clinical and encephalographic seizure activity is widely reported, ranging from 20-70%.[14,17] However, the timing and type of abnormality are not consistent. Strikingly, only 2% of the CNMC cohort had a diagnosis of epilepsy at age 5, in spite of the relatively high rate of brain injury (40%) on neonatal CT scan. It is still plausible, however, that ECMO children may have a lower seizure threshold which could become evident around age 7 or with adolescence.

Auditory deficits

Hearing screening is routine for all neonates at the time of NICU discharge and is particularly relevant for the ECMO population. Elevated brainstem auditory evoked response (BAER) thresholds are reported in more than 25% of ECMO infants at initial testing.[18] The majority of these cases are mild (25-40 dB) and eventually resolve. Follow-up behavioral testing at 1 year of age is warranted for all patients even if the neonatal screening was passed, due to questions regarding sensitivity/specificity of the BAER test and the documented high occurrence of progressive sensorineural hearing loss among non-ECMO infants with similar underlying diseases (persistent pulmonary hypertension and CLD). The rate of bilateral hearing loss requiring amplification was 5% among the CNMC 5-year-old ECMO cohort. The hearing loss was diagnosed on the initial BAER and recorded on the discharge summary, but the essential follow-up by the primary care physicians was inconsistent. Progressive hearing loss has also been reported.[19]

Factors which have been associated with sensorineural hearing loss in non-ECMO patients include asphyxia, hyperventilation, hypocapnia, and prolonged diuretic usage. There is no evidence to date that the ECMO procedure increases the risk for hearing loss, but children who had CDH as a primary diagnosis appear to be at greater risk.[20]

Visual deficits

Visual deficits are rare among ECMO-treated neonates, but isolated cases have been reported. For example, one center reported blindness of unknown etiology in an otherwise normal infant. The patient developed bilateral retinal detachments that were not diagnosed as retinopathy of prematurity (ROP). Progressive blindness first diagnosed at 1 year of age was seen in a patient with a complex coagulopathy being treated with heparin and aspirin. Visual loss followed obstruction of the right ophthalmic artery but the left eye retained normal vision.

Cases of cortical visual impairment are rare but would be expected to follow posterior brain injury. In spite of a fairly bleak clinical picture in the immediate neonatal period, visual function typically improves. In one case, an ECMO neonate sustained cortical infarct over the entire posterior portion of her brain. At 8 years of age, the patient was able to read words, but had difficulty stringing words together on a page. Her verbal skills were in the low/average range. Better recovery is expected following unilateral infarct in the visual cortex. Cortical visual impairment is also consistent with cases of severe periventricular leukomalacia. Routine cortical visual-evoked response testing is not recommended.

In a prospective study of 58 ECMO patients who received routine ophthalmic examinations prior to hospital discharge, the ocular findings included 2 incidences of optic nerve pallor and 2 of retinal hemorrhage. This incidence is not sufficient to support universal screening.[21] Select ocular abnormalities were identified among infants who had other congenital anomalies. The early concern about ROP due to hyperoxia associated with ECMO has not been borne out. ROP is related to the degree of immaturity of the retinal vasculature, and the occurrence among ECMO neonates >2 kg is uncommon. Mild ROP has occasionally been detected, but is not

expected to result in visual deficits. The recommendations may change if a greater number of preterm infants are being treated. If ECMO is used to treat neonates <2 kg or <34 weeks gestational age, then ophthalmic exams prior to hospital discharge should be considered to rule out ROP. Otherwise, routine ophthalmic exams during or after ECMO are not recommended.

Predictors of mental and motor disability

Based on logistic regression analysis of our ECMO cohort (n=152), the single overriding factor associated with disability in early childhood was the extent and severity of neonatal neuroimaging abnormality.[22] The power of this single factor is captured in the odds ratio for disability by injury severity as depicted in Table 2. A slight elevation of disability risk was present for ECMO children with either no identified brain injury or mild injury on neonatal CT scan, compared to the normal controls (n=53).

Multiple other single factors have also been reported to be associated with poorer neurodevelopmental status, including low birth weight, a pre-ECMO diagnosis other than meconium aspiration, the need for CPR prior to cannulation, the presence of 2 or more abnormal EEGs, a long hospital stay, the presence of CLD after ECMO, and socioeconomic status.[11,16,22-25] Outcomes vary between institutions.

Finally, special circumstances also need to be considered. Reviewing data from 1984-1999 from the ELSO Registry, Southgate et al.

Table 2. Odds ratios for disability at age 5 by severity of neonatal neuroimaging relative to normal control children.

Severity of abnormality	n	Abnormal (%)	OR	95% CI	P
Normal control	53	1 (1.89)			
None	88	9 (10.23)	5.924	0.73-48.16	0.090
Mild	38	5 (13.16)	7.879	0.88-70.46	0.078
Moderate	12	4 (33.33)	26.00	2.57-263.06	0.003
Severe	14	8 (57.14)	69.33	7.351-653.91	<0.0001

reported that 91 neonates with a diagnosis of Trisomy 21 were treated with ECMO for respiratory failure.[26] The survival rate to decannulation was similar to non-Trisomy 21 infants, but survival to discharge was poorer. Non-ECMO children with Trisomy 21 have an average IQ of 50. The impact of ECMO on neurodevelopmental outcome in this subset of the population remains to be determined.

Specific neuropsychologic deficits

By 5 years of age, the majority of ECMO-treated neonates are functioning in the normal range on standard measures of IQ, although the group mean is significantly lower than the mean for normal controls.[5] There is no consistent neuropsychological profile that identified the "ECMO child". Instead, the neuropsychological profile appears to be related to the severity of the brain injury, as depicted in Figure 1. Furthermore, ECMO 5-year-old children with normal neuroimaging had a neuropsychological profile parallel and just below to that of normal controls.

Even among the non-handicapped ECMO children, the risk for learning problems at school age appears to be as high as 50%. Most of the ECMO children in the CNMC cohort who were

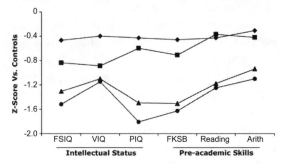

Figure 1. Brain injury severity on neonatal US/CT scan and neurocognitive outcome at age 5 (n=152). Z-scores computed from normal control data (n=53), thus control group mean = 0. FSIQ=Full Scale IQ, VIQ=Verbal IQ, PIQ=Performance IQ. FKSB=Florida Kindergarten Screening Battery.[19]

identified as "at risk" at age 5 were receiving special educational services by the end of first grade. Five children who had not been identified as at academic risk at age 5 were also receiving special educational services by the end of first grade; 4 of these had significant behavior problems.

Although normal cognitive status at age 2 is predictive of normal IQ at age 5, apparent disability at age 2 is not sufficiently predictive for disability at age 5. For example, among the CNMC 5-year cohort, 70 children had Bayley testing at age 2, with 51 children (73%) scoring in the normal range (MDI >84). Of those, 92% had Full Scale IQ scores >84 at age 5, 9 children scored below 70 on the Bayley at age 2, but only 6 (66%) had an IQ below 70 at age 5. The shift in disability status is important, but does not account for learning disability at school age.

Psychosocial morbidity

Behavioral problems are commonly reported among children who have had complex neonatal courses accompanied an increase in parental stress. There are limited data regarding behavior adjustment and family stress among ECMO survivors. Early studies of temperament and behavior in ECMO toddlers have been reported, but these studies lacked normal controls. Although isolated incidences of severe psychopathology (e.g., autism) have been reported, this appears to reflect the incidence in the general population, and there is no evidence that ECMO survivors are at increased risk.

Behavioral adjustment

Behavioral problems are a significant concern and may often be detected early. In the CNMC cohort, parents of non-retarded 5-year-old ECMO survivors report higher levels of social and attention problems on the Child Behavior Checklist than parents of normal control children, and elevated ratings on the

Conners' Hyperactivity Index.[5] Overall, ECMO parents were nearly 3 times more likely to report clinically significant levels of behavioral problems (primarily social problems and attention/hyperactivity) among their children compared to normal controls (42% vs. 16%). Among the ECMO children, 24% had both behavior problems and neuropsychologic deficits, compared to 8% of the control children. Hypothesized causes of behavior problems include subtle neurologic injury affecting behavioral control, secondary effects of family stress, and/or differences in parenting styles when the child is perceived as "vulnerable". A relationship between behavior difficulties and school failure is common in the general population and supports the need for early intervention for both developmental and behavioral issues.

Family stress

The often unexpected and acute crisis precipitating ECMO therapy is a traumatic event for parents, and can be very disruptive to families. Clinical observations and parent surveys suggest that the impact can be long lasting.[27,28] Family function at 1 year post-ECMO has been reported as similar to that of preterm infants. ECMO mothers were no more likely than mothers of normal controls to report clinically significant levels of parenting stress on a standardized questionnaire. However, in a semi-structured interview, it was common for ECMO parents to express intense emotions while recalling the NICU experience even 5 years later. Standardized measures of parent stress may not capture the lingering emotional impact of the neonatal crisis. Therefore, it is prudent to provide early and sustained emotional support for parents of ECMO patients, even if the infant appears to be doing well.

ECMO follow-up

Prior to NICU discharge, the neonatologist should discuss with the parent(s) the type of follow-up needed and expectations. A CT or MRI scan prior to discharge should be routine, as should a hearing screening.

Developmental follow-up at each ECMO institution is essential. It provides important feedback to the ECMO team and important support for vulnerable parents. A guideline for neonatal ECMO follow-up is available on the ELSO website. Comprehensive multidisciplinary follow-up is required for those children who have chronic medical issues, particularly the CDH children. Communication across multiple disciplines (e.g., Surgery, Neonatology, Pulmonary, GI/Nutrition, Neurology, and Developmental Specialists) is often problematic, underscoring the role of a team approach and case management to prioritize the needs of the child and communicate directly to the parent and the child's pediatrician.

Summary

As a general rule of thumb, a given ECMO child's risk for developmental disability is probably parallel to their pre-ECMO mortality risk (by diagnostic group), whether they required pre-ECMO CPR, the degree of prematurity, and particularly the presence of neuroimaging abnormality for that ECMO center. Chronic pulmonary issues and prolonged hospital stay are also markers of poor outcome. Feeding issues warrant special attention.

As a general expectation, virtually all ECMO-treated neonates approaching discharge (~1 month of age) exhibit signs of general CNS depression, including lethargy, hypotonia (particularly evident in head control), and weak primitive reflexes, consistent with mild to moderate hypoxic-ischemic encephalopathy. By 4 months of age, the typical ECMO infant is functioning in the normal range on standard developmental assessment (e.g., Bayley Scales). Mild hypotonia or asymmetry persists in approximately 25% of the infants. Mild motor delay typically accompanies the hypotonia. The prognosis is generally good. By 1-2 years of age significant developmental delay and/or neuro-logic abnormality is reported in approximately 10-15% of the infants. By 3 years of age, the rate of apparent disability is fairly stable at around 15%, but more subtle problems that may be related to learning disabilities later in school begin to emerge, particularly in the areas of language or visual/perceptual functioning and persistent behavior problems. This general clinical picture persists into school age. Parenting issues may not be apparent, but are typically present, even into childhood, and affect both the home life and the child's adaptation to school.

References

1. Grimm P. Feeding difficulties in infants treated with ECMO. *CNMC ECMO Symposium* 1993:25.
2. Nield T, Hallway M, Fodera C, et al. Outcome in problem feeders post ECMO. *CNMC ECMO Symposium* 1990:79.
3. Glass P. Patient neurodevelopmental outcomes after neonatal ECMO. In: Arensman R & Cornish J, eds. *Extracorporeal life support*. Boston, MA: Blackwell Scientific Publications, 1993.
4. Van Meurs KP, Robbins ST, Reed VL, et al. Congenital diaphragmatic hernia: long-term outcome in neonates treated with extracorporeal membrane oxygenation. *J Pediatr* 1993; 122:893-899.
5. Glass P, Wagner A, Papero P, et al. Neurodevelopmental status at age five years of neonates treated with extracorporeal membrane oxygenation. *J Pediatr* 1995; 127:447-457.
6. Walsh-Sukys M, Bauer R, Cornell D, Friedman H, Stork E, Hack M. Severe respiratory failure in neonates: mortality and morbidity rates and neurodevelopmental outcomes. *J Pediatr* 1994; 125:104-110.
7. Weitzman M, Gortmaker S, Sobol A, Perrin J. Recent trends in the prevalence and severity of childhood asthma. *JAMA* 1992; 268:2673-2677.
8. Boykin AR, Quivers ES, Wagenhoffer KL, et al. Cardiopulmonary outcome of neonatal extracorporeal membrane oxygenation at ages 10-15 years. *Crit Care Med* 2003; 31(9):2380-2384.
9. Vaucher YE, Dudell GG, Beiar R, et al. Predictors of early childhood outcome in candidates for ECMO. *J Pediatr* 1996; 128:109-117.
10. Doski J, Butler J, Louder D, Dickey L, Cheu H. Outcome of infants requiring cardiopulmonary resuscitation before extracorporeal membrane oxygenation. *J Pediatr Surg* 1997; 32:1318-1321.
11. Revenis M, Glass P, Short B. Mortality and morbidity rates among lower birth weight infants (2000 to 2500 grams) treated with extracorporeal membrane oxygenation. *J Pediatr* 1992; 121:452-458.
12. Hofkosh D, Thompson A, Nozza R, Kemp S, Bowen A, Feldman H. Ten years of ECMO: neurodevelopmental outcome. *Pediatrics* 1991; 87:549-555.
13. Towne B, Lott I, Hicks D, Healey T. Long-term follow-up of infants and children treated with ECMO: a preliminary report. *J Pediatr Surg* 1985; 20:410-414.
14. Wildin S, Landry S, Zwischenberger J. Prospective, controlled study of developmental outcome in survivors of ECMO: the first 24 months. *Pediatrics* 1994; 93:404-408.
15. Scher M, Kosaburo A, Beggarly M, Hamid M, Steppe D, Painter M. Electrographic seizures in preterm and full-term neonates: clinical correlates, associated brain lesions, and risk for neurologic sequelae. *Pediatrics* 1993; 91:128-134.
16. Hahn J, Vaucher Y, Bejar R, Coen R. Electroencephalographic and neuroimaging findings in neonates undergoing extracorporeal membrane oxygenation. *Neuropediatrics* 1993; 24:19-24.
17. Graziani L, Streletz L, Baumgart S, Cullen J, McKee L. Predictive value of neonatal electroencephalograms before and during

extracorporeal membrane oxygenation. *J Pediatr* 1994; 125:969-975.

18. Desai S, Stanley C, Graziani L, McKee L, Baumgart S. Brainstem auditory evoked potential screening (BAEP) unreliable for detecting sensori-neural hearing loss in ECMO survivors: a comparison of neonatal BAEP and follow-up behavioral audiometry. *CNMC ECMO Symposium* 1994:62.

19. Cheung PY, Robertson CM. Sensorineural hearing loss in survivors of neonatal extracorporeal membrane oxygenation. *Pediatr Rehabil* 1997:Apr-Jun; 1(2):127-130.

20. Lund D, Mitchell J, Kharasch V. Congenital diaphragmatic hernia: the hidden morbidity. *J Pediatr Surg* 1994; 29:258-264.

21. Haney B, Thibeault D. Ocular findings in infants treated with ECMO—Followup of 3 year prospective study. *CNMC ECMO Symposium* 1997:45.

22. Glass P, Bulas D, Wagner A, et al. Severity of brain injury following neonatal extracorporeal membrane oxygenation and outcome at age 5 years. *Dev Med Child Neurol* 1997; 39:441-448.

23. Allare M, Shwer M, Waggoner J, et al. Is CPR or medical resuscitation a contraindication to neonatal ECMO? Long-term outcomes of neonates post resuscitation and ECMO: the Phoenix Experience. *CNMC ECMO Symposium* 1993:31.

24. Kornhauser MS, Baumgart S, Desai SA, et al. Adverse neurodevelopmental outcome after extracorporeal membrane oxygenation among neonates with bronchopulmonary dysplasia. *J Pediatrics* 2000; 113:307-311.

25. Kumar P, Shankaran S, Bedard MP, et al. Identifying at risk infants following neonatal extracorporeal membrane oxygenation. *Journal of Perinatology* 1999; 19:367-372.

26. Southgate MW, Annibale DJ, Hulsey TC, et al. International experience with Trisomy 21 infants placed on extracorporeal membrane oxygenation. *Pediatrics* 2001; 107:549-552.

27. Caron E, White J, Curley M. Concerns of parents whose children were supported on extracorporeal membrane oxygenation. *CNMC ECMO Symposium* 1993:15.

28. Landry S, Frost-Westin M, Cherin J, Griffith P, Allison P, Zwischenberger J. Outcome across the first two years for neonates receiving ECMO and for their caretakers. *CNMC ECMO Symposium* 1990:18.

22

Acute Hypoxic Respiratory Failure in Children

Desmond Bohn, M.B., F.R.C.P.C.

Introduction

The management of acute hypoxic respiratory failure (AHRF) has changed radically since mechanically assisted ventilation using negative pressure was first introduced in the 1930s. Although these devices were remarkably effective in the treatment of diseases associated with weakness or paralysis of the respiratory muscles (pump failure), they were not effective in diseases involving the pulmonary parenchyma (lung failure). The demonstration that positive pressure ventilation was effective for the treatment of AHRF occurred 40 years ago during the poliomyelitis epidemic in Europe and Scandinavia when patients were tracheostomized and manually ventilated with gases delivered by a simple anesthetic circuit.[1] This, in turn, led to the development of the first mechanical positive pressure ventilators (PPV) by Engstrom in Scandinavia and Emerson in North America and ushered in the era of intensive care medicine. The succeeding interval has seen major technological advances in ventilator design without similar improvement in the survival of the pulmonary disease processes they were designed to treat. We are now in an era where we have a vast array of choices of ventilator management strategies for the treatment of AHRF in both adults and children. It is difficult to evaluate the efficacy of these therapies because few have undergone clinical trials and most published experience is based on rescue therapy in a high mortality group of patients with hypoxia and pulmonary barotrauma.

While it is disappointing that the advances in ventilator technology have not resulted in improved survival in AHRF, we have come to recognize that when it comes to dealing with patients with the type of parenchymal lung disease typified by diffuse atelectasis and hypoxemia, PPV is as likely to be part of the problem as part of the solution. One of the basic principles adopted in PPV in the past 40 years is to attempt to mimic normal physiology. This has not been taken into account when choosing ventilator settings until recently. The objective was to achieve normocarbia and normoxia with tidal volumes and respiratory rates which were appropriate for the normal lung. While this strategy is fundamentally sound and without hazard in the normal lung, the same does not apply to a diseased lung. With the realization of the importance of ventilator-induced lung injury, alternative ventilation strategies are being explored in the management of AHRF. These are based more on the recognition that the ventilation strategy should be adapted to the underlying pathophysiology of the lung rather than simply mimicking normal lung physiology. This new approach demands that we rethink some of the traditional teaching about normal respiratory physiology and concentrate on understanding the underlying pathophysiology. In addition, an awareness of the increasing evidence for secondary lung injury produced by mechanical ventilation is required.

The pathophysiology of acute lung injury

For the purposes of this review, we will ignore AHRF caused by neuromuscular or central nervous system diseases which come under the broad heading of failure of respiratory "pump", are typified by elevations in $PaCO_2$, involve minimal if any intrapulmonary shunting, and are easily managed with conventional ventilation settings. We will concentrate instead on diseases that produce acute "lung failure" which are typically associated with diffuse atelectasis, permeability edema, low lung compliance, and intrapulmonary shunting. We shall use as our paradigm adult (now correctly termed acute) respiratory distress syndrome (ARDS) following the agreed European/North American Consensus Conference definition of bilateral infiltrates on chest radiograph, absence of cardiac failure, and a PaO_2/FiO_2 ratio <200.[2]

In the non-diseased state, the total cardiac output passes through the pulmonary capillaries which are either juxtaposed to the alveoli (intra-alveolar) or contained within the interstitial space (extra-alveolar) with minimal leakage of fluid. The junctions between the capillary endothelial cells are permeable to fluid flux and they are impermeable to protein and solutes in the normal state. The small amount of fluid that leaks into the interstitial space is reabsorbed by the lymphatics. The epithelial lining is impermeable to both fluid and solutes. This normal state can be perturbed by inhalational injury to the epithelial lining (e.g., aspiration, smoke inhalation), by systemic diseases that damage the integrity of the endothelium (e.g., sepsis, trauma, embolism), or by primary surfactant deficiency, which results in a number of pathological changes within the lung. Any of these insults can activate neutrophils and cause them to migrate to the lung where they attach to the endothelium and open the tight junctions, resulting in leakage of fluid and protein initially into the interstitial space and subsequently into the alveolus. The leakage of this material containing fibrin results in inhibition of surfactant activity, and formation of hyaline membranes around the alveolar lining. Epithelial injury results in damage to the surfactant producing type 2 cells. Frequently there is plugging of the pulmonary microcirculation with platelet thrombi, and this, together with the release of thromboxane, produces a rise in pulmonary vascular resistance and pulmonary hypertension. This phase of ARDS is frequently referred to as the exudative phase. The gradual leakage of fluid into the interstitial space causes the lung to lose some of its elasticity; the earliest symptom being tachypnea as functional residual capacity (FRC) falls and the lung becomes stiffer. The initial blood gas abnormalities are characteristically hypoxemia and hypocarbia, with $PaCO_2$ only rising above normal later in the progression of illness as respiratory muscle fatigue begins. A second proliferative phase of ARDS follows which is characterized by fibroblast infiltration into the interstitial space and the deposition of fibrous tissue, and the resulting development of chronic lung disease (CLD). At this stage, there is gross destruction of air spaces and dilatation of terminal bronchi leading to a honeycomb appearance to the lung.

In the 1970s, pathologists frequently referred to this constellation of findings as "respirator lung". Clinicians argued that the ventilator allowed time for the full expression of the underlying disease and that these lesions had little to do with the ventilator. The only damage that was unequivocally due to the ventilator was the constellation of air leak syndromes known collectively as barotrauma. All other symptoms were attributed to oxygen toxicity. In reality, it is difficult for a pathologist viewing a section of lung tissue to define where the primary lung disease stops and ventilator-induced injury begins. A rebuttal to the argument about the ventilator being responsible for these pathological changes was provided in a paper by Nash entitled "Respirator lung: A misnomer".[3] In this study normal goats were ventilated for 2 weeks with either air or 100% oxygen; those on oxygen died, while those on air all survived without damage. They concluded that "mechanical PPV, at physiological inspiratory pressures, does not in and of itself cause morphologic pulmonary alterations." An error inherent to this conclusion is that the term "physiological inspiratory pressures" meant a peak inspiratory pressure (PIP) of 12 cm H_2O, and diseased lungs need substantially higher pressures.

It has taken a long time to recognize the potential dangers of PPV; it is difficult to believe when using PPV to treat pulmonary edema that it also causes pulmonary edema. The evidence is now overwhelming that PPV produces severe pathology in the normal lung and contributes substantially to the pathology in the abnormal lung. More importantly, having at least partially understood the cause of the injury, we are developing tactics to minimize the damage. In order to understand the rationale for the use of non-conventional ventilation strategies, we should first review the evolution of PPV as well as the now abundant evidence for positive pressure-induced lung damage in both normal and injured lungs.

The evolution of PPV in acute respiratory failure

Since the early days of mechanical ventilation, it has been recognized that positive pressure respiration does not mimic normal breathing. If this were so, patients with normal lungs could be ventilated on a FiO_2 of 0.21 at the same tidal volumes and respiratory rates seen in spontaneous breathing. It was Bendixen[4] in 1963 who showed that during general anesthesia, mechanical ventilation in patients with normal lungs was associated with a fall in PaO_2 and a rise in $PaCO_2$. He ascribed this change to the development of atelectasis due to the loss of the normal intermittent "sighing" present in the unanesthetized spontaneously breathing human. He proposed the use of an intermittent large tidal volume breath or "sigh" to overcome this problem which then became a design feature of ventilators of that period. It was not until a decade later that Froese and Bryan[5] showed that the major cause of atelectasis with the induction of anesthesia and muscle relaxation was a loss in lung volume due to the cephalad movement of the diaphragm. To compensate for this physiological aberration the inspired oxygen concentration and delivered tidal volumes have been increased to well in excess of those used in spontaneous respiration. However, in diseased lungs, what seemed like a medical imperative (i.e., to normalize blood gases in patients with diffusely atelectatic, low compliant lung disease by using ever larger tidal volumes) rarely resulted in survival. It was not until the 1970s that it was first shown that by maintaining a positive end expiratory pressure (PEEP) oxygenation could be improved. Ashbaugh[6] showed that PEEP was effective in ventilated adult patients with ARDS, and Gregory[7] went on to show that a similar strategy could be used successfully in spontaneously breathing newborns with hyaline membrane disease. During the subsequent 20 years the use of PPV with PEEP has proved successful in improving oxygenation in both ARDS and respiratory distress syndrome (RDS). The correct amount of PEEP is the amount that improves oxygenation without adverse effect on hemodynamics. Suter and Fairley[8] increased PEEP until they achieved the highest compliance; which varied from 0-15 cm H_2O, depending on the severity of the loss of lung compliance. Further increases in PEEP decreased both the compliance and oxygen transport.

One of the major difficulties in setting a PEEP level or any ventilatory parameter in ARDS is the non-homogeneity of the disease process. In ARDS, the disease looks diffuse on the plain film, but on the CT scan there is a collection of densities in the dependent parts of the lung, with the non-dependent lung looking close to normal.[9,10] Furthermore, these densities, which presumably represent atelectatic or flooded units, are mobile as their location changes with posture. It is clear that the pressures required to open the dependent regions of the lung may over-distend the non-dependent regions. Although the application of PEEP is consistently associated with improved oxygenation in AHRF, the recognition that mortality from oxygenation failure has not decreased significantly in the past twenty years, despite major improvements in ventilator technology, has led to a search of alternate rescue therapy. In order to evaluate whether these innovations represent a useful option in AHRF, the role that PPV plays in the development of acute lung injury must be explored.

Ventilator-induced lung injury

The term barotrauma is used most commonly to describe damage to the lung from the ventilator and is usually understood to refer to a constellation of air leak syndromes, the incidence of which rises almost linearly with the PIP. The word barotrauma does not adequately reflect the subtle but serious epithelial and endothelial injury leading to pulmonary edema and protein leak induced by mechanical ventilation and high inspired oxygen levels. The first clear study of the problem was a classic paper by Webb and Tierney.[11] Rats with normal lungs were mechanically ventilated with room air for a target period of 1 hour. Those ventilated at pressures of 45/0 cm H_2O developed severe hypoxemia, decreased compliance, and died with post-mortem evidence of extensive alveolar and perivascular edema. Those ventilated at 30/0 cm H_2O had reasonable gas exchange, no change in compliance, and survived. Animals ventilated at 14/0 cm H_2O showed no

abnormality. Thus, a clear dose response was established for the induction of lung injury. Dreyfuss[12] added a time dimension; in normal animals after 5 minutes of PPV at 45/0 cm H_2O there was perivascular edema with no visible epithelial lesions. After 20 minutes at the same pressure there was widespread alveolar flooding with swelling and disruption of the epithelium. These animal studies are not directly comparable to human subjects because of the differences in species, the fact that the animals used had highly compliant chest walls, the studies were performed in animals with open chests. However, Kolobow[13] studied normal sheep ventilated at 50/0 cm H_2O and showed severe and often lethal lung damage within 24 hours. These studies appear to use unreasonably high pressures, but they were done in normal lungs, attempting to simulate what would happen in the sick lung where the injury is by no means uniform, and the regions of relatively normal lung tissue are frequently subjected to high peak airway pressures. If half the alveoli are closed, the distention of the open units has to more or less double to maintain normocarbia. Tsuno[14] showed that ventilating sheep at 30/0 cm H_2O for 48 hours resulted in severe (not lethal) lung damage. Dreyfuss[15] showed that protein leak into the lung was similarly produced when the same tidal volume was generated by negative pressure ventilation as with positive pressure. Furthermore, he demonstrated that when high positive pressures were used, but the volume expansion of the lung was restricted by a body cast, there was no protein leak. The study concluded that it was the volume distention of the lung that was important in producing the lung injury. Similarly, Hernandez[16] produced a protein leak in an isolated rabbit lung using trivial pressures (15 cm H_2O) while it required 45 cm H_2O to produce a similar leak in the intact rabbit, and again, this could be prevented by limiting expansion with a body cast.[17]

A significant body of experimental data suggests that in normal animals, cyclical lung distention delivered by PPV with PIP of ≥30 cm H_2O can produce permeability edema and pathological changes which are similar to ARDS, and that these changes can be at least partially prevented by PEEP. Given the fact that patients with this type of lung disease require positive intrathoracic pressure to reverse their hypoxemia, these studies suggest that the ideal strategy to prevent ongoing injury would be to prevent lung over-distention by limiting the PIP while maintaining a lung volume at an end expiration with PEEP sufficient to prevent alveolar derecruitment. There are several experimental studies comparing the degree of injury using low tidal volume/high PEEP with high tidal volume ventilation/low PEEP, high PEEP, and low PEEP strategies. Corbridge[18] in an acid aspiration model showed a significantly lower shunt fraction and less pulmonary edema with a high PEEP (10 cm H_2O) low tidal volume strategy, compared to a normal tidal volume low PEEP (3 cm H_2O), with the same peak pressure. Sandhar[19] had positive results in a surfactant depletion model created by repetitive lung lavage. First, the inflection point on the pressure/volume (P/V) curve was measured which is the pressure at which lung volume starts to increase (around 11 cm H_2O). Then the PEEP was set above the measured inflection point on the inflation limb of the P/V curve and this was compared to a 3 cm H_2O PEEP group. Mean airway pressures were matched by altering the I:E ratio. Improved gas exchange and few, if any, hyaline membranes were found in the high PEEP group. The problem with this high PEEP strategy is that in the abnormal lung the "opening pressure" is about 10-15 cm H_2O. If peak pressure is also limited, the tidal volume may be insufficient to control $PaCO_2$. Therefore, both Corbridge and Sandhar had to increase respiratory rate to maintain normocarbia. Thus, there is a possibility that the differences in lung damage may be due to other factors such as alteration in pulmonary hemodynamics or cardiac output. This issue was addressed by Muscedere[20] who

injured the lung by surfactant depletion and brief mechanical ventilation. The animals were sacrificed and a static P/V curve measured to define the inflection point on the inflation limb of the curve (~15 cm H_2O). The lungs were then ventilated in air with a fixed tidal volume of 2 ml for 2 hours. One group was ventilated with no PEEP, the next with a PEEP of 4 cm H_2O (i.e., below the inflection point), and the next had a PEEP set above the inflection point. A control group had no post-mortem ventilation and were statically inflated for 2 hours. Those with no PEEP or PEEP below the inflection point had a marked decrease in compliance, whereas those ventilated above the inflection point had a significant increase in compliance. The pathology was of particular interest as both animals ventilated without PEEP or with PEEP below the inflection point had severe hyaline membrane formation, with an important difference in distribution; those with no PEEP had lesions mainly in respiratory and membranous bronchioles, whereas those with PEEP below the inflection had lesions predominantly in the alveolar ducts. In marked contrast, those ventilated above the inflection had no more damage than the control group who received no post-mortem ventilation. However, in those ventilated above the inflection point there was a small but significant increase in pneumothorax. Two conclusions can be drawn from this study: first, injury is clearly related to the degree of end-expiratory pressure; and second, those subjected to the highest pressures had the greatest volutrauma, while those ventilated above the inflection point had the least injury.

Apart from direct injury to the lung, there are important remote effects due to cytokine release associated with PPV. There is now experimental data which shows that lung over-distention itself results in the release of cytokines which may be responsible for multi-organ injury and dysfunction.[21] Although very high airway pressures were used in this animal model, a protective effect with PEEP is demonstrated. Finally, it should be pointed out that the important variable is not airway pressure but transpulmonary pressure; that is, the difference in pressure between the alveolus and the pleural space. It should be noted that mouth pressure does not necessarily equal alveolar pressure because of flow resistive pressure drops in the small airways. In instances where intra-abdominal pressure is high or the chest wall is stiff, higher airway pressures may be required to achieve adequate alveolar ventilation without being injurious to the lung.

Pulmonary oxygen toxicity

Although most of the attention has been focused on positive pressure in the development of secondary lung injury, high inspired oxygen concentrations also play an important role. There are numerous studies in primate models that show prolonged exposure to high inspired oxygen concentrations results in a proliferation of type II epithelial cells and increased endothelial permeability.[22-31] In human disease it is difficult to separate the primary disease process from the effects of exposure of the injured lung to high oxygen concentrations. However, a study on normal human lungs showed that an FiO_2 of 0.95 for 17 hours resulted in an increase in the albumin concentration in bronchoalveolar lavage fluid, and development of permeability edema.[32] Therefore, it would seem logical that an essential part of any ventilation strategy in patients with acute lung injury would include measures to minimize high oxygen concentrations, as well as to recruit and retain lung volume.

Epidemiology and markers of severity of acute lung injury

The term acute respiratory distress syndrome was first coined by Ashbaugh[6] in an article in Lancet in 1967 which described the acute onset of tachypnea, hypoxemia, and loss of

compliance in 11 previously healthy adults and 1 child, 7 of whom died. At autopsy all had diffuse atelectasis, alveolar hemorrhage, and edema together with hyaline membrane formation. The similarity to the lungs of premature infants with hyaline membrane disease prompted the authors to name it "adult" respiratory distress syndrome. Among the treatments described as being "therapeutic trials of apparent value" was the use of PEEP. In the ensuing near 40 years, a large body of literature has been published on this topic which reports mortality rates as low as 30% and as high as 80%. Since ARDS is a syndrome rather than a disease entity, mortality may be significantly influenced by the underlying disease process. Patients with sepsis and immunodeficiency tend to have higher mortality rates. Gattonini[33] divided ARDS into pulmonary and extrapulmonary causes and demonstrated different responses to PEEP. In adult studies, the overall mortality in large cohort studies was ~60%,[34-40] whereas in the control arm of several controlled trials the mortality was lower, in the range of 40-50%.[41-45] This difference can be partially accounted for by the large number of patients excluded from these studies based on the likelihood of death from non-pulmonary causes. Factors that have been shown to negatively influence survival include the development of multi-organ failure, use of low PEEP, increasing FiO_2 requirement, and ventilation with high tidal volumes.[35-37,41,45]

Epidemiological data on ARDS/acute lung injury (ALI) in pediatric patients is hard to come by. Data from studies on children requiring mechanical ventilation published in the 1980s and 1990s suggested that the mortality is similar to adult ARDS.[46–49] However, recently published studies in an era in which where there has been an increasing focus on ventilation-induced lung injury (VILI) has shown that the mortality is in the range of 20-30%.[50-55] Attempts have been made to predict outcome in order to select patients for alternative ventilation strategies, including ECMO, using either physiological scoring systems or measures of the severity of the oxygenation defect (Table 1).

In hypoxic newborns, the oxygenation index (OI) has proved to be a reasonably robust predictor of mortality and is widely accepted as an indicator for the initiation of ECMO. In older children, where oxygenation failure is frequently part of multi-organ failure, the OI was thought to be less reliable. In a multi-center retrospective study of outcomes in 470 ventilated patients, including those treated with ECMO and HFOV, the combination of the OI, PIP, PEEP, age, FiO_2, and PRISM score were the best predictors of outcome.[56] A subsequent publication using this data which analyzed the outcome of ECMO-eligible patients suggested that the use of ECMO resulted in improved sur-vival.[57] This formed the basis for the design of a prospective multi-center randomized controlled trial (RCT) comparing ECMO with a pressure-limited lung protective ventilation strategy. This study was terminated after enrolling 406 patients when the mortality in the ECMO-eligible patients was 18% compared to the predicted rate of 40%.[51]

The relationship between outcome, measured by mortality, and duration of ventilation using the severity of the oxygenation defect (OI and PaO_2/FiO_2), as well as non-pulmonary organ dysfunction has been confirmed by two more recent studies.[52,54] The difference in mortality between adult and pediatric studies may be accounted for by the fact that ARDS/ALI in children, like lung disease of prematurity, is frequently a single organ disease. This is especially true in the first 2

Table 1. Predictors of outcome in AHRF.

Study	Design	Inclusion criteria	Patients	Mortality
Rivera[47]	1990	FiO_2 0.9, PIP >25 cm H_2O	42	55%
Timmons[49]	1991	FiO_2 0.5, PEEP >6 cm H_2O	44	75%
Tamburro[48]	1991	FiO_2 0.6, PaO_2 <60 mm Hg	37	46%
Davis[46]	1993	Lung injury score >2.5	60	60%
Timmons[56]	1995	FIO_2 ≥0.5 PEEP ≥6 cm H_2O x 12 hr.	470	43%
Fackler[51]	1997	FiO_2 ≥0.5 PEEP ≥6 cm H_2O x 12 hr.	161	20%
Peters[53]	1998	PaO_2/FiO_2 <200	110	22%
Dahlem[50]	2003	P/F <300	44	27%
Trachsel[54]	2005	FiO_2 ≥0.5 PEEP ≥6 cm H_2O x 24 hr.	131	27%
Flori[52]	2005	P/F <300	328	22%

P/F ratio = PaO_2/ FiO_2 ratio, PEEP = peak end expiratory pressure, PIP = peak inspiratory pressure

Table 2. Alternative ventilation strategies.

Ventilation mode	Flow	Airway pressure	Main features	Disadvantages
Volume control (VC)	Variable according to rate of gas flow; commonly rapid constant with plateau but can be decelerating at slow gas flow	Compliance- and resistance-dependent; gradual rise to peak followed by plateau	Guaranteed MV	Not leak-compensated; high airway pressures in severe lung disease
Pressure control (PC)	Decelerating	Square wave; preset pressure	More even distribution of gas flow; leak-compensated	Varying TV and MV according to compliance
Pressure control inverse ratio ventilation (PC-IRV)	Decelerating	Square wave	Lower PIP	Auto-PEEP; cardiovascular compromise
Pressure regulated volume control	Decelerating	Square wave	Lowest airway pressure with guaranteed minute volume	PIP can vary below preset level
Pressure-limited ventilation	Decelerating	Square wave	Low tidal volume Reduced secondary injury	Hypercapnia
Intratracheal pulmonary ventilation (ITPV)	High constant gas flow		Reduce dead space	High gas flow can lead to humidifier "blow out"
Airway release ventilation (ARV)	High constant gas flow	CPAP with intermittent release	Spontaneous respiration	Useful only in mild lung injury
High frequency ventilation (HFV)	High constant gas flow	Sustained MAP	Very low TV; reduced secondary injury	Underestimation of MAP and less than ideal humidity on HFJV

CPAP = continuous positive airway pressure, HFJV = high frequency jet ventilation, MAP = mean airway pressure, MV = minute ventilation, PEEP = peak end expiratory pressure, PIP = peak inspiratory pressure, TV = tidal volume years of life. The question should be raised as to whether these patients should be classified as AHRF rather than ARDS.[54,58] Where ECMO fits in the treatment algorithm for children with isolated pulmonary failure in an era of lung-protective ventilation strategies remains unclear, and can only be judged on a case-by-case basis.

Alternative ventilation strategies

The non-conventional ventilation strategies available for the treatment of AHRF include those that use standard tidal volumes and rates but vary the inspiratory time (prolonged I:E ratio), and those that use reduced PIP and tidal volume while maintaining a normal $PaCO_2$ by either ventilating dead space (high frequency ventilation [HFV]), reducing the dead space (intratracheal pulmonary ventilation) or allowing the $PaCO_2$ to rise (pressure-limited ventilation permissive hypercapnia). In addition to these, there are adjuncts to mechanical ventilation (surfactant and nitric oxide [NO]) as well as PPV by mask (non-invasive ventilation). Finally, one can eliminate the secondary injury altogether by removing the ventilator and providing extracorporeal oxygenation. The characteristics of these various alternative strategies are summarized in Table 2. The more commonly used ventilation strategies will be discussed in detail.

Pressure limited ventilation (permissive hypercapnia)

The traditional approach to mechanical ventilation has always been one targeted to the objective of a normal PaO_2 and $PaCO_2$; the accepted practice has been to use tidal volumes of 10-15 ml/kg. With the increasing recognition that high volumes can injure the already damaged lung has come the realization that it may be safer to ventilate with reduced tidal volume and a pressure-limited target rather than targeting $PaCO_2$. The origin of this revolutionary approach can be traced back to a landmark study by Darioli and Perret[59] published in 1984 entitled "Mechanical controlled hypoven-

tilation in status asthmaticus". A series of adult patients is described that are ventilated using the volume control mode, but with tidal volumes of 8-12 ml/kg, a low inspiratory flow rate, and a rate of 6-10 cycles/min. with the maximum PIP set at 50 cm H_2O. If this was exceeded with the initial settings, the tidal volume was reduced further and the $PaCO_2$ allowed to rise. The duration of ventilation was short (<3 days). All patients survived in an era where 10-20% mortality was the norm for ventilatory support in status asthmaticus. Even more importantly, the principle was established that normocarbia should not be the objective in this situation as the measures required to achieve it are potentially harmful if not lethal. The objective is to correct the hypoxemia while accepting hypercarbia.

The next important study supporting this position was a study by Hickling.[60] He hypothesized that simply reducing the tidal volume and allowing the CO_2 to rise would be equally effective in preventing the ventilation-induced lung injury. This revolutionary concept was tested in 50 patients with ARDS as defined by a Lung Injury Score of >2.5 and a PaO_2/FiO_2 ratio of <150. The ventilation strategy used was synchronized intermittent mandatory ventilation (SIMV), volume-controlled ventilation with the target of PIP <30 cm H_2O when this could be easily achieved, and always <40 cm H_2O with a tidal volume of as low as 5 ml/kg. In many instances, this resulted in significant hypercarbia but no attempt was made to correct this. Sodium bicarbonate was not used to correct the acidosis. The oxygenation strategy used was to increase the PEEP with the objective of reducing the FiO_2 to <0.6. Patients were allowed to breathe spontaneously. The remarkable result was that the hospital mortality in this series was 16% compared with a predicted mortality of 39%. Despite criticism that this was retrospective data and did not conform to the proof of a randomized controlled clinical trial, no single study has done more to influence ventilation practices in the past 20 years. Both of these studies have used the volume control mode with limitation of tidal volume as a method of reducing the PIP. The alternative option as a method of preventing volume distention of the injured lung is to use the pressure control mode with limitation of the PIP. It has been suggested that this may be preferable since, in addition to allowing for a decelerating gas flow pattern, it guarantees that the pre-set PIP will not be exceeded. This has led to a renewed interest from adult intensivists in a mode of ventilation that was abandoned 20 years ago except in neonatal acute respiratory failure (ARF). In fact, the credit for the development of the permissive hypercapnia approach in the AHRF really belongs to Wung[61] who advocated it in the management of persistent pulmonary hypertension (PPHN) in 1985.

Based on the accumulated experimental data from animals and the admittedly limited human experience, a pressure-limited permissive hypercapnia strategy would seem to make good sense as long as we accept that hypercarbia itself, while not desirable, is not intrinsically harmful. While most would agree that modest elevations of $PaCO_2$ in the range of 50 mm Hg are of little concern, levels of >100 mm Hg cause great anxiety to a generation of critical care physicians trained to strict adherence to the physiological norm.

What then are the basis for these concerns, and how do we weigh them against the potential for doing harm by continuing the practice of ventilating to a normal $PaCO_2$? Acute elevations in CO_2 result in the rapid development of an intracellular acidosis. A rising hydrogen ion concentration produces an increase in pulmonary vascular resistance and in cerebral blood flow, which may cause cerebral injury or pulmonary hypertension. Apart from this, there is little evidence that pH levels as low as 7.2 have any adverse effect on myocardial performance or tissue oxygen delivery, while hypocapnia has the opposite effect.[62,63] Indeed, experimental evidence would suggest the contrary. In animal models of ischemia, reperfusion of the lung, and sepsis; hypocapnia has been shown to worsen, while hypercarbia and acidosis have been shown to attenuate the injury.[64-69] In a clinical setting, as long as the kidneys are functioning

normally, patients can compensate for pH levels that drop as low as 7.1 with effective bicarbonate retention by the kidney. In both of the permissive hypercapnia series reported above, there was effective renal compensation, and bicarbonate was not used to correct respiratory acidosis. In Hickling's study, CO_2 levels over 100 mm Hg were permitted with the pH dropping as low as 7.1 without the administration of bicarbonate.[60] The notably improved survival would suggest that acidosis had little adverse effect on myocardial performance. There is also evidence in the literature that in children, levels of $PaCO_2$ >200 mm Hg are not associated with adverse consequences as long as oxygenation is maintained.[70]

If we accept that pressure-limited ventilation with low tidal volumes and hypercapnia is unlikely to be harmful and is at least as effective as pressure control in ARDS, do we have any evidence to prove that it may, in fact, lower mortality? Although the retrospective studies published to date suggest this is true, there are now four published prospective studies in adults comparing this approach with standard ventilation technique. Amato,[41] in a randomized controlled clinical trial in adult patients with ARDS, compared a standard volume control mode with a ventilation strategy that used a low tidal volume combined with PEEP level set above the inflection point in order to reduce the FiO_2 to <0.5. They were able to demonstrate an improved survival to ICU discharge in the lung protective group. Although this would suggest that reduced tidal volume ventilation will reduce mortality in AHRF, this cannot be interpreted as the definitive study given the fact that the tidal volumes of 10-15 ml/kg used in the conventional arm of this study resulted in $PaCO_2$ levels of 35-38 mm Hg, which would not be in keeping with current conventional practice. Three other randomized controlled trials[42-44] also failed to demonstrate a beneficial effect using tidal volume reduction in ARDS patients, but none used the aggressive lung recruitment strategies advocated by Amato. However, building on the observations made in the experimental study of Tremblay[21] which demonstrated the release of cytokines associated with lung distention, Ranieri demonstrated a reduction in mediators of injury in a randomized trial of a low-stretch vs. conventional tidal volume ventilation in adults with ARDS with a trend toward improved survival.[71]

The single most influential study on ventilation-induced lung injury in ARDS was the ARDSNet randomized trial of 6 ml/kg vs. 12 ml/kg tidal volume.[45] A relative risk reduction in mortality in the low tidal volume group of 22% was seen in this study of 800 randomized patients. Although this is a landmark study, it cannot be assumed that 6ml/kg tidal volume should be adopted as the standard ventilator setting. A large number of patients were screened for study entry but not included. Secondly, it has been subsequently pointed out that a significant number of patients in the 12 ml/kg arm of the study actually had their tidal volumes increased following randomization,[72] which begs the question as to whether at least part of the outcome difference was due to injurious ventilation in that group rather than a protective effect of a lower tidal volume. Clearly, it would be unwise to assume that this low tidal volume represents a standard that should be adopted for all patients with ARDS.[73] Rather, the study should be interpreted as showing that high tidal volume ventilation contributes to mortality in ARDS and that tidal volume reduction with hypercarbia is safe and may improve outcome. A second ARDSNet study comparing a high lung volume recruitment strategy with low PEEP did not show a survival benefit.[74]

Algorithm for a lung protective ventilation strategy in acute hypoxic respiratory failure

The following is an outline of a lung protective strategy for the management of pediatric patients with severe oxygenation failure (Figure 1). The algorithm is based on data from pediatric patients which suggest that the requirement for $FiO_2 \geq 0.5$ and a PEEP ≥ 6 cm H_2O for more than 12 hours predicts a mortality of 40%.[56] It has as its foundation the prevention of lung over-distention by the use of low tidal volumes and PEEP together with the objective of reducing the FiO_2 to the lowest level compatible with adequate oxygenation. A balance has to be struck between what would be desirable in all situations (low PIP and low FiO_2) and what would be tolerable in situations of severe lung disease in order to prevent further increase in lung injury. This approach clearly separates ventilation dictated by PIP and ventilator rate (Figure 2) from oxygenation which is determined by PEEP and FiO_2 (Figure 3).

	Objective	Tolerance
Ventilation	PIP ≤30 cm H_2O normal pH	PIP ≤35 cm H_2O
	or	
	compensated respiratory acidosis (pH >7.2)	Ph 7.1
Oxygenation	FiO_2 ≤0.5 SaO_2 90%	SaO_2 85%

STRATEGY

- Pressure-limited ventilation to a maximum PIP of 35 cm H_2O

- Ignore hypercarbia and target the pH rather than the $PaCO_2$ with the objective of a compensated respiratory acidosis (pH >7.2) but a tolerance for a pH down to 7.1

- Increase the PEEP to a level that enables you to reduce the FiO_2 to 0.5 or less, compatible with a saturation of 90% (PaO_2 60 mm Hg)

Figure 1. Lung protective ventilation strategy in pediatric AHRF.

Objective: **pH >7.2** **PIP <30 cm H$_2$O**
Tolerance: **pH >7.1** **PIP <35 cm H$_2$O**

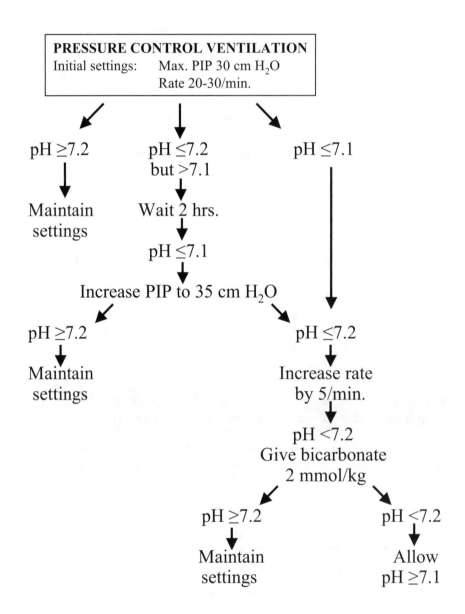

PRESSURE CONTROL VENTILATION
Initial settings: Max. PIP 30 cm H$_2$O
                          Rate 20-30/min.

pH ≥7.2   pH ≤7.2   pH ≤7.1
                     but >7.1

Maintain   Wait 2 hrs.
settings
                     pH ≤7.1

Increase PIP to 35 cm H$_2$O

pH ≥7.2   pH ≤7.2

Maintain   Increase rate
settings   by 5/min.

                                     pH <7.2
                              Give bicarbonate
                                  2 mmol/kg

               pH ≥7.2   pH <7.2

              Maintain   Allow
              settings   pH ≥7.1

Figure 2. Ventilation algorithm for the management of pediatric AHRF.

Objective: SaO$_2$ >90%   FiO$_2$ <0.5

Tolerance: SaO$_2$ >85-90%

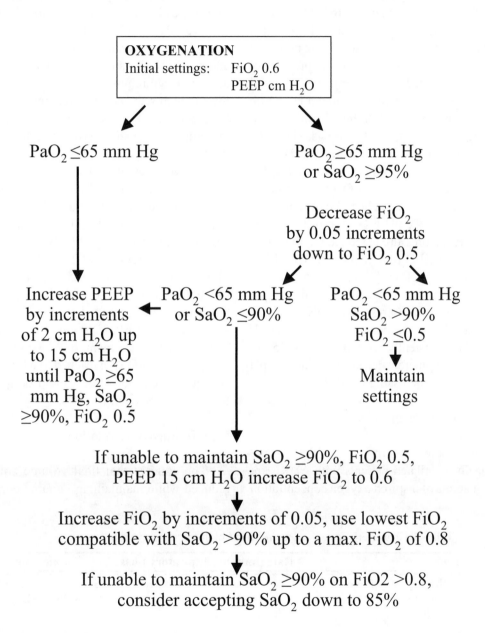

Figure 3. Oxygenation algorithm for the management pediatric AHRF.

Ventilation strategy

Ventilation is controlled by PIP and respiratory rate. The objective in this strategy is to limit PIP to a maximum of 35 cm H_2O, ignoring the $PaCO_2$ as long as there is an appropriate pH compensation (pH >7.2). Patients are managed with a pressure-limited mode (pressure control or pressure-limited volume control). The initial pressure setting objective is ≤30 cm H_2O with a ventilation rate of 20-40 breaths/minute, depending on age. If the first blood gas shows an uncompensated respiratory acidosis (pH <7.2) on 2 consecutive readings 2 hours apart, the PIP is increased to 35 cm H_2O. Once the target PIP of 35 cm H_2O is reached, the pH and PaO_2 is measured. If the pH is >7.2 at or below the target PIP, the pressure is reduced to the target PIP of 30 cm H_2O regardless of $PaCO_2$ level. If the pH falls below 7.2 on PIP 35 cm H_2O, the respiratory rate may be increased by 5 per minute. If this fails to restore the pH to >7.2, 2 mmol/kg of IV bicarbonate may be given. If the pH is consistently <7.2 at a PIP of 35 cm H_2O, consider increasing the tolerance to pH 7.1 rather than increasing the PIP.

Oxygenation strategy

The principal determinants of PaO_2 in mechanically ventilated patients with AHRF are combinations of inspired oxygen concentration and PEEP. The combination of PEEP and inspiratory time dictate the mean airway pressure (MAP). As high inspired oxygen concentrations have been identified as causing secondary lung injury, the objective is to use the lowest FiO_2 to achieve a PaO_2 >55 mm Hg or an arterial saturation >90%. To guarantee adequate oxygenation at the outset of the study, the FiO_2 is initially set at 0.8 with a minimum PEEP of 6 cm H_2O. The FiO_2 is then reduced in increments of 0.05 as long as the PaO_2 remains above 55 mm Hg or the saturation remains above 90%, to maintain the FiO_2 of ≤0.5. If the FiO_2 cannot be reduced to this level without PaO_2 dropping to <55 mm Hg or the saturation to <90%, the FiO_2 is maintained at the lowest level possible while PEEP in increments of 2 cm H_2O is added until PaO_2 increases to >55 mm Hg. PEEP will continue to be added in increments of 2 cm H_2O while the FiO_2 is reduced to at least 0.5 up to a maximum PEEP level of ≤20 cm H_2O. If the PaO_2 cannot be maintained >55 mm Hg or the saturation >90% with a PEEP of 20 cm H_2O, FiO_2 may be increased in increments of 0.05 until a target PaO_2 and saturation are reached. If a FiO_2 >0.70 is required, consideration should be given to tolerating an SaO_2 of 85-90%.

High frequency ventilation

The concept that tidal volume could be reduced while maintaining minute ventilation

Table 3. Characteristics of various forms of high frequency ventilation.

Type	Rate (/min.)	Expiratory phase	Application
High Frequency Positive Pressure Ventilation (HFPPV)	60-120	Passive	Surgical procedures, RDS, ARDS
High Frequency Oscillatory Ventilation (HFOV)	60-900	Active	RDS, ARDS in children
High Frequency Jet Ventilation (HFJV)	60-300	Passive	RDS, ARDS

RDS: respiratory distress syndrome
ARDS: acute respiratory distress syndrome

with rapid rates was first introduced in the 1970s as a ventilatory support technique for surgical procedures involving the upper airway which benefited from a relatively motionless surgical field. This was subsequently redesigned as a support mode for the management of patients with AHRF as a way of mitigating the effects of pulmonary barotraumas. It proved particularly useful in the management of patients with bronchopleural fistula. There are various forms of HFV now being used in clinical medicine, the characteristics of which are summarized in Table 3. This review will concentrate on the two most commonly used: high frequency oscillatory ventilation (HFOV) and high frequency jet ventilation (HFJV). Both have been used to treat patients with RDS and ARDS with the objective of minimizing lung injury by using small tidal volume ventilation while maintaining oxygenation using a high volume, open lung volume strategy.

There is little rationale for considering HFV as just "another ventilator" which happens to operate at faster rates and lower airway pressures than conventional ventilators, without a clear understanding of the clinical situations in which these features may provide a considerable advantage. There are several situations for which HFV can be considered in preference to conventional mechanical ventilation (CMV):

- To improve oxygenation by recruiting lung volume while avoiding cyclical lung distention with high PIP (the "open lung" strategy)
- To achieve more effective CO_2 elimination in situations where this may be particularly important (e.g., PPHN)
- To minimize the effect of secondary or therapy-induced lung injury in situations of diffuse parenchymal lung disease with hypoxia
- To minimize the effect on cardiovascular function by reducing airway pressure

- To improve operating conditions for certain procedures on the airway and lung

High frequency oscillatory ventilation

The discovery that a high frequency sine wave was capable of moving CO_2 out of the lung was first made serendipitously during experiments in paralyzed animals designed to measure thoracic impedance. Following this original observation, the same technique was shown to produce excellent gas exchange in normal animals using tidal volumes well below dead space. The principle that oxygen would diffuse down a concentration gradient had been well established 20 years before when it was shown that arterial oxygen saturation could be maintained over periods of apnea as long as 20 minutes if a high flow of gas was delivered directly into the airway. This technique, known as apneic oxygenation, was used during anesthesia for laryngeal surgery where oxygen and volatile agents at high flows were delivered via a catheter placed through the vocal cords. The technique was limited in duration by the inevitable rise in $PaCO_2$ (3-6 mm Hg/min) that occurred with apnea. However, it was noted that some CO_2 elimination would occur due to the washout of dead space, and that elimination improved the nearer the catheter was placed to the carina. It was also demonstrated that cardiac contraction enhanced the diffusion of CO_2 up the trachea towards the carina, a phenomenon referred to as cardiogenic mixing. The application of the high frequency sine wave to the airway solved the problem of hypercarbia by further enhancing the diffusion of CO_2 due to extremely efficient mixing of gases within the lung. Although the delta P (difference between peak and end expiratory pressures) is high when measured at the peak of the airway in this system, this does not reflect alveolar pressure, which is much lower. Although there is some bulk flow, this is insufficient for alveolar ventilation, and the enhanced gas exchange is accounted for by accelerated diffusion. The first oscillators used to demonstrate this were either adapted from a loudspeaker design or engineering prototypes using a piston within a cylinder driven by a high speed electric motor at speeds of up to 25 Hz. The original animal experiments were performed at 15 Hz (900/min) with fresh gas flows in the circuit of up to 10-15 l/min with attempts to use an expiratory valve in the circuits.

HFOV has progressed from being a physiological curiosity to an alternative mode of ventilation with potential advantages in the management of AHRF. The conventional ventilator cycle not only produces a convective flow of gas to sweep CO_2 out of the lung, but it has to produce a pressure within the lung in excess of alveolar "opening pressure" in order to achieve oxygen exchange. In the low compliant, atelectatic lung, as seen in acute lung injury, airway pressure during the expiratory phase of the respiratory cycle falls below closing pressure unless high levels of PEEP are used. It is this constant opening and closing of terminal airway units under high pressure that result in further injury to the already damaged lung. HFOV offers an entirely different ventilation strategy for dealing with this form of lung disease. High volume cycling is not necessary to eliminate CO_2. Increasing airway pressure by adjusting fresh gas flow can be used to raise MAP above alveolar opening pressure and maintain lung volume at that level, where the small airway pressure swings around the mean and is less injurious to the lung, and the continual cycle of inflation and collapse of terminal lung units is avoided.

In order to establish whether or not HFOV is less injurious to the lung, several groups of investigators have attempted to develop an animal model of acute lung injury and assess the effects of ventilation on the damaged lung. The Toronto group has chosen to use the surfactant depleted lung produced by repeated lavage.[75] They have been able to show quite conclusively

both by blood gas and pathological criteria, that HFOV causes less damage to the injured lung than CMV at matched MAPs, using "open lung strategy". They found that with lavage and surfactant depletion, the lungs were poorly compliant. They were unable to demonstrate any difference between the modes of ventilation until they used a sustained inflation or "sigh" maneuver of 30 cm H_2O for 15 seconds. They were able to achieve excellent oxygenation in the HFOV group of animals while in the CMV group, the animals again became hypoxic and went on to die from pressure-related complications. Postmortem histology of the lungs in this study also showed some striking differences. Those treated with CMV had changes consistent with severe lung damage as seen in ARDS, namely hyaline membrane formation, polymorphonuclear infiltration, and edema formation, while the lung histology in the HFOV group was normal. This study led to an appreciation that in the presence of the diffusely atelectatic lung, either mode of ventilation was equally injurious unless the lung volume was increased above its opening pressure by a sustained inflation and maintained at that level. In the case of HFOV, this was readily achieved, but the lung became rapidly atelectatic on CMV despite the use of PEEP.

The group from San Antonio, Texas chose to use another model of lung injury similar to RDS.[76] Their model was the premature baboon with the characteristics of RDS and severe hyaline membrane formation in the lung. They compared the outcome in HFOV-treated baboons and those treated with CMV. The mortality was clearly higher in CMV-treated animals, which typically showed the effects of severe pulmonary barotrauma on post-mortem examination. The HFOV-treated animals, on the other hand, survived much longer with better gas exchange, required lower FiO_2 and airway pressures, and had little evidence of pulmonary barotrauma at post-mortem. The importance of this approach has been emphasized in the study by McCulloch[77] in the animal lung lavage model, which showed HFOV at a high lung volume produced superior gas exchange and less barotrauma when compared to both HFOV at low lung volume or CMV. In addition, hysteresis and compliance were better in the HFOV group at a high volume based on analysis of the P/V curve.

Following these animal studies, many prospective RCTs comparing HFOV with conventional ventilation in preterm infants[78-84] as well as rescue studies in term infants have been performed.[85-86] These have shown that HFOV is an effective form of ventilation which may reduce the incidence of CLD and the need for ECMO.

The use of HFOV has now extended outside the newborn period with the demonstration of its efficacy as a rescue therapy for older children (up to 35 kg) with AHRF complicated by pulmonary barotrauma.[87] A RCT was designed to compare CMV and HFOV in children outside the newborn period with hypoxemia despite high MAPs or airleak.[88] The study was a randomized crossover design and the HFOV strategy used the open lung approach with a MAP setting 5 cm H_2O above that used on conventional ventilation. However, the conventional ventilation group did define a lung protective strategy. The survival was higher in the HFOV group; however, this was a small study (n=58) and it would be difficult to show an outcome benefit in a study of this size. Also, there was a prolonged period of time on CMV before randomization which makes this more of a rescue study than a true evaluation of two different ventilation strategies. In contrast to this, an RCT of early intervention with HFOV in adults with ARDS showed a definite trend to lower mortality in patients randomized to HFOV, although the study was underpowered and did not reach statistical significance.[89] The study design included pressure-limited, permissive hypercapnia in the conventional arm and a lung recruitment strategy in the HFOV arm.

Despite the lack of a high level of evidence that the use of HFOV influences outcome in pediatric patients with ARDS, it has been widely adopted as an effective rescue strategy.[90] There is also the recognition that it needs to be combined with a lung recruitment strategy that requires the use of high MAPs to open up the lung to improve oxygenation and decrease the FiO_2. Therefore, the strategy requires that initial MAP settings be 2-5 cm H_2O above that used on the conventional ventilator with increment increases until there are signs of lung recruitment as evidenced by the ability to reduce the FiO_2 while maintaining the same or improved SaO_2. This can be confirmed radiologically by counting 9 or more posterior ribs. Mean airway pressures of 35 cm H_2O or higher are frequently required and can be tolerated as long as hemodynamic instability does not occur.

High frequency jet ventilation

HFJV was first developed in clinical anesthesia to provide small tidal volume ventilation for procedures involving the larynx and tracheobronchial tree where the ability to achieve a normal CO_2 with low airway pressures provided ideal operating conditions. Although HFJV and HFOV operate on the same physiological principles using very small tidal volumes delivered at high rates, they should not be considered as merely variations on a theme. HFJV uses a high pressure gas source to deliver small tidal volumes at frequencies of 1-5 Hz. Apart from the slower rates used in HFJV, the other major difference is that expiration is passive with HFJV while it is active in HFOV. The published experience with HFJV in AHRF is considerably less than HFOV and mostly documents its use as rescue therapy in adult patients with either hypoxemia despite high PEEP or established air leak. The rationale for use is usually the avoidance of further barotrauma by the use of smaller tidal volumes while maintaining a high mean airway pressure, with lower peak airway pressures. Most of the published experience consists of anecdotal reports where this strategy has proved successful. The evidence that the same objective could not have been achieved with conventional ventilation is not convincing. Improvements in oxygenation can be obtained by increasing the MAP, but this usually involves some cardiovascular compromise because of the transmitted pressure. The single, randomized, crossover trial comparing HFJV with CMV in adults with AHRF showed no difference in survival.[91] There are, however, trials in children which suggest a benefit. A rescue study published by Smith[92] has shown comparable gas exchange with lower measured airway pressures when patients with ARDS complicated by barotrauma were switched from CMV to HFJV. A randomized, controlled clinical trial of HFJV in neonates with pulmonary interstitial emphysema (PIE) has shown an improvement in PIE and lower mortality rate in infants treated with HFJV compared to CMV.[93]

There are some technical safety concerns when utilizing HFV concerning the adequacy of humidification as well as reported cases of necrotizing tracheobronchitis. In addition, the airway pressures measured from the catheter within the trachea during HFJV probably represent a serious underestimate of true MAP because of the Bernoulli effect and there is likely to be a significant amount of auto-PEEP present.

Prone position ventilation

The current standard supine position for nursing the critically ill patient may be less than ideal in patients with AHRF. Froese and Bryan showed over twenty years ago that during PPV there was a cephalad movement of the dorsal part of the diaphragm and loss of lung volume with normal lungs ventilated in the supine position,[5] and Bryan advocated ventilating in the prone position.[94] With PPV in the supine position, there is preferential perfusion of dependent lung regions, and CT images of ARDS patients have shown that this is the most prominent area for hemorrhage and edema formation.[9,10] Several studies have now described the practice of turning hypoxic patients with AHRF to the prone position with improvement in oxygenation and decreases in intrapulmonary shunt, although this finding is not universal.[95] The proposed mechanisms for this improvement are increased FRC, change in regional diaphragm motion, redistribution of blood flow to less injured lung units, and improved secretion clearance. Studies of experimental lung injury have shown that when turning to the prone position preferential perfusion does not shift to the ventral part of the lung and that edema is more uniformly distributed along the gravitational axis. There were also no changes in FRC or regional diaphragm movement. The explanation for the decreased shunting seen with the prone position seems to be that the gravitational distribution of pleural pressure is much more uniform in the prone position. In the supine position the gravitational forces result in pleural pressure becoming positive in the dependent lung regions and dorsal lung units are below closing volume. This finding suggests that transpulmonary pressure may not exceed airway pressure in this region resulting in lung collapse. The gravitational pleural pressure differences in the thorax are much less in the prone position, resulting in less of the lung being below closing volume, and decreased shunt.

The clinical and physiological studies suggest that there may be a benefit to gas exchange with changing from supine to prone position when ventilating patients with hypoxemia due to ARDS.[96-102] Translating this into an outcome benefit has proven more challenging. In the largest study in adults where patients with a P/F ratio were randomized to prone position ventilation for ≥6 hours of 24, there was no difference in outcome, although there was a consistent and reproducible improvement in oxygenation.[103] However, a subgroup analysis showed that there was a significant reduction in mortality (20 vs. 40%) in those patients with the worst oxygenation defect defined as P/F <82.

There are few studies of prone positioning in children with ARDS or AHRF. Prospective case series demonstrate a high response rate in terms of improvement in oxygenation[104-106] and Korencki[107] found a similar effect in a small, randomized trial. However, the clinical studies would suggest that prone position ventilation, while not benefiting all patients, should be included in the algorithm for the management of patients with severe hypoxemia.

Adjuncts to positive pressure ventilation

Surfactant replacement therapy

Surfactant deficiency in premature newborn infants was first described over 30 years ago. A lack of surfactant causes an increase in surface tension at the alveolar level as well as causing the diffusely atelectatic lung that is typically seen in this disease. If these surface tension forces are reduced with the administration of surfactant, then the tendency for these alveoli to collapse will be reduced and ventilation can be applied at lower peak airway pressures. With the development of naturally occurring and synthetic surfactants, this has now become a reality. Few therapies in the treatment of AHRF in any age group have undergone such extensive study as surfactant replacement therapy in RDS. There are now over 30 published RCTs of either synthetic or natural surfactant given at the time of delivery or shortly thereafter. These have been reviewed in a meta-analysis by Jobe[108] which concluded that surfactant replacement therapy has reduced the mortality in premature infants with RDS. Most controlled trials have been able to demonstrate a reduction in the complications associated with ventilating the lung of the premature infant such as pneumothorax, intraventricular hemorrhage, and patent ductus arteriosus. The data on the incidence of bronchopulmonary dysplasia is less convincing. Some studies have shown a reduction in the incidence while others have not. Even so, surfactant replacement therapy remains one of the few unqualified success stories in the treatment of neonates with RDS over the past 20 years.

The use of surfactant replacement therapy outside the newborn age group is less clear. Since the first descriptions of ARDS in the 1960s it has been recognized that there were surfactant abnormalities without clear evidence of deficiency. There is abundant experimental and clinical evidence to show that surfactant is inactivated in ARDS, probably secondary to the protein leak into the alveolus. Samples of broncho-alveolar lavage fluid taken from adult patients with ARDS and post-mortem lung lavage studies have shown changes in the surfactant protein and phospholipid concentration and altered surface tension behavior of the fluid.[109] Although the administration of surfactant can be shown to improve oxygenation and compliance in experimental models of ARDS, demonstrating a benefit in humans with AHRF has proved more problematic. A RCT of nebulized Exosurf in adult patients with sepsis-induced ARDS demonstrated no benefit.[110] Although this result was disappointing, it may be premature to dismiss surfactant replacement therapy as ineffective. Not all surfactants are equally efficacious and the synthetic varieties which do not have any of the surfactant proteins (A, B, or C) may be less than ideal in this situation. A prospective, randomized, open-label RCT of bovine surfactant in adult patients with ARDS showed superior gas exchange and improved survival in the surfactant-treated patients.[111] However, a larger prospective RCT of recombinant surfactant replacement therapy in ARDS showed no benefit.[112]

The situation is somewhat more promising in children. Case series and randomized studies suggest that some patients with AHRF may see an improvement in oxygenation with surfactant replacement therapy.[113-115] In a recent RCT of a natural surfactant containing both proteins B and C (Infasurf, Forest Laboratories, Inc., New York, NY) Willson found that mortality was lower in those patients receiving surfactant (19 vs. 36%) without any difference in ventilator-free days.[55] The greatest difference in mortality was seen in those patients who were less than 12 months old. This again implies that the epidemiology of ARDS/ALI in this age group is more likely to be single system lung disease where lung-specific therapy will have the greatest impact on outcome. Dramatic responses to surfactant replacement therapy have been reported in immunosuppressed children with pneumocystis pneumonitis.[113,114,116]

Inhaled nitric oxide

Few therapies in critical care medicine in the past 20 years have generated the interest and enthusiasm as that surrounding the medical use of inhaled NO (iNO). Experiments in the 1970s first described the vital role played by the intact endothelium with inducing vascular dilatation. NO was subsequently identified as the endothelial derived relaxing factor, and experimental studies which demonstrated that iNO is a highly selective pulmonary vasodilator led quickly to its introduction into clinical medicine. It has now become evident that NO is a biologically important compound with ubiquitous actions that involve multiple organ systems. NO is synthetized from L-arginine by the enzyme nitric oxide synthetase (NOS). NO is then diffused rapidly from the endothelial cell into the vascular smooth muscle where it stimulates guanylate cyclase to produce cyclic guanosine monophosphate (cGMP), a potent vasodilator. The systemic nitrodilators currently used operate by a similar mechanism but their pulmonary vasodilator effects cannot be separated from the systemic. In the case of iNO, the vasodilator properties are confined to the pulmonary circulation because the marked affinity of NO for hemoglobin results in its rapid binding and inactivation as soon as it crosses the alveolar capillary membrane. NO is an unstable molecule which reacts with oxygen to form higher oxides of nitrogen, the most toxic

of which is nitrogen dioxide. The speed of this reaction is proportional to both the concentration of oxygen and the duration of exposure and is greatly enhanced by high inspired oxygen concentrations. The initial animal experiments with NO demonstrated its remarkable ability to selectively dilate the pulmonary vascular bed after pulmonary vasoconstriction had been induced by either inhalation of a hypoxic gas mixture or the infusion of the potent vasoconstrictor thromboxane. In these studies, there seemed to be a dose-dependent vasodilator effect as the inhaled concentration was increased from 10 to 80 ppm.

There has also been increasing experience in the use of iNO as part of the ventilatory management of both pediatric and adult patients with ARDS. In this situation, pulmonary hypertension is secondary to the inflammatory-mediated release of pulmonary vasoconstrictors, the development of pulmonary microthrombi, and areas of local ventilation-perfusion mismatch, rather than being the primary pathophysiological disturbance. Again, the published studies document its use as rescue therapy in non-controlled clinical trials, often as an adjunct to other alternative ventilation therapies. Most of these show a pulmonary vasodilator effect with a fall in pulmonary vascular resistance (PVR) in the range of 20-30% and an improvement in oxygenation secondary to improved ventilation-perfusion matching.[117-123] Although the introduction of iNO frequently allows for weaning of ventilator settings to less injurious levels, it remains to be seen whether there will be a reduction in mortality in syndromes associated with multi-organ failure and where hypoxemia is frequently not the cause of death. There are also concerns about the safety of adding iNO in situations where sepsis is often the underlying etiology, given the fact that septic shock has been shown to be associated with the overproduction of endogenous NO. The conversion of NO to peroxynitrite, which has been shown to damage type 2 alveolar epithelial cells, is also potentially hazardous in the already injured lung.[124]

There are now at least six published RCTs of iNO in adult patients with ARDS.[125-130] While most have shown an improvement in oxygenation, in a significant number of patients this is frequently not sustained and none has shown a benefit in terms of increased survival. The most recent study randomized 385 patients with hypoxemia and P/F <250 to receive either 5ppm iNO or placebo gas, having excluded patients with sepsis and multi-organ failure.[128] There was no difference in outcome as measured by survival and length of assisted ventilation. Randomized studies and case series in pediatric patients with AHRF have reached similar conclusions.[117-120,131-133] Having said this, iNO may still have a place in the treatment algorithm for severe hypoxemia because there is a small minority of patients that demonstrate dramatic improvement in oxygenation. Perhaps the most effective mode of gas delivery is to use it in combination with HFOV. Studies in both adults and children suggest that this technique of lung recruitment allows for more effective delivery of iNO at the alveolar level than with conventional ventilation.[134,135] A summary of the published literature would support a short trial of iNO in severe hypoxemia and discontinuation if no response is seen, bearing in mind that the therapy is expensive and not without potential harmful effects. However, there clearly is no benefit from the routine use of iNO in this patient population.[136,137]

Non-invasive ventilation

One of the most important innovations in mechanical ventilation in the past 10 years has been the widespread use of non-invasive ventilation (NIV) in AHRF. First introduced into clinical medicine as CPAP by Gregory[7] in 1971 for the management of RDS, it has only been recently reintroduced into the management of older children and adults with AHRF.[138,143] The potential advantages include avoidance of endotracheal intubation and the need to use sedating and paralyzing drugs, and the reduction in the incidence of sinusitis, sepsis, and nosocomial pneumonia. In patients with heart failure, NIV also has a beneficial effect on cardiac function by decreasing the left ventricular afterload.[144] There have been a number of randomized trials in adults comparing the early use of NIV in acutely ill patients with AHRF with standard care consisting of oxygen by face mask, endotracheal intubation, and PPV. The results of these have been somewhat conflicting. Most show improvement in oxygenation with the use of NIV, but in terms of intubation rates, duration of ICU stay, and mortality some suggest benefit and others are neutral.[145-147] Studies of the use of NIV in the management of adult patients who fail extubation show that it does not decrease the need for re-intubation.[148,149] However, there seems to be a more clearly demonstrated benefit in immunocompromised patients and those with malignancies where case series and randomized trials have shown that early intervention improves outcome.[145,150-152] A summary of the accumulated experience with NIV in ICU patients indicates that early intervention in patients who are tachypneic and hypoxemic before they develop hypercarbia and multi-organ dysfunction increases the likelihood for the avoidance of intubation and a potential outcome benefit.[140,143,153]

There is far less published pediatric experience with NIV, which mostly consists of case series, but there is accumulating experience which would suggest that in selected patients its early use may avoid the need for intubation.[141,154-157]

Extra-pulmonary therapies in acute respiratory distress syndrome

Steroids and fluids

Since ARDS is a multi-organ syndrome rather than a lung-specific disease it stands to reason that there are a number of non-pulmonary interventions that may have an important impact on outcome. Meduri et al. published a number of non-randomized clinical studies of the use of steroids in the late "proliferative" phase of ARDS.[158] Patients are typically beyond the first week of their illness and have signs of inflammation with fever, elevated white cell counts, and evidence of fibroblast infiltration on lung biopsy. In a randomized, placebo-controlled trial, Meduri showed improved survival and a reduced incidence of organ dysfunction in a study of only 26 patients.[159] This finding has to be interpreted with some caution because it has not been confirmed in a much larger multicenter study, and the routine use of steroids cannot be recommended in patients with ARDS.

One of the features of ARDS in any age group is the increased degree of endothelial permeability that leads to the leakage of protein-rich fluid into the alveolar space, resulting in atelectasis. A standard approach to this problem has been fluid restriction and the use of diuretic therapy. Clinical studies in adults have suggested that this approach may improve oxygenation without any measurable impact on survival.[160,161] Martin, in a randomized trial of patients who were hypoproteinemic, has shown that the combination of albumin and lasix improves gas exchange and fluid balance.[162] The potential flaw is sacrifice of non-pulmonary organ function in order to achieve a better PaO_2. If the net effect is volume contraction, reduced cardiac output, and decreased tissue oxygen delivery, there is no net gain for the patient. Furthermore, the overenthusiastic use of diuretics and fluid restriction may push patients into renal failure, which would have a negative impact on outcome. Therefore the issue of the "wet" vs. "dry" lung is unresolved.

Acute hypoxic respiratory failure–a treatment algorithm based on assessment of severity and indications for ECMO

Although the mortality of AHRF in children is approximately half of that in adults, there are still groups of patients where the outcome is poor. These include patients with immunosup-

pression and suspected sepsis who frequently have multi-system organ dysfunction, where the cause of death may not be hypoxemia. However, changes in ventilation strategies can have a significant impact on survival. Survival in bone marrow transplant patients, for example, has increased from 10% to greater than 40% in some series.[163-171] This leads to a reconsideration of whether ECMO is indicated for this patient group.[172] A second group with a poor prognosis are infants with pertussis and pulmonary hypertension where ECMO has been particularly unsuccessful.[173-177] Ventilation strategy should be guided by a ventilation algorithm based on the severity of the oxygenation defect. Both the OI and the P/F ratio have been shown to be predictive of outcome and extubation success in pediatric studies of AHRF.[52,54] Therefore, a rising OI or a falling P/F ratio should be used to track the severity of the oxygenation defect and trigger the next step in the ventilation algorithm, similar to the one described by Ullrich for adults with ARDS.[178] A similar protocol for pediatric patients would include the early use of NIV, pressure-limited ventilation with high PEEP, HFOV, prone position ventilation, iNO, surfactant replacement therapy and ECMO when the patient remains hypoxemic with an OI that is rising. Also, cooling febrile, hypoxemic patients in order to decrease oxygen consumption can be an effective strategy.[179]

The place of ECMO in the management algorithm of AHRF of children outside the newborn period is difficult to define. Outcome figures from the ELSO Registry suggest an overall survival of around 40-50%, with single institution survival as high as 70-80%.[180-183] The problem with interpreting this data is that they are center-specific and do not account for wide variations in ventilation practices. While there is no debate that ECMO can be life-saving therapy, the difficulty lies in defining oxygenation failure in an era of multiple alternative ventilation strategies. The data on ventilator-induced lung injury suggests that, at times, the patient is being rescued from the therapy rather than the disease. The most successful ECMO outcomes will be in those patients with single system lung disease and the worst will be in those with hypoxia and multiple organ failure.

Summary

This review of pediatric AHRF has as its premise the frequently overlooked fact that ventilators do not cure lung disease, in fact they do the opposite. For too long, mechanical ventilation has been guided by normal lung physiology with escalations in volume and pressure to achieve "normal" blood gases. We must now recognize that this approach may be inherently harmful and that the ventilator strategy must be adapted to match the underlying pathophysiology of the lung. Limitation of airway pressure with tolerance of hypercarbia is already improving survival in the management of status asthmaticus, where mortality rates in the 1970s were 25-50% in patients requiring ventilation. In ARDS, the "open lung" strategy with prevention of over-distention would seem to have the most to offer. This is particularly true with HFOV where the early application of an aggressive volume recruitment strategy followed by a reduction of MAP can be highly effective.

Demonstrating improvement in outcome of patients with AHRF from changes in ventilation practice will prove difficult, as it is a syndrome with a multiplicity of causes rather than a single disease entity. Non-conventional ventilation techniques probably have the most to offer patients with hypoxia due to single system pulmonary failure, while patients with immunosuppression and multi-organ dysfunction would be expected to benefit least. Given the multiplicity of therapies now available, there is a need for large well-designed multicenter studies in children to determine what techniques are truly effective and at what stage in the disease process they should be introduced.

References

1. Lassen HCA. A preliminary report on the 1952 epidemic of poliomyelitis in Copenhagen with special reference to the treatment of acute respiratory insufficiency. *Lancet* 1953; 1:37-41.

2. Bernard GR, Artigas A, Brigham KL, et al. The American-European Consensus Conference on ARDS. Definitions, mechanisms, relevant outcomes, and clinical trial coordination. *Am J Respir Crit Care Med* 1994; 149:818-824.

3. Nash G, Bowen JA, Langlinais PC. "Respirator Lung" a misnomer. *Arch Pathol* 1971; 91:234-240.

4. Bendixen HH, Hedley-Whyte J, Laver MB. Impaired oxygenation in surgical patients during general anaesthesia with controlled ventilation. *N Engl J Med* 1963; 269:991-996.

5. Froese A, Bryan AC. Effects of anaesthesia and paralysis on diaphragmatic mechanics in man. *Anesthesiology* 1974; 41:242-255.

6. Ashbaugh DG, Bigelow DB, Petty TL, Levine BE. Acute respiratory distress in adults. *Lancet* 1967; 2:319-323.

7. Gregory GA, Kitterman JA, Phibbs RH, Tooley WH, Hamiliton WK. Treatment of the idiopathic respiratory-distress syndrome with continuous positive airway pressure. *N Engl J Med* 1971; 284:1333-1339.

8. Suter PM, Fairley HB, Isenberg MD. Optimum end expiratory airway pressure in patients with acute pulmonary failure. *N Engl J Med* 1975; 292:284-289.

9. Gattinoni L, Pelosi P, Vitale G, Presenti A, D'Andrea L, Mascheroni D. Body position changes redistribute lung computed-tomographic density in patients with acute respiratory failure. *Anesthesiology* 1991; 74:15-23.

10. Gattinoni L, Pesenti A, Bombino M, et al. Relationships between lung computed tomographic density, gas exchange, and PEEP

in acute respiratory failure. *Anesthesiology* 1988; 69:824-832.

11. Webb HH, Tierney DF. Experimental pulmonary edema due to intermittent positive pressure ventilation with high inflation pressures. Protection by positive end-expiratory pressure. *Am Rev Respir Dis* 1974; 110:556-565.

12. Dreyfuss D, Basset G, Soler P, Saumon G. Intermittent positive pressure hyperventilation with high inflation pressures produces pulmonary microvascular injury in rats. *Am Rev Respir Dis* 1985; 132:880-884.

13. Kolobow T, Moretti MP, Fumagalli R, et al. Severe impairment in lung function induced by high peak airway pressure during mechanical ventilation. *Am Rev Respir Dis* 1987; 135:312-331.

14. Tsuno K, Prato P, Kolobow T. Acute lung injury from mechanical ventilation at moderately high airway pressures. *J Appl Physiol* 1990;69:956-961.

15. Dreyfuss D, Soler P, Basset G, Saumon G. High inflation pulmonary edema: effects of high airway pressure, high tidal volume and positive end-expiratory pressure. *Am Rev Respir Dis* 1988; 137:1159-1164.

16. Hernandez LA, Coker PJ, May S, Thompson AL, Parker JC. Mechanical ventilation increases microvascular permeability in oleic acid-injured lungs. *J Appl Physiol* 1990; 69:2057-2061.

17. Hernandez LA, Peevy KJ, Moise AA, Parker JC. Chest wall restriction limits high airway pressure-induced lung injury in young rabbits. *J App Physiol* 1989; 66:2364-2368.

18. Corbridge TC, Wood LDH, Crawford GP, Chudoba MJ, Yanos J, Sznajder JI. Adverse effects of large tidal volume and low PEEP in canine acid aspiration. *Am Rev Respir Dis* 1990; 142:311-315.

19. Sandhar BK, Niblett DJ, Argiras EP, Dunnill MS, Sykes MK. Effects of positive end expiratory pressure on hyaline membrane

formation in a rabbit model of the neonatal respiratory distress syndrome. *Intensive Care Med* 1988; 14:538-546.

20. Muscedere JG, Mullen JB, Gan K, Slutsky AS. Tidal ventilation at low airway pressures can augment lung injury. *Am J Respir Crit Care Med* 1994; 149:1327-1334.

21. Tremblay L, Valenza F, Ribeiro S, Li J, Slutsky A. Injurious ventilatory strategies increase cytokines and c-fos m-RNA expression in an isolated rat lung model. *J Clin Invest* 1997; 99:944-952.

22. Coalson JJ. Experimental models of bronchopulmonary dysplasia. *Biol Neonate* 1997; 71 Suppl 1:35-38.

23. Coalson JJ, King RJ, Winter VT, et al. O_2- and pneumonia-induced lung injury. I. Pathological and morphometric studies. *J Appl Physiol* 1989; 67:346-356.

24. Coalson JJ, Kuehl TJ, Prihoda TJ, deLemos RA. Diffuse alveolar damage in the evolution of bronchopulmonary dysplasia in the baboon. *Pediatr Res* 1988; 24:357-366.

25. Crapo JD, Hayatdavoudi G, Knapp MJ, Fracica PJ, Wolfe WG, Piantadosi CA. Progressive alveolar septal injury in primates exposed to 60% oxygen for 14 days. *Am J Physiol* 1994; 267:L797-806.

26. de los Santos R, Coalson JJ, Holcomb JR, Johanson WG, Jr. Hyperoxia exposure in mechanically ventilated primates with and without previous lung injury. *Exp Lung Res* 1985; 9:255-275.

27. de los Santos R, Seidenfeld JJ, Anzueto A, et al. One hundred percent oxygen lung injury in adult baboons. *Am Rev Respir Dis* 1987; 136:657-661.

28. Delemos RA, Coalson JJ, Gerstmann DR, Kuehl TJ, Null DM, Jr. Oxygen toxicity in the premature baboon with hyaline membrane disease. *Am Rev Respir Dis* 1987; 136:677-682.

29. Fracica PJ, Knapp MJ, Piantadosi CA, et al. Responses of baboons to prolonged hyper-

oxia: physiology and qualitative pathology. *J Appl Physiol* 1991; 71:2352-362.

30. Sackner MA, Landa J, Hirsch J, Zapata A. Pulmonary effects of oxygen breathing. A 6-hour study in normal men. *Ann Intern Med* 1975; 82:40-43.

31. Yusa T, Crapo JD, Freeman BA. Hyperoxia enhances lung and liver nuclear superoxide generation. *Biochim Biophys Acta* 1984; 798:167-174.

32. Davis WB, Rennard SI, Bitterman PB, Crystal RG. Pulmonary oxygen toxicity. Early reversible changes in human alveolar structures induced by hyperoxia. *N Engl J Med* 1983; 309:878-883.

33. Gattinoni L, Pelosi P, Suter PM, Pedoto A, Vercesi P, Lissoni A. Acute respiratory distress syndrome caused by pulmonary and extrapulmonary disease. Different syndromes? *Am J Respir Crit Care Med* 1998; 158:3-11.

34. Doyle RL, Szaflarski N, Modin GW, Wiener-Kronish JP, Matthay MA. Identification of patients with acute lung injury. Predictors of mortality. *Am J Respir Crit Care Med* 1995; 152:1818-1824.

35. Estenssoro E, Dubin A, Laffaire E, et al. Incidence, clinical course, and outcome in 217 patients with acute respiratory distress syndrome. *Crit Care Med* 2002; 30:2450-2456.

36. Ferguson ND, Frutos-Vivar F, Esteban A, et al. Airway pressures, tidal volumes, and mortality in patients with acute respiratory distress syndrome. *Crit Care Med* 2005; 33:21-30.

37. Monchi M, Bellenfant F, Cariou A, et al. Early predictive factors of survival in the acute respiratory distress syndrome. A multivariate analysis. *Am J Respir Crit Care Med* 1998; 158:1076-1081.

38. Roupie E, Lepage E, Wysocki M, et al. Prevalence, etiologies and outcome of the acute respiratory distress syndrome among hypoxemic ventilated patients. SRLF Col-laborative Group on Mechanical Ventilation. Societe de Reanimation de Langue Francaise. *Intensive Care Med* 1999; 25:920-929.

39. Suchyta MR, Clemmer TP, Elliott CG, Orme JF, Jr., Weaver LK. The adult respiratory distress syndrome. A report of survival and modifying factors. *Chest* 1992; 101:1074-1079.

40. Zilberberg MD, Epstein SK. Acute lung injury in the medical ICU: comorbid conditions, age, etiology, and hospital outcome. *Am J Respir Crit Care Med* 1998; 157:1159-1164.

41. Amato MBP, Barbas CSV, Medeiros DM, et al. Effect of a protective-ventilation strategy on mortality in the acute respiratory distress syndrome. *N Engl J Med* 1998; 338:347-354.

42. Brochard L, Roudot-Thoraval F, Roupie E, et al. Tidal volume reduction for prevention of ventilator-induced lung injury in acute respiratory distress syndrome. The Multicenter Trail Group on Tidal Volume reduction in ARDS. *Am J Respir Crit Care Med* 1998; 158:1831-1838.

43. Brower RG, Shanholtz CB, Fessler HE, et al. Prospective, randomized, controlled clinical trial comparing traditional versus reduced tidal volume ventilation in acute respiratory distress syndrome patients. *Crit Care Med* 1999; 27:1492-1498.

44. Stewart TE, Meade MO, Cook DJ, et al. Evaluation of a ventilation strategy to prevent barotrauma in patients at high risk for acute respiratory distress syndrome. Pressure- and Volume-Limited Ventilation Strategy Group. *N Engl J Med* 1998; 338:355-361.

45. The Acute Respiratory Distress Syndrome Network. Ventilation with lower tidal volumes as compared with traditional tidal volumes for acute lung injury and the acute respiratory distress syndrome. *N Engl J Med* 2000; 342:1301-1308.

46. Davis SL, Furman DP, Costarino AT. Adult respiratory distress syndrome in children: Associated disease, clinical course, and predictors of death. *J Pediatr* 1993; 123:35-45.

47. Rivera RA, Butt W, Shann F. Predictors of mortality in children with respiratory failure: possible indications for ECMO. Anaesth Intensive Care 1990; 18:385-389.

48. Tamburro RF, Bugnitz MC, Stidham GL. Alveolar-arterial oxygen gradient as a predictor of outcome in patients with non-neonatal pediatric respiratory failure. *J Pediatrics* 1991; 119:935-938.

49. Timmons OD, Dean JM, Vernon DD. Mortality rates and prognostic variables in children with adult respiratory distress syndrome. *J Pediatr* 1991; 119:896-899.

50. Dahlem P, van Aalderen WM, Hamaker ME, Dijkgraaf MG, Bos AP. Incidence and short-term outcome of acute lung injury in mechanically ventilated children. *Eur Respir J* 2003; 22:980-985.

51. Fackler JC, Bohn D, Green TP, et al. ECMO for ARDS; stopping a RCT. *Am J Respir Crit Care Med* 1997; 155(A504).

52. Flori HR, Glidden DV, Rutherford GW, Matthay MA. Pediatric acute lung injury: prospective evaluation of risk factors associated with mortality. *Am J Respir Crit Care Med* 2005; 171:995-1001.

53. Peters MJ, Tasker RC, Kiff KM, Yates R, Hatch DJ. Acute hypoxemic respiratory failure in children: case mix and the utility of respiratory severity indices. *Intensive Care Med* 1998; 24:699-705.

54. Trachsel D, McCrindle BW, Nakagawa S, Bohn DJ. Oxygenation index predicts outcome in children with acute hypoxemic respiratory failure. *Am J Respir Crit Care Med* 2005; 15:206-211.

55. Willson DF, Thomas NJ, Markovitz BP, et al. Effect of exogenous surfactant (calfactant) in pediatric acute lung injury: a randomized controlled trial. *JAMA* 2005; 293:470-476.

56. Timmons OD, Havens PL, Fackler JC. Predicting death in pediatric patients with acute respiratory failure. Pediatric Critical Care Study Group. Extracorporeal Life Support Organization. *Chest* 1995; 108:789-797.

57. Green TP, Timmons OD, Fackler JC, Moler FW, Thompson AE, Sweeney MF. The impact of extracorporeal membrane oxygenation on survival in pediatric patients with acute respiratory failure. Pediatric Critical Care Study Group. *Crit Care Med* 1996; 24:323-329.

58. Sokol J, Jacobs SE, Bohn D. Inhaled nitric oxide for acute hypoxemic respiratory failure in children and adults (Cochrane Review). *Cochrane Database Syst Rev* 2003:CD002787.

59. Darioli R, Perret C. Mechanical controlled hypoventilation in status asthmaticus. *Am Rev Respir Dis* 1984; 129:385-387.

60. Hickling KG, Walsh J, Henderson S, Jackson R. Low mortality rate in adult respiratory distress syndrome using low-volume, pressure-limited ventilation with permissive hypercapnia: a prospective study. *Crit Care Med* 1994; 22:1568-1578.

61. Wung JT, James LS, Kilchevsky E, James E. Management of infants with severe respiratory failure and persistence of the fetal circulation, without hyperventilation. *Pediatrics* 1985; 76:488-494.

62. Laffey JG, Kavanagh BP. Carbon dioxide and the critically ill--too little of a good thing? *Lancet* 1999; 354:1283-1286.

63. Laffey JG, Kavanagh BP. Hypocapnia. *N Engl J Med* 2002; 347:43-53.

64. Shibata K, Cregg N, Engelberts D, Takeuchi A, Fedorko L, Kavanagh BP. Hypercapnic acidosis may attenuate acute lung injury by inhibition of endogenous xanthine oxidase. *Am J Respir Crit Care Med* 1998; 158:1578-1584.

65. Laffey JG, Engelberts D, Duggan M, Veldhuizen R, Lewis JF, Kavanagh BP. Carbon dioxide attenuates pulmonary impairment resulting from hyperventilation. *Crit Care Med* 2003; 31:2634-2640.

66. Laffey JG, Engelberts D, Kavanagh BP. Injurious effects of hypocapnic alkalosis in the isolated lung. *Am J Respir Crit Care Med* 2000; 162:399-405.

67. Laffey JG, Engelberts D, Kavanagh BP. Buffering hypercapnic acidosis worsens acute lung injury. *Am J Respir Crit Care Med* 2000; 161:141-146.

68. Laffey JG, Jankov RP, Engelberts D, et al. Effects of therapeutic hypercapnia on mesenteric ischemia-reperfusion injury. *Am J Respir Crit Care Med* 2003; 168:1383-1390.

69. Laffey JG, Tanaka M, Engelberts D, et al. Therapeutic hypercapnia reduces pulmonary and systemic injury following in vivo lung reperfusion. *Am J Respir Crit Care Med* 2000; 162:2287-2294.

70. Goldstein B, Shannon DC, Todres ID. Supercarbia in children: Clinical course and outcome. *Crit Care Med* 1990; 18:166-168.

71. Ranieri VM, Suter PM, Tortorella C, et al. Effect of mechanical ventilation on inflammatory mediators in patients with acute respiratory distress syndrome: a randomized controlled trial. *JAMA* 1999; 282:54-61.

72. Eichacker PQ, Gerstenberger EP, Banks SM, Cui X, Natanson C. Meta-analysis of acute lung injury and acute respiratory distress syndrome trials testing low tidal volumes. *Am J Respir Crit Care Med* 2002; 166:1510-1514.

73. Parshuram CS, Kavanagh BP. Positive clinical trials: understand the control group before implementing the result. *Am J Respir Crit Care Med* 2004; 170:223-226.

74. Brower RG, Lanken PN, MacIntyre N, et al. Higher versus lower positive end-expiratory pressures in patients with the acute respiratory distress syndrome. *N Engl J Med* 2004; 351:327-336.

75. Hamilton PP, Onayemi A, Smyth JA, et al. Comparison of conventional and high-frequency ventilation: oxygenation and lung pathology. *J Appl Physiol* 1983; 55:131-138.

76. Delemos RA, Coalson JJ, Gerstmann DR, et al. Ventilatory management of infant baboons with hyaline membrane disease: the use of high frequency ventilation. *Pediatr Res* 1987; 21:594-602.

77. McCulloch PR, Forkert PG, Froese AB. Lung volume maintenance during HFO in surfactant deficient rabbits. *Am Rev Respir Dis* 1988; 137:1185-1192.

78. Clark RH, Gerstmann DR, Null DM, deLemos RA. Prospective randomised comparison of high-frequency oscillatory and conventional ventilation in respiratory distress syndrome. *Pediatrics* 1992; 89:5-12.

79. Gerstmann DR, Minton SD, Stoddard RA, et al. The provo multicenter early high-frequency oscillatory ventilation trial: improved pulmonary and clinical outcome in respiratory distress syndrome. *Pediatrics* 1996;98:1044-1057.

80. HIFI Study Group. High-frequency oscillatory ventilation compared with conventional mechanical ventilation in the treatment of respiratory failure in preterm infants. *N Engl J Med* 1989; 320:88-93.

81. HiFO Study Group. Randomised study of high-frequency oscillatory ventilation in infants with severe respiratory distress syndrome. *J Pediatr* 1993; 122:609-619.

82. Ogawa Y, Miyasaka K, Kawano T, et al. A multicenter randomized trial of high frequency oscillatory ventilation as compared with conventional mechanical ventilation in preterm infants with respiratory failure. *Early Hum Dev* 1993; 32:1-10.

83. Rettwitz-Volk W, Veldman A, Roth B, et al. A prospective, randomized, multicenter trial

of high-frequency oscillatory ventilation compared with conventional ventilation in preterm infants with respiratory distress syndrome receiving surfactant. *J Pediatr* 1998; 132:249-254.

84. Kinsella JP, Truog WE, Walsh WF, et al. Randomized, multicenter trial of inhaled nitric oxide and high-frequency oscillatory ventilation in severe, persistent pulmonary hypertension of the newborn. *J Pediatr* 1997; 131:55-62.

85. Clark RH. High-frequency ventilation in acute pediatric respiratory failure. *Chest* 1994; 105:652-653.

86. Carter JM, Gerstmann DR, Clark RH, et al. High-frequency oscillatory ventilation and extracorporeal membrane oxygenation for the treatment of acute neonatal respiratory failure. *Pediatrics* 1990; 85:159-164.

87. Arnold JH, Truog RD, Thompson JE, Fackler JC. High-frequency oscillatory ventilation in pediatric respiratory failure. *Crit Care Med* 1993; 21:272-278.

88. Arnold JH, Hanson JH, Toro-Figuero LO, Gutierrez J, Berens RJ, Anglin DL. Prospective, randomized comparison of high-frequency oscillatory ventilation and conventional mechanical ventilation in pediatric respiratory failure. *Crit Care Med* 1994; 22:1530-1539.

89. Derdak S, Mehta S, Stewart TE, et al. High-frequency oscillatory ventilation for acute respiratory distress syndrome in adults: a randomized, controlled trial. *Am J Respir Crit Care Med* 2002; 166:801-808.

90. Arnold JH, Anas NG, Luckett P, et al. High-frequency oscillatory ventilation in pediatric respiratory failure: a multicenter experience. *Crit Care Med* 2000; 28:3913-3919.

91. Carlon GC, Howland WS, Ray C, Miodownik S, Griffin JP, Groeger JS. High-frequency jet ventilation. A prospective randomized evaluation. *Chest* 1983; 84:551-559.

92. Smith DW, Frankel LR, Derish MT, et al. High-frequency jet ventilation in children with the adult respiratory distress syndrome complicated by pulmonary barotrauma. *Pediatr Pulm* 1993; 15:279-286.

93. Keszler M, Ryckman FC, McDonald JV, Jr., et al. A prospective, multicenter, randomized study of high versus low positive end-expiratory pressure during extracorporeal membrane oxygenation. *J Pediatr* 1992; 120:107-113.

94. Bryan AC. Conference on the scientific basis of respiratory therapy.Pulmonary physiotherapy in the pediatric age group. Comments of a devil's advocate. *Am Rev Respir Dis* 1974; 110:143-144.

95. Albert RK, Leasa D, Sanderson M, Robertson HT, Hlastala MP. The prone position improves arterial oxygenation and reduces shunt in oleic-acid-induced acute lung injury. *Am Rev Respir Dis* 1987; 135:628-633.

96. Blanch L, Mancebo J, Perez M, et al. Short-term effects of prone position in critically ill patients with acute respiratory distress syndrome. *Intensive Care Med* 1997; 23:1033-1039.

97. Chatte G, Sab JM, Dubois JM, Sirodot M, Gaussorgues P, Robert D. Prone position in mechanically ventilated patients with severe acute respiratory failure. *Am J Respir Crit Care Med* 1997; 155:473-478.

98. Douglas WW, Rehder K, Beynen FM, Sessler AD, Marsh HM. Improved oxygenation in patients with acute respiratory failure: the prone position. *Am Rev Respir Dis* 1977; 115:559-566.

99. Fridrich P, Krafft P, Hochleuthner H, Mauritz W. The effects of long-term prone positioning in patients with trauma- induced adult respiratory distress syndrome. *Anesth Analg* 1996; 83:1206-1211.

100. Jolliet P, Bulpa P, Chevrolet JC. Effects of the prone position on gas exchange and hemodynamics in severe acute respiratory

distress syndrome. *Crit Care Med* 1998; 26:1977-1985.

101. Langer M, Mascheroni D, Marcolin R, Gattinoni L. The prone position in ARDS patients: a clinical study. *Chest* 1988; 94:103-107.

102. Pappert D, Rossaint R, Slama K, Gruning T, Falke KJ. Influence of positioning on ventilation-perfusion relationships in severe adult respiratory distress syndrome. *Chest* 1994; 106:1511-1516.

103. Gattinoni L, Tognoni G, Pesenti A, et al. Effect of prone positioning on the survival of patients with acute respiratory failure. *N Engl J Med* 2001; 345:568-573.

104. Casado-Flores J, Martinez de Azagra A, Ruiz-Lopez MJ, Ruiz M, Serrano A. Pediatric ARDS: effect of supine-prone postural changes on oxygenation. *Intensive Care Med* 2002; 28:1792-1796.

105. Curley MA, Thompson JE, Arnold JH. The effects of early and repeated prone positioning in pediatric patients with acute lung injury. *Chest* 2000; 118:156-163.

106. Murdoch IA, Storman MO. Improved arterial oxygenation in children with the adult respiratory distress syndrome: the prone position. *Acta Paediatr* 1994; 83:1043-1046.

107. Kornecki A, Frndova H, Coates AL, Shemie SD. A randomized trial of prolonged prone positioning in children with acute respiratory failure. *Chest* 2001; 119:211-218.

108. Jobe AH. Pulmonary surfactant therapy. *N Engl J Med* 1993; 328:861-868.

109. Gregory TJ, Longmore WJ, Moxley MA, et al. Surfactant chemical composition and biophysical activity in acute respiratory distress syndrome. *J Clin Invest* 1991; 88:1976-1981.

110. Anzueto A, Baughman RP, Guntupalli KK, et al. Aerosolized surfactant in adults with sepsis-induced acute respiratory distress syndrome. Exosurf Acute Respiratory Distress Syndrome Sepsis Study Group. *N Engl J Med* 1996; 334:1417-1421.

111. Gregory TJ, Steinberg KP, Spragg R, et al. Bovine surfactant therapy for patients with acute respiratory distress syndrome. *Am J Respir Crit Care Med* 1997;155:1309-1315.

112. Spragg RG, Lewis JF, Walmrath HD, et al. Effect of recombinant surfactant protein C-based surfactant on the acute respiratory distress syndrome. *N Engl J Med* 2004; 351:884-892.

113. Creery WD, Hashmi A, Hutchison JS, Singh RN. Surfactant therapy improves pulmonary function in infants with Pneumocystis carinii pneumonia and acquired immunodeficiency syndrome. *Pediatr Pulmonol* 1997; 24:370-373.

114. Herting E, Moller O, Schiffmann JH, Robertson B. Surfactant improves oxygenation in infants and children with pneumonia and acute respiratory distress syndrome. *Acta Paediatr* 2002; 91:1174-1178.

115. Moller JC, Schaible T, Roll C, et al. Treatment with bovine surfactant in severe acute respiratory distress syndrome in children: a randomized multicenter study. *Intensive Care Med* 2003; 29:437-446.

116. Marriage SC, Underhill H, Nadel S. Use of natural surfactant in an HIV-infected infant with Pneumocystis carinii pneumonia. *Intensive Care Med* 1996; 22:611-612.

117. Abman SH, Griebel JL, Parker DK, Schmidt JM, Swanton D, Kinsella JP. Acute effects of inhaled nitric oxide in children with severe hypoxemic respiratory failure. *J Pediatr* 1994; 124:881-888.

118. Day RW, Allen EM, Witte MK. A randomised, controlled study of the 1-hour and 24-hour effects of inhaled nitric oxide therapy in children with acute hypoxemic respiratory failure. *Chest* 1997; 112:1324-1331.

119. Day RW, Guarin M, Lynch JM, Vernon DD, Dean JM. Inhaled nitric oxide in children

with severe lung disease: results of acute and prolonged therapy with two concentrations. *Crit Care Med* 1996; 24:215-221.

120. Nakagawa TA, Morris A, Gomez RJ, Johnston SJ, Sharkey PT, Zaritsky AL. Dose response to inhaled nitric oxide in pediatric patients with pulmonary hypertension and acute respiratory distress syndrome. *J Pediatr* 1997; 131:63-69.

121. Goldman AP, Haworth SG, Macrae DJ. Does inhaled nitric oxide suppress endogenous nitric oxide production? *J Thorac Cardiovasc Surg* 1996; 112:541-542.

122. Rossaint R, Falke KJ, Lopez F, Slama K, Pison U, Zapol WM. Inhaled nitric oxide for the adult respiratory distress syndrome. *N Engl J Med* 1993; 328:399-405.

123. Rossaint R, Gerlach H, Schmidt-Ruhnke H, et al. Efficacy of inhaled nitric oxide in patients with severe ARDS. *Chest* 1995; 107:1107-1115.

124. Haddad IY, Gyorgy P, Hu P, Galliani C, Beckman JS, Matalon S. Quantification of nitrotyrosine levels in lung sections of patients and animals with acute lung injury. *J Clin Invest* 1994; 94:2407-2413.

125. Dellinger RP, Zimmerman JL, Taylor RW, et al. Effects of inhaled nitric oxide in patients with acute respiratory distress syndrome: results of a randomized phase II trial. Inhaled Nitric Oxide in ARDS Study Group. *Crit Care Med* 1998; 26:15-23.

126. Lundin S, Mang H, Smithies M, Stenqvist O, Frostell C. Inhalation of nitric oxide in acute lung injury: results of a European multicentre study. The European Study Group of Inhaled Nitric Oxide. *Intensive Care Med* 1999; 25:911-919.

127. Michael JR, Barton RG, Saffle JR, et al. Inhaled nitric oxide versus conventional therapy: effect on oxygenation in ARDS. *Am J Respir Crit Care Med* 1998; 157:1372-1380.

128. Taylor RW, Zimmerman JL, Dellinger RP, et al. Low-dose inhaled nitric oxide in patients with acute lung injury: a randomized controlled trial. *JAMA* 2004; 291:1603-1609.

129. Troncy E, Collet JP, Shapiro S, et al. Inhaled nitric oxide in acute respiratory distress syndrome: a pilot randomized controlled study. *Am J Respir Crit Care Med* 1998; 157:1483-1488.

130. Meade MO, Granton JT, Matte-Martyn A, et al. A randomized trial of inhaled nitric oxide to prevent ischemia-reperfusion injury after lung transplantation. *Am J Respir Crit Care Med* 2003; 167:1483-1489.

131. Demirakca S, Dotsch J, Knothe C, et al. Inhaled nitric oxide in neonatal and pediatric acute respiratory distress syndrome: dose response, prolonged inhalation, and weaning. *Crit Care Med* 1996; 24:1913-1919.

132. Goldman AP, Tasker RC, Hosiasson S, Henrichsen T, Macrae DJ. Early response to inhaled nitric oxide and its relationship to outcome in children with severe hypoxemic respiratory failure. *Chest* 1997; 112:752-758.

133. Dobyns EL, Cornfield DN, Anas NG, et al. Multicenter randomized controlled trial of the effects of inhaled nitric oxide therapy on gas exchange in children with acute hypoxemic respiratory failure. *J Pediatr* 1999; 134:406-412.

134. Dobyns EL, Anas NG, Fortenberry JD, et al. Interactive effects of high-frequency oscillatory ventilation and inhaled nitric oxide in acute hypoxemic respiratory failure in pediatrics. *Crit Care Med* 2002; 30:2425-2429.

135. Mehta S, MacDonald R, Hallett DC, Lapinsky SE, Aubin M, Stewart TE. Acute oxygenation response to inhaled nitric oxide when combined with high-frequency oscillatory ventilation in adults with acute respiratory distress syndrome. *Crit Care Med* 2003; 31:383-389.

136. Sokol J, Jacobs SE, Bohn D. Inhaled nitric oxide for acute hypoxic respiratory failure

in children and adults: a meta-analysis. *Anesth Analg* 2003; 97:989-998.

137. Adhikari N, Granton JT. Inhaled nitric oxide for acute lung injury: no place for NO? *JAMA* 2004; 291:1629-1631.

138. Abou-Shala N, Meduri U. Noninvasive mechanical ventilation in patients with acute respiratory failure. *Crit Care Med* 1996; 24:705-715.

139. Antonelli M, Pennisi MA, Conti G. New advances in the use of noninvasive ventilation for acute hypoxaemic respiratory failure. *Eur Respir J Suppl* 2003; 42:65s-71s.

140. Brochard L. Mechanical ventilation: invasive versus noninvasive. *Eur Respir J Suppl* 2003; 47:31s-37s.

141. Fortenberry JD. Noninvasive ventilation in children with respiratory failure. *Crit Care Med* 1998; 26:2095-2096.

142. Teague WG. Noninvasive ventilation in the pediatric intensive care unit for children with acute respiratory failure. *Pediatr Pulmonol* 2003; 35:418-426.

143. Wysocki M, Antonelli M. Noninvasive mechanical ventilation in acute hypoxaemic respiratory failure. *Eur Respir J* 2001; 18:209-220.

144. Bradley TD. Continuous positive airway pressure for congestive heart failure. *CMAJ* 2000; 162:535-536.

145. Antonelli M, Conti G, Bufi M, et al. Noninvasive ventilation for treatment of acute respiratory failure in patients undergoing solid organ transplantation: a randomized trial. *JAMA* 2000; 283:235-241.

146. Delclaux C, L'Her E, Alberti C, et al. Treatment of acute hypoxemic nonhypercapnic respiratory insufficiency with continuous positive airway pressure delivered by a face mask: A randomized controlled trial. *JAMA* 2000; 284:2352-2360.

147. Ferrer M, Esquinas A, Leon M, Gonzalez G, Alarcon A, Torres A. Noninvasive ventilation in severe hypoxemic respiratory failure: a randomized clinical trial. *Am J Respir Crit Care Med* 2003; 168:1438-1444.

148. Esteban A, Frutos-Vivar F, Ferguson ND, et al. Noninvasive positive-pressure ventilation for respiratory failure after extubation. *N Engl J Med* 2004; 350:2452-2460.

149. Keenan SP, Powers C, McCormack DG, Block G. Noninvasive positive-pressure ventilation for postextubation respiratory distress: a randomized controlled trial. *JAMA* 2002; 287:3238-3244.

150. Conti G, Marino P, Cogliati A, et al. Noninvasive ventilation for the treatment of acute respiratory failure in patients with hematologic malignancies: a pilot study. *Intensive Care Med* 1998; 24:1283-1288.

151. Hilbert G, Gruson D, Vargas F, et al. Noninvasive ventilation in immunosuppressed patients with pulmonary infiltrates, fever, and acute respiratory failure. *N Engl J Med* 2001; 344:481-487.

152. Meert AP, Close L, Hardy M, Berghmans T, Markiewicz E, Sculier JP. Noninvasive ventilation: application to the cancer patient admitted in the intensive care unit. *Support Care Cancer* 2003; 11:56-59.

153. Liesching T, Kwok H, Hill NS. Acute applications of noninvasive positive pressure ventilation. *Chest* 2003; 124:699-713.

154. Akingbola OA, Hopkins RL. Pediatric noninvasive positive pressure ventilation. *Pediatr Crit Care Med* 2001; 2:164-169.

155. Akingbola OA, Simakajornboon N, Hadley Jr EF, Hopkins RL. Noninvasive positive-pressure ventilation in pediatric status asthmaticus. *Pediatr Crit Care Med* 2002; 3:181-184.

156. Cheifetz IM. Invasive and noninvasive pediatric mechanical ventilation. *Respir Care* 2003; 48:442-453.

157. Fortenberry JD, Del Toro J, Jefferson LS, Evey L, Haase D. Management of pediatric acute hypoxemic respiratory insufficiency with bilevel positive pressure (BiPAP) na-

sal mask ventilation. *Chest* 1995; 108:1059-1064.

158. Meduri GU, Chinn AJ, Leeper KV, et al. Corticosteroid rescue treatment of progressive fibroproliferation in late ARDS. Patterns of response and predictors of outcome. *Chest* 1994; 105:1516-1527.

159. Meduri GU, Headley AS, Golden E, et al. Effect of prolonged methylprednisolone therapy in unresolving acute respiratory distress syndrome. *JAMA* 1998; 280:159-165.

160. Mitchell JP, Schuller D, Calandrino FS, Schuster DP. Improved outcome based on fluid management in critically ill patients requiring pulmonary artery catheterization. *Am Rev Respir Dis* 1992; 145:990-998.

161. Schuster DP. The case for and against fluid restriction and occlusion pressure reduction in adult respiratory distress syndrome. *New Horiz* 1993; 1:478-488.

162. Martin GS, Mangialardi RJ, Wheeler AP, Dupont WD, Morris JA, Bernard GR. Albumin and furosemide therapy in hypoproteinemic patients with acute lung injury. *Crit Care Med* 2002; 30:2175-2182.

163. Ben-Abraham R, Paret G, Cohen R, et al. Diffuse alveolar hemorrhage following allogeneic bone marrow transplantation in children. *Chest* 2003; 124:660-664.

164. Diaz de Heredia C, Moreno A, Olive T, Iglesias J, Ortega JJ. Role of the intensive care unit in children undergoing bone marrow transplantation with life-threatening complications. *Bone Marrow Transplant* 1999; 24:163-168.

165. Feickert HJ, Schepers AK, Rodeck B, Geerlings H, Hoyer PF. Incidence, impact on survival, and risk factors for multi-organ system failure in children following liver transplantation. *Pediatr Transplant* 2001; 5:266-273.

166. Hagen SA, Craig DM, Martin PL, et al. Mechanically ventilated pediatric stem cell transplant recipients: effect of cord blood transplant and organ dysfunction on outcome. *Pediatr Crit Care Med* 2003; 4:206-213.

167. Hayes C, Lush RJ, Cornish JM, et al. The outcome of children requiring admission to an intensive care unit following bone marrow transplantation. *Br J Haematol* 1998; 102:666-670.

168. Keenan HT, Bratton SL, Martin LD, Crawford SW, Weiss NS. Outcome of children who require mechanical ventilatory support after bone marrow transplantation. *Crit Care Med* 2000; 28:830-835.

169. Lamas A, Otheo E, Ros P, et al. Prognosis of child recipients of hematopoietic stem cell transplantation requiring intensive care. *Intensive Care Med* 2003; 29:91-96.

170. Rossi R, Shemie SD, Calderwood S. Prognosis of pediatric bone marrow transplant recipients requiring mechanical ventilation. *Crit Care Med* 1999; 27:1181-1186.

171. Warwick AB, Mertens AC, Shu XO, Ramsay NK, Neglia JP. Outcomes following mechanical ventilation in children undergoing bone marrow transplantation. *Bone Marrow Transplant* 1998; 22:787-794.

172. Leahey AM, Bunin NJ, Schears GJ, Smith CA, Flake AW, Sullivan KE. Successful use of extracorporeal membrane oxygenation (ECMO) during BMT for SCID. *Bone Marrow Transplant* 1998; 21:839-840.

173. Halasa NB, Barr FE, Johnson JE, Edwards KM. Fatal pulmonary hypertension associated with pertussis in infants: does extracorporeal membrane oxygenation have a role? *Pediatrics* 2003; 112:1274-1278.

174. Pooboni S, Roberts N, Westrope C, et al. Extracorporeal life support in pertussis. *Pediatr Pulmonol* 2003; 36:310-315.

175. Skladal D, Horak E, Fruhwirth M, Maurer H, Simma B. Successful treatment of ARDS and severe pulmonary hypertension in a child with Bordetella pertussis infection. *Wien Klin Wochenschr* 2004; 116:760-762.

176. Sreenan CD, Osiovich H. Neonatal pertussis requiring extracorporeal membrane oxygenation. *Pediatr Surg Int* 2001; 17:201-203.

177. Williams GD, Numa A, Sokol J, Tobias V, Duffy BJ. ECLS in pertussis: does it have a role? *Intensive Care Med* 1998; 24:1089-1092.

178. Ullrich R, Lorber C, Roder G, et al. Controlled airway pressure therapy, nitric oxide inhalation, prone position, and extracorporeal membrane oxygenation (ECMO) as components of an integrated approach to ARDS. *Anesthesiology* 1999; 91:1577-1586.

179. Manthous CA, Hall JB, Olson D, et al. Effect of cooling on oxygen consumption in febrile critically ill patients. *Am J Respir Crit Care Med* 1995; 151:10-14.

180. Moler FW, Custer JR, Bartlett RH, et al. Extracorporeal life support for severe pediatric respiratory failure: an updated experience 1991-1993. *J Pediatr* 1994; 124:875-880.

181. Vats A, Pettignano R, Culler S, Wright J. Cost of extracorporeal life support in pediatric patients with acute respiratory failure. *Crit Care Med* 1998; 26:1587-1592.

182. Weber TR, Kountzman B. Extracorporeal membrane oxygenation for nonneonatal pulmonary and multiple-organ failure. *J Pediatr Surg* 1998; 33:1605-1609.

183. Swaniker F, Kolla S, Moler F, et al. Extracorporeal life support outcome for 128 pediatric patients with respiratory failure. *J Pediatr Surg* 2000; 35:197-202.

23

Management of Pediatric Respiratory Failure on ECLS

Björn Frenckner, M.D., Ph.D. and Palle Palmer, M.D.

Introduction

Pediatric ECLS and pediatric ECMO are terms used for extracorporeal life support in children older than 1 month. This distinction from "neonatal" ECLS is made because of the different pathophysiology and diagnoses encountered in newborns. Conditions treated with ECMO during the first month of life are congenital or acquired at birth. The most common indications for ECMO in newborns are meconium aspiration syndrome (MAS), pulmonary hypoplasia with or without congenital diaphragmatic hernia (CDH), pneumonia/septicemia, and persistent pulmonary hypertension of the newborn (PPHN). These conditions are characterized by increased pulmonary vascular resistance causing pulmonary hypertension. Since the fetal shunts are still open in newborns, right-to-left shunts with further deterioration in oxygenation are seen when pulmonary pressure exceeds systemic pressure.

In patients beyond the neonatal period, conditions which require treatment with ECLS are acquired after birth. The fetal shunts are closed and there is no right-to-left shunting. Viral pneumonia, bacterial pneumonia, ARDS, and aspiration are the most common diagnoses encountered.[1] Cases of intrapulmonary hemorrhage and pneumocystis carinii infection have also been reported. Many patients have conditions that are rare or difficult to place into diagnostic categories. Consequently, many pediatric patients in the ELSO Registry are reported as having "other" diagnoses.

Despite the differences in pathophysiology between neonatal and pediatric patients, the basic principles of ECLS are the same. Desaturated blood is withdrawn from a central vein or the right atrium and pumped through a membrane oxygenator and a heat exchanger before it is returned to the patient. In the oxygenator, the blood is oxygenated and carbon dioxide is removed. If the blood is returned to a central artery, the process is referred to as venoarterial (VA) ECMO, whereas if the blood is returned to a major vein, the bypass is referred to as venovenous (VV) ECMO. The physiology and advantages of the different modes of ECLS are described in Chapters 2 and 5.

Successful use of ECLS was first reported in adult patients in 1972[2] and was followed by other encouraging reports.[3-5] The first successful treatment of a newborn was reported in May of 1975 by Bartlett et al. in Irvine, California,[6] and was followed by other successful neonatal cases.[7] An NIH-sponsored multi-center study of adult ECLS was performed in 1979.[8] The results of that study were disappointing; less than 10% of patients in either the ECLS or the control group survived. Results of ECLS in neonatal patients were more encouraging and in

1980 Bartlett's group had treated 45 newborns, of which over 50% survived.[9] During the following years, neonatal ECLS was adopted by an increasing number of centers, and survival increased to about 80%.[1] Encouraged by the results in neonates, several centers started to offer ECLS to older children with acquired pulmonary conditions. The number of pediatric cases reported to the ELSO Registry is still significantly less than the number of neonatal cases (Figure 1).

All patients receiving ECLS are in critical condition. Their chance of survival with so-called "conventional treatment" is regarded as minimal. Regardless of the underlying condition, these patients have been subjected to aggressive ventilation with high oxygen concentrations and high airway pressures for a number of days. In order to maintain adequate tissue perfusion, many patients are fluid overloaded and often have vascular leakage. Urinary output is often low. Some patients exhibit multi-organ failure. Coagulopathy is often present with coagulation factor deficiencies.[10] It is important to consider that ECLS only supports the patient by providing gas exchange while the lungs are incapable of doing so. Further iatrogenic barotrauma and

hyperoxic trauma to the lungs can be avoided with ventilator settings and oxygen concentrations at non-injurious levels. Meticulous intensive care must be provided to these critically ill patients in order to be successful in achieving survival with low morbidity.

Circuit design

The circuit design is essentially the same in neonatal, pediatric, and adult ECLS. The characteristics of the components are discussed in Chapter 6. The necessary blood flow through the circuit for adequate ECLS support and the necessary dimensions of the different components are determined by the weight of the patient (Table 1).

Oxygenator

The most widely used membrane lung for ECLS is manufactured by Medtronic Inc. (Minneapolis, MN). It is a silicone rubber membrane and has proven suitable for long-term extracorporeal use. Although its gas exchange is not as efficient in terms of gas exchange per square meter (m^2) as the more modern hollow fiber

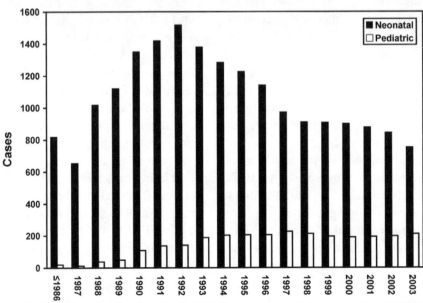

Figure 1. Number of neonatal and pediatric ECLS cases reported by year to the ELSO Registry.

Table 1. Size of different components of the circuit based on the patient's weight.

Weight (kg)	2-8	8-12	12-20	20-30	>30
Tubing size (in.)	1/4	3/8	3/8	3/8	1/2
Raceway tubing (in.)	1/4	3/8	3/8	3/8	1/2
Bladder (in.)	1/4	3/8	3/8	3/8	3/8
Oxygenator:					
Medtronic (m^2)	0.8	1.5	2.5	3.5	4.5*
Medos Hilite LT	0800	2400	2400	7000	7000
Venous cannula†	10-14	16	18	20	22
Arterial cannula†	8-10	12	14	16	20

*In larger children, 2 oxygenators may be necessary.
†Figures refer to minimum size of cannulas.

membranes, it is a true membrane with no plasma leakage from the blood to the gas phase during long-term use. This membrane oxygenator is the only one approved by the FDA for long-term use.

The Medtronic oxygenators are available in sizes from 0.4 to 4.5 m^2, however, membranes smaller than 0.8 m^2 are not recommended for standard ECLS. In children >30 kg and in adults, 1 or 2 size 4.5 m^2 oxygenators are necessary. These can be assembled in parallel or in series. A parallel circuit will yield a lower pre-oxygenator circuit pressure and allow the oxygenators to be changed without interrupting the ECLS flow. The smallest oxygenators are equipped with 1/4-inch connectors while the larger ones have 3/8-inch connectors.

The Medos Hilite LT (Medos Medizintechnik, Stolberg, Germany) is a hollow fiber oxygenator designed for long-term use with a non-silicone diffusion membrane and minimal plasma leakage. These membranes are available as follows:

Model No.	Surface area (m^2)	Blood flow (ml/min)	Prime volume (ml)
0800	0.32	800	55
2400	0.65	2400	95
7000	1.90	7000	275

All three sizes have an integrated heat exchanger. The Medos Hilite LT membranes are not FDA approved and are, therefore, not routinely used in the U.S., but have been used in Europe for several years.

Heat exchanger

The most commonly used heat exchanger in pediatric ECLS is manufactured by Medtronic. It is a long, narrow, cylindrical device in which blood flows through stainless steel tubes immersed in warm water with a countercurrent flow. The larger Medtronic oxygenators (2.5, 3.5, and 4.5 m^2) contain a built-in heat exchanger, but in circuits containing smaller oxygenators, a separate device is needed. Ideally, the blood should flow downward in the heat exchanger, so the device will serve as a final bubble trap before the oxygenated blood returns to the patient.

Tubing

As with all other components, the size of the tubing should be determined by patient size. Tubing that is too narrow will give a high resistance, decreasing drainage capacity on the venous side. On the arterial side, it will cause high circuit pressure, which will increase the risks of hemolysis and circuit rupture. On the other hand, tubing that is too large will cause low flow velocity, which will increase the risk for clot formation. The recommended size (Table 1) must match the size of the connectors on the other circuit components.

Pump

Most ECLS centers use roller pumps; these can accommodate different sizes of raceway tubing most commonly, ¼-, ⅜-, and ½-inch. The pump flow at a given speed, measured in revolutions per minute (rpm), is directly proportional to the cross-sectional area of the tubing. When the size of the raceway tubing is changed, the pump must be calibrated in order to deliver the correct flow rate, measured in liters per minute (lpm). With newer, computerized pumps, calibration is unnecessary, but the size of the tubing must be entered.

Centrifugal pumps generate flow via a spinning rotor magnetically coupled to a motor in a disposable pump head. The pump head has 2 connectors: one for blood inlet and one for blood outlet. The pump heads are manufactured in different sizes with either ¼-inch or ⅜-inch connectors.

The M pump is a fairly new device that has recently been approved by the FDA. It is a non-occlusive roller pump resembling the Rhône-Poulenc pump used by Chevalier et al.[11] The raceway segment is a flaccid silicone rubber chamber which fills passively. If venous return is inadequate, the chamber collapses and no negative pressure is generated. Raceway segments are only available in one size which is suitable for large children and adults. Although an interesting concept, the M pump has not gained widespread use.

Bladder

When a conventional roller pump is used, a device to avoid negative pressure on the venous side is essential; without such a device, hemolysis or cavitation of air into the circuit may result when the pump speed exceeds the venous return from the patient. The conventional device employed for this purpose is a collapsible silicone rubber bladder in the circuit, located just before the pump. The bladder is placed in a specially designed bladder box in which a microswitch will stop the pump should the bladder collapse.

Bladders and bladder boxes are manufactured by Medtronic Inc. (Minneapolis, MN) and OriGen Biomedical (Austin, TX) in two sizes to fit ¼-inch and ⅜-inch connectors. Some centers use a bridge of tubing across the bladder in older patients in order to decrease flow resistance; however, the resulting decrease in flow velocity may increase the risk of clotting in the bladder.

Cannulation technique

Traditionally VA ECLS has been the most frequently utilized mode of ECLS in children and accounts for 60% of the cases listed in the ELSO Registry.[1] However, there is an increasing trend toward the use of VV bypass. In 2004, only half of the pediatric respiratory ECLS cases used VA ECLS.

In ECLS, blood is drained from a major vein or from the right atrium. Most commonly, a catheter is inserted through the right internal jugular vein and passed down to the right atrium, where it drains desaturated blood into the circuit. Drainage may also be achieved by cannulation of a femoral vein with the catheter placed either in the femoral vein or in the inferior vena cava. Direct cannulation of the right atrium is a also an option, and is generally used during open chest cannulations in cardiac patients. It is essential that the drainage capacity is adequate, as this determines the maximum extracorporeal blood flow attainable and thereby, also the maximal extracorporeal support. The venous cannula must be of adequate size (Table 1) and placed in the correct position. If drainage remains inadequate despite volume replacement and optimal catheter position, an additional venous cannula may be required. This is easily connected to the drainage tubing with a Y-connector.

In VA ECLS, the oxygenated blood is returned to the patient through a cannula inserted into a major artery. The common carotid artery, which in children is the largest extrathoracic artery, is often used. In neonates, it may be repaired by a simple closure of the arteriotomy or by resection and anastomosis.[12] Cannulation of the common carotid artery requires ligation of the vessel, which has been of some concern, especially in older children. Some centers perform carotid artery reconstruction after ECMO, but the long-term outcome remains unclear.[13] Oxygenated blood may also be returned via the femoral artery. Due to the relatively sparse collateral circulation, this usually requires distal cannulation. Another disadvantage of femoral artery cannulation is that oxygenated blood is delivered far from the aortic root. The head and the coronary arteries will be perfused by desaturated blood unless the extracorporeal circuit drains nearly all blood returned to the right atrium. Another possibility is to use a very long femoral cannula and to position the tip in the aortic root; however, the flow resistance of that cannula would be relatively high secondary to the length. Cannulation of the subclavian artery is another possibility that has been well described, even in neonates;[14] to date, it has not been widely used. Direct cannulation of the aortic root requires an open thoracotomy and is not the preferred method of ECLS for respiratory support.

VV ECLS can be performed with a double or single cannula system. In the double cannula system, blood is drained by one cannula and returned to the patient via another cannula inserted into a major vein. Commonly, blood is drained from the right atrium via a cannula inserted in the right internal jugular vein as in VA ECLS, and is returned to the femoral vein, although the opposite (drainage from the femoral vein and return to the right atrium) may be used.[15] A double cannula VV ECLS technique has been used in 20% of pediatric ECLS cases to date. A single cannula VV system can either involve a double lumen cannula or a single lumen cannula with a tidal flow system. Double lumen cannulas are manufactured by Jostra (Maquet Cardiopulmonary, Hirrlingen, Germany) (sizes 12F and 15F) and by OriGen (sizes 12F, 15F, and 18F). These cannulas provide one large lumen

for drainage and a narrower lumen for infusion. Several side holes allow for venous drainage. The double lumen cannulas are inserted in the right internal jugular vein and positioned in the right atrium. The infusion hole is directed towards the tricuspid valve in order to minimize recirculation. Initially, the double lumen cannula was used only in neonates,[16,17] but has more recently been used in smaller children.[18] The 18F OriGen cannula allows adequate venous drainage in children up to 10-12 kg. When larger cannulas become available, single cannula VV ECLS will also be possible in larger children. Of the pediatric ECLS cases reported to the ELSO Registry to date, 10% were performed with a double lumen cannula. In 2004, however, this technique accounted for almost 20% of treatments. A single cannula tidal flow ECLS system has been widely used by Chevalier et al. in neonates.[11] This circuit involves a non-occlusive pump, valves, and a raceway of silicone rubber acting as a small reservoir (Chapter 6). The single cannula is connected to the drainage tubing and the infusing tubing with an Y-connector. While blood is being drained, the infusion tubing is closed. When the pump segment is filled, the drainage tubing is closed and the infusion line is opened. A similar system has been used in the pediatric age group, but details have not been reported.[19,20]

VA ECLS can be converted to VV ECLS and vice versa during the run. If a patient on VA ECLS improves but the run is estimated to continue for a considerable time, this may be an indication for conversion to VV, as the risk of complications on VV ECLS is lower. For example, the consequences of an accidental embolus from the circuit are considerably more serious if the patient is on VA bypass. On the other hand, a patient initially put on VV bypass may need conversion to VA bypass if the support is found to be inadequate. Increased pulmonary vascular resistance, pulmonary hypertension, and right heart failure may also be indications for conversion from VV to VA bypass. In the

ELSO Registry, 6% of pediatric patients were converted from VV to VA (of which 45% survived); very few were converted from VA to VV. In adult patients, 11% were converted from VA to VV (of which 82% survived) and 7% converted from VV to VA (none survived).[21]

Vascular access may be achieved by a direct cutdown, via a percutaneous technique, or by a semipercutaneous technique. When the neck vessels are cannulated, a towel is placed under the shoulders to extend the neck. The head is turned slightly to the left and the right side of the neck is scrubbed. If an open technique is used, an oblique incision along the anterior border of the sternocleidomastoid muscle or a low transverse incision above the clavicle is performed. Use of electrocautery may help to minimize bleeding. The vessels are mobilized by dissection anterior to the sternocleidomastoid muscle. The omohyoid muscle is divided if necessary. If a standard cutdown procedure is performed, the vessel is encircled both centrally and peripherally. Care should be taken not to injure the vagal nerve. Any bleeding should be controlled before the patient is heparinized, after which the vessel is ligated in the distal direction. A vascular clamp is placed centrally, and the vessel is incised. When cannulating the common carotid artery it is essential to gain control of the intima, which is easily done with two 5-0 Prolene sutures. Stay sutures can be used to lift the wall of the internal jugular vein so that the cannula may be more easily advanced. As soon as the cannula has entered the vessel, the vascular clamp is released and the cannula is advanced to the desired position. The venous cannula should be advanced quickly to avoid bleeding that would otherwise occur through the side holes. Ideally the tip of the arterial cannula should be positioned where the innominate artery enters the aortic arch. The venous cannula should be placed with its tip in the lower part of the right atrium. As a rule of thumb, the position of the tip of the arterial cannula corresponds to the border between the upper and middle thirds

of the sternum, and the position of the tip of the venous cannula corresponds to the border between the middle and lower third of the sternum. The vessel is tied over the cannula. A small piece of a vessel loop between the ligature and the vessel will facilitate cutting the ligature when the patient is decannulated. The cannulas must be secured to ensure that accidental decannulation does not occur. Meticulous hemostasis is essential before closing the wound with running sutures. Placement of fibrin glue may provide further hemostasis. The internal jugular vein may also be cannulated in the distal direction and connected with a Y-connector in order to increase venous drainage and avoid increased venous pressure.

If the semipercutaneous technique[22] is used, the internal jugular vein is prepared as described above. A percutaneous puncture of the vessel is performed under direct visualization and the cannula is introduced with a modified Seldinger technique. The wound is closed as described previously. Percutaneous cannulation of the internal jugular vein with a modified Seldinger technique has been used successfully for several years in adult, pediatric patients, and also recently in neonates.[23] Immediate availability of a surgical team is mandatory, however, if percutaneous access to the vein is not achieved or if the vein is accidentally lacerated during the percutaneous procedure.

Cannulation of the femoral vessels is performed with essentially the same technique as for the neck vessels. Distal ligation of the femoral vein may be performed in neonates and small children if a traditional cutdown procedure is performed. In older children, the base of the saphenous vein may be used for placement of the cannula, making ligation of the femoral vein unnecessary. Percutaneous or semipercutaneous technique makes femoral vein ligation unnecessary. Ligation of the femoral artery is not recommended because of inadequate collateral circulation. Instead, the artery can be cannulated in both directions. In adults, the femoral artery has been cannulated percutaneously, avoiding the need for distal perfusion.[21]

As soon as the cannulas are in position and have been adequately secured, they are connected to the ECLS circuit. Air must be evacuated carefully, after which the extracorporeal circulation is initiated. If venous return is adequate, the venous cannula is likely in the correct position. If the venous return is inadequate, the cannula may be incorrectly placed. Chest radiograph and/or ultrasound will provide the desired information, as well as information regarding the position of the arterial cannula in cases of VA ECMO. The arterial cannula should be withdrawn if it is close to the aortic valve in order to avoid damaging the valve or interfering with left ventricular emptying.

Daily management

The daily management of pediatric ECLS patients is essentially the same as that of neonatal or adult patients with respect to extracorporeal support.

Patient monitoring

The ECLS patient should be monitored by a bedside ECLS specialist 24 hours a day. The ECLS specialist must be familiar with the principles of ECLS and must have an in-depth knowledge of the technical equipment and management of patients on ECLS. The ECLS specialist must also be capable of managing emergency situations until an ECLS-trained physician is available. The specialist may be an ICU nurse, nurse anesthetist, respiratory therapist, or perfusionist; has been trained in-house, and is referred to as the "ECLS specialist" or "ECMO technician".

In addition to technical support, continuous clinical observation of the patient is essential. Visual observation of the color of the blood (i.e., the light red blood entering the patient and the dark color of blood drained) is a simple bedside test that the patient is being adequately oxygen-ated by the ECLS machine. In some centers the ECLS specialist is also responsible for general patient care, but in the majority of ECLS centers, a separate ICU nurse will have the responsibility for general patient care. In all instances, the ECLS specialist is responsible for the continuous surveillance of the ECLS machine and the extracorporeal support.

Anticoagulation

In order to avoid coagulation, heparin is continuously infused into the circuit. The usual heparin dose is 20-50 units/kg/hr and the rate is adjusted to keep the activated clotting time (ACT) in the range of 180-200 seconds (depending on the ACT device used) as determined by hourly sampling. When the levels are unstable, more frequent sampling may be required.

Platelet count should be checked at least daily. ECLS patients routinely become thrombocytopenic due to platelet inactivation, predominantly in the membrane lung. Ideally the platelet count should be maintained above 100,000/mm³. The heparin infusion rate will often need to be increased during platelet transfusions or, alternatively, when a heparin bolus administered.

Apart from ACT levels, monitoring of the coagulation system varies between centers. Fibrin monomers, D-dimers, fibrinogen, and AT III are monitored daily in some ECLS centers. Increased levels of fibrin monomers and D-dimers may be early signs of a consumptive process in the circuit. This is called circuit "disseminated intravascular coagulation" (circuit DIC) and is often accompanied by lower heparin requirements and bleeding problems, which may resolve after change of the circuit.

Antibiotics

Normally all ECLS patients are kept on antibiotics. A popular combination is an aminoglycoside and a penicillin. If the patient is already on antibiotics prior to initiation of ECLS, an individual assessment is made to determine if the regimen should be continued, combined with additional antibiotics, or changed.

Cultures from blood, urine, the trachea, and other areas of interest are regularly taken. If tests for bacterial growth are positive, the antibiotic regimen is altered accordingly. Fungal growth may occur during long-term treatment with broad-spectrum antibiotics. Immunocompromised children are at special risk. Fungal prophylaxis and treatment is individually based.

Sedation

Pediatric patients who need extracorporeal support have usually been ventilated for some period. At initiation of ECLS, they are normally sedated and often paralyzed. All children will continue to require significant sedation and analgesia for the first days on bypass. Pharmacological paralysis is only rarely needed. After the first few days, the need for sedation varies. The general management of pain and sedation during ECLS is outlined in Chapter 34. As in all ICU patients, usual causes of anxiety must be considered before routine sedation is given. Pain is best controlled with analgesics. Hypercarbia and hypoxemia should ideally be alleviated by adjusting ECLS flow and gas flow to the oxygenator. Establishing a close relationship between staff and the patient may decrease the need for pharmacological sedation. Gentle patient care, frequent verbal communication, and physical contact are often effective sedatives. For most children it is essential to have a parent at bedside most of the time. Storytelling and book reading can help calm the patient. Many children prefer to be entertained with television or games. Most children will only require mild pharmacological sedation by the end of the ECLS run and are able to communicate to some extent with parents and staff. When needed, opiates and benzodiazepines are frequently used for phar-macological sedation in these patients and for pain management.

Nutrition

Total parenteral nutrition (TPN) with amino acids, fat, and glucose has been the standard nutritional support for ECLS patients. In neonates, there has been concern that enteral feeding might increase the risk for necrotizing enterocolitis.[9] The possibility that there has been prior ischemic insult to the gut, in combination with use of vasopressors, has led to concerns regarding enteral feeding in older patients. These critically ill patients may also have gastrointestinal dysmotility resulting in adynamic ileus.[24,25] Nevertheless, absence of enteral feeding and support of the patient with total parenteral nutrition will result in hypoplasia of intestinal villi, risk for bacterial translocation, and risk for TPN-associated cholestasis. Pettignano et al. reported the use of total enteral nutrition in 13 pediatric patients on VA or VV ECLS.[26] These patients also received metaclopropamide or cisapride to increase gastric motility. The authors concluded that enteral feeding was well-tolerated without complications. Early enteral feeding in adult ECLS patients has also been successful.[21,27]

Cardiac support

All patients placed on ECLS have suffered from some period of hypoxemia, which may have affected the myocardium. Many patients have required inotropic drugs before initiation of ECLS. As soon as the patient is on bypass, oxygenation will immediately improve and, unless the myocardium has suffered irreversible damage, cardiac performance will improve allowing inotropic support to be gradually withdrawn. Severe cardiac dysfunction on ECLS will result in a low pulse pressure and low cardiac output (referred to as "cardiac stun").[28]

VV ECLS generally yields a higher saturation in the coronary arteries than VA ECLS, as oxygenated blood is infused in the right atrium or the inferior vena cava. The best coronary oxygenation in VV ECLS will occur with femoro-atrial bypass or when a double lumen cannula is used and the infusion line is directed correctly toward the tricuspid valve. However, VV ECLS obviously does not support cardiac function, and patients on VV bypass may initially need inotropic support while on bypass. If myocardial performance is still inadequate, conversion to VA bypass may be necessary. VA ECLS supports both cardiac and pulmonary function; however, the coronary arteries are perfused with blood at low saturation as long as blood is ejected from the left ventricle.

Renal

As previously mentioned, patients placed on ECLS often have capillary leakage and have been fluid overloaded in order to maintain an adequate blood volume and pressure. During the first days on bypass this may continue. Patients may need large volumes of fluid to maintain adequate venous return, and they may initially become more edematous. When capillary leakage subsides, extracellular fluid returns to the vascular compartment and diuresis will increase. In general, the patients should be kept as dry as possible and administration of diuretics such as furosemide is required. A low dose infusion of dopamine can also be beneficial.

Inadequate urinary output despite acceptable blood pressure and diuretics may be a sign of renal dysfunction. Hemofiltration or hemodialysis is easily initiated in patients on bypass and is directly connected to the extracorporeal circuit. Indications are mainly fluid overload and hyperkalemia (see Chapter 32).

Pulmonary therapy

ECLS alone does not cure the underlying pulmonary disease; instead, it provides gas exchange until pulmonary recovery occurs. Therefore, it is important to provide optimal pulmonary therapy during the ECLS course. There

is little scientific data concerning pulmonary management on ECLS and the current strategy is based mostly on clinical experience.

Prior to bypass, patients have been managed with high ventilator settings, including high pressure and oxygen concentration. These conditions are injurious to the lungs and cause further damage if continued. As soon as ECLS has started, it is essential to decrease oxygen concentration and peak pressure to non-traumatic levels. The oxygen concentration is reduced to approximately 40% or lower and peak inspiratory pressures (PIP) should be limited to 20 cm H_2O in infants and 30 cm H_2O in older children. A high positive end expiratory pressure (PEEP) (8-14 cm H_2O) has been shown to reduce lung opacification after initiation of ECLS in neonates, and the length of the ECLS run in general.[29] Some centers advocate a high PEEP in older children as well.

Pulmonary toilet must be performed properly while the patient is on ECLS. If secretions are abundant, suctioning should be done frequently. Instillation of saline in the entotracheal tube may facilitate evacuation of mucus. Generally, the suction catheter should not pass beyond the endotracheal tube in order to avoid injury to the trachea or bleeding. Bronchoscopy can be performed easily when the patient is on bypass and should be done if there is any suspicion of bronchial obstruction from mucus or other material.

As in other ICU patients, it is beneficial to change the patient's position in order to facilitate drainage of different parts of the lungs. Prone positioning may be used in order to recruit lung tissue and improve ventilation-perfusion matching.[30] When the patient's position is changed, great attention must be paid to the cannulas so that bleeding from the cannulation site or accidental decannulation does not occur. In a study of 95 pediatric ECMO patients, 63 received intermittent prone positioning. There were no complications from this practice and survival was 82%.[31]

It may be advantageous to keep patients on spontaneous pressure-supported ventilation by increasing $PaCO_2$ or decreasing pH if the patient is alkalotic. This approach requires the patient to be awake or only mildly sedated (see Chapter 34). Although not scientifically proven, pressure-supported spontaneous ventilation seems beneficial compared to standard positive pressure ventilation. This strategy yields larger tidal volumes and improves gas exchange. Further studies are needed to determine the optimal mode to ventilate patients on ECLS.

ECLS is a costly and highly invasive procedure with significant complications. The duration of ECLS should be as short as possible. Weaning from ECLS must be delayed until pulmonary function recovers enough to provide adequate gas exchange. Pulmonary therapy and lung management during ECLS are, therefore, crucial.

Weaning and decannulation

As soon as the patient is stable on bypass, ventilator settings are decreased to non-injurious levels. After cannulation, lung compliance is extremely low; decreasing the ventilator pressures will diminish the tidal volume significantly, in many cases close to zero. At the onset of ECLS, there is often increased capillary leakage. The patient may need substantial fluid replacement, and will exhibit poor urinary output. General body and pulmonary edema will often increase during the first days on ECLS. Pulmonary radiographs will demonstrate increased atelectasis and only small segments of the lungs will be aerated. Measurements of end tidal pCO_2 will show values close to zero as the alveoli are essentially non-ventilated and there is very little gas exchange taking place.

Increased diuresis is one of the first signs of clinical improvement, and will be followed by resolving edema. Ideally, at this time, compliance will increase, and the tidal volume will increase either on ventilator-induced breaths or on spontaneous pressure-supported breaths. Breath sounds can be heard by auscultation. End tidal CO_2 measurement will show increasing values, indicating that there is gas exchange. Improvement will also be visible on a chest radiograph, although this is often delayed at least 24 hours following signs of clinical improvement. Pulmonary improvement will be reflected by an increased mixed venous saturation. At a constant circuit flow rate, an increased mixed venous saturation (SvO_2) means decreased extracorporeal oxygen delivery, as the delivered oxygen is directly proportional to [Q x (1 – SvO_2 ÷ 100)], where Q is the extracorporeal flow rate. Assuming that the total oxygen consumption of the patient is not changed, decreased extracorporeal oxygen delivery means increased oxygen uptake by the lungs.

Once pulmonary function improves, the extracorporeal flow may be decreased. When the patient is on VA bypass, weaning of extracorporeal flow may be guided by monitoring the SvO_2. The latter reflects hemoglobin-bound oxygen which has not been extracted by the tissue when the arterial blood passes through the capillaries to the venous side. A SvO_2 >65-70% indicates that there is adequate oxygen delivery. Extracorporeal flow can be decreased in small increments as long as the SvO_2 is kept above 65-70%. In lengthy ECLS runs where the patient is difficult to wean, lower values of SvO_2 may need to be tolerated until improvement is seen. After further improvement in pulmonary function, and when the ECLS machine is contributing only minimally to the patient's gas exchange (i.e. the flow rate is down to ~20-30 cc/kg/min for small children; ~10 cc/kg/min in older children), the patient is probably ready for discontinuation of ECLS.

There are several options for discontinuation of VA bypass:

- The patient is decannulated if the ECLS run has been fairly short, the weaning process has been uneventful, and if the patient is stable after several hours on minimal ECLS flow.

- If there has been a long ECLS run or if there is uncertainty whether the patient will tolerate removal from ECLS, the circuit may be disconnected, the cannulas connected with short pieces of tubing through a roller pump, and blood is circulated through this A-V shunt at a minimal flow rate.

- Similar to the situation above, some centers cut away the circuit and keep the cannulas patent by infusing a heparinized solution.

- If a bridge is used between the arterial and venous lines in the circuit, the cannulas can be clamped, filled with a heparinized solution, and the bridge opened. The blood is then circulated through the circuit now isolated from the patient. The catheters are "flashed" to prevent clot formation.

The last three alternatives leave the cannulas in place while ECLS is discontinued. In this way, a trial off ECLS may be carried out for up to 24 hours before decannulation. If this is not tolerated, the patient is easily placed back on bypass.

If the patient is on VV bypass, SvO_2 measurements are not as accurate because of the variable degree of recirculation. Instead, weaning is performed by monitoring clinical parameters such as: arterial blood gases, vital signs, tidal volumes, compliance, and end tidal CO_2. When the patient is on minimal support and is ready for a trial off ECLS, this is accomplished in the short-term by disconnecting the gas supply to the oxygenator. If a longer test off ECLS is required, the circuit may be disconnected from the patient as described previously and the cannulas connected to each other via a roller pump resulting in a VV shunt, or by infusing heparinized solution into the cannulas.

Cannulas inserted with a percutaneous or a semipercutaneous technique can be simply removed without a surgical procedure. Bleeding is controlled by a skin suture and simple pressure at the cannulation site. Cannulas inserted with

an open technique require a surgical procedure for removal. Some patients do not tolerate positive pressure ventilation and can only be maintained off ECLS on spontaneous pressure-supported ventilation. The decannulation procedure is, therefore, performed using only sedation and a local anesthetic. Removal of the venous cannula should be done quickly while briefly increasing the airway pressure. Otherwise, if there is negative intrathoracic pressure when the side hole of the venous cannula is outside the vessel, air can be aspirated into the superior vena cava causing an air embolism.[32]

ECLS termination

Unfortunately, not all ECLS runs are successful. Termination of ECLS may be necessary because of various complications. Cerebral hemorrhage or infarction may lead to cerebral edema and subsequent brain death, making further ECLS pointless. Life-threatening bleeding complications, which cannot be controlled surgically, may also prompt discontinuation of ECLS and if this occurs when the patient is totally dependent on ECLS, death will be unavoidable. If lung function is present, it may be possible to transition off ECLS to high ventilator settings. If necessary, ECLS may be reinstituted when bleeding has been controlled.

A controversial question is the duration of the ECLS run if the patient's lung function does not improve. Open lung biopsy on ECLS has been recommended in order to determine if the lungs show irreversible damage.[33-35] However, this procedure cannot be performed without at least some risk for bleeding. Evaluation of pulmonary prognosis from a single biopsy specimen is also problematic. The difficulty of discontinuing ECLS is further illustrated by Green et al.[36] who, in a multi-center study of 382 patients treated with ECLS, found that the probability of survival was the same in children with ECLS courses >2 weeks compared with those treated after shorter periods. ECLS was terminated in some patients for pulmonary futility at durations of ECLS associated with survival in a substantial number of patients in whom ECLS was continued.[36] Nevertheless, if lung function does not improve, termination of ECLS must be considered at some point unless pulmonary transplantation is feasible. The possibility that the lungs will not recover should be discussed with the parents ideally before initiation of ECLS.[37]

Results

In neonates, it is now generally accepted that ECLS is a life-saving procedure. Three randomized studies have shown significant improvement in patients treated with ECLS compared to patients given conventional treatment.[38-40] In pediatric patients, there are no randomized studies comparing ECLS treatment with conventional treatment. In a retrospective multi-center study involving 331 patients from 32 hospitals, ECLS was compared with conventional treatment. In 53 diagnosis- and risk-matched pairs, there was a significantly lower mortality among the ECLS patients (26% vs. 47%).[41] The authors concluded that ECLS was responsible for the improved survival, as there was no association of outcome with the use of other tertiary technologies. They stressed the need for prospective randomized studies to determine if ECLS improves survival in the pediatric patient with respiratory failure.

In July 2004, a total of 2,810 pediatric ECLS runs had been reported to the ELSO Registry, with an overall survival rate of 55%. Survival has increased slightly over time; the first third of the 2,810 ECLS runs were reported before 1994 with a mean survival of 52%, while the following two thirds had survivals of 58% and 57%, respectively. This is a significant difference, based on Chi square analysis, but it is not possible to conclude if this represents a difference in patient selection or improved ECLS survival. Survival is highest in cases of aspiration pneumonia (65%), viral pneumonia (63%), and post-operative or post-traumatic ARDS (63%) (Table 2).

The largest single center experience was published by the University of Michigan[42] and involved 128 pediatric patients treated with ECLS between 1985 and 1998. Overall survival to hospital discharge was 71%. Mean pre-ECLS PaO_2/FiO_2 ratio was 58, indicating the critical condition of the patients. The average ECLS duration was 288 hours with a maximum of 47 days in a surviving patient. An excellent survival was also seen in a series of 82 pediatric ECLS patients mainly supported by VV bypass.[43] The overall survival to hospital discharge was 77%. Median PaO_2/FiO_2 ratio was 61 in the 68 patients on VV support and 46 in those on VA support. Peek and Sosnowski have reported the treatment of 81 pediatric ECLS patients with a survival rate of 77%.[18] The average time on ECLS was 191 hours. In the Stockholm experience, 46 pediatric patients have been treated

Table 2. Number of patients and survival to hospital discharge or transfer in different primary diagnoses in pediatric ECLS.[1]

Primary diagnosis	Total	Survived	(%)
Bacterial pneumonia	290	157	(54)
Viral pneumonia	728	457	(63)
Aspiration	168	110	(65)
Pneumocystis	22	9	(41)
ARDS, post-op/trauma	70	44	(63)
ARDS, non-post-op/trauma	278	144	(52)
Acute resp. failure, non-ARDS	605	286	(47)
Other	649	350	(54)

with 30 survivors to discharge (65%). The average time on ECLS was 355 hours with 1 survivor after an ECMO run of 48 days.

Respiratory failure is one of the most common causes of death in pediatric burn patients. It may be caused by direct smoke inhalation injury, ARDS, or pneumonia/septicemia. A few series of ECLS treatments of these patients have been published. Out of a total of 25 patients, 17 (68%) survived, although one was severely handicapped.[34,44-47]

Pulmonary hemorrhage is a rare but potentially fatal condition when treated with conventional therapy. In spite of anticoagulation and impaired homeostasis due to the extracorporeal circulation, the ECLS survival is good. Positive outcomes have been reported in neonates and adults, including 1 patient with profuse bleeding from several mycotic aneurysms leading to hypovolemic shock.[48-50] In a report of 8 children with pulmonary hemorrhage and a PaO_2/FiO_2 ratio between 33 and 70 on mechanical ventilation, all survived to hospital discharge after VV or VA ECLS.[51]

Due to concern about increased bleeding, pulmonary failure after major trauma was previously considered a contraindication for ECLS. Encouraging results with adult trauma patients have stimulated centers to use ECLS for pediatric trauma patients when they meet traditional ECLS criteria.[25,52] A total of 70 patients has been reported to the ELSO Registry with diagnoses of post-operative or post-traumatic ARDS with a survival to hospital discharge rate of 63% (Table 3). In a recently published report, 5 children were treated with ECLS after motor vehicle accidents and major injuries, of which 4 required major surgery. The PaO_2/FiO_2 ratio before ECLS was 23-109. Of the five children, four survived to hospital discharge.[53]

Severe Bordetella pertussis infection in infants is associated with extremely high mortality. Initial reports of ECLS treatment were disappointing and the value of ECLS treatment of patients with pertussis infection was questioned.[54]

In a single-center series of 12 infants there were 7 deaths.[55] The authors concluded that in spite of the high mortality, ECLS support should be offered to infants with severe pertussis meeting conventional ECLS criteria. A retrospective chart review of the ELSO Registry revealed a total of 61 children with pertussis placed on ECLS support between 1990 and 2002.[56] The mean age of the patients was 88 days, and the overall mortality was 70%. Mortality was significantly higher in infants younger than 6 weeks (84%) compared to children older than 6 weeks (61%).

Pneumocystis carinii pneumonia mainly occurs during immunosuppressive treatment in patients with malignancies and is a severe complication with a poor prognosis if mechanical ventilation is required. In the ELSO Registry, only 22 cases have been reported, out of which 9 (41%) survived. A single-center experience was more optimistic with 3 of 4 patients surviving.[57]

Complications

ECLS is a particularly invasive procedure in extremely ill patients. Complications are frequently seen and involve both the patient and the ECMO equipment.

The most serious complication is a total brain infarction. Theoretically, this is the only condition which can cause death in a patient on VA bypass. Total brain infarction is generally the result of cerebral edema caused by a focal process such as a cerebral hemorrhage or local cerebral infarction, or a generalized injury such as hypoxemia. Ideally, patients should be placed on ECLS before they become so hypoxemic that brain injury has occurred.

Patients on VA bypass are at greater risk of developing cerebral infarctions or hemorrhage than patients on VV bypass due to the direct arterial infusion. Any emboli from the circuit (air or clots) may occlude the small end arteries in the cerebral circulation. The infarcted area in the brain is at risk for subsequent hemorrhage, which, if it occurs, may become extensive because of the heparinization and the ECLS induced coagulopathy.

The most common complication is bleeding. It occurs most frequently at the cannulation site. If the patient has had surgery during or prior to ECLS, bleeding may occur at the surgical site. Meticulous hemostasis during cannulation and other surgical procedures are essential to avoid bleeding. Gastrointestinal bleeding, urinary tract bleeding, and tracheal bleeding may be the result of generalized coagulopathy, especially if occurring simultaneously at several sites. Signs of ECLS-induced coagulopathy include abnormal coagulation parameters such as increased D-dimers and fibrin monomers. Heparin requirements may be decreased, and changing the ECLS circuit will often dramatically improve the coagulopathy.

To avoid infectious complications, patients on ECLS are routinely given antibiotics. Despite this, infectious complications are occasionally seen, especially in long runs. Symptoms may include a non-specific patient deterioration with worsening pulmonary function, increased C-reactive protein, and positive blood cultures. Individual treatment will depend on the causative organism.

Mechanical complications can occur in the ECLS circuit. Some may be severe and require instant response by the bedside ECMO technician, nurse, or physician. Tubing rupture will cause immediate exsanguination if not promptly addressed. Air in the circuit will require temporary termination of bypass, evacuation of air from the circuit, and correction of the underlying problem. Accidental decannulation is probably the most serious mechanical complication if the patient is totally dependent on bypass. Some mechanical complications are so common that it is questionable if they should be regarded as complications. Oxygenator failure occurs so commonly in long ECLS runs that oxygenator changes can be regarded as a routine procedure in ECLS.

Cannula malfunction is regarded as a mechanical complication. The position of the drainage cannula (most commonly in the right atrium) is crucial as it will determine the maximal flow. If the flow is inadequate when ECLS is started, it is commonly caused by a malposition of the drainage cannula. Radiographic or ultrasound examination will usually provide the necessary information. High pressure in the circuit may be caused by a malposition of the arterial cannula when the tip is positioned against the aortic wall. If the ligature around the carotid artery and the arterial cannula is tied too tight, it may compress the cannula, causing the cannula lumen to narrow, resulting in high circuit pressure.

Mechanical and patient complications reported to the ELSO Registry are listed in Table 3.

Summary

Pediatric ECLS refers to extracorporeal support in children who are beyond the neonatal period. A different pathophysiology is encountered in children compared to neonates. The fetal shunts are closed. Increased pulmonary vascular resistance leading to pulmonary hypertension will therefore not lead to right to left shunting. Instead the patients may develop right heart failure.

Conditions that require treatment with ECLS are all acquired after birth. The most common diagnoses are viral pneumonia, bacterial pneumonia, ARDS, and aspiration.

The basic principles of ECLS are the same as in neonates and in adults. Desaturated blood is withdrawn from a central vein or the right atrium and pumped through a membrane oxygenator and a heat exchanger before it is returned to a central artery (VA ECLS) or to a central vein (VV ECLS). The size of the dif-

Table 3. Mechanical and patient complications in 2,810 pediatric ECLS patients reported to the ELSO Registry.

	Reported	(%)	Survived	(%)
Mechanical:				
Oxygenator failure	387	(13.8)	172	(44)
Raceway rupture	20	(0.7)	7	(35)
Other tubing rupture	107	(3.8)	50	(47)
Pump malfunction	87	(3.1)	41	(47)
Heat exchanger malfunction	18	(0.6)	7	(39)
Clots: oxygenator	190	(6.8)	101	(53)
bridge	118	(4.2)	63	(53)
bladder	158	(5.6)	83	(53)
hemofilter	86	(3.1)	36	(42)
other	206	(7.3)	105	(51)
Air in circuit	56	(2)	29	(52)
Cracks in pigtail connectors	28	(1)	16	(57)
Cannula problems	398	(14.2)	193	(48)
Hemorrhagic:				
Cannulation site bleeding	259	(9.2)	156	(60)
Surgical site bleeding	451	(16)	211	(47)
Hemolysis (Hb >50 mg/dl)	247	(8.8)	103	(42)
DIC	79	(2.8)	23	(29)
Neurologic:				
Brain death clinically determined	170	(6)	—	—
Seizures: clinically determined	205	(7.3)	71	(35)
EEG determined	40	(1.4)	15	(38)
CNS infarction by US/CT	90	(3.2)	36	(40)
CNS hemorrhage by US/CT	134	(4.8)	35	(26)
Renal:				
Creatinine 1.5–3.0	281	(10)	79	(28)
Creatinine >3.0	139	(4.9)	39	(28)
Dialysis required	521	(18.5)	164	(31)
Hemofiltration required	400	(14.2)	163	(41)
CAVHD required	86	(3.1)	25	(29)
Cardiovascular:				
Inotropes on ECLS	1206	(42.9)	523	(43)
CPR required	164	(5.8)	31	(19)
Myocardial stun by echo	27	(1)	7	(26)
Cardiac arrhythmia	227	(8.1)	76	(33)
Hypertension requiring meds	320	(11.4)	188	(59)
PDA: right to left	2	(0.1)	—	—
left to right	5	(0.2)	1	(20)
bidirectional	2	(0.1)	2	(100)
Tamponade: blood	29	(1)	11	(38)
serous	3	(0.1)	2	(67)
air	6	(0.2)	1	(17)
Pulmonary:				
Pneumothorax requiring Tx	370	(13.2)	148	(40)
Pulmonary hemorrhage	124	(4.4)	36	(29)
Infectious:				
Culture-proven infection	585	(20.8)	271	(46)
WBC <1500	91	(3.2)	30	(33)
Metabolic:				
Glucose <40	25	(0.9)	6	(24)
Glucose >240	250	(8.9)	92	(37)
pH <7.20	119	(4.2)	29	(24)
pH >7.60	49	(1.7)	33	(67)
Hyperbilirubinemia (>2 direct or >15 total)	86	(3.1)	22	(26)

ferent components of the circuit is determined by the weight of the patient and the anticipated extracorporeal flow. The patients may be cannulated through an open cut down procedure, by a semipercutaneous procedure, or by a percutaneous technique.

During ECLS the patient is monitored 24 hours a day by an ECLS specialist. Pulmonary care and treatment of the underlying disease is of utmost importance as ECLS alone does not cure the patient. A successful outcome relies upon adequate pulmonary recovery occurring during extracorporeal support.

The overall survival of 2,810 pediatric ECLS patients reported to the ELSO Registry was 55%. In a large single institution material the survival to hospital discharge was 77%. There are no prospective randomized studies in the pediatric age group comparing survival with ECLS vs. conventional treatment, but in a retrospective multicenter study ECLS survival was 47%, compared to 26% in the matched control group. Survival is highest in patients with aspiration pneumonia, viral pneumonia and post-traumatic ARDS.

References

1. ELSO Registry. Ann Arbor, MI: Extracorporeal Life Support Organization; July 2004.

2. Hill JD, O'Brien TG, Murray JJ, et al. Extracorporeal oxygenation for acute post-traumatic respiratory failure (shock-lung syndrome): Use of the Bramson Membrane Lung. *N Engl J Med* 1972; 286:629-634.

3. Schulte HD. Membrane oxygenators in prolonged assisted extracorporeal circulation. *Dtsch Med Wochenschr* 1973; 98:508-513.

4. Geelhoed GW, Adkins PC, Corso PJ, Joseph WL. Clinical effects of membrane lung support for acute respiratory failure. *Ann Thorac Surg* 1975; 20:177-187.

5. Gille JP, Bagniewski AM. Ten years of use of extracorporeal membrane oxygenation (ECMO) in the treatment of acute respiratory insufficiency (ARI). *Trans Am Soc Artif Intern Organs* 1976; 22:102-109.

6. Bartlett RH, Gazzaniga AB, Jefferies MR, Huxtable RF, Haiduc NJ, Fong SW. Extracorporeal membrane oxygenation (ECMO) cardiopulmonary support in infancy. *Trans Am Soc Artif Intern Organs* 1976; 22:80-93.

7. Bartlett RH, Gazzaniga AB, Huxtable RF, Schippers HC, O'Connor MJ. Extracorporeal circulation (ECMO) in neonatal respiratory failure. *J Thorac Cardiovasc Surg* 1977; 74:826-833.

8. Zapol WM, Snider MT, Hill JD, et al. Extracorporeal membrane oxygenation in severe respiratory failure. *JAMA* 1979; 242:2193-2196.

9. Bartlett RH, Andrews AF, Toomasian JM, Haiduc NJ, Gazzaniga AB. Extracorporeal membrane oxygenation (ECMO) for newborn respiratory failure: 45 cases. *Surgery* 1982; 92:425-433.

10. McManus ML, Kevy SV, Bower LK, Hickey PR. Coagulation factor deficiencies during initiation of extracorporeal membrane oxygenation. *J Pediatr* 1995; 126:900-904.

11. Chevalier JY, Couprie C, Larroquet M, Renolleau S, Durandy Y, Costil J. Veno-venous single lumen cannula extracorporeal lung support in neonates: A five year experience. *ASAIO J* 1993; 39: M654-M658.

12. Moulton SL, Lynch FP, Cornish JD, Bejar RF, Simko AJ, Krous HF. Carotid artery reconstruction following neonatal extracorporeal membrane oxygenation. *J Pediatr Surg* 1991; 7:794-799.

13. Adolph V, Bonis S, Falterman K, Arensman R. Carotid artery repair after pediatric extracorporeal membrane oxygenation. *J Pediatr Surg* 1990; 25:867-870.

14. McGough EC, McGough S, Hawkins JA. Subclavian artery cannulation for infant

extracorporeal membrane oxygenation. *Ann Thorac Surg* 1993; 55:787-788.

15. Pesenti A, Gattinoni L, Kolobow T, Damia G. Extracorporeal circulation in adult respiratory failure. *ASAIO Trans* 1988; 34:43-47.

16. Anderson HL, Otsu T, Chapman RA, Bartlett RH. Veno-venous extracorporeal life support in neonates using a double lumen catheter. *Trans Am Soc Artif Intern Organs* 1989; 35:650-653.

17. Perreult T, Mallahoo K, Morneault L, Johnston A, Adolph V. Use of a 12 french double lumen catheter in a newborn supported with extracorporeal membrane oxygenation. *ASAIO J* 1994; 40:100-102.

18. Peek GJ, Sosnowski AW. Extra-corporeal membrane oxygenation for pediatric respiratory failure. *Br Med Bull* 1997; 53:745-756.

19. Trittenwein G, Furst G, Golej J, et al. Single needle venovenous extracorporeal membrane oxygenation using a nonocclusive roller pump for rescue in infants and children. *Artif Organs* 1997; 21:793-797.

20. Trittenwein G, Golej J, Burda G, et al. Neonatal and pediatric extracorporeal membrane oxygenation using nonocclusive blood pumps: the Vienna experience. *Artif Organs* 2001; 25:994-999.

21. Kolla S, Awad SA, Rich PB, Schreiner FJ, Hirschl RB, Bartlett RH. Extracorporeal Life Support for 100 Adult Patients With Severe Respiratory Failure. *Ann Surg* 1997; 226:544-566.

22. Peek GJ, Firmin RK, Moore HM, Sosnowski AW. Cannulation of neonates for veno-venous extracorporeal life support. *Ann Thorac Surg* 1996; 61:1851-1852.

23. Reickert CA, Schreiner RJ, Barntlett RH, Hirschl RB. Percutaneous access for venovenous extracorporeal life support in neonates. *J Pediatr Surg* 1998; 33:365-369.

24. Cataldi-Betcher EL, Seltzer MH, Slocum BA. Complications occurring during enteral nutrition support: A prospective study. *J Parenter Enteral Nutr* 1983; 7:546-552.

25. Anderson HL, Shapiro MB, Delius RE, Steimie CN, Chapman RA, Bartlett RH. Extracorporeal life support for respiratory failure after multiple trauma. *J Trauma* 1994; 37:266-274.

26. Pettignano R, Heard M, Deavis R, Labuz M, Hart M. Total enteral nutrition versus total parenteral nutrition during pediatric extracorporeal membrane oxygenation. *Crit Care Med* 1998; 26:358-363.

27. Lindén V, Palmér K, Reinhard J, et al. High survival in adult patients with ARDS treated by extracorporeal membrane oxygenation, minimal sedation and pressure supported ventilation. *Intensive Care Med* 2000; 26:1630-1637.

28. Martin GR, Short BL, Abbott C, O'Brien AM. Cardiac stun in infants undergoing extracorporeal membrane oxygenation. *J Thorac Cardiovasc Surg* 1991; 101:607-611.

29. Keszler M, Ryckman FC, McDonald Jr. JV, et al. A prospective, multicenter, randomized study of high versus low positive end-expiratory pressure during extracorporeal membrane oxygenation. *J Pediatr* 1992; 120:107-113.

30. Langer M, Mascheroni D, Marcolin R, Gattinoni L. The prone position in ARDS patients. A clinical study. *Chest* 1988; 94:103-107

31. Haefner SM, Bratton SL, Annich GM, Bartlett RH, Custer JR. Complications of intermittent prone positioning in pediatric patients receiving extracorporeal membrane oxygenation for respiratory failure. *Chest* 2003; 123:1589-1594.

32. Krummel TM, Greenfield LJ, Kirkpatrick BV, Mueller DG, Ormazabal M, Salzberg AM. Clinical use of an extracorporeal membrane oxygenator in neonatal pulmonary failure. *J Pediatr Surg* 1982; 17:525-531.

33. Egan TM, Duffin J, Glynn MF, et al. Ten-year experience with extracorporeal membrane

oxygenation for severe respiratory failure. *Chest* 1988; 94:681-687.

34. Ombrellaro M, Goldthorn JF, Harnar TJ, Shires GT. Extracorporeal life support for the treatment of adult respiratory distress syndrome after burn injury. *Surgery* 1994; 115:523-526.

35. Bond SJ, Lee DJ, Stewart DL, Buchino JJ. Open lung biopsy in pediatric patients on extracorporeal membrane oxygenation. *J Pediatr Surg* 1996; 31:1376-1378.

36. Green TP, Moler FW, Goodman DM. Probability of survival after prolonged extracorporeal membrane oxygenation in pediatric patients with acute respiratory failure. *Crit Care Med* 1995; 23:1132-1139.

37. Paris JJ, Schraber MD, Statter M, Arensman R, Siegler M. Beyond autonomy—physicians' refusal to use life-prolonging extracorporeal membrane oxygenation. *N Engl J Med* 1993; 329:354-357.

38. Bartlett RH, Roloff DW, Cornell RG, Andrews AF, Dillon PW, Zwischenberger JB. Extracorporeal circulation in neonatal respiratory failure: a prospective randomized study. *Pediatrics* 1985; 76:479-487.

39. O'Rourke PP, Crone RK, Vacanti JP, et al. Extracorporeal membrane oxygenation and conventional medical therapy in neonates with persistent pulmonary hypertension of the newborn: a prospective randomized study. *Pediatrics* 1989; 84:957-963.

40. UK collaborative randomised trial of neonatal extracorporeal membrane oxygenation. UK Collaborative ECMO Trial Group. *Lancet* 1996; 348:75-82.

41. Green TP, Timmons OT, Fackler JC, Moler FW, Thompson AE, Sweeney MF. The impact of extracorporeal membrane oxygenation on survival in pediatric patients with acute respiratory failure. *Crit Care Med* 1996; 24:323-329.

42. Swaniker F, Kolla S, Moler F, et al. Extracorporeal life support outcome for 128 pediatric patients with respiratory failure. *J Pediatr Surg* 2000; 35:197-202.

43. Pettignano R, Fortenberry JD, Heard ML, et al. Primary use of the venovenous approach for extracorporeal membrane oxygenation in pediatric acute respiratory failure. *Pediatr Crit Care Med* 2003; 4:291-298.

44. Pierre EJ, Zwischenberger JB, Angel C, et al. Extracorporeal membrane oxygenation in the treatment of respiratory failure in pediatric patients with burns. *J Burn Care Rehabil* 1998; 19:131-134.

45. Lessin MS, El-Eid SE, Klein MD, Cullen ML. Extracorporeal membrane oxygenation in pediatric respiratory failure secondary to smoke inhalation injury. *J Pediatr Surg* 1996; 31:1285-1287.

46. Goretsky MJ, Greenhalgh DG, Warden GD, Goretsky MJ, Ryckman FC, Warner BW. The use of extracorporeal life support in pediatric burn patients with respiratory failure. *J Pediatr Surg* 1995; 30:620-623.

47. Kane TD, Greenhalgh DG, Warden GD, Goretsky MJ, Ryckman FC, Warner BW. Pediatric burn patients with respiratory failure: predictors of outcome with the use of extracorporeal life support. *J Burn Care Rehabil* 1999; 20:145-150.

48. Daimon S, Umeda T, Michishita I, Wakasugi H, Genda A, Koni I. Goodpasture's-like syndrome and effect of extracorporeal membrane oxygenator support. *Intern Med* 1994; 33:569-573.

49. Siden HB, Sanders GM, Moler FW. A report of four cases of acute, severe pulmonary hemorrhage in infancy and support with extracorporeal membrane oxygenation. *Pediatr Pulmonol* 1994; 18:337-341.

50. Larsson J, Frenckner B, Lindén V, Palmér K. Management, including embolization, of multiple mycotic pulmonary artery aneurysms causing critical lung hemorrhages during VA ECMO. In: The 20th

Annual CNMC Symposium; February 20-24, 2004; Keystone, CO.

51. Kolovos NS, Schuerer DJ, Moler FW, et al. Extracorporal life support for pulmonary hemorrhage in children: a case series. *Crit Care Med* 2002; 30:577-580.

52. Michaels AJ, Schriener RJ, Kolla S, et al. Extracorporeal life support in pulmonary failure after trauma. *J Trauma* 1999; 46:638-645.

53. Fortenberry JD, Meier AH, Pettignano R, Heard M, Chambliss CR, Wulkan M. Extracorporeal life support for posttraumatic acute respiratory distress syndrome at a children's medical center. *J Pediatr Surg* 2003; 38:1221-1226.

54. Williams GD, Numa A, Sokol J, Tobias V, Duffy BJ. ECLS in pertussis: does it have a role? *Intensive Care Med* 1998; 24:1089-1092.

55. Pooboni S, Roberts N, Westrope C, et al. Extracorporeal life support in pertussis. *Pediatr Pulmonol* 2003; 36:310-315.

56. Halasa NB, Barr FE, Johnson JE, Edwards KM. Fatal pulmonary hypertension associated with pertussis in infants: Does extracorporeal membrane oxygenation have a role? *Pediatrics* 2003; 112:1274-1278.

57. Linden V, Karlen J, Olsson M, et al. Successful extracorporeal membrane oxygenation in four children with malignant disease and severe Pneumocystis carinii pneumonia. *Med Pediatr Oncol* 1999; 32:25-31.

24

Neurologic Outcome Following ECLS in Pediatric Patients with Respiratory or Cardiac Failure

Heidi J. Dalton, M.D. and Susan E. Day, M.D.

Introduction

There are numerous studies which address neurodevelopmental outcomes for neonates with respiratory failure who have been treated with ECMO.[1-8] Long-term follow-up studies of neonatal ECMO patients have provided important information regarding development, school performance, commonly observed learning disabilities, and behavioral issues. In contrast, studies on the pediatric population are few in number, with the majority focusing on the patients treated with ECLS following surgery for congenital heart disease. This chapter will focus on the information that is available on the neurologic outcome of the pediatric patient placed on ECLS for respiratory or cardiac failure.

ELSO Registry data on neurologic complications

The ELSO Registry provides data on neurologic compromise, reported as a complication during the ECLS period, including brain death, seizures, and cerebral infarct or cranial hemorrhage diagnosed by neuroimaging. These data do not provide a complete picture of outcome following ECMO because many patients do not have imaging studies or neurologic examinations prior to ECMO initiation, making it impossible to determine whether the abnor-malities are attributable to pre-existing conditions or to ECMO therapy. In addition, some ECMO patients do not receive brain imaging prior to hospital discharge, leading to potential under-reporting of intracranial hemorrhage and cerebral infarct. Finally, the absence of seizures or central nervous system abnormality on head computed tomography (CT) or magnetic resonance imaging (MRI) does not predict normal neurologic outcome.

According to the July 2005 ELSO Registry,[9] a total of 3,064 pediatric patients (age >30 days and <18 years) have received ECMO for respiratory failure. Of this group, 6% expired due to brain death, and 9% had seizures while on bypass. Ultrasound or CT imaging studies revealed infarction in 3% and hemorrhage in 5% of the pediatric patients.

A total of 3,265 pediatric patients (>30 days and <16 years of age) have received ECMO for cardiac indications. Brain death was reported in 6% of these patients, seizures were noted in 11%, cerebral infarcts in 4%, and intracranial hemorrhage in 4%. Among pediatric cardiac patients, the incidence of brain death was highest (9%) among patients >1 year of age at time of ECLS cannulation. The incidence of seizures was 14% in cardiac ECMO patients >30 days and <1 year old, while 8% of ECLS cardiac patients between 1-16 years old had seizures reported. The incidence of cerebral infarct for cardiac patients was 4% in all groups, while intracranial hemorrhage was 5% in those >30 days and <1 year and 3% in patients 1-16 years old (Table 1).

The Registry data are useful as a description of short-term neurologic complications which place the patient at risk for long-term developmental problems. The incidence of brain death is higher for pediatric ECMO patients than for neonatal patients. Hemorrhage and infarct are reported more frequently in neonates, but this is possibly due to the ease of obtaining ultrasound in this age group. The most commonly described complication for all age groups is seizures, and some studies suggest that abnormal EEG during or after ECMO is predictive of poor neurologic outcome.[10-12] One encouraging fact is that the incidence of short-term neurologic complications does not appear to be rising in any group. An exception is the increase in cerebral hemorrhage reported in cardiac patients <30 days of age over the last 5 years. The rate of intracranial hemorrhage in neonatal cardiac patients treated with

ECMO increased from 4-8% in the 1990s to 10-18% currently.[13] It is unknown whether this is a result of the greater complexity of neonatal cardiac diagnoses, an increase in the number of patients imaged, differences in coagulation status at time of ECLS, or other factors.

Changes in ECLS patient diagnoses

Once viewed primarily as a therapy of last resort for neonates with respiratory failure, ECLS has evolved into a tool that is being used in more varied situations.[14] Increasing numbers of neonates with hypoplastic left heart syndrome and other complex cardiac diseases are being supported with ECLS.[15-17] These children are extremely fragile and may have multiple organ system dysfunction with poor neurologic outcome independent of their need for ECLS. Similarly, pediatric patients with respiratory failure now include those with trauma or those who have failed multiple other therapeutic modalities, including inhaled nitric oxide, high

Table 1. Comparison of neonatal and pediatric ECLS outcome and complications by diagnosis.[9]

Diagnosis and patient population	Cumulative number treated with ECLS	% survival to discharge or transfer	% Neurologic complications (% occurrence in total patients reported)			
			Brain death	Seizure (determined clinically or by EEG)	Infarct (determined by ultrasound or CT)	Hemorrhage (determined by ultrasound or CT)
Neonatal respiratory*	19,939	77	1	11	9	6
Pediatric respiratory†	3,064	64	6	9	3	5
Neonatal cardiac*	2,617	37	1	12	3	10
Pediatric cardiac‡	3,265	43	6	11	4	4
Age >30 days and < 1 yr	1,765	42	5	14	4	5
Age 1-16 yrs	1,500	44	9	8	4	3

* Age ≤ 30 days at cannulation
† Age > 30 days and <18 years at cannulation
‡ Age > 30 days and <16 years at cannulation

frequency ventilation, and prone positioning.[18-20] These pre-ECMO events may impact the rate and severity of neurologic deficits observed and reported.

The recent increase in rapid-deployment ECLS for patients in cardiac arrest and the use of ECLS for patients following transplantation, sepsis, burns, trauma and other previously excluded diagnoses illustrates how the application of ECLS has evolved with accumulating experience and improvements in techniques and equipment. The impact of these changes and the fact that the majority of pediatric ICU patients have underlying illnesses, in addition to their acute illness, makes it more challenging to identify which factors impact neurologic function and long-term quality-of-life.[21]

Two areas where the use the ECLS has expanded significantly are the use as a bridge to transplantation and for resuscitation from cardiac arrest. Early literature on pediatric cardiac ECLS discouraged its use to bridge patients to heart transplantation because of concerns about the long waiting time for organ availability and the complications known to occur with prolonged ECLS use. Many clinicians counseled against offering ECLS because of the likelihood that complications would cause ECLS to be discontinued before an organ would become available. As ECMO techniques improved and longer successful runs were reported, the use of ECLS as a bridge to transplantation increased.[22-24] According to the ELSO Registry in July 2005, a total of 332 patients have been bridged to heart transplantation with ECMO, with an overall survival of 46%.[9] Neonates comprised 16% of the total of 561, while 69% were pediatric patients (>30 days and <16 years) and 15% were adult (≥16 years). Survival rates to discharge or transfer for these neonatal, pediatric, and adult patients were 50%, 34%, and 42%, respectively. In one recent report by Bae et al., 300 patients were listed for transplantation at a single center between 1984-2003, and 21 required ECMO as a bridge to transplantation, with a survival of 60%.[25] These results have changed the attitude toward the use of ECLS as a bridge to heart transplantation.

Early reports of severe neurologic injury or non-recovery discouraged the use of ECLS for acute cardiac arrest. As resuscitation techniques improved and techniques to implement ECMO emergently developed (termed "rapid deployment ECMO" or "eCPR"), the acceptable survival of such patients was reported. To date, 384 pediatric patients (age >30 days) have received ECLS for cardiac arrest, with 39% surviving to discharge.[9] This represents a dramatic increase in the reported survival of patients placed on ECLS for resuscitation as compared to patients who are treated conventionally. In a review of 200 in-hospital pediatric arrests from a single site, overall survival was 26%, with 10% of patients experiencing poor neurologic function.[26] In one report of 11 patients who were placed on ECLS during cardiac arrest overall survival was 64%. No long-term sequelae were noted in survivors, although no specific neurologic testing was reported.[27] It is premature to conclude that rapid deployment ECLS for cardiac arrest is superior to conventional resuscitation; long-term follow-up studies of survivors are needed.

Neurologic outcome for pediatric respiratory ECLS

Pediatric ICU survivors are not routinely seen in follow-up and there are few long-term outcome studies of ECLS-treated patients. Descriptions of the neurologic outcome of pediatric ICU patients have generally reported their status at the time of hospital discharge. The available data have demonstrated correlation between diagnoses known to impact neurologic status and overall neurologic function, at least for patients with impairment. Those patients who suffer stroke, hemorrhage or other defined injury such as hypoxic-ischemic events are found to have neurologic or motor impairment prior to discharge. However, more subtle morbidities, such as behavior problems, poor school performance, or learning disabilities, are less likely to be identified prior to discharge. Only a few small studies have reported the long-term neurodevelopmental outcome of post-ECMO respiratory failure patients (Table 2).

Heulitt noted that of 15 pediatric and 4 adult patients supported with ECLS for respiratory failure at Children's Hospital of Arkansas, 58% survived to discharge.[28] The Pediatric Cerebral Performance Category (PCPC), a measure of cognitive impairment, was used with the 11 survivors, of whom 64% were normal, 27% had mild disability, and 9% had moderate disability. Using the Pediatric Overall Performance Category (POPC), a measure of functional morbidity, for the same 11 patients, 27% were normal, 45% had mild disability, 18% had moderate disability, and 9% were severely disabled.

In another small series, Fajardo et al. reported on 26 pediatric patients who were evaluated 1-3 years following ECMO.[29] In the 13 preschool age children, 38% were normal, 31% had abnormalities prior to ECMO (cortical atrophy,

Goldenhar's syndrome, Trisomy 21, and child abuse) and remained at pre-ECMO baseline, and 31% were abnormal following ECMO. None of these patients had evidence of cerebral hemorrhage or infarct on CT examination, although cortical atrophy with mild hydrocephalus was present in some patients. Whether the abnormalities observed following ECMO were related to pre-ECMO hypoxemia or ischemia or to ECMO is not known. In the 13 school age children, parents described 77% as normal, 8% as above average, and 15% as below average. Of the 5 patients over 5 years of age at cannulation, 4 (80%) were normal with no CT abnormalities. The child identified with development delay had head CT evidence of hypoxic-ischemic encephalopathy.

Amigoni et al. prospectively evaluated 12 neonates and 9 children who received ECMO for respiratory failure with age-appropriate neurodevelopmental testing, electroencephalogram (EEG), auditory evoked potentials, visual evoked potentials, somatosensory evoked potentials, and head ultrasound or CT scans at conclusion of ECLS at 6, 12, 24, and 36 months after ECLS.[30]

Table 2. Long-term neurologic outcome of pediatric patients treated with ECMO for respiratory failure.

Author, Year	Population	Time/type of follow-up	Normal or unchanged	Impaired
Heulitt et al. (1993)[28]	11 survivors out of 19 ECMO patients (15 children and 4 adults)	PCPC and POPC	64% (PCPC) 27% (POPC)	36% (PCPC) 63% (POPC)
Fajardo (1975)[29]	26 children (13 pre-school, 13 school-age)	1-3 years following ECMO	Preschool: 69% School age: 85%	Preschool: 31% School age: 8%
Amigoni et al. (2005)[30]	9 pediatric, ages 4-162 months	Developmental exam, EEG, BAEP, SEP, neuroimaging at 6, 12, 24, and 36 months after ECMO	66%	34%

PCPC = Pediatric Cerebral Performance Category (cognitive), POPC = Pediatric Overall Performance Category (functional), EEG = Electroencephalogram, BAEP = Brainstem auditory evoked potential, SEP = Somatosensory evoked potential

Pre-ECMO variables, including oxygenation index (OI), pH, and PaO_2, and ECMO variables, including pH, PaO_2, length of ECMO course, activated clotting time (ACT), and EEG were collected. The Glasgow outcome score (GOS) was used to classify neurologic outcome in 1 of 5 levels: good recovery, moderate disability, severe disability, persistent vegetative state, or death. An outcome other than "good recovery" was coded as "negative" or "abnormal." The purpose of the study was to identify pre-ECMO and ECMO predictors of long-term neurologic outcome. Of the 9 pediatric patients, 3 had abnormal outcomes by GOS at 12 months after ECMO, including 1 with developmental delay and 2 with hemiparesis with epilepsy. When tested at 12 months following ECMO, 6 of 9 pediatric patients had complete normalization of tests performed. EEG, neuroimaging or evoked potential exams were abnormal at 12 months in 3 pediatric patients and did not change over subsequent evaluations. Some tests performed either before, during, or after ECMO showed a degree of correlation. Specifically, the worst EEG during ECMO (P=0.017), the first EEG after ECMO (P=0.028), the first somatosensory evoked potentials following ECMO (P=0.014), and the neuroimaging score at the conclusion of bypass (P=0.016) correlated with long-term neurologic sequelae. Physiologic variables occurring before and during ECMO, such as oxygenation index, pH, PaO_2, or ACT, did not correlate with neurologic outcome. The authors concluded that long-term follow-up is needed in pediatric and neonatal ECLS patients because of the progressive improvement seen in the 12 months following ECMO. They suggest that somatosensory evoked potentials may have utility as an early predictor of long-term neurologic outcome.

Neurologic outcome for pediatric cardiac ECLS

Patients with congenital heart disease, particularly those with right to left shunts, are at risk for neurologic complications such as venous thrombosis, arterial infarction, brain abscess, seizures, and developmental delay.[31,32] The overall incidence of neurologic abnormalities in children following cardiopulmonary bypass is largely unknown. A number of perioperative risk factors have been identified, including duration of deep hypothermic cardiac arrest (DHCA).[33,34] Long-term follow up studies of children following cardiopulmonary bypass (CPB) are few in number and difficult to interpret due to small sample sizes, limited pre- and post-operative evaluation, and poor follow-up for neurologic and neurodevelopmental status.

Several studies of infants and children supported post-operatively with ECLS report neurologic outcome data, with only two conducting long-term follow-up. The findings of those studies are summarized in Table 3. In a study of 64 pediatric patients treated with ECMO at the University of Michigan for post-operative cardiac dysfunction between 1981-95, Kulik et al. reported that neurologic complications were noted in 28 (44%) prior to hospital discharge.[35] Seizures occurred in 18 patients (28%), three patients (5%) had embolus or thrombus, nine patients (14%) had an intraventricular hemorrhage greater than grade II, and 13 patients (20%) had anoxic encephalopathy. In 19 (68%) of patients with neurologic complications, hemodynamic compromise had occurred prior to ECMO and 5 patients (18%) had evidence of neurologic complication prior to ECMO. Eight (30%) of patients with neurologic complications had received CPR prior to ECMO, and 4 (14%) had several hours of low cardiac output prior to ECMO. Sixty-nine percent of patients who were electively removed from ECMO had neurologic and/or multisystem organ failure. No long-term follow-up was performed. A more recent study by Kolovis et al. reported survival of 50% for 74 pediatric cardiac patients treated with ECLS after surgery at the University of Michigan between 1995-2001, but did not include data on neurologic outcome.[36]

Hamrick et al. studied neurodevelopmental outcome in 53 infants who required ECMO after cardiac surgery.[37] The age at cannulation ranged from 1-362 days with a median age of 27 days. Survival was 32%. Of the 36 non-survivors, 58% had support discontinued; the reasons for discontinuation were neurologic complications (26%), poor cardiac function (58%), and multiple organ system failure (16%). Of the 17 survivors, 14 were seen in follow-up (1 lost to follow-up and 2 late deaths). Of the 14, 72% had normal neuromotor outcome when seen following discharge at 1, 1.5, 2.5, and 4.5 years of age. Cognitive function as measured by age-appropriate testing was normal in 50%, with 29% being described as abnormal ($\geq$2 standard deviations below the mean, or IQ <69) and 21% having suspect cognitive outcome (1-2 standard deviations below the mean, or IQ 70-75). Ten patients received MRIs, with 5 having evidence of hypoxic-ischemic injury. All patients with normal MRIs had a normal outcome. The authors found that factors such as pre-ECMO cardiac arrest, longer aortic cross-clamp time, and need for hemofiltration correlated with poor outcome. No survivors with an aortic cross-clamp time >40 minutes had a normal outcome. Non-survivors were more likely than survivors to have had cardiac arrest as an indication for ECMO, longer aortic cross-clamp time, or requirement for hemofiltration. The authors note that rapid-response ECMO was not available during this study period. Other variables such as age, weight, diagnosis, duration of bypass, or length of ECMO run were not associated with survival. MRIs performed on 10 patients showed several with evidence of hypoxic-ischemic injury in addition to the usual hemorrhagic and thrombotic findings seen in ECMO survivors. Although the survival was low (32%), 72% of survivors had normal neuromotor outcome and 50% had normal cognitive outcome.

Ibrahim et al. from Children's Hospital in Boston recently reported on the long-term follow-up of children with cardiac disease who required mechanical circulatory support over a ten year period.[38] This group included patients with pre- and post-op cardiac failure, cardiac

Table 3. Neurologic outcome of pediatric patients treated with ECLS for cardiac failure.

Author (year)	Population	Type of ECLS support	Time/type of follow-up	Normal or unchanged	Impaired (suspect or abnormal)
Kulik et al. (1996)[35]	64 children	ECMO for post-op cardiac surgery	At discharge	56%	44% (of which 68% had hemodynamic compromise prior to ECMO)
Hamrick et al. (2003)[37]	53 infants	ECMO for post-op cardiac surgery	1, 1.5, 2.5, 4.5 yrs Developmental exam	Motor 72% Cognitive 50 %	Motor 28% Cognitive 50%
Ibrahim et al. (2000)[38]	37 children (26 ECMO, 11 VAD)	Pre/post op, arrest, bridge to transplantation	11-92 months Parental interview	41% (ECMO) 80% (VAD)	59% (ECMO) 20% (VAD)
Morris et al. (2004)[39]	21 children	Rapid deployment ECLS for cardiac arrest	At discharge	50%	50%

arrest, cardiomyopathy and bridge to transplant. Overall survival to hospital discharge was 41%, and there was 1 death following discharge in the VAD and ECMO group. The indication for circulatory assist in the VAD group was predominantly failure to wean from CPB (70%) while ECMO indications were predominantly hypoxia (36%) and cardiac arrest (28%). Thirty-seven children (26 ECMO and 11 ventricular assist device [VAD] survivors) were followed for an average of 42 months. The follow-up data presented in this study consisted of telephone interviews of parents and written questionnaires sent to pediatricians and cardiologists. Eighty percent of the patients in both groups were described as exhibiting good to excellent general health. Neurologic follow-up was completed for 21 ECMO long-term survivors, all of whom were considered neurologically normal at time of cannulation. Neurologic impairment of moderate to severe degree was noted in 59% of the ECMO patients and 20% of the VAD survivors. Poor neurologic outcome was associated with low weight at the time support was originally instituted and with the duration of hypothermic circulatory arrest. The majority of patients with these characteristics were supported with ECMO as opposed to VAD. Adverse neurologic outcomes were not associated with pre-support cardiac arrest, carotid cannulation or carotid reconstruction, or in-hospital neurologic complications. The authors conclude that those infants surviving to hospital discharge after requiring mechanical circulatory assistance have good long-term survival and overall general health. However, the neurologic outcome for these survivors is concerning.

ECLS for resuscitation from cardiac arrest is a relatively new use. The ELSO Registry reports survival to discharge in approximately 40%. Several small series report higher rates of survival and have been summarized by Morris et al.[39] (Table 4). Morris reported on 66 patients resuscitated with rapid-deployment ECLS at Children's Hospital of Philadelphia from 1995-

2002. Of the 66 patients, 50% were decannulated and 33% survived to discharge. Prior to discharge, the Pediatric Cerebral Performance Category (PCPC) and Pediatric Overall Performance Category (POPC) were determined for survivors who were greater than 2 months old. Five out of 10 patients had no change in PCPC or POPC when compared with admission. Of patients with CPR duration of >60 minutes prior to ELCS, neurologic function was grossly normal in 3 (50%). When compared to patients suffering cardiac arrest within a 2 year period who were not resuscitated with ECLS, no survivors were noted if CPR duration was >30 minutes. The authors concluded that "extracorporeal cardiopulmonary resuscitation can be used to successfully resuscitate selected children following refractory in-hospital cardiac arrest, and can be implemented during active cardiopulmonary resuscitation."

The use of ECLS for stabilization of infants following Stage I Norwood hypoplastic left heart has been reported by Ungereider et al.[40] Eighteen infants from 2 centers were placed on VADs in the OR following CPB. The survival to hospital discharge was 89% with mean time on mechanical support of 3 days with low rate of bleeding complications (11%). Neurodevelopmental testing of 8 infants showed normal outcome using the Mullen Scales of Early Learning and the Vineland Adaptive Behavior Scales.

Summary of pediatric ECMO outcome

Among pediatric respiratory failure patients who receive ECMO, survival to hospital discharge is presently 50-60%, while pediatric cardiac survival is ~ 40%. There are few studies reporting long-term neurologic and neuropsychologic function in children who have undergone ECMO for these indications. The information available regarding long-term neurologic outcome in pediatric ECMO is not nearly as detailed as the neonatal literature, and although the rates of neuromotor impairment are low, the rates of abnormal cognitive outcome are concerning.

Because of the availability of alternative therapies for support of respiratory failure and improvements in cardiac surgery techniques, patients placed on ECMO today appear to be more critically ill than in the past. ECMO runs are longer, and complications increase with the length of ECLS treatment. An ongoing examination of neurodevelopmental outcome, resource use, and health care cost is needed for pediatric patients treated with ECLS.

References

1. Dalton HJ, Thompson AE. Extracorporeal membrane oxygenation. In: Fuhrman BP, Zimmerman JJ, eds. *Pediatric Critical Care.* 2nd ed. St.Louis, MO: Mosby; 1998:562-575.

2. Towne BH, Lott IT, Hicks DA, Healey T. Long-term follow-up of infants and children treated with extracorporeal membrane oxygenation (ECMO): a preliminary report. *J Pediatr Surg* 1985; 20:410-414.

.3. Boykin AR, Quivers ES, Wagenhoffer KL, et al. Cardiopulmonary outcome of neonatal extracorporeal membrane oxygenation at ages 10-15 years. *Crit Care Med* 2003; 31:2380-2384.

4. Glass P, Coffman C, Kenworthy L, et al. Longitudinal neurocognitive status following neonatal ECMO. Pediatr Res 1999; 45:243A.

5. Lott IT, McPherson D, Towne B, Johnson D, Starr A. Long-term neurophysiologic outcome after neonatal extracorporeal membrane oxygenation. *J Pediatr* 1990; 116:343-349.

6. Hofkosh D, Clouse H, Smith-Jones J, et al. Ten years of extracorporeal membrane oxygenation: neurodevelopmental outcome. *Pediatrics* 1991; 87:549-555.

7. Bulas D, Glass P. Neonatal ECMO: neuroimaging and neurodevelopmental outcome. *Semin Perinatol* 2005; 29:58-65.

Table 4. Summary of literature reporting survival following extracorporeal cardiopulmonary resuscitation (eCPR) in children.[39]

Author (year)	Population	Number of successful cannulations	Number (%) decannulated to sustained spontaneous circulation	Survivors (%)	Duration of CPR in mins: median (range) or mean ±sd
Aharon et al. (2001)	Pediatric postcardiotomy	10	NR	8 (80)	42 (5–110)
Dalton et al. (1993)	Pediatric cardiac	17	NR	11 (65)	42 (5–140)
del Nido (1996)	Pediatric postcardiotomy	11	7 (64)	6 (55)	65 ±9
Duncan et al. (1998)	Pediatric cardiac	11	9 (82)	6 (55)	55 (20–103)
Morris et al. (2004)[39]	Neonatal and pediatric cardiac	66	33 (50)	21 (33)	50 (5-105)
Parra et al. (2000)	Pediatric cardiac	4	4 (100)	4 (100)	16 (12–20)
Posner et al. (2000)	Pediatric ER	2	1 (50)	1 (50)	50, 90

8. Rais-Bahrami K, Wagner AE, Coffman C, Glass R, Short BL. Neurodevelopmental outcome in ECMO vs near-miss ECMO patients at 5 years of age. *Clin Pediatr* 2000; 39:145-152.

9. Extracorporeal Life Support Organization. *ECLS Registry report of the Extracorporeal Life Support Organization (ELSO)*. Ann Arbor, MI: University of Michigan; July 2005.

10. Cheung RT. Neurological complications of heart disease. Bailllieres Clin Neurol. 1997;6:337-355.

11. Campbell LR, Bunyapen C, Gangarosa ME, Cohen M, Kanto WP. Significance of seizures associated with extracorporeal membrane oxygenation. J Pediatr 1991;119;789-92.

12. Graziani LJ, Streletz LJ, Baumgart S, Cullen J, McKee LM. Predictive value of neonatal electroencephalogram before and during extracorporeal membrane oxygenation. J Pediatr 1994;125;969-75.

13. Extracorporeal Life Support Organization. *ECLS complications trend report of the Extracorporeal Life Support Organization (ELSO)*. Ann Arbor, MI: University of Michigan; January 2005.

14. Hintz SR, Benitz WE, Colby CE, Sheehan AM, Rycus P, Van Meurs KP. Utilization and outcomes of neonatal cardiac extracorporeal life support: 1996-2000. *Pediatr Crit Care Med* 2005;6:33-38.

15. Connor JA, Arons RR, Figueroa M, Gebbie KM. Clinical outcomes and secondary diagnoses for infants born with hypoplastic left heart syndrome. *Pediatrics* 2004; 114: e160-5.

16. Ungerleider RM, Shen I, Yeh T, et al. Routine mechanical ventricular assist following the Norwood procedure--improved neurologic outcome and excellent hospital survival. *Ann Thorac Surg* 2004; 77:18-22.

17. Kulik T, Moler F, Palmisano J. Outcome-associated factors in pediatric patients treated with extracorporeal membrane oxygenator after cardiac surgery. *Circulation* 1996; 94: II63-68.

18. O'Toole G, Peek G, Jaffe W, Ward D, Henderson H, Firmin RK. Extracorporeal membrane oxygenation in the treatment of inhalation injuries. *Burns* 1998; 24:562-565.

19. Michaels AJ, Schreiner RJ, Kolla S, et al. Extracorporeal life support in pulmonary failure after trauma. *J Trauma* 1999; 46:638-645.

20. Goldman A, Kerr S, Butt W, et al. Extracorporeal support for intractable cardiorespiratory failure due to meningococcal disease. *Lancet* 1997; 349:466-469.

21. PALISI Network. Effect of mechanical ventilator weaning protocols on respiratory outcomes in infants and children: a randomized controlled trial. *JAMA* 2002; 288:2561-2568.

22. Delius RE, Zwischenberger JB, Cilley R, et al. Prolonged extracorporeal life support of pediatric and adolescent cardiac transplant patients. *Ann Thorac Surg* 1990; 50:791.

23. Duncan B, Hraska V, Jonas R, et al. Mechanical circulatory support in children with cardiac disease. *J Thorac Cardiovasc Surg* 1999; 117:529-542.

24. Reddy SL, Hasan A, Hamilton LR, Smith JH, et al. Mechanical versus medical bridge to transplantation in children. What is the best timing for mechanical bridge? *Eur J Cardiothorac Surg* 2004; 25:605-609.

25. Bae JO, Frischer JS, Waich M, Stolar CJ, et al. Extracorporeal membrane oxygenation in pediatric cardiac transplantation. *J Pediatr Surg* 2005; 40:1051-1056.

26. Reis AG, Nadkarni V, Perondi MB, Grisi S, Berg RA. A prospective investigation into the epidemiology of in-hospital pediatric cardiopulmonary resuscitation using the international Utstein reporting style. *Pediatrics*.2002; 109:200-209.

27. del Nido PJ, Dalton HJ, Thompson AE, Siewers RD. Extracorporeal membrane oxygenator rescue in children during cardiac arrest after cardiac surgery. *Circulation* 1992; 86:II300-304.

28. Heulitt MJ, Moss MM, Walker WM. Morbidity and mortality in pediatric patients with respiratory failure. Presented before the *Extracorporeal Life Support Organization,* 1993; Ann Arbor Michigan.

29. Fajardo EM. Outcome and follow-up of children following extracorporeal life support in ECMO. In: Zwischenberger JB, Barlett RH, eds. *Extracorporeal cardiopulmonary support in critical care.* Ann Arbor, MI: Extracorporeal Life Support Organization; 1996: 373-381.

30. Amigoni A, Pettenazzo A, Biban P, et al. Neurologic outcome in children after extracorporeal membrane oxygenation: prognostic value of diagnostic tests. *Pediatr Neurol* 2005; 32:173-179.

31. Cheung RT. Neurological complications of heart disease. *Baillieres Clin Neurol* 1997; 6:337-355.

32. du Plessis AJ, Chang AC, Wessel DL, et al. Cerebrovascular accidents following the Fontan operation. *Pediatr Neurol* 1995; 12:230-236.

33. Kirkham FJ. Recognition and prevention of neurological complications in pediatric cardiac surgery. Pediatr Cardiol 1998; 19:331-345.

34. Wypij D, Newburger JW, Rappaport LA, et al. The effect of duration of deep hypothermic circulatory arrest in infant heart surgery on late neurodevelopment: the Boston Circulatory Arrest Trial. *J Thorac Cardiovasc Surg* 2003; 126:1397-1403.

35. Kulik TJ, Moler FW, Palmisano JM, et al. Outcome-associated factors in pediatric patients treated with extracorporeal membrane oxygenator after cardiac surgery. *Circulation* 1996; 94:II63-68.

36. Kolovos NS, Bratton SL, Moler FW, et al. Outcome of pediatric patients treated with extracorporeal life support after cardiac surgery. *Ann Thorac Surg* 2003; 76:1435-1442.

37. Hamrick SEG, Gremmels DB, Keet CA, et al. Neurodevelopmental outcome of infants supported with extracorporeal membrane oxygenation after cardiac surgery. *Pediatrics* 2003; 111:e671-675.

38. Ibrahim AE, Duncan BW, Blume ED, Jonas RA. Long-term follow-up of pediatric cardiac patients requiring mechanical circulatory support. *Ann Thorac Surg* 2000; 69:186-192.

39. Morris MC, Wernovsky G, Nadkarni VM. Survival outcomes after extracorporeal cardiopulmonary resuscitation instituted during active chest compressions following refractory in-hospital pediatric cardiac arrest. *Pediatr Crit Care Med* 2004; 5:440-446.

40. Ungerleider RM, Shen I, Yeh T Jr, et al. Routine mechanical ventricular assist following the Norwood procedure—improved neurologic outcome and excellent hospital survival. *Ann Thorac Surg* 2004; 77:18-22.

25

ECLS for Adult Respiratory Failure: Etiology and Indications

Giles J. Peek, M.D., F.R.C.S., C.Th., Ravindranath Tirouvopaiti, M.B.B.S., F.R.C.S., and Richard K. Firmin, M.B.B.S., F.R.C.S.

Introduction

Although the perception is that ECMO is used primarily in neonatal patients, it is interesting to remember that the first successful use of ECLS was for post-traumatic acute respiratory distress syndrome (ARDS) in an adult patient.[1] The first randomized controlled trial of ECMO was also in adults.[2] Adult ECMO represents a small fraction of the total number of cases in the ELSO Registry, but along with cardiac ECLS it is an area in which case numbers are growing rather than declining. It seems likely that centers which exclusively offer neonatal respiratory support will find it hard to maintain case numbers unless they expand their services to include cardiac patients as well as pediatric and adult respiratory patients.

The Conventional Ventilation or ECMO for Severe Adult Respiratory Failure (CESAR) trial[1] is due for completion by the end of 2006, and will hopefully define the place of ECMO in the management of adult respiratory failure (ARF). If a survival advantage for ECMO over conventional management is found, it is likely to stimulate increased interest in adult ECLS. It is estimated that there are at least 350 patients per year in the U.K. alone with ARDS and/or pneumonia that might benefit from ECMO. Acute asthma with a relative risk of death increased by 1.48 may also be an indication for

ECMO.[4] This equates to ~3,500 patients with ARDS and pneumonia in the U.S. each year who would be potential ECMO candidates. In this chapter, the evidence for using ECLS in ARF will be discussed and compared to outcomes with conventional treatment of the same patient group, providing a framework for case selection.

Evidence for use of ECLS in ARF

ECMO was shown to have no impact on survival in adults in the 1970s and again in 1994.[2,5] However, it is important to examine both of these trials in some detail, as well as a number of cohort studies to understand why ECMO may still be a rational treatment option for adults.

The 1970s NIH ECMO trial

Following the success of Bartlett and Hill in 1971, ECMO seemed like the magic bullet to combat the relatively new disease of ARDS.[1] Investigators moved quickly to perform a multicenter, randomized, controlled trial. In this trial, all patients with respiratory failure as defined as the need for positive pressure ventilation with an inspired oxygen concentration >50 were entered into a database. There were 90 patients with severe respiratory failure who fulfilled

ECMO criteria (fast entry criteria: PaO_2 <50 mm Hg with FiO_2 1, and PEEP >5 cm H_2O; slow entry criteria: PaO_2 <50 mm Hg for >12 hours with FiO_2 >0.6, PEEP >5 cm H_2O, and shunt fraction >30%). They were randomized to receive either ECMO or to continue conventional treatment. The trial was curtailed prematurely because of high mortality in both treatment groups (91.7% in the conventional arm vs. 86.4% in the ECMO arm).

However, there were a number of important differences in both the case selection and the manner in which ECMO was conducted in this era which make comparisons with modern day treatment inaccurate. First, all the patients were supported with venoarterial (VA) cannulation via the femoral vessels, in contrast to modern practice which is almost exclusively venovenous (VV). Second, the current practice of lung rest was unknown at the time; therefore, patients were maintained on high-pressure ventilation (mostly volume cycled) in 100% oxygen throughout their ECMO course. In fact, it was the poor outcome of patients in this study which inspired Theodore Kolobow to investigate ventilator-induced lung injury (VILI)[6-8] which has led to the development of lung-protective ventilation strategies. Finally, significant bleeding complications were associated with ECMO at an average rate of 3.8 liters on the first day of treatment.[9] This was felt to be mostly related to largely untested institutional protocols as 6 of the 9 centers had no ECMO experience prior to the trial. Heparin dose and target activated clotting times (ACTs) were much closer to those used in cardiopulmonary bypass (CPB) rather than those used in ECMO patients. Patients selected for the study retrospectively were determined to have had end-stage terminal lung disease at randomization[9] with evidence of hyaline membranes, thrombosis, and fibrosis on histology. One factor was the duration of high-pressure ventilation prior to randomization, which averaged 9.6 days. It is now known that survival

in adults supported with ECMO is a direct function of both age and duration of pre-ECLS ventilation, which determine the amount of VILI they have sustained.[10] These changes are usually irreversible after 7-9 days depending on the age of the patient, with younger patients being more resilient. The 1970s NIH ECMO trial taught a fundamental lesson about VILI, heparin management, and case selection; but, it did not determine the role of ECMO in adult respiratory failure. Unfortunately it stifled the use of ECMO in adults for 10-15 years. The development of neonatal ECMO by Dr. Bartlett and others continued,[11] but adult ECMO was not actively pursued following the trial.

Extracorporeal carbon dioxide removal

Kolobow, Gattinoni, and Bartlett developed the concept of VV ECMO to target CO_2 removal (extracorporeal carbon dioxide removal [$ECCO_2R$]) allowing apneic oxygenation at low ventilator rates, thereby reducing sheer stress and lung injury.[7,12-15] Gattinoni applied this to patients with severe ARF of parenchymal origin. CO_2 was cleared through a low flow VV bypass using a specially designed double lumen cannula inserted into the femoral vein. To avoid lung injury from conventional mechanical ventilation, the lungs were maintained "at rest" with 3-5 breaths/min, and a peak airway pressure of 35-45 cm H_2O, considered low at the time. Lung function improved in 31 of 43 patients (72.8%), and 21 patients (48.8%) survived to discharge. The mean time on bypass for the survivors was 5.4 ±3.5 days. Improvement in lung function, when present, occurred within 48 hours. Blood loss averaged 1800 ±850 ml/day, a great improvement on the 1970s, but still greater than what is considered acceptable today. The survival of nearly half the patients when 90% of them were expected to die was unprecedented, and stimulated a resurgence of interest in adult ECLS, both with ECMO and $ECCO_2R$.

Randomized, controlled trial of ECCO$_2$R vs. pressure-controlled inverse ratio ventilation

Gattinoni's work was proof that ECLS was possible in adults with an acceptable survival rate, but failed to prove that there was a survival advantage with ECCO$_2$R compared to conventional treatment. Morris set out to duplicate the work of Gattinoni and designed a study where patients would be randomized to either ECCO$_2$R or the best conventional treatment, which at the time was pressure-controlled inverse ratio ventilation (PCIRV) using a computer-controlled algorithm.[5] Pesenti from Gattinoni's group attempted to duplicate the clinical protocols, but the study was initiated before Morris' team had accumulated sufficient expertise, and it proved difficult for Pesenti to change prior practices. Forty patients with severe ARDS who met the 1970s ECMO entry criteria were randomized. The main outcome measure was survival at 30 days following randomization. Survival was not significantly different in the mechanical ventilation arm (n=19) and ECCO$_2$R (n=21) patients (42% vs. 33%, respectively, P=0.8). All the deaths occurred within 30 days of randomization, and the overall patient survival was 38%, 4 times higher than expected from the historical data of the 1970s study (P= 0.0002). The survival of the ECCO$_2$R group was not significantly different from that documented by Gattinoni. The PCIRV group survival was significantly higher than the 12% expected from the 1970s study (P= 0.0001). As there was no significant difference in survival between the mechanical ventilation and the ECCO$_2$R groups, Morris concluded that there was no justification for the use of ECCO$_2$R in ARDS. There were significant complications in the ECCO$_2$R group with patients being removed from ECLS for both thrombosis and hemorrhage. It also proved impossible to maintain adequate oxygenation in the ECCO$_2$R group necessitating a significant increase in peak airway pressure with higher levels in the ECLS group than the conventional arm. Inexperience with ECCO$_2$R undoubtedly contributed to these problems. If the team had gained experience with ECCO$_2$R before embarking on RCT, it is possible that the outcome would have been different. Morris' higher than expected survival with conventional ventilation leads to an alternative conclusion to this study; namely, that ECLS performed by an inexperienced team was comparable to the best mechanical ventilation. Morris' experience and difficulty in maintaining apneic oxygenation was not unusual. Most ECLS centers that used adult ECLS in the mid- to late 1980s had similar experiences and ultimately abandoned ECCO$_2$R in favor of ECMO which supports oxygenation as well as CO$_2$ removal.

Adult ECMO in the modern era

Adult respiratory ECMO, as practiced today, was pioneered by Bartlett and his team at the University of Michigan in Ann Arbor in 1988. The concept was to first select patients with potentially reversible disease and then, second, to use VV cannulation configured to give enough extracorporeal flow to support oxygenation and CO$_2$ removal. The third key principle was to reduce the level of ventilation to allow lung rest.[16] With this approach Bartlett documented 50% survival in a group of patients with a 90% expected mortality, a great improvement compared with the 20% survival in the NIH ECMO trial. This approach was used in the U.K. by Firmin and Sosnowski in 1989 in Leicester, U.K. The Leicester group documented 66% survival for their first 50 patients, using selection criteria similar to Bartlett's.[17] This approach to adult respiratory ECMO was duplicated by several other groups including teams in Stockholm,[18] Galveston, Shreveport,[19] and Wake Forest. As of July 2005 the ELSO Registry recorded 1,105 adult respiratory cases with an overall ECLS survival of 60% and survival of 53% to discharge or transfer.[20]

Survival with conventional treatment

With reasonable survival figures for adults with severe but potentially reversible respiratory failure, we must now determine whether similar outcomes can be obtained with conventional intensive care. The answer to this question must await the outcome of the CESAR trial, but there are a number of case series that can be used to determine the outcome in groups of similar patients.

An historical series

The group at Cardiopulmonics in Salt Lake City, Utah, conducted a prospective cohort study of adults receiving intensive care for ARF in 25 of the world's leading ICUs (11 in the U.S., 14 in Europe) between 1992-92.[21] The study group included all patients receiving ventilation with >50% oxygen for >24 hours. 1,426 patients with ARF were studied. The hospital survival was only 55.6%. The results were further analyzed for patients who were hypoxic or hypercarbic on study entry (group A, n=375 patients), and those who were not (group B, n=1,051 patients). Hospital survival rate was 33.3% for group A patients and 63.6% for group B. The severity of lung injury at the time of entry into the survey was a major prognostic factor, with hospital survival rates varying from 18% for patients with ARF with advanced lung injury, to 67% for patients with ARF with less severe lung injury. Survival rates <20% were seen if the mechanical ventilator FiO_2 was 0.80-1.0. Peak inspiratory pressure (PIP) >50 cm H_2O at entry into the survey was associated with <20% survival, while PIP <30 cm H_2O was associated with a survival rate of 60%. ARF patients with multi-organ failure had lower survival rates (10%) than those with pulmonary dysfunction alone (45%). Significant changes in intensive care management have taken place since 1992; however, the survival in patients who were hypoxic, hypercarbic, with multi-system failure

was very low (<20%). Since these patients make up the majority of cases referred for ECMO, we need to focus on recent studies of this subset of patients.

Databases

Based on the NIH ARDS Network database, a 70% mortality would be anticipated in patients who are currently placed on ECMO if they continued on conventional treatment.[22] The Case Mix Programme Database, which is the national comparative audit of patient outcomes coordinated by the Intensive Care National Audit and Research Centre (ICNARC) in the U.K., also supports this estimated mortality.[23] The mortality of the 1,506 patients with a PaO_2/FiO_2 ratio of ≤100 mm Hg in this database was 61.6%. The mean PaO_2/FiO_2 ratio in the patients referred for ECMO in Leicester was 65 ±37 mm Hg. It seems reasonable, therefore, to consider using ECMO in this group of adults, as they are at a high risk of death with continued conventional treatment.

Prone ventilation

Prone positioning has become a popular treatment modality for patients with ARF.[24] Oxygenation improves 60-70% of the time, but the effect on survival is unknown. Gattinoni et al. conducted a multi-center, randomized trial to compare conventional supine ventilation in patients with acute lung injury or ARDS with a predefined strategy of placing patients in a prone position for >6 hrs/day for 10 days.[25] 304 patients were enrolled with 152 in each arm. The mean PaO_2/FiO_2 ratio was 122 mm Hg in the supine group and 117 mm Hg in the prone group. The average number of non-pulmonary, failed organs was 1.4 for the overall supine group and 1.3 for the prone group. The mortality rate was 23% during the 10-day study period, 49.3% at the time of discharge from the ICU, and 60.5 % at 6 months. The relative risk of death in the prone group as compared with the supine group was 0.84 at the end of the study period (95% confidence interval, 0.56-1.27), 1.05 at the time of discharge from the ICU (95% confidence interval, 0.84-1.32), and 1.06 at 6 months (95% confidence interval, 0.88-1.28). During the study period, the increase in the PaO_2/FiO_2 ratio was greater in the prone than the supine group (63.0 ±66.8 vs. 44.6 ±68.2, P= 0.02). There was no increase in complications associated with prone ventilation such as accidental extubation. The authors concluded that there was improvement in physiology without an associated effect on outcome with prone ventilation. It is noteworthy that the patients in this study had mostly single system failure and were less hypoxic than patients who are referred for ECMO; thus, we have only 50% survival in a group of patients with less severe disease than those placed on ECMO.

These data confirm that severe ARF in adults has a high associated mortality rate, particularly when accompanied by multi-organ failure. The use of ECLS in these patients is therefore reasonable. In the next section, we will discuss case selection, which depends on the identification of patients who have potentially reversible disease and have not sustained terminal VILI.

Potentially reversible disease

While patients referred for adult respiratory support can be broadly divided into those with pneumonia and those with ARDS, obtaining a successful outcome depends on the assessment of the reversibility of their condition. Cannulating a patient with non-reversible disease will not change the outcome; the patient will still die, but it will take longer, be more expensive, and prove more traumatic for the family. Three factors underpin the assessment of reversibility, these are the pre-morbid condition of the patient, the etiology of the respiratory failure, and the duration of ventilation.

Pre-morbid condition of the patient

It is sometimes difficult to obtain accurate information about the patient's pre-morbid condition and the presence of chronic diseases during the referral process. This may be due to the fact that the intensive care staff referring the patient does not have the information or because they are omitting facts so as not to discourage acceptance of the patient for ECMO. Patients need a reasonable level of pre-morbid health in order to survive severe respiratory failure. On the whole, they should have been independently mobile, able to climb stairs normally, and not on home oxygen. The elderly should be of normal capacity with respect to their activities of daily living (i.e., self care). Patients with malignancy who have undergone surgery, chemotherapy, and/or bone marrow transplant should have a reasonable prognosis (i.e., 5-year expected survival of ≥50%) according to the oncologist. Patients with sudden ARDS or pneumonia at the time of a bone marrow transplant who are acutely neutropenic or have a poor prognosis require particular care before being selected for ECMO. Patients with HIV need to be considered in a similar way. Patients presenting with sudden onset of AIDS with pneumocystis pneumonia have a poorer prognosis than a patient whose viral load has been reduced by anti-retroviral medication. Expert opinion from the infectious diseases team should be sought and the prognosis balanced against the risk to the ECMO team and other patients in the ICU. It is not standard practice to offer ECMO to HIV positive patients who have a marginal prognosis, as ECMO is unlikely to change their outcome. One of the features of running an ECMO program is having patients referred from a wide range of disciplines. One must not be afraid to ask the referring physician (or an independent expert) for information on the natural history and prognosis of the underlying condition.

Etiology of respiratory failure

Patients with aspiration pneumonia tend to do particularly well, while patients with pregnancy-associated ARDS tend to have a lower survival. Other common etiologies include bacterial (pneumococcal, staphylococcal), atypical (legionella, mycoplasma), and viral pneumonia (chickenpox, influenza A). Tuberculosis is becoming increasingly common even in patients who are not immunocommpromised. Common causes of ARDS include trauma, pancreatitis, and sepsis. Other diagnoses which have a good prognosis, with ECMO support include asthma, Wegener's Granulomatosis, and pulmonary embolism.

Duration of ventilation

Total duration of ventilation not to exceed 7 days was originally a standard exclusion and rigidly followed. This is a very effective strategy for selecting cases with a good prognosis; however, as worldwide experience has increased, it has become clear that it is the duration of high pressure/high FiO_2 ventilation that is most important along with patient age in regards to VILI (Figure 1). Younger patients can be successfully managed with ECMO after as many as 9 days ventilation,[21] while the elderly probably should not be offered support if they have been ventilated for >5 days. The CESAR trial selection criteria (Tables 4 and 5) regarding the length of ventilation and the severity of respiratory failure is useful for decision making for including or excluding a patient for consideration of ECMO therapy.

Leicester, U.K. case series

Between August 1989 and May 2004, a total of 269 adult patients (≥18 years old) received ECMO at Groby Road/Glenfield Hospital, Leicester, U.K. The indication for use of ECMO was severe but potentially reversible respiratory failure refractory to conventional management. ECMO was used for cardiac support in patients with cardiac failure refractory to maximal medical treatment, in patients who were difficult to wean from CPB following cardiac surgery, and for patients with pulmonary embolism. ECMO complications were classified as mechanical if the complication was related to the ECMO circuit or as patient-related.

ECMO was used for respiratory failure in 94% (Table 1) and cardiac failure in 6% of patients (overall survival was 65%). Complete data on complications were available in 222 patients and the remainder (n=47) were excluded from further analysis.

Patient- and mechanical-related complications

Multiple logistic regression analysis of the complications (Table 2) revealed that cannulation site bleeding, hypertension, cardiac arrhythmias, and pulmonary complications were independently associated with mortality, but none of the mechanical complications (Table 3) were associated with mortality.

CESAR Trial

CESAR (conventional ventilation or ECMO for severe adult respiratory failure) is a national randomized controlled trial in the U.K. funded

Table 1. ECMO used for respiratory failure and cardiac failure.

Complication	Patients affected (%)
Respiratory failure	94
Pneumonia	54.6
Primary ARDS	14.5
Secondary ARDS	8
Status asthamaticus	1.86
Other	15
Cardiac failure	6
Overall survival	>65

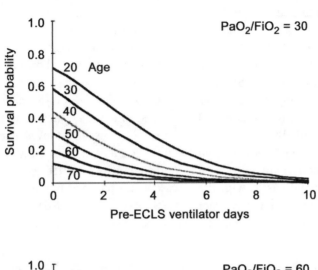

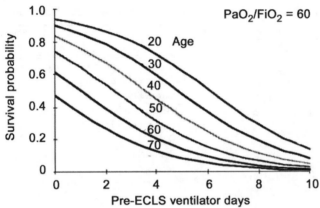

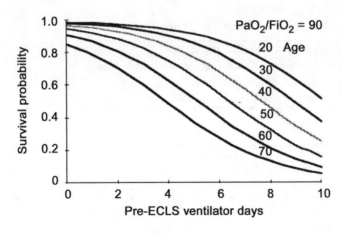

Figure 1. Graphical representation of the effect of pre-ECLS ventilator days and age on probability of survival shown for 3 PaO_2/FiO_2 ratios as derived from multiple logistic regression model of pre-ECLS variables.[9]

by the National Health Service and the Health Technology Assessment agency. The hypothesis is that ECMO will improve survival without severe disability 6 months post randomization for adults with severe, but potentially reversible respiratory failure. The inclusion and exclusion criteria are given in tables 4 and 5. Suitable patients can be entered from any of the 96 participating U.K. hospitals and are randomized to either transfer to Glenfield Hospital for consideration of ECMO or continued conventional management. The conventional care is provided in the original center in most cases, with the exception of a minority of smaller intensive care units where patients are transferred to larger hospitals to ensure equivalent care. The conventional care is not controlled, but the NIH ARDS-net protocol is recommended. The primary end point is survival without severe disability measured by an independent observer in the patients' home. The first patient was entered on July 23, 2001 and as of July 31, 2005, 145 patients have been recruited with a sample size of 180 patients. The trial is blinded in that the outcome in the conventional arm is not known to the investigators in the ECMO unit. The survival in the ECMO arm is similar to our previously reported experience; indeed the case series reported in this chapter contains the CESAR patients enrolled to date. Trial completion is expected by the end of 2006.

Table 2. Incidence of mechanical complications.

Complication	Patients affected n	(%)
Oxygenator failure	51	(23)
Pump malfunction	15	(6.8)
Race way/tubing rupture	4	(1.8)
Cracks on connectors	18	(8.1)
Air in circuit	2	(0.9)
Cannula problems	13	(5.9)
Clots in bridge	47	(21.2)
Clots in bladder	55	(25.8)
Clots in oxygenator	94	(42.3)

Table 3. Patient-related complications.

Complication	Patients affected n	(%)
Gastrointestinal hemorrhage	15	(6.8)
Cannula site bleeding	32	(14.4)
Clinical brain death	8	(3.6)
Cerebral infarction	2	(0.9)
Intracranial bleeding	2	(0.9)
Renal	102	(45.9)
Pulmonary	29	(13.1)
Inotropes	115	(51.8)
Arrhythmias	50	(22.5)
Hypertension	6	(2.7)
Infection	60	(27.0)
Metabolic	32	(14.4)

Table 4. CESAR trial entry criteria.

- Adult patients (18-65 years)
- Severe, but potentially reversible respiratory failure
- Murray score ≥ 3.0
- Uncompensated hypercapnia with pH <7.2

Table 5. CESAR trial exclusion criteria.

- Duration of high pressure and high FiO_2 ventilation >7 days (defined as either/or FiO_2 >80% or plateau pressure >30 cm H_2O)
- Severe trauma within the last 24 hrs., intracranial bleeding and any other contraindication to limited heparinization (trauma or operation in the last 24 hrs. is not an absolute contraindication if the bleeding is controlled or controllable)
- Patients who are moribund and have any contraindication to the continuation of active treatment

Conclusion

Case selection for adult respiratory ECLS hinges upon the accurate identification of reversible disease. The two main facets of this decision are 1) exclusion of patients who have a chronic disease with a poor pre-morbid condition, and 2) the determination that a patient has been ventilated for too long a period and has suffered terminal ventilator-induced lung injury. The literature to date indicates that ECLS in this group of patients is a reasonable treatment that is certainly no worse than continued conventional ventilation. We await the outcome of the CESAR trial in 2006 to determine if there is a survival or cost-efficient advantage.

References

1. Hill JD, O'Brien TG, Murray JJ, et al. Prolonged extracorporeal oxygenation for acute post-traumatic respiratory failure (shock-lung syndrome). Use of the Bramson membrane lung. *N Engl J Med* 1972; 286:629-634.

2. Zapol WM, Snider MT, Hill JD, et al. Extracorporeal membrane oxygenation in severe acute respiratory failure. A randomized prospective study. *JAMA* 1979; 242:2193-2196.

3. Conventional Ventilation or ECMO for Severe Adult Respiratory Failure. The CESAR trial. Available at http://cesar-trial.org. Accessed July 6, 2005.

4. Vandentorren S, Baldi I, Annesi M, et al. Long-term mortality among adults with or without asthma in the PAARC study. *Eur Respir J* 2003; 21:462-467.

5. Morris AH, Wallace CJ, Menlove RL, et al. Randomized clinical trial of pressure-controlled inverse ratio ventilation and extracorporeal CO_2 removal for adult respiratory distress syndrome. *Am J Respir Crit Care Med* 1994; 149:295-305.

6. Kolobow T. Acute respiratory failure. On how to injure healthy lungs (and prevent sick lungs from recovering). *ASAIO Trans* 1988; 34:31-34.

7. Kolobow T, Moretti MP, Fumagalli R, et al. Severe impairment in lung function induced by high peak airway pressure during mechanical ventilation. An experimental study. *Am Rev Respir Dis* 1987; 135:312-315.

8. Mascheroni D, Kolobow T, Fumagalli R, Moretti MP, Chen V, Buckhold D. Acute respiratory failure following pharmacologically induced hyperventilation: an experimental animal study. *Intensive Care Med* 1988; 15:8-14.

9. Hill JD, Rodvien R, Snider MT, Bartlett RH. Clinical extracorporeal membrane oxygenation for acute respiratory insufficiency. *Trans Am Soc Artif Intern Organs* 1978; 24:753-763.

10. Kolla S, Awad SS, Rich PB, Schreiner RJ, Hirschl RB, Bartlett RH. Extracorporeal life support for 100 adult patients with severe respiratory failure. *Ann Surg* 1997; 226:544-564.

11. Bartlett RH, Gazzaniga AB, Jefferies MR, et al. Extracorporeal membrane oxygenation (ECMO) cardiopulmonary support in infancy. *Trans Am Soc Artif Intern Organs* 1976; 22:80-93.

12. Borelli M, Kolobow T, Spatola R, Prato P, Tsuno K. Severe acute respiratory failure managed with continuous positive airway pressure and partial extracorporeal carbon dioxide removal by an artificial membrane lung. A controlled, randomized animal study. *Am Rev Respir Dis* 1988; 138:1480-1487.

13. Kolobow T, Borelli M, Spatola R, Tsuno K, Prato P. Single catheter venous-venous membrane lung bypass in the treatment of experimental ARDS. *ASAIO Trans* 1987; 33:561-564.

14. Zwischenberger JB, Toomasian JM, Drake K, Andrews AF, Kolobow T, Bartlett RH.

Total respiratory support with single cannula veno-venous ECMO: Double lumen continuous flow vs. single lumen tidal flow. *Trans Am Soc Artif Organs* 1985; 31:610-615.

15. Gattinoni L, Pesenti A, Mascheroni D, et al. Low-frequency positive-pressure ventilation with extracorporeal CO_2 removal in severe acute respiratory failure. *JAMA* 1986; 256:881-886.

16. Anderson HL3, Delius RE, Sinard JM, et al. Early experience with adult extracorporeal membrane oxygenation in the modern era. *Ann Thorac Surg* 1992; 53:553-563.

17. Peek GJ, Moore HM, Moore N, Sosnowski AW, Firmin RK. Extracorporeal Membrane Oxygenation for Adult Respiratory Failure. *Chest* 1997; 112:759-764.

18. Linden V, Palmer K, Reinhard J, et al. High survival in adult patients with acute respiratory distress syndrome treated by extracorporeal membrane oxygenation, minimal sedation, and pressure supported ventilation. *Intensive Care Med* 2000; 26:1630-1637.

19. Scott LK, Boudreaux K, Thaljeh F, et al. Early enteral feedings in adults receiving venovenous extracorporeal membrane oxygenation. *JPEN J Parenter Enteral Nutr* 2004; 28:295-300.

20. ELSO Data Registry Report: International Summary. University of Michigan, Ann Arbor, MI, July 2002.

21. RH Bartlett, multiple personal communications, 1995-2005.

22. Vasilyev S, Schaap RN, Mortensen JD. Hospital survival rates of patients with acute respiratory failure in modern respiratory intensive care units. An international, multicenter, prospective survey. *Chest* 1995; 107:1083-1088.

23. CESAR: Protocol for a collaborative randomised controlled trial, February 2003. Available at: http://www.cesar-trial.org. Accessed July 25, 2005.

24. Rossaint R, Lewandowski K, Pappert D, Slama K, Falke K. Therapy of ARDS. 1. Current therapeutic strategy including extracorporeal gas exchange. *Anaesthesist* 1994; 43:298-308.

25. Gattinoni L, Tognoni G, Pesenti A, et al. Effect of prone positioning on the survival of patients with acute respiratory failure. *N Engl J Med* 2001; 345:568-573.

26

Management of ECLS in Adult Respiratory Failure

Robert H. Bartlett, M.D.

Introduction

When, how, and why should ECLS be used for respiratory support in adults? ECLS can sustain life during a period when there is little or no lung function. Thus, it is a reasonable treatment option in patients with acute lung disease that is potentially lethal, but reversible within a few weeks. Neither the devices nor the technique are experimental; ECLS will support life when native lung function will not. ECLS does not directly treat acute lung disease, but simply allows time for spontaneous recovery, pharmacologic management, or other direct lung treatments while avoiding mechanical ventilator settings which can be injurious. ECLS should be considered when acute lung disease is lethal but reversible, following tight protocols that permit evaluation of the methods and the outcome.

In Chapter 25, Firmin and Peek discussed the identification of adult patients who have a high risk of death or disability despite optimal therapy. At the University of Michigan the criterion of refractory hypoxemia despite optimal therapy is used to select patients in this high-risk group. Standard optimal therapy includes: 1) pressure controlled inverse-ratio ventilation (PC IRV), with inspiratory plateau pressure limited to 30-40 cm H_2O (accepting hypercarbia if hypoventilation results from this pressure limit);

2) FiO_2 limited to 0.6 (accepting hypoxemia if it results from this limitation); 3) optimizing oxygen delivery (DO_2) /oxygen consumption (VO_2) >4:1 ratio by monitoring mixed venous saturation; 4) optimizing lung function by prone positioning and diuresis to dry weight; 5) normal hematocrit, normal weight, normal nutrition. (Table 1).[1] ECLS is used for patients who have been on mechanical ventilation for <7 days and fail to improve. In this chapter, the University of Michigan protocol will be described in detail, with rationale, justification, and comment about other methods of which there is some controversy.[1-5]

Patient approach

The first approach to the ECLS patient is to institute standard therapy as described above. This is often difficult or impossible to achieve at the referring hospitals so patients are transferred using a transport ventilator and helicopter transport team. If the patient can not be managed with the transport ventilator on maximal settings, instituting ECLS in the referring hospital is considered for safe transport. Transport on ECLS is necessary in ~10% of the adult patients who are referred for ECLS (See Chapter 9). Several steps should be taken in any patient who is being considered for ECLS, preferably before transfer. The right

Table 1. Goals and conditions for ARDS patient management.

	Pre-ECLS (failure to improve is indication for ECLS)	During ECLS (lung rest with systemic treatment)	Weaning from ECLS (after lung recovery)	Weaning from ventilation
Ventilator Settings				
FiO$_2$	0.6-1.0	0.2-0.4	<0.5	<0.4
Mode	PCIRV	PCIRV	PCIRV	IMV + pressure support
Pi	35	<30	25-30	15→5
Pe	10-20	10	5-10	0-5
TV	measure	measure	measure	measure
I:E ratio	1.5-2:1	2:1	1:1	1:2
Rate	15-25	6	8-12	<20 spontaneous
Blood gases				
SaO$_2$	>90	>85*	>90	>90
PaCO$_2$	<80	40	<50	<50
Oxygen delivery (DO$_2$)				
DO$_2$/VO$_2$	4:1	>4:1	>4:1	>4:1
Hematocrit	>40	>45	>40	>40
CI	>3	>3	>3	>3
SvO$_2$	>70	>80**	>70	>70
Fluid Balance	5-10% over dry weight	dry weight no edema	dry weight no edema	dry weight no edema
Nutrition (enteral if possible)				
Calories	30 cal/kg/day	30 cal/kg/day	30 cal/kg/day	30 cal/kg/day
Protein	1 g/kg/day	1 g/kg/day	1 g/kg/day	1 g/kg/day
Position	prone q6h	prone q6h	sitting	sitting
ACT	normal	1.5 x normal	1.5 x normal	normal
Platelet count	normal	>100,000	>100,000	rebound >300,000
Sedatives	full anesthesia	least possible	minimal	none
Paralytics	if needed to ↓ VO$_2$	none	none	none
Airway	ETT	ETT or tracheostomy	tracheostomy	tracheostomy

PCIRV=pressure-controlled inverse-ratio ventilation, CI=cardiac index, Pi=inspiratory pressure, Pe=expiratory pressure, TV=tidal volume, I:E ratio=inspiratory to expiratory ratio, DO$_2$/VO$_2$=oxygen delivery/oxygen consumption, SvO$_2$=mixed venous saturation, SaO$_2$=arterial oxygen saturation, PaCO$_2$=partial pressure arterial CO$_2$, ETT=endotracheal tube
*SaO$_2$ on VV is 80-85% if no lung function.
**SvO$_2$ on VV is 80-85%, SaO$_2$ on VA >95%.

In the first column, typical ventilator settings and blood gases for severe ARDS are shown, along with other goals of management. Patients who have severe respiratory failure of this fashion treated with the algorithm usually improve and recover without needing ECLS. If recovery does not occur or if the patient deteriorates despite optimal management then ECLS is used to decrease ventilator pressure rate and inspired oxygen concentration. The rest of management remains the same and the ventilator settings during ECLS are shown in the second column. In the third column ventilator settings which would indicate significant lung recovery and weaning from ECLS are shown. Other aspects of management remain the same with the exception of decreasing sedation and analgesics. After ECLS progressive recovery occurs and when gas exchange is adequate at lower ventilator settings, as shown in the fourth column, the patient is usually ready to be weaned from mechanical ventilation.

internal jugular and right femoral vein may be needed for ECLS cannulation. Any type of IV access in these vessels will allow placement of a wire and percutaneous cannulation; therefore, placement or maintenance of IV in the right internal jugular and right femoral is desirable. An Oximetrix (Abbott Critical Care Systems, North Chicago, IL) pulmonary artery catheter should be placed for mixed venous saturation and pressure monitoring. This catheter will interfere with right jugular cannulation, so it should be placed through the left internal jugular or left subclavian vein. An intraarterial catheter should be placed for pressure monitoring and blood access. The patient may require venoarterial (VA) access; therefore, a right femoral artery catheter should be placed. A separate arterial monitoring catheter should be placed using a radial artery. The mechanical ventilator should have the option of pressure-controlled, inverse-ratio ventilation with full monitoring of pulmonary mechanics. End tidal CO_2 monitoring is also desirable.

The approach to general management and transportation is explained to family members and the risks and benefits of ECLS are discussed. A packet of written information is given to the family and the spouse, parent, or other designated person signs a consent form, even ECMO is only a possibility. This is done so the family is informed ahead of time and so emergency management can proceed if necessary. The ECLS consent form includes emergency procedures such as re-operation for bleeding or chest tube placement as well as elective procedures such as bronchoscopy and cannula adjustment. During this time, any research protocols are explained and the family is asked to sign consent forms.

Vascular access

Venovenous access

Venovenous (VV) access is the method of choice when cardiac function is adequate. The inferior vena cava (IVC) via the femoral vein for venous drainage is used and arterialized blood is returned to the right atrium via the right internal jugular.[5] Percutaneous access originally described by Pesenti and Gattinoni has been a major advantage.[6] Specially designed, thin-walled, wire wound, BioMedicus (Medtronic, Minneapolis, MN) catheters are used exclusively. These catheters are designed for long-term support and can be placed over a wire using the Seldinger technique. A 38 centimeter long 23F catheter is used for internal jugular and femoral vein access. The M number on this catheter is 2.4, and it delivers 5 l/min at 100 cm H_2O siphon (see Chapter 6). This is adequate support for most adult patients. Larger catheters with lower M numbers are available for use in patients >100 kg. Smaller diameter catheters can be used for infusion, but a 23F for both IVC and superior vena cava (SVC) are used at University of Michigan in case the flow needs to be reversed as discussed below. The experience has shown that percutaneous placement can be achieved in >90% of patients. However, if the catheter can not be placed or if there are complications during attempted percutaneous cannulation, direct cutdown access is required. Since cutdown access is only used when percutaneous access has failed, it is always performed emergently, and is a difficult operation. The intended vein has already been punctured if not lacerated, and proximal and distal control while gaining direct exposure is impossible. The surgeon must be able to gain access and achieve cannulation quickly, without excessive blood loss, a procedure that requires a high level of skill and experience. For this reason, it is essential to have a readily available surgeon who is capable of performing this operation particularly when percutaneous access is planned. In the future, jugular cannulation alone will be the access method of choice using a double lumen catheter or a tidal flow system.[7] With any type of VV access, recirculation occurs and increases as flow increases.

Nonetheless, VV access is always adequate for CO_2 removal and is almost always adequate for oxygenation.

Venoarterial access

VA access is reserved for those cases involving profound cardiac failure (e.g., myocarditis, post-cardiac surgical patients, resuscitation). The requirement for inotropic drugs is not in itself an indication for VA bypass. When VA access is required, the right internal jugular is preferred for venous drainage. The choices for arterial return are the common carotid artery, the axillary, or the femoral artery. In the past, the carotid was preferred because it can be ligated distally, distal perfusion is not required or desirable, and it delivers arterialized blood directly into the aortic root. However, 15% of adult patients have ischemic injury following carotid ligation, particularly if the carotid is ligated while the patient is hypoxemic and hypotensive. Most adult patients going on VA ECLS are hypoxemic and hypotensive; consequently the right femoral artery is the arterial access of choice for these patients. However, when the femoral artery is used, distal collateral circulation is often inadequate and separate distal perfusion is often required. In addition, the infused blood does not reach the aortic root or arch, so the heart and brain may be perfused with desaturated blood if the patient has concomitant respiratory and cardiac failure.

Femoral access can usually be gained by percutaneous techniques, placing a 17F, 19F, or 21F catheter over a wire. In 30-50% of patients with femoral artery perfusion, collateral circulation to the distal leg is inadequate or becomes inadequate because of catheter-induced spasm. Because of the high incidence of leg ischemia, some centers place a superficial femoral artery distal perfusion catheter in every ECLS patient. This requires direct cutdown on the groin after bypass has been established and the patient is stabilized. At the University of Michigan, every patient cannulated via the femoral artery has a catheter placed by cutdown in the posterior tibial artery at the ankle after the patient is stabilized. If the pressure in the posterior tibia is consistently >50 mm Hg, distal perfusion is not required. If the pressure is <50 mm Hg, then a perfusion catheter is attached to the main infusion line and the leg is perfused via the posterior tibial catheter at the rate of 1-200 cc/min. This technique avoids the potential consequences of leg ischemia.

Venoarterial venous access

Sometimes the blood drainage for VA access is from the IVC via the femoral vein to the femoral artery. In this situation, the SVC blood passes through the lungs and perfuses the coronaries, right arm, and head, mixing with the femoral arterial perfusate blood in the aortic arch or descending aorta. If the patient has severe respiratory failure, the blood in the upper circulation is not well oxygenated. A two-circulation syndrome results with hypoxemic blood circulating in the upper part of the body and well-oxygenated blood circulating in the lower part of the body. One approach is to use a long arterial catheter to reach the root of the aorta, but the resistance to flow is very high. This situation can be addressed by placing a right atrial infusion catheter via the right internal jugular vein and directing the infused blood into both the femoral artery and into the right atrium. This mode of vascular access is called venoarterial venous (VAV) access. VAV is sufficient to support both cardiac and lung function. Once the native lungs recover, the right atrial catheter is used for additional venous drainage.

ECLS circuit

The circuit should be designed to be capable of providing at least 50 cc/kg/min blood flow and at least 6 cc/kg/min oxygen delivery. To accomplish this level of blood flow, the drainage catheter should be the catheter which will fit into the access vein, and the venous drainage tubing should be ½-inch diameter. Blood return tubing can be ⅜-inch or even ¼-inch diameter keeping in mind that the post-pump circuit pressures will be higher if smaller tubing is used. One oxygenator designed for adult cardiopulmonary bypass (CPB) will be sufficient in most cases (e.g., Kolobow 4.5 m^2 spiral coil oxygenator [Medtronic, Minneapolis, MN]). Two adult-size oxygenators are arranged parallel in order to have a large surface area for gas exchange in the event membrane lung function deteriorates or a second oxygenator is added if the initial device loses function.

The circuit hardware is essentially the same as that used for pediatric or neonatal ECMO. The pump is adjusted to use ½-inch super Tygon (Saint-Gobain Performance Plastics, Portage, WI) tubing. A large servo-regulation bladder with ⅜-inch connectors is used or a neonatal bladder is used in conjunction with large bypass tubing connected by Y-connectors around the side of the bladder. A centrifugal pump can be used; however, hemolysis is a major potential complication.

An adult-size circuit prepared and assembled on a standard ECMO cart is kept available for use. To use the circuit, it is primed in the same fashion as for a neonatal circuit: CO_2 followed by crystalloid salt solution (until all bubbles are removed), then albumin is added for surface coating. Calcium chloride (1 gram) is added to maintain normal ionized calcium levels while going on bypass. In adult patients, bypass is started with this clear prime and subsequently a combination of packed red blood cell (PRBC) transfusion and diuresis is used to restore the hematocrit to normal. It is possible to use a blood-primed circuit with adults, but the extra steps required to do this are usually unnecessary. Circuit monitors always include an on-line mixed venous saturation monitor in the venous drainage line, pre- and post-oxygenator pressure monitors, flow measurement (usually simple rpm counting on the roller pump is adequate), and a device for measuring whole blood activated clotting time (ACT).

ECLS management on bypass

Gas exchange and perfusion

Once the circuit is primed and adequate bypass is achieved, flow is progressively increased until venous return is limited by venous drainage. With an appropriately sized venous drainage catheter, venous return in the range of 5 l/min should be possible for most adult patients. If the venous return is significantly less than that, and blood volume is adequate, then the circuit must be evaluated for a problem with kinking, placement of the venous access catheter, or high intrathoracic or intraperitoneal pressures. All of these possibilities are investigated until high flow VV support is achieved. It is important to make these adjustments after turning the ventilator pressure down to rest settings (typically 35/10 cm H_2O at respiratory rate 6 breaths/min). When ventilator pressure and rate have been decreased (allowing improved intrathoracic venous return), extracorporeal flow is gradually decreased from the maximum possible level, following arterial and venous saturation. Flow is decreased until arterial saturation is in the range of 90%, and FiO_2 is then decreased to levels below 0.5. During this time, diuresis has been instituted, and transfusion of packed red blood cells (PRBCs) is started to return the hematocrit from its diluted level to 45%. Thereafter, VV flow is maintained to sustain drainage blood saturation at 80-85%, which will result in arterial saturation between 80-90%. As long as the hematocrit and cardiac output are normal, this will result in adequate systemic oxygen delivery. If the native lung has no function, and the metabolic demand (VO_2) is high, even high flow VV ECLS may not be able to achieve adequate oxygen delivery. In this circumstance, arterial saturation as low as 75% is tolerated for days at a time. However, an arterial saturation >80% is preferred. To achieve this, the drainage and infusion catheters are repositioned and oxygen consumption is decreased with paralysis and hypothermia if necessary. When native lung function begins to return, an increase in arterial saturation (above mixed venous saturation) will be evident, and VV flow rate can be decreased to maintain arterial saturation ~90%. When the VV flow is decreased to levels of approximately 2 l/min, the patient is ready for a trial off bypass.

Recirculation

Recirculation invariably occurs during VV access, particularly with the two-catheter technique currently in use. This is addressed in part by the use of double lumen catheters in adult sizes or by the use of tidal flow VV access, which minimizes the effect of recirculation. Nonetheless, for the present time recirculation remains a significant problem. It is helpful to have an Oximetrix pulmonary artery catheter in place; major recirculation is identified if pulmonary artery saturation is considerably lower than venous drainage saturation. This circumstance is most likely to occur when the catheter position results in perfusate blood being selectively siphoned into the venous drainage catheter, allowing coronary sinus and caval blood to selectively enter the right ventricle. When this occurs, significant recirculation is present and can be corrected by re-positioning the catheters, and checking pulmonary artery and venous drainage saturation until they equilibrate.

CO_2 clearance always exceeds oxygen transfer. Adjusting the sweep flow rate to the membrane lungs regulates blood CO_2. In general, the PCO_2 is maintained at ~40 mm Hg. The major concern is respiratory alkalosis caused by excessive CO_2 removal. Usually this is controlled simply by decreasing the gas flow rate to the membrane lung (a ratio of 1 liter gas flow: 1 liter blood flow is normally adequate).

However, long periods of low gas flow to the membrane lungs may result in water accumulation and membrane lung dysfunction. When this happens, the gas flow is increased and CO_2 is added to maintain normocarbia.

Patient management on bypass

Extracorporeal management and general patient management are both performed by the ECLS specialist and the nurse at the bedside. Decisions for blood samples, blood infusion, platelet infusion, heparin maintenance, diuretics, and nutritional management are made by the bedside team, under a general set of physician orders. The goals during ECLS are shown in Table 1.

While on bypass, standard vital signs such as including pulmonary artery pressure, systemic and mixed venous saturation, end tidal CO_2, ventilator pressures and tidal volume, urine output, daily weight, hemoglobin and hematocrit, and creatinine and bilirubin are monitored every day or every other day. Cardiac output can be measured by thermal dilution using modified catheters which have an injection port in the right ventricle. Even with this technique, some tricuspid regurgitation and false values are possible. Thermal dilution cardiac output measurement with catheter injection port in the right atrium is not possible during ECLS because the injectant disappears into the venous drainage catheter. The circuit is monitored by continuously measuring blood flow, inlet and outlet pressure from each membrane lung, direct inspection for signs of wear or thrombosis, and coagulation measurements as described above.

Ventilator management

After ECLS is initiated and the patient is stabilized on bypass, ventilator settings are decreased to pressure 30/10 cm H_2O, rate 6 breaths/min, FiO_2 0.5. The ventilator is maintained at these settings, and oxygenation and CO_2 are regulated by blood flow and gas flow to the membrane lung. The hematocrit is maintained between 45 and 48% to facilitate oxygen delivery and ease the requirement for high cardiac output. Inotropic drugs can usually be discontinued within 1-2 days. Pulmonary function is assessed by monitoring the saturation of venous drainage blood, pulmonary arterial blood, and arterial blood with a pulse oximeter. Blood gases are usually measured in arterial and venous blood 1-2 times/day, but more frequent blood gas measurements are usually not necessary. Lung function is continually measured by the difference between pulmonary artery and arterial blood oxygen saturation and end tidal CO_2. Standard treatment for severe lung dysfunction is continued during ECLS including bronchoscopy when necessary, prone positioning, and diuresis to dry weight. Although it is not necessary for management, native lung VO_2 and CO_2 consumption (VCO_2) and membrane lung VO_2 and VCO_2 daily, are monitored for several reasons. The total VO_2 is determined and used for indirect calorimetry for purposes of nutritional planning.[8] In addition, the total patient VCO_2 is determined and the respiratory quotient calculated, again for nutritional planning. The percentage of total VO_2 achieved through the native lung is calculated. If the percentage is less than 25% of total VO_2 after the first week on support, the prognosis for lung recovery is poor.

Lung management

Some aspects of airway management can be undertaken which are unique to the ECLS patient because the patient is on extracorporeal support and does not have to breathe. If there is a large broncho-pleural fistula, it can be managed by selectively ventilating the opposite lung, and selectively occluding the injured bronchus with a balloon catheter for 1-2 days, or stopping ventilation altogether while the air leak seals. Once the air leak has been sealed for 48

hours, the atelectatic lung is re-recruited with continuous static airway pressure in the range of 20-30 cm H_2O. If the primary problems include excessive exudate or occlusion of the airways, bronchoscopy is performed with lengthy periods devoted to airway cleaning and lavage. The use of perfluorocarbon liquid ventilation in these patients to lavage the airways and to improve alveolar recruitment and oxygenation has great potential for future treatment.[9] Generally early tracheostomy is favored in respiratory failure patients because of the decreased incidence of nosocomial pneumonia from pharyngeal bacteria and due to the easier airway access and ventilator weaning. If tracheostomy has not already been performed prior to ECLS, it is performed by percutaneous access on the first or second day of bypass. However, this does introduce the risk of bleeding at the tracheal stoma site; therefore, if it appears the patient will be weaned off bypass within a few days, tracheostomy is delayed until then.

Acute lung injury resolves into severe pulmonary fibrosis in a short time, particularly if the patient has been on high-pressure, high-oxygen ventilation for several days. Meduri showed that this fibrosis can be treated and perhaps prevented by high-dose solumedrol.[10] His findings were corroborated by the randomized trial conducted by the NIH-ARDS Network. The Meduri protocol is used for patients who are not improving after the first 5-7 days. As reported by Meduri, ~75% of patients have a prompt response with recovery of lung function and decreasing pulmonary vascular resistance.

Occasionally, ECLS has been used for the management of patients with severe airway obstruction secondary to status asthmaticus or airway occlusion due to blood clots or other foreign material.[11] In these circumstances, oxygenation is usually adequate and the primary problem is CO_2 retention, high intrathoracic pressures, cardiovascular collapse, or barotrauma. Relatively low flow ECLS is used for CO_2 removal (extracorporeal carbon dioxide removal, or $ECCO_2R$) and to permit decreasing ventilator settings to low, non-damaging settings. VV access is sufficient for these patients, and bronchoscopy, lung lavage, and direct airway management can be carried out at a later time. These patients usually recover promptly and are successfully managed with ECLS.

Anticoagulation and bleeding

During cannulation 100 units/kg of heparin is given if the patient does not have major coagulopathy or ongoing bleeding. Usually this results in adequate anticoagulation for cannulation. Whole blood ACT returns near normal after 1-2 hours. Thereafter, dilute heparin solution is infused continuously to maintain the whole blood ACT at approximately 180 seconds (1.5 times normal). For reasons discussed elsewhere in this book, it is important to follow whole blood ACT rather than heparin levels or coagulation studies. Whole blood ACT is measured hourly or more frequently if necessary. The ECLS specialist titrates the heparin dose to maintain ACT within the desired range. Adult ECLS patients are maintained on bypass for days or even weeks with ACTs at 180 seconds with no bleeding, clotting, or embolization. Thrombocytopenia often occurs, platelets are transfused to maintain the platelet count at ~100,000/mm³, although most adult patients will level off at 30-40,000/mm³ platelets without platelet transfusion. The platelet count is maintained at a higher level because it has been found to decrease the incidence of bleeding considerably. However, a smaller number of highly functional platelets is preferred over a large number of transfused platelets that have compromised function. Aprotinin or tranexamic acid appear to enhance platelet function in the laboratory,[12,13] and it may be preferable to use these drugs with lower platelet counts rather than to arbitrarily infuse platelets.

If bleeding occurs at these levels of anticoagulation and platelet infusion, the standard algorithm is to decrease heparin to an ACT of 140 seconds, transfuse platelets until the count is >100,000/mm³, and consider adding aprotinin to the drug regimen. The dose of aprotinin is the same as for cardiac operations (10,000 units as a test dose followed by 100,000 units/hr), although a lower dose may be as effective. If these methods do not stop bleeding in a few hours (or if transfusion is necessary) then surgical intervention is considered. Usually, bleeding is from the site of recent operation or recently placed chest tubes. The decision to operate for uncontrolled bleeding is based to some extent on the site of the bleeding. If the bleeding is into the GI tract, avoiding operating on the patient is paramount and endoscopic coagulation is used instead, if possible. If the bleeding is into the free peritoneal cavity, immediate operation to provide free blood drainage and remove clots is performed, and there is a low threshold to go to full exploration for an attempt at direct control of the bleeding site. If bleeding occurs from chest tubes or in the thoracic cavity, and there has been a recent thoracotomy operation such as a cardiac operation or lung transplant operation, the threshold is low for opening the incision and exploring the chest directly in the ICU. If the bleeding is from a chest tube site, directly from the lung, or from a chest tube puncture and there has been no recent thoracotomy, several steps are taken to determine if bleeding is coming from the chest wall and there is an attempt to control it at that level. First, the chest tubes are removed and replaced, the access site is explored under direct vision with good lighting and exposure, the tissue around the chest tube is extensively cauterized, and a balloon catheter is placed in an attempt to tamponade bleeding from intercostal vessels. If these steps do not solve the problem, then bleeding is coming directly from the lung or some other site inside the chest, and bedside thoracotomy is performed. If a laparotomy or thoracotomy are necessary for bleeding control, the incisions are left open all the way to the thorax or abdomen and the entire wound is covered with adherent plastic dressing to permit frequent re-exploration, which is often necessary. Once the bleeding has completely stopped and the patient is stable off bypass, all levels of the surgical incision are closed.

From time to time it is necessary to conduct a surgical operation while patients are on ECLS. Usually this is an elective tracheostomy or is related to active bleeding in the chest or abdomen. However, on occasion operations such as liver transplantation, lung transplantation, heart transplantation, or evacuation of intracranial hematoma is performed on ECLS patients. Tracheostomy, chest, and abdominal exploration are usually done at the bedside in the ICU with a full operating team and sterile precautions in place. Other operations are performed in the OR. When elective or emergent operations on bypass are done, the heparin dose is decreased until the whole blood ACT is 140 seconds, platelets are administered until the count is >100,000/mm³, and preparations to use autotransfusion are conducted, if necessary. A variety of operations with this regimen have been successfully carried out without major bleeding or complications.

When managing the patient at low ACT and high platelet count, either for operations or to control bleeding, thrombosis may occur in the circuit. The circuit is carefully monitored by examining directly for clots and monitoring pressure drop across the membrane lung. Usually the first sign of clotting in the circuit is an increase in pressure drop and loss of function in the membrane lung. If this occurs, the lung can be changed. More commonly the entire circuit is changed to a fresh circuit. When managing a patient with low heparin, and high platelet counts, an identical full circuit is standing by for rapid replacement if necessary.

Hemodynamics

Hemodynamics and cardiac status are monitored by pulse contour, pulmonary capillary wedge pressure, systemic blood pressure, and signs of systemic perfusion. Mixed venous saturation which is useful as an indicator of the adequacy of oxygen delivery is distorted in the VV access patient because of re-circulation. Nonetheless, once the patient is on a stable level of VV bypass, changes in delivery:consumption ratio will be reflected as a change in venous saturation, and this is a useful guide to determine the adequacy of systemic perfusion. As mentioned above, it is possible to measure the cardiac output by thermal dilution whenever necessary. With all these monitors, perfusion is expected to be maintained at adequate levels throughout the course of ECLS. If there is any question about ventricular dysfunction, valvular dysfunction, clots in the heart, or pericardial tamponade, the heart is evaluated by echocardiography. Usually it is possible to wean off inotropic drugs within a 1-2 days of starting ECLS. If there is severe myocardial dysfunction that is unresponsive to small doses of inotropes, conversion to VA access is performed, usually by a direct cutdown approach to the right common carotid artery. If VA bypass is started in order to transport the patient or because of severe hemodynamic instability, the conversion to VV access is made as soon as adequate myocardial function is demonstrated.

Nutrition

Nutrition is managed as it is for any critically ill patient, using total parenteral nutrition leading rapidly to enteral nutrition when possible. In most ECLS patients it is possible to feed via the intestine, using conventional tube feeding formulas. Nutrition with caloric support based on indirect calorimetry is used and protein support is based on the direct measurement of total nitrogen loss. The goal is to provide fat and carbohydrates in amounts approximately 10% in excess of daily resting energy expenditure (REE), and to sustain positive nitrogen balance throughout the course of ECLS.[13]

Fluid, electrolyte, and renal management

Fluid, electrolyte, and renal management is also conducted as it would be in any critically ill patient. Almost all ECLS patients have a gross increase in extracellular fluid. If a diuretic regimen has not already been instituted, high doses of diuretics are used to achieve dry weight within a few days of initiation of ECLS. If renal function is inadequate to achieve that goal, continuous hemofiltration is instituted. This is a simple technique accomplished by simply attaching the hemofilter to the extracorporeal circuit and removing extracellular fluid at a rate necessary to achieve fluid balance at dry weight. Renal failure is managed in a conventional fashion and usually returns to normal when hemofiltration is discontinued.

Sedation and paralysis

Usually, patients who are started on ECLS have been heavily sedated and perhaps paralyzed to facilitate ventilator management. Often, the status of brain function has been unknown for several days. As soon as stable ECLS is achieved, all sedative and paralytic drugs are stopped or actively reversed until the status of brain function is determined. Most of these patients have had prolonged periods of hypoxia, usually associated with low blood flow, and may not return to normal consciousness during initial testing. However, one would expect to see the patient moving all extremities, eyes, and tongue, and to be able to respond to simple commands. Once we have verified that level of neurologic function, minimal sedation is provided using morphine and/or benzodiazepines titrated to apparent patient comfort. Frequently patients are paralyzed, particularly during the early phases when the ventilator is managed with a very long inspiratory phase and short expiratory phase, which appears uncomfortable for many patients. In addition, paralysis is sometimes necessary when patient agitation and activity increases VO_2 beyond the capability of our delivery system. However, it is preferable to not keep patients paralyzed, but to keep them as awake and alert as possible during prolonged support. If the patient is paralyzed and heavily sedated, the agents are reversed every 1-2 days in order to evaluate brain function.

If in the course of this testing it is apparent that the patient has sustained a significant decrease in brain function, head CT scanning is conducted with a relatively low threshold, and keeping in mind the potential for diffuse swelling secondary to hypoxic ischemic encephalopathy preceding ECLS treatment, localized intracranial bleeding, or infarction. Although unusual, severe brain dysfunction has been seen from each of these causes. When it is apparent that severe brain damage has occurred, and it does not rapidly improve within ~24 hours, ECLS is discontinued.

On occasion, the diagnosis of cortical brain death can be made by physical examination after reversing pharmacologic agents (e.g., by lack of spontaneous movement, pupillary reflexes, and response to cold caloric stimulation of the ears). In such a case, head CT or EEG is unnecessary to confirm the diagnosis, although these studies are often reassuring to team members or the patient's family before discontinuing ECLS.

Complications

Systemic complications such as sepsis, renal failure, liver failure, and nosocomial pneumonia are managed as they would be in any ICU patient. Complications which require an operation, even a small one, must be carefully evaluated before any procedures are undertaken. Venous cutdown, central vein or peripheral arterial puncture, chest tube placement, and pericardial drainage can all lead to uncontrolled bleeding if performed at the wrong time by inexperienced personnel. Even complications such as tension pneumothorax and total airway occlusion can be managed for hours at a time on ECLS while carefully preparing for an elective chest tube or bronchoscopic procedure. It is important that all members of the team understand this and understand the potential serious consequences of emergency procedures.

Although the risk of infection is high, the actual incidence of systemic sepsis in ECLS patients is quite low. Even when systemic sepsis is the presenting symptom (e.g., streptococcal pneumonia) severe infections usually subside quickly in response to appropriate antibiotics and drainage. If the patient has continuing bacteremia despite all appropriate treatment, it is not possible to simply change vascular access lines. Antibiotics are continued until the systemic infection is cleared without changing lines. If this is unsuccessful and sepsis it is the major complicating factor in patient management, then the entire circuit is changed, on the rationale that some thrombi in the circuit may have become infected. If this is not successful, then vascular monitoring lines are changed over wires.

Weaning and decannulation

When native lung function begins to improve, ECLS flow is decreased until the native lung is supporting 50-80% of total gas exchange. At this point the patient is ready for a trial off ECLS. This is usually done at FiO_2 1.0, ventilator pressure 30/10 cm H_2O, and rate of 10 breaths/min. On VV bypass, the membrane lung is simply capped off from gas flow and extracorporeal blood flow is continued to allow venous saturation monitoring and to avoid the need for separate heparinization of the patient and the circuit. If gas exchange and hemodynamics are adequate on these settings, then the FiO_2 is rapidly decreased. When the patient can sustain adequate gas exchange at FiO_2 0.5 or less at these low ventilator pressures, then ECLS can be discontinued (Table 1). Usually this is accomplished simply by removing the vascular access catheters. When the catheters

have been placed percutaneously, they can be removed and bleeding can be controlled by local pressure for ~1 hour. If the catheters have been placed by direct cutdown access, then operative removal is required. It is possible to repair the neck vessels at this time, but it is rarely done. If the femoral vessels were used for cutdown access, they must be repaired. It is preferred to do the vascular repairs in the OR.

During the trial off ECLS, if lung recovery has been recent and the patient appears to be unstable, extracorporeal support is continued for 24 hours to re-verify adequate lung function. An intermediate step is to disconnect the circuit leaving the catheters in place with continued heparinization to avoid clotting in the catheters. On occasion it has been necessary to return quickly to extracorporeal support, and it is much easier to do this if the catheters are in place. Once the patient has been removed from extracorporeal support, continued ventilator management follows the standard protocol. The patient is maintained as awake as possible, continuing prone and sitting positions and weaning down to low ventilator settings as rapidly as possible. If a tracheostomy was not placed during ECLS, it is placed as soon as the patient is weaned off extracorporeal support to facilitate rapid ventilator weaning and to avoid nosocomial pneumonia.

As mentioned in Chapter 2, a progressive increase in pulmonary vascular resistance toward systemic levels is an ominous sign and usually represents progressive and irreversible fibrosis in the lung parenchyma.[14] When the mean pulmonary artery pressure is consistently greater than two-thirds that of systemic pressure, the risk of right ventricular failure is high, and arrhythmias leading to ventricular tachycardia and fibrillation may occur. It is possible to support the circulation by converting to VA access at this point, but this situation has been uniformly fatal because of progressive lung injury. Consequently, we consider right ventricular failure after days or weeks of VV support to be a sign of irreversibility and do not even attempt cardiac resuscitation if it occurs. Conversely, if the patient has been on ECLS for 3-4 weeks with no sign of lung improvement, but pulmonary artery pressure is less than half that of systemic pressure, extracorporeal support is continued with the expectation of recovery, which does occur in many such patients.

If the patient has recovered from severe pulmonary parenchymal damage caused by pneumonia, over distention, or pulmonary embolism, lung function will typically demonstrate the effects of small and large pneumatoceles where some alveoli used to be. These pneumatoceles can be visualized by CT scan and sometimes on chest radiograph. This will result in a pattern of very large, dead-space ventilation, resulting in CO_2 retention despite high minute ventilation on the ventilator. Usually oxygenation is quite good in these patients because the pneumatoceles have no blood supply and the normal alveoli have adequate blood flow. It is likely that microthrombosis in some pulmonary capillaries also contributes to this picture of large alveolar dead space.[14] This physiologic pattern appears to be quite ominous in the post-ECLS period; however, it is almost always transient and resolves within a period of weeks. Resolution occurs because fibrosis in the wall of the pneumatoceles occurs, resulting in contraction of these small areas of dead space. In addition, pulmonary capillary flow returns to areas where thrombosis or embolism has limited pulmonary flow to normal alveoli. Both of these changes are associated with obvious worsening of the chest radiograph. The best prognostic sign in a post-ECLS patient is improving physiology with worsening chest radiograph. As pulmonary circulation improves, pulmonary vascular resistance should fall even further, and it is important to continuously monitor pulmonary artery pressures until the patient is off the ventilator.

Late follow-up of these patients has been reported in many studies.[15,16] Patients have essentially normal pulmonary function by 6-12 months following the episode of acute respiratory failure. Detailed pulmonary function reveals a slight restrictive pattern, and often these patients have airways which are very reactive to cold, exercise, or other stimuli. Late neurologic complications are rare in adults and almost all patients are rehabilitated to full function. Late follow-up is discussed in more detail in Chapter 27.

Results

Following this algorithm for patient management, the survival rate for adult patients treated with ECLS for severe respiratory failure at the University of Michigan is 52% (Table 2).[17] Approximately half of patients have ARDS following primary lung injury, usually pneumonia. The other half of these patients have secondary lung injury following shock, trauma, sepsis, pancreatitis, or other cause. Death results from irreversible pulmonary fibrosis, brain injury, or from multiple-organ failure or sepsis. In recent years, the survival rate at U of M is 60-70%.

Table 2. The University of Michigan experience with ECLS for severe ARDS.

	Survival to discharge	
	n	(%)
Primary lung injury		
Pneumonia		
Bacterial	79	(57)
Viral	33	(65)
Aspiration	13	(62)
Fungal	7	(29)
Vasculitis	6	(17)
Pulmonary hemorrhage	3	(67)
Chemical injury	3	(67)
Secondary lung injury		
Trauma	32	(44)
Sepsis	22	(50)
Cardiogenic	16	(63)
Post-lung transplant	16	(44)
Pancreatitis	9	(67)
Post-operative	8	(38)
Other	8	(38)
Overall	255	(52)

It is important to note that patients with severe respiratory failure referred for ECLS often improve and recover when managed with the algorithm described in Table 1. Therefore, the overall survival rate for patients referred for ECLS is approximately 85%. The mortality risk of these patients at the time of referral is 80-90%, so the value of the treatment algorithm and ECLS, if needed, seems well justified. However, there is currently a prospective, randomized trial of ECLS in adult respiratory failure underway in the U.K. to evaluate this conclusion.[18]

Summary

ECLS is considered for adults with acute respiratory failure when the risk of death or disability is >80%. Protocol-driven ventilator care emphasizing position, diuresis, oxygen delivery, and low peak pressure results in recovery and survival in many of patients referred for ECLS. Patients who fail on this regimen or are too unstable to attempt this regimen are supported with ECLS, with a 54% survival. The technique of ECLS management includes optimizing oxygen delivery, careful anticoagulation, prevention and management of complications, and a thorough protocol for all aspects of critical care.

References

1. Shanley CJ, Bartlett RH. The management of acute respiratory failure. *Curr Opin Gen Surg*; 1994; :7-16.
2. Anderson H 3rd, Steimle C, Shapiro M, et al. Extracorporeal life support for adult cardiorespiratory failure. *Surgery* 1993; 114:161-172.
3. Chapman RA, Bartlett RH. *Extracorporeal Life Support Manual for Adult and Pediatric Patients*. Ann Arbor, MI: The University of Michigan Medical Center; 1991.
4. Pranikoff T, Hirschl RB, Steimle CN, Anderson HL, Bartlett RH. Efficacy of extracorporeal life support in the setting of adult cardiorespiratory failure. *ASAIO J* 1994; 40: M339-343.
5. Rich PB, Younger J, Soldes OS, Awad SS, Bartlett RH. Use of extracorporeal life support for adult patients with respiratory failure and sepsis. *ASAIO J* 1998; 44:263-266.
6. Pesenti A, Gattinoni L, Bombino M. Long term extracorporeal respiratory support: 20 years progress. *Int Crit Care Digest* 1993; 12:15-18.
7. Kolla S, Crotti S, Lee A, et al. Total respiratory support with tidal flow extracorporeal circulation in adult sheep. *ASAIO J* 1997; 43:M811-816.
8. Bartlett RH, Dechert RE, Mault JR, Ferguson SK, Kaiser AM, Erlandson EE. Measurement of metabolism in multiple organ failure. *Surgery* 1982; 92:771-779.
9. Hirschl RB, Croce M, Gore D, et al. Prospective, randomized, controlled pilot study of partial liquid ventilation in adult acute respiratory distress syndrome. *Am J Respir Crit Care Med* 2002; 165:781-787.
10. Meduri GU, Headley AS, Golden E, et al. Effect of prolonged methylprednisolone therapy in unresolving acute respiratory distress syndrome: a randomized controlled trial. *JAMA* 1998; 280:159-165.
11. Shapiro MB, Kleaveland AC, Bartlett RH. Extracorporeal life support for status asthmaticus. *Chest* 1993; 103:1651-1654.
12. Havel MD, Griesmacher A, Weigel G, et al. Aprotinin increases release of von Willebrand factor in cultured human umbilical vein endothelial cells. *Surgery* 1992; 112:573-577.
13. Plotz FB, von Oeveren W, Aloe LS, et al. Prophylactic administration of tranexamic acid preserves platelet numbers during extracorporeal circulation in rabbits. *ASAIO Trans* 1991; 37:M416-417.
14. Zapol WM, Snider MT. Pulmonary hypertension in severe acute respiratory failure. *N Engl J Med* 1977; 296:476-480.

15. Fallat RJ, Tucker HJ, Sigcova L. Lung function in long-term survivors of severe ARDS. *Am Rev Resp Dis* 1976; 113:181.

16. McHugh LG, Miberg JA, Whitcomb ME, Schoene RB, Maunder RJ, Hudson LD. Recovery of function in survivors of the acute respiratory distress syndrome. *Am J Respir Crit Care Med* 1994; 150:90-94.

17. Hemmila MR, Rowe SA, Boules TN, et al. Extracorporeal Life Support for Severe Acute Respiratory Distress Syndrome in Adults. *Ann Surg* 2004; 240:595-607.

18. Conventional Ventilation or ECMO for Severe Adult Respiratory Failure. Comparing conventional ventilation methods with ECMO for treatment of severe ARF in adults. Available at http://www.cesar-trial.org. Accessed April 12, 2004.

27

Long-term Results of ECMO for Adult Respiratory Failure

Nikki Jones, M.B.Ch.B., A.F.R.C.S.(Ed), Samantha Harris, M.Sc., and Chris Cordle, Ph.D.

Introduction

This chapter discusses the long-term results of ECMO for respiratory support in adults. Long-term problems experienced by patients following critical illness can be largely categorized as respiratory, neuromuscular, and psychological. These problems are discussed broadly before reporting specifically about the follow-up of adult ECMO patients from Glenfield Hospital in Leicester, U.K.

Background

Adult respiratory distress syndrome (ARDS) is defined as a reduction in lung compliance, low PaO_2/FiO_2 ratio (<200 mm Hg) and bilateral alveolar infiltrates seen on chest radiograph. It is a pulmonary manifestation of systemic inflammatory response syndrome (SIRS). The term severe adult respiratory failure (SARF) includes all causes of respiratory failure such as severe asthmatic episodes and pneumonia, as well as ARDS. The actual incidence of ARDS is unknown and some estimates are as high as 71 in 100,000.[1,2] More recent, and perhaps more reliable, estimates of 4.5 per 100,000 take into account stricter diagnostic criteria and better databases.[3] This patient population is sizable, utilizing a large amount of resources. The overall cost is substantial and often the outcome is poor, particularly as ARDS has a high mortality, with <40% survival at 6 months, despite optimal conventional therapy.[4] Much has been done to investigate the etiology and optimal treatments to improve survival, but little is known of the long-term clinical and psychological outcome of those that survive.

Clinical research on ICU patients has traditionally focused on mortality and hospital discharge as outcome measures. However post-discharge survival and functional capacity are very important as well. In the U.K., the development of ICU follow-up clinics has facilitated research which is now focusing on the long-term outcome of patients treated in the ICU, looking at whether survivors have a reasonable quality-of-life. A problem with such studies is that it is difficult to differentiate whether the effects are due to the initial underlying pathology, ICU management, drug therapy, or other therapies such as inhaled nitric oxide (iNO), high frequency jet ventilation (HFJV), or ECMO.

Pulmonary problems

Patients develop severe pulmonary fibrosis and ventilator lung injury related to volutrauma, barotrauma, and oxygen toxicity resulting from aggressive ventilation at high pressure, volume, and oxygen concentration. It is now widely accepted that low volume/low pressure ventilation reduces the incidence of pulmonary fibrosis, multi-organ failure, and increases survival.[5]

Some studies report that patients develop pulmonary fibrosis during the early stages of recovery[6-8] despite the use of low volume/low pressure, but these changes are dynamic with alveolar structures actively remodeled. This has been verified by progressive improvements in pulmonary function tests with little or no abnormalities seen up to 12 months after treatment.[8-10] Others report that patients still have a degree of pulmonary fibrosis at 1 year, with an improvement after discharge, but with no return to baseline pulmonary function. There are little data on pulmonary function 1 year after the initial illness.

In the NIH ECMO trial published in 1979, patients treated with venoarterial (VA) ECMO were reported as showing significant functional abnormalities at follow-up.[11,12] This led to the theory that ECMO may predispose the lungs to abnormal repair. Many possible causes for this have been hypothesized with the prevailing theories being that changes in the pulmonary blood flow or the ventilation strategies employed during the NIH adult ECMO trial played a fundamental role in altering long-term repair.

One major limitation of such retrospective studies is the lack of data on the patients' pre-morbid condition. Thus, we can only assume that pulmonary function tests, CT scans, and chest radiographs would have been normal and any subsequent changes are due to the illness or treatment. These assumptions may not be valid. A study by Ferrer et al. which looked at quality-of-life scores in the St. Georges questionnaire indicated that a control group had some of the same problems as a group of respiratory patients, thus suggesting that these "norms" should be considered when evaluating any patient with respiratory problems.[13]

Psychological and neuromuscular problems

In addition to pulmonary effects, there are reported neurological, psychological, and physical effects. Post-traumatic stress disorder (PTSD), ICU psychosis, polyneuropathies, and fixed flexion deformities are widely recognized as complications of illness and prolonged sedation.

The main neurological and musculoskeletal complications appear to be polyneuropathies and myopathies.[14,15] It is likely that these have multiple causes with drugs, immobility, and nutrition having a role. In a study by the Toronto group,[16] muscle wasting was a major cause of significant deterioration in quality-of-life and functional ability at least 1 year after discharge. The muscle wasting, myopathy, and/or polyneuropathy experienced by these patients may also be responsible for some respiratory problems such as shortness of breath, which can occur despite relatively normal pulmonary function tests and imaging.[16-18]

An additional and unexpected side effect of prolonged illness is alopecia. This has been reported in pediatric ECMO patients,[19] but it is also recognized in adult ICU survivors.[20] The mechanism for this is unclear, but, again, nutrition and drugs may have roles.

There are numerous psychological assessment tools available, but most studies use the SF-36 questionnaire,[21] the Hospital Anxiety and Depression Scale (HADS)[22] score, and a disease-specific quality-of-life questionnaire, in addition to assessment by a clinical psychologist. The main psychological problem reported is PTSD, commonly presenting as flashbacks and hallucinations. In one study, it was reported that patients who were conscious on ICU admission tended to have the most significant PTSD.[23] Those with chronic illness such as chronic obstructive pulmonary disease (COPD) fared better psychologically compared to those that suffered trauma and subsequently ARDS.

Little is known about the effects of venovenous (VV) ECMO on respiratory, neurological, psychological, or physical function. We believe that lung rest on ECMO and gentle ventilation following ECMO decannulation should prevent long-term pulmonary sequelae, but there is little evidence to support this hypothesis.

Adult ECMO follow-up study

A retrospective study carried out at Glenfield Hospital studied the pulmonary, neurological, physical, and psychological sequelae of SARF in adults who had been treated with VV ECMO. Since this was a retrospective study and patients admitted for ECMO with SARF were not assessed with these tests prior to their illness, it is difficult to make a comparison or draw conclusions regarding the long-term effects of ECMO. We can only assume that prior assessments would have been normal.

Patients

The 202 study patients managed with VV ECMO for SARF between 1989 and 2001 met the following criteria:

- 18-69 years of age
- Potentially reversible respiratory failure
- Absence of cardiopulmonary edema
- >2 quadrants with alveolar infiltrates
- PaO_2/FiO_2 <200 mm Hg or uncompensated hypercapnea with pH <7.2
- Ventilated for <7 days
- No contraindication to heparinization or continuing active treatment

The results were as follows: 72% (145 patients) were discharged from the ECMO unit and 50.5% (102) survived to hospital discharge. Of the 102 patients, 79% (81) were successfully contacted and 39% (40) agreed to participate and were seen in follow-up. Mean length of time from admission to follow-up was 43.2 ±20.1

months (range 12-92 months) (Figure 1). Patient demographics are shown in Table 1. Diagnoses included ARDS secondary to trauma (8), bacterial pneumonia (15), viral pneumonia (7), and other SARF (10). Only 1 patient failed to complete any of the evaluations.

Methodology

Patients were assessed by an independent physician; underwent pulmonary function tests (PK Morgan Benchmark equipment, MDAS version 3, 1990) and chest CT scans; completed a breathing problem questionnaire (BPQ),[24,25] a Hospital Anxiety and Depression Scale (HADS)[22] and a Functional Limitations Profile (FLP);[26] and were evaluated by a clinical psychologist. The BPQ is a 33-item, COPD-specific, quality-of-life questionnaire. A problems score is obtained, with a maximum of 103. High scores indicate poor health status. The HADS is a standardized and widely used rating scale for assessing anxiety and depression in non-psychiatric patient groups. It is easy to complete and was designed for use as a screening test in general medical clinics. The FLP is a British version of the widely used American Sickness Impact Profile.[23] The aim of the scale is to assess changes in physical and psychological function due to ill health. It consists of 136 items arranged in 12 categories of activity. Higher scores indicate more limitation of function. Two dimension scores can be calculated – the physical dimension and the psychosocial dimension.

Table 1. Patient demographics.

Patient demographics	n=40
Male	18 (45%)
Age	34.5 ±SD
Smoker	22 (55%)
Length of ventilation (days)	19.4 ±0.5
ECMO duration (hrs.)	166.4 ±108.4
Time to follow-up (mos.)	44.2 ±20.1

Data Analysis

Data were analyzed using the SPSS computer package (SPSS Inc., Chicago, IL). Multivariable analysis was carried out for all data on respiratory findings. Since there are multivariables with many large, absolute numbers, especially for the pulmonary function tests, our results are summarized in tables with only the P values to demonstrate significance. The P value criterion for retention of variables was ≤0.05.

Physical findings

Pulmonary function

The most common abnormality was a decrease in residual volume (RV) that was seen in 18 patients (49%); 11 of these 18 (30%) also had a functional residual capacity (FRC) <80% predicted, indicative of a mild restrictive pattern. Of the patients, 10 (27%) had a per-second forced expiratory volume (FEV_1) <80% predicted, 4 patients (11%) had a forced vital capacity (FVC) <80% predicted, and 5 (14%) had a total lung capacity (TLC) <80% predicted. A restrictive pattern was seen in 3 patients (8%) with normal FEV_1 and FVC. An obstructive pattern was seen in 3 (8%); 2 were known smokers and 2 were known to have asthma/COPD. The pulmonary function abnormalities comparing smokers and non-smokers are summarized in Table 2.

The reduced diffusion capacity (KCO) appears to be influenced by sex (higher in males), history of smoking (P=0.01), and the etiology of SARF (higher in trauma P=0.00). Trauma patients had surprisingly poor pulmonary function tests, with significant abnormalities in FEV_1, FVC, and TLC, as well as KCO (Table 3).

All of these findings, with the exception of TLC, improved over time. Trauma patients with resulting rib fractures had a reduction in TLC, whereas only those sustaining pulmonary contusions and no rib fractures had a normal TLC. Conversely, patients with bacterial pneumonia had a better pulmonary outcome, the majority having normal pulmonary function tests. The TLC was significantly higher in this

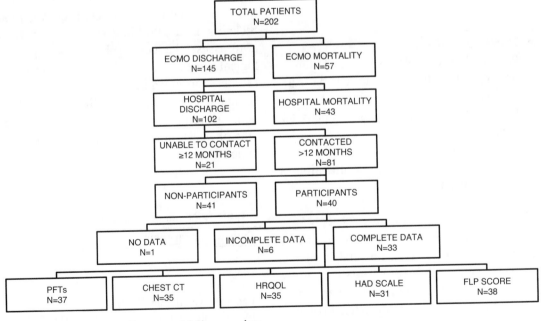

Figure 1. Patient enrollment and follow-up data.

group compared to the trauma group. Females had a better TLC compared to males; however, further analysis revealed that this may be due to the fact that most of the trauma patients were male and a majority of the bacterial pneumonia patients were female (Table 4). There was no significant difference in time to follow-up for all groups.

The gas transfer (TL) was the only pulmonary function test to be influenced by the length of the ECMO run. The shorter the time on ECMO, the better the gas transfer value at follow-up.

Chest CT scan

CT scans at follow-up showed atelectasis in 15 (43%), bronchiectasis in 11 (31%), and parenchymal scarring in 16 (46%). Other abnormalities relating to bronchovascular structures were seen in 18 (51%). Fibrosis was seen in 6 (17%), and emphysema was noted in 3 (9%). PFTs were essentially normal in these patients, with only a reduction in RV. One patient had pulmonary fibrosis on CT scan, but PFTs were normal. Normal CT scans were seen in 3 (9%).

Table 2. Pulmonary function tests: smoking/non-smoking results.

Pulmonary function	Smoker n (%)		Non-smoker n (%)	
Did not complete PFT	3	(8%)	0	—
Normal pulmonary function	3	(8%)	6	(15%)
Abnormal gas transfer (TL)	6	(15%)	4	(10%)
Abnormal diffusion capacity (KCO)	4	(10%)	0	—
≥5 abnormalities	2	(5%)	1	(3%)

Table 3. Trauma vs. non-trauma.

Lung function parameter	Intermediate term			Long term		
	Non-trauma n=18	Trauma n=4	P	Non-trauma n=12	Trauma n=3	P
%FEV$_1$	0.96	0.74	0.03	0.90	0.75	0.05
%FVC	1.03	0.85	0.05	1.00	0.77	0.01
%FEV$_1$/FVC	0.99	0.90	0.20	0.96	1.01	0.42
%PEFR	0.99	0.80	0.04	1.07	0.98	0.31
%TLC PRED.	0.97	0.88	0.20	0.94	0.7133*	0.01
%FRC PRED.	0.90	0.77	0.20	0.90	0.68	0.04
%RV PRED.	0.88	0.85	0.86	0.82	0.63	0.20
%TL PRED.	0.92	0.95	0.82	0.83	0.96	0.04
%KCO PRED.	1.06	1.22	0.14	1.00	1.38	0.003

Table 4. %TLC Predicted Factors.

Factor	Significance	r^{2}a	ANOVA p
(constant)	0	0.07	0.11
Sex (male)	0.04	–	–
(constant)	0	0.08	0.09
Bacterial pneumonia	0.03	–	–
(constant)	0	0.15	0.02
Trauma	0.01	–	–

Atelectasis appears to be dependent on the duration of ventilation and correlates with trauma and age. It is most common in the early period following ECMO, and a decline in incidence is seen over time, with a plateau reached at 4 years post-ECMO.

The incidence of bronchiectasis was more prevalent in patients with a diagnosis of viral pneumonia and long ECMO runs (Table 5). There appears to be a relationship between the primary diagnosis and development of fibrosis as seen on CT scan at long-term follow-up. Patients with bacterial pneumonia were not prone to develop late fibrosis when compared to other diagnostic categories (P=0.06).

Health-related quality-of-life questionnaire

Patients' symptoms as reported in the BPQ were unrelated to either their CT scan results or PFTs, with 28 patients (80%) scoring below 16. The highest score (indicative of poor health status) was 52 in a patient with FEV_1, RV, and FRC <80% predicted and a normal CT scan. Of the 7 patients (20%) that scored relatively highly in the questionnaire (i.e., a score >16), 2 (6%) had normal PFTs and 5 (14%) were smokers. The factor most predictive of a high score on the BPQ was older age (P=0.05).

Musculoskeletal and neurological findings

Musculoskeletal complaints were relatively common and consisted of joint pain (11), poor mobility (11), and neuropathy (6). Of the patients with poor mobility, 3 (8%) had a stroke (CVA). Fatigue was reported in 14 (35%). Of

Table 5. Variables for bronchiectasis.

Variable	Sig.	r^2a
Follow-up time	0.90	0.29
Viral pneumonia	0.02	—
ECMO (hrs.)	0.01	—
Constant	0.01	—

the 3 that had a CVA, 2 developed this diagnosis 3 months post-discharge. Of the patients, 1 underwent amputations for ischemic gangrene while on ECMO. Since we were unable to test objectively for polyneuropathy, we inquired instead about symptomology, which was deemed to be adequate since the patients' subjective findings are more relevant when determining quality-of-life. Interestingly, 4 of the 7 patients who scored >16 in the BPQ also complained of fatigue, suggesting a direct relationship between their breathlessness and muscle fatigue. Despite these complaints, 32 of 39 (82%) patients were able to return to work.

Other physical findings

Alopecia was noted by 1 patient, another reported their fingernails falling out, and others reported a difference in hair color and texture. These findings are uncommon, but they are recognized as either a response to severe stress or to drugs administered and are found in other ICU patients as well.

Psychological

The HADS was completed in 31 patients (78%). A summary of the scores for these patients can be seen in Table 6. A threshold score of 11 was used for both scales to define cases of significant morbidity. This has been found to identify those subjects who have a high probability of suffering from a mood or anxiety disorder with the lowest rate of false positives.[21] The majority of participants were not clinically anxious or depressed. Suicidal thoughts were expressed by 1 patient. These findings are similar to those found in a larger study involving 143 ICU survivors where scores >8 were considered significant.[20]

An FLP was completed by 38 participants. The mean score was 1153 ±1330, (median 567, range 0-4968). There was a wide range of functional disability across the sample, although overall the participants were functioning well. The scores were generally higher (indicating greater disability) on the social dimension compared with the physical dimension.

Following discharge from the ECMO center, 40 ECMO survivors returned and were interviewed 1-8 years later. The questions centered on the patients' memories, experiences, and recovery. Half of the interviews were carried out by a clinical psychologist and the remainder by a senior ECMO specialist. The interviews were analyzed using descriptive statistics for closed questions and thematic content analysis for open-ended questions and explanations. The sample size and distribution were not adequate for statistical testing. From the data, 3 themes arose: memories/reflection, recovery, and support.

Memories/reflection

Of the participants, 24 (59%) claimed to have vivid memories of their time on ECMO including confusion (34%), fear/anxiety (19%), paranoia (19%), with 20% remembering feelings of being violated, trapped, angry, lonely, and/or isolated. Previous ICU studies have not reported patients' specific memories, so these results cannot be compared.

Little or no memory of their ECMO experience was reported by 5 (12%) participants, but

Table 6. HAD scores.

HAD Score		Total N=31 n (%)	
Anxiety			
0-7	Not clinically significant	18	58
8-10	Borderline anxiety	7	23
11-21	Clinically significant	6	19
Range of scores:	1-16		
Depression			
0-7	Not clinically significant	27	87
8-10	Borderline anxiety	3	10
11-21	Clinically significant	1	3
Range of scores:	0-15		

anxiety was expressed about being asked to recall it. This contrasts with another study which found 58% of patients reported no memory of their illness.[27] A small number of patients recalled memories of specific events such as a power failure. Although these events may have actually occurred, patients may have confused them with events in a dream or hallucination, as 28 (70%) patients reported suffering nightmares about their experience on ECMO. The occurrence of these dreams/hallucinations ranged from rarely (8, 20%) to frequently (13, 33%). The contents of these nightmares were recalled by 22 patients (55%); common themes included deceased friends/family (18%), their own death or a threat to their life (7%), and physical violation (5%). There was a definite deficit in the participants' ability to distinguish between true memories and dreams.

Many participants (77%) stated that they thought about their ECMO experience fairly frequently, but their involvement in the follow-up study was mentioned as a major trigger for many of them to reflect upon their hospital experience. For 15 patients (47%), this reflection resulted in feeling lucky or gratified to be alive; 9 (29%) reported negative feelings (e.g., about their scars, having nightmares, or experiencing panic attacks). Ongoing problems related to memory or concentration was reported by 22 (54%).

Recovery

Mood problems

Problems with changes in mood following ECMO were experienced by 28 (70%) patients. The most common symptoms were irritability (61%), depression (61%), anxiety (46%), mood swings (43%), and others (21%) including panic attacks, tiredness, and feelings of stress. This is similar to a smaller study[27] which found 42% of patients post-ICU discharge showing evidence of mood changes, ranging from frustration and anger to depression.

Personality changes

A profound change in personality following ECMO treatment was reported by 28 (70%). Some patients (10%) claimed to be more "laid back" prior to their illness while others (18%) felt they were more "laid back" after. Increased nervousness was reported by 6 (15%) and 2 (5%) reported feeling "more daring". 2 patients felt they were less sociable than before their illness while 1 had become more sociable. Four patients considered themselves to be more emotional and sensitive in general since their illness.

Social well-being and physical fitness

The avoidance of certain activities or places following ECMO was reported by 7 (42%) patients. Exercise that had been previously enjoyed was avoided by 6 (15%), because they felt physically limited (e.g., experienced tiredness upon walking). Half of the patients, indicated it was due to fear rather than any real physical problems.

Avoidance of social situations was reported by 9 patients (29%) with panic attacks and agoraphobia reported by 4 (10%). Anger over what had happened was attributed as the cause in 1 patient; another spoke of avoiding activities which triggered memories of being ill. This avoidance reaction is symptomatic of PTSD. Patients with this condition often avoid situations which trigger memories of a traumatic event to avoid feelings of fear, helplessness, and horror.[28-30]

Interestingly, there was no reported clinically significant change in alcohol consumption since the patients' critical illnesses with 27 (68%) reporting no change, 3 (7%) admitting an increase in consumption, and 8 (19%) stating that their consumption had decreased.

Sexual function

Although not specifically questioned about their sexual functions, 3 male patients volun- teered the information that since their critical illness there was a change in their sex life. Of these 3, 2 attributed these sexual changes to body image concerns resulting from their surgical scars. It is possible that more patients experienced these problems, but did not confide this information to the interviewer. Sexual dysfunction has been identified in previous studies, with male impotence and erectile dysfunction being cited as the main problems.[20,28,31] No information is available on whether women patients experienced any changes in sexual functioning.

Professional Support

10 (25%) of patients had seen a psychologist or psychiatrist following ECMO; only 4 (10%) had seen one prior to ECMO. The reasons for seeking professional counseling were not provided, however, 2 (5%) reported being diagnosed with PTSD, 2 were examined as part of a compensation claim process, and 2 patients reported depression. The remaining 4 patients who utilized mental health services did not state why they had been referred for professional counseling.

After leaving the hospital, the majority of patients (78%) were generally satisfied with the medical care they had received. Specifically, 28 (70%) were satisfied with their general practitioner (GP) and 25 (63%) were satisfied with their attending doctor. For those who did report dissatisfaction, it was directed at GPs or physiotherapists who they felt had no understanding of their experience. This may illustrate a problem with the information provided to community services when ECMO patients are discharged from the hospital.

Although not specifically queried, 14 (35%) patients felt that it was important to have ongoing contact with the ECMO service. Contact with other ECMO patients through an ECMO support group was reported by 13 patients (33%), but how helpful this was is unknown, as this question was not posed. The contact was not found to be helpful by 2 patients (5%).

Family Support

The patients stated that the support they received from their friends and family was excellent (family 91%, friends 85%). The effect of their illness and ECMO treatment on their family members caused distress for 5 of the patients and 3 patients (7%) said their children were worried or frightened whenever they subsequently fell ill. Hall-Smith in 1997 reported that patients expressed feelings of guilt for the stress experienced by their families due to their illness.[27] Although no patients in the ECMO study talked specifically about feelings of guilt, patients were aware of how stressful the experience had been for their family.

Discussion

Due to the retrospective nature of this study and the fact that patients admitted for ECMO with SARF did not have PFTs, BPQ, or CT scans prior to illness, it is difficult to draw conclusive evidence of long-term pulmonary effects. Another major limitation of this study is that only half of the survivors were assessed. We assume that the results would have been similar with the entire cohort, but it is possible that patients who declined follow-up may have had physical or psychological problems which precluded their participation, so we exercise caution when interpreting the results.

Similar to previous studies, we found that patients had minor reductions in pulmonary function, with evidence of mild restrictive abnormalities.[6-12,32-38] Knoch et al. and Stoll et al.[39,40] found that patients with ARDS who were treated with ECMO had changes in their lung function tests, with the predominant abnormality being diminished KCO at long-term follow-up. It has been suggested previously that the reduction in KCO may be due to the chronic vascular

obstruction or vascular remodeling that occurs during the recovery phase of ARDS;[12] however, evidence of this was not supported by CT scan results. The % TLC predicted was better in those with bacterial pneumonia and worse in patients with trauma, both statistically significant.

Trauma has not been previously reported as a significant factor in poor pulmonary function tests or abnormal CT scan findings. Indeed, all other studies report that trauma patients have normal pulmonary function tests after 1 year, although they have evidence of scarring on radiological examination.[41-46] Most of our trauma patients had abnormal pulmonary function tests which improved over time. It is difficult to explain why this group does not fare as well as others in the intermediate period. There may be a difference in the inflammatory response and, consequently, different sequelae compared to patients with infection or ARDS. It has been reported that in early trauma there is an increase in polymorphonuclear neutrophilic (PMN) response compared to patients with sepsis or pneumonia; this may also be the cause for the findings seen.[47] There may be some other factor that has led to abnormal lung tissue repair or delayed healing that resolves over time. It is known that along with lung fibrosis, neuromuscular weakness causes a decline in pulmonary function.[16-18] It is possible that post-ECMO patients have poor muscle strength or are inhibited by fear of perceived pain, resulting in shallow breathing and subsequent poor pulmonary function. It is interesting to note that the trauma patients who sustained rib fractures had a reduction in TLC. Perhaps this reduction may be due to a restriction from the chest wall injury or scar tissue.

Surprisingly, patients with bacterial pneumonia appear to have a better outcome when compared to other diagnostic categories. It is not clear why these patients had no evidence of fibrosis on CT scan compared to other patients and had a higher % TLC predicted values. There was no difference in time on ECMO, severity of illness, or time to follow-up. All patients were ventilated using the low volume/low pressure strategy. Again, perhaps there is an unknown mechanism at the cellular level that can explain these results. It is known that patients with bacterial pneumonia do not develop the anti-Ia (HLA-DR) or Leu 10 (HLA-DS) monoclonal antibodies seen in patients with viral, myco-bacterial, or pneumocystic lung disease or in cases of idiopathic pulmonary fibrosis.[48,49] This difference in host response may explain why patients with bacterial pneumonia do not have radiologic evidence of fibrosis or abnormal pulmonary function tests.

It is well documented that patients treated for severe respiratory failure often have radio-logical evidence of fibrosis.[50-53] In our study, we found fibrosis in only 17% of our patients; atelectasis and pulmonary scarring were more predominant (43% and 46%, respectively). This may be due to the lung-protective strategy used in our ECMO patients.

The development of atelectasis as a result of muscle paralysis during general anesthesia is well studied, particularly when the diaphragm is affected.[54-58] In patients >12 months after admission for severe respiratory failure, it may be that the finding of atelectasis could be attributed to the continued diaphragmatic and chest wall muscle weakness from prolonged illness and mechanical ventilation. This may also explain the reduction in atelectasis on CT scan with time as muscle strength returns. Older patients are more likely to have atelectasis and this could, again, be due to muscle weakness, but other factors such as impaired function of surfactant may be involved. We did not perform lung biopsies and broncho-alveolar lavage in these otherwise healthy patients at follow-up to identify these factors. Interestingly, we did not see any correlation in atelectasis with a reduced FEV_1, FVC, or RV as reported in other studies.[32-37] Pulmonary function may return to normal while radiological imaging continues to show signs of atelectasis. The clinical significance of

atelectasis on CT imaging is still unknown and we advise performing pulmonary function tests in addition to chest CT scans.

Nearly all patients scored low on the BPQ, indicating a good quality-of-life with little or no breathing difficulties. The most commonly answered question that resulted in a score of at least 1 consistently in all age groups was pa-tients' rating of energy level compared to other people their own age. Age was a significant factor in BPQ score, with older patients scor-ing higher. Smokers were also more likely to have a high score. BPQ scores did not correlate with reductions in pulmonary function tests or changes seen on CT scans. At clinical review by an independent physician, most patients rate themselves as asymptomatic with a good qual-ity-of-life. This may be due to the fact that most feel they might have died if they had not been treated with ECMO and feel grateful.

Although the majority of patients in this study were not clinically anxious or depressed, a minority were significantly traumatized by their ECMO treatment and continued to expe-rience psychological problems several years later. The most common problems experienced were recurrent dreams or nightmares, upsetting memories, mood/personality changes, and prob-lems with socializing or recreation. Delusional memories and nightmares have also been re-ported elsewhere.[20,59-62] It has been hypothesized that the dreams and nightmares represent real or symbolic reminders of their time in the ICU and these are experienced by survivors of critical illness in an attempt to rationalize their illness.[27] The high incidence of dreams or nightmares in patients following intensive care treatment have prompted units to examine their sedation practices.[27,63,64] Sedation has been highlighted as a problem area with ECMO patients and merits further research.

It is known that during a patient's stay in intensive care, the family members, especially the spouse, exhibit significant symptoms of anxiety and/or depression which may not be apparent until after the patient is discharged when it is manifested as overprotective behavior by family members.[65,66] The word "over-protective" was used by 3 patients in the ECMO study to describe the attitudes of their family members following their illness. It is clearly important to ensure that multidisciplinary follow-up addresses the needs of the whole family during the patient's rehabilitation.[67,68]

Conclusion

Our results, like other studies, show that ECMO-treated patients experience little significant long-term pulmonary sequelae after their recovery from SARF. There is no apparent correlation between pulmonary function, radiological findings, and patient symptoms. Most patients were asymptomatic, but prior smokers were more likely to be symptomatic and have abnormal PFTs. The initial underlying cause for the SARF is significant, with trauma patients exhibiting prolonged symptoms. In general, the patients appear to have a good quality-of-life. Most patients were functioning well socially and, although some were unable to resume their previous job, most were able to return to some form of work. Our study shows that patients with SARF should be treated with ECMO if appropriate and that the long-term clinical and functional outcome is good. The use of VV ECMO does not appear to predispose the lungs to abnormal repair.

As previously mentioned, the major limitation of this study was its retrospective nature and varying length in follow-up time. Therefore, the follow-up results from the Conventional ventilation or ECMO for Severe Adult Respiratory Failure (CESAR) trial are eagerly awaited. The Department of Health study entitled "Comprehensive Critical Care- A Review of Adult Critical Care Services" in the U.K. recommended that "NHS Trusts review the provision of follow-up services and ensure that there is appropriate provision for those patients

who will benefit."[69] The initial results from our study, in conjunction with the results from the Conventional Ventilation or ECMO for Severe Adult Respiratory Failure (CESAR) trial, will enable follow-up services to be designed to meet the specific needs of adult ECMO patients and their families.

References

1. Reynolds HN, McCunn M, Borg U, Habashi N, Cottingham C, Bar-Lavi Y. Acute respiratory distress syndrome: estimated incidence and mortality rate in a 5 million-person population base. *Crit Care* 1998; 2:29-34.

2. National Heart and Lung Institute, National Institutes of Health. *Respiratory Distress Syndromes: Task Force Report on Problems, research approaches, needs.* Washington, DC: US Government Printing Office; DHEW Publication No (NIH) 73-432 1972: 165-180.

3. Webster NR, Cohen AT, Nunn JF. Adult respiratory distress syndrome-how many cases in the UK? *Anaesthesia* 1988; 43:923-926.

4. Prone-Supine Study Group. Effect of prone positioning on the survival of patients with acute respiratory failure. *N Engl J Med* 2001; 345:568-573.

5. The Acute Respiratory Distress Syndrome Network. Ventilation with lower tidal volumes as compared with traditional tidal volumes for acute lung injury and the acute respiratory distress syndrome. *N Engl J Med* 2000; 342:1301-1308.

6. Peters JI, Bell RC, Prihoda TJ, Harris G, Andrews C, Johanson WG. Clinical Determinants of abnormalities in pulmonary functions in survivors of the adult respiratory distress syndrome. *Am Rev Respir Dis* 1989; 139:1163-1168.

7. Waanders H, Meinders AE. Long-term sequelae on pulmonary function in survivors

of the adult respiratory distress syndrome. *Neth J Med* 1991; 38:177-182.

8. Elliot CG. Morris AH, Cengiz M. Pulmonary function and exercise gas exchange in survivors of adult respiratory distress syndrome. *Am Rev Respir Dis* 1981; 123:492-495.

9. Ghio AJ, Elliot GC, Crapo RO, Berlin SL, Jensen RL. Impairment after ARDS. *Am Rev Respir Dis* 1989; 139:1158-1162.

10. McHugh LG, Milberg JA, Whitcomb ME, Schoene RB, Maunder RJ, Hudson LD. Recovery of function in survivors of the acute respiratory distress syndrome. *Am J Respir Crit Care Med* 1994; 150:90-94.

11. Zapol WM, Treslstad RL, Coffey JW, et al. Extra-corporeal membrane oxygenation in severe acute respiratory failure. A randomised prospective study. *JAMA* 1979; 242:2193-2196.

12. Ingbar DH, Matthay RA. Pulmonary sequelae and lung repair in survivors of the adult respiratory distress syndrome. *Crit Care Clin* 1986; 2:629-665.

13. Ferrer M, Villasante C, Alonso J, et al. Interpretation of quality of life scores from the St Georges Respiratory Questionnaire. *Eur Respir J* 2002; 19:405-413.

14. Garnacho-Montero J, Madrazo-Osuna J, Garcia-Garmendia JL, et al. Critical illness polyneuropathy: risk factors and clinical consequences. A cohort study in septic patients. *Int Care Med* 2001; 27:1288-1296.

15. Berek K, Margreiter J, Willeit J, Berek A, Schmutzhard E, Mutz NJ. Polyneuropathies in critically ill patients: a prospective evaluation. *Int Care Med* 1996; 22:849-855.

16. Canadian Critical Care Trials Group. One-year outcomes in survivors of the acute respiratory distress syndrome. *N Engl J Med* 2003; 348:683-693.

17. Hudson LD, Lee CM. Neuromuscular sequelae of critical illness. *N Engl J Med* 2003; 348:745-747.

18. Survivors of the acute respiratory distress syndrome- letters to editor. *N Engl J Med* 2003; 348:2149-2150.

19. Pettignano R, Heard ML, Labuz MD, Wagoner SF, Fortenberry J. Hair loss after extracorporeal membrane oxygenation. *Paed Crit Care Med* 2003; 4:363-366.

20. Eddleston JM, White P, Guthrie E. Survival, morbidity and quality of life after discharge from intensive care. *Crit Care Med* 2000; 28:2293-2299.

21. Ware JJ, Sherbourne CD. The MOS 36-item short-form health survey (SF-36). I. Conceptula framework and item selection. *Medical Care* 1992; 30:473-483.

22. Zigmond SS, Snaith RP. The Hospital Anxiety and Depression Scale. *Acta Psychiatr Scand* 1983; 67:361-370.

23. Perrins J, King N, Collings J. Assessment of long-term psychological well-being following intensive care. *Intensive Crit Care Nurs* 1998; 14:108-116.

24. De Bruin AF, De Wittel LP, Stevens F, Diedricks JPM. Sickness Impact Profile: the state of the art of a generic functional status measure. *Social Science and Medicine* 1992; 35:1003-1014.

25. Hyndland ME, Bott J, Singh S, Kenyon AP. Domains, constructs and the development of the breathing problems questionnaire. *Qual Life Res* 1994; 3:245-256.

26. Hyndland ME, Singh SJ, Sodergren SC, Morgan MPL. Development of a shortened version of the Breathing Problems Questionnaire suitable for use in a pulmonary rehabilitation clinic: a purpose-specific, disease specific questionnaire. *Qual Life Res* 1998; 7:227-233.

27. Hall-Smith J, Ball C, Coakley J. Follow-up services and the development of a clinical nurse specialist in intensive care. *Int Crit Care Nursing* 1997;13:243-248.

28. Waldman C, Gaine M. The intensive care follow-up clinic. *Care of the Critically Ill* 1996; 12:118-121.

29. Yehuda R. Current concepts: post-traumatic stress disorder. *N Engl J Med* 2002; 346:108-114.

30. Jones C, Griffiths RD, Humphris G, Skirrow PM. Memory, delusions, and the development of acute posttraumatic stress disorder-related symptoms after intensive care. *Crit Care Med* 2001; 29:573-580.

31. Quinlan J, Waldmann C. Sexual dysfunction after intensive care. *B J Anaes* 1998; 81:809.

32. Orme J, Romney JS, Hopkins RO, et al. Pulmonary function and health-related quality of life in survivors of acute respiratory distress syndrome. *Am J Respir Crit Care Med* 2002;167:690-694.

33. Aggarwal AN, Gupta D, Behera D, Jindal SK. Analysis of static pulmonary mechanics helps to identify functional defects in survivors of acute respiratory distress syndrome. *Crit Care Med* 2000; 28:3480-3483.

34. Luhr O, Aardal S, Nathorst-Westfelt U, et al. Pulmonary function in adult survivors of severe acute lung injury treated with inhaled nitric oxide. *Acta Anaesthesiol Scand* 1998; 42:391-398.

35. Yahav J, Leiberman P, Molho M. Pulmonary function following the adult respiratory distress syndrome. *Chest* 1978; 74:247-250.

36. Schelling G, Stoll C, Vogelmeier C, et al. Pulmonary function and health-related quality of life in a sample of long-term survivors of the acute respiratory distress syndrome. *Int Care Med* 2000; 26:1304-1311.

37. Suchyta MR, Elliott CG, Jensen RL, Crapo RO. Predicting the presence of pulmonary function impairment in adult respiratory distress syndrome survivors. *Respir* 1993; 60:103-108.

38. Yernault JC, Englert M, Sergysels R, Degaute JP, De Coster A. Follow-up of pulmonary function after "shock lung". *Bull Eur Physiopathol Respir* 1977; 13:241-248.

39. Knoch M, Kukule I, Muller E, Holtermann W. Pulmonary function one year after extracorporeal lung assist. A long-term follow-up of patients with acute adult respiratory distress syndrome. Abstract. *Anaesthesiol Intensivemend Notfallmed Schmerzther* 1992; 27:477-482.

40. Stoll C, Haller M, Briegel J, et al. Health related quality of life in long-term survivors after treatment with extracorporeal membrane oxygenation (ECMO) for the acute respiratory distress syndrome (ARDS). Abstract *Der Anaesthesist.* 1998; 47:24-29.

41. Hirshberg B, Oppenheim-Eden A, Pizov R, et al. Recovery from blast lung injury- one year follow-up. *Chest* 1999; 116:1683-1688.

42. Livingston DH, Richardson JD. Pulmonary disability after severe blunt chest trauma. *J Trauma* 1990; 30:562-567.

43. Horovitz JH, Carrico CJ, Shires GT. Pulmonary response to major injury. *Arch Surg* 1974; 108:349-355.

44. Kishikawa M, Yoshioka T, Shimazu T, Sugimoto H, Yoshioka T, Sugimoto T. Pulmonary contusion causes long-term respiratory dysfunction with decreased functional residual capacity. *J Trauma* 1991; 31:1203-1210.

45. Landercasper J, Cogbill TH, Lindesmith LA. Long-term disability after flail chest injury. *J Trauma* 1984; 24:410-414.

46. Svennevig JL, Vaage J, Westheim A, Hafsahjl G, Refsum HE. Late sequelae of lung contusion. *Inj: B J Acc Surg* 1989; 20:253-256.

47. Pallister I, Dent C, Topley N. Increased neutrophil migratory activity after major trauma: a factor in the etiology of acute respiratory distress syndrome? *Crit Care Med* 2002; 30:1717-1721.

48. Jakab GJ. Sequential virus infections, bacterial superinfections and fibrogenesis. *J Clin Pathol* 1987; 40:725-733.

49. Kallenberg CG, Schilizzi BM, Beaumont F, De Leij L, Poppema S, The TH. Expression of class II major histocompatibility complex antigens on alveolar epithelium in interstitial lung disease: relevance to pathogenesis of idiopathic pulmonary fibrosis. *Am Rev Respir Dis* 1983; 128:730-739.

50. Nobauer-Huhmann IM, Eibenberger K, Schaefer-Prokop C, et al. Changes in lung parenchyma after acute respiratory distress syndrome (ARDS): assessment with high-resolution computed tomography. *Eur Radiol* 2001; 11:2436-2443.

51. Desai SR, Wells AU, Rubens MB, Evans TW, Hansell DM. Acute respiratory distress syndrome: CT abnormalities at Long-term follow-up. *Radiol* 1999; 210:29-35.

52. Puybasset L, Cluzel P, Chao N, Slutsky AS, Coriat P, Rouby J-J. The CT scan ARDS study Group. A computed tomography scan assessment of regional lung volume in acute lung injury. *Am J Respir Crit Care Med* 1998; 158:1644-1655.

53. Howling SJ, Evans TW, Hansell DM. The significance of bronchial dilation on CT in patients with adult respiratory distress syndrome. *Clin Radiol* 1998; 53:105-109.

54. Tokics L, Strandberg A, Brismar B, Lundquist H, Hedenstierna G. Computerized tomography of the chest and gas exchange measurements during ketamine anaesthesia. *Acta Anaesthesiol Scand* 1987; 31:684-692.

55. Tokics L, Hedenstierna G, Svensson L, et al. V/Q distribution and correlation to atelectasis in anaesthetized paralyzed humans. *J Appl Physiol* 1996; 81:1822-1833.

56. Lindberg P, Gunnarsson L, Tokies L, et al. Atelectasis and lung function in the post-operative period. *Acta Anaesthesiol Scand* 1992; 36:546-553.

57. Tokics L, Henenstierna G, Strandberg A, Brismar B, Lundquist H. Lung collapse and gas exchange during general anaesthesia: effects of spontaneous breathing, muscle paralysis and positive end-expiratory pressure. *Anaesthesiology* 1987; 66:157-167.

58. Brismar B, Hedenstierna G, Lundquist H, Strandberg A, Svensson L, Tokies L. Pulmonary densities during anesthesia with muscular relaxation- a proposal of atelectasis. *Anaestheiology* 1985; 62:422-428.

59. Griffiths RD, Jones C. Recovery from intensive care. *BMJ* 1999; 319:427-429.

60. Crocker C. A multidisciplinary follow-up clinic after patients discharge from ITU. *B J Nursing* 2003; 12:910-914.

61. Chaboyer W, Grace J. Following the path of ICU survivors: a quality-improvement activity. *Nursing in Critical Care* 2003; 8:149-155.

62. Jones, C, O'Donnell C. After intensive care-what then? *Int Crit Care Nursing* 1994; 10:89-92.

63. Robson WP. The physiological after-effects of critical care. *Nursing in Critical Care* 2003; 8:165-171.

64. Lane M, Cadman B, Park G. Learning to use remifentanil in the critically ill. *Care of the Critically Ill* 2002; 18:140-143.

65. Pochard F, Azoulay E, Chevret S, et al. Symptoms of anxiety and depression in family members of intensive care unit patients: ethical hypothesis regarding decision-making capacity. *Crit Care Med* 2001; 29:1893-1897.

66. Jones C, Griffiths RD, Macmillan RR, Palmer TEA. Psychological problems occurring after intensive care. *B J Int Care* 1994; 2:46-53.

67. Covinsky KE, Goldman L, Cook F, et al. The impact of serious illness on patient's families. *JAMA* 272:1839-1844.

68. Lange P. Family stress in the intensive care unit. *Crit Care Med* 2001; 29:2025-2026.

69. Department of Health. Comprehensive Critical Care. A Review of Adult Critical Care Services. London, England: The Stationary Office; 2000.

28

Pediatric Cardiac Failure: Management and Use of ECLS

Brian W. Duncan, M.D.

Introduction

Mechanical circulatory support has become increasingly common in the therapeutic approach for patients with cardiac disease when other forms of treatment fail. For adults in the acute setting, left ventricular failure due to coronary artery disease has been managed with intra-aortic balloon pumping (IABP) and left ventricular assist device (LVAD) insertion. For chronic circulatory support, implantable LVAD systems have demonstrated a survival advantage over drug therapy in adult patients with end-stage heart failure.[1,2] In children, however, isolated left ventricular failure is relatively rare while right ventricular failure, pulmonary hypertension, and hypoxemia often contribute significantly to circulatory failure in pediatric heart disease. Due to these physiologic differences, isolated support of the left ventricle by IABP or LVAD has limited applicability in children. ECMO provides biventricular cardiopulmonary support and remains the primary modality of mechanical circulatory assistance in children with heart disease for whom conventional medical treatment has failed. This chapter will address the current status of ECMO in these patients by examining historical aspects of its development, technical issues related to management of the

circuit, clinical features such as indications and contraindications for this treatment, and special situations unique to ECMO support in children with cardiac disease.

Historical aspects

The development of ECMO for pediatric cardiac support

The use of ECMO to provide support for circulatory failure arose as a natural follow-up to work in the 1970s that established the efficacy of ECMO in the treatment of respiratory failure. Work by pioneering investigators in this field remains interesting and inspiring. Baffes et al. is credited with the first use of prolonged extracorporeal circulation for congenital heart disease.[3] The duration of support was relatively brief for the patients in this study; however, significant innovations were introduced including the use of an ECMO circuit for resuscitation after cardiac arrest and for perioperative stabilization at the time of palliative cardiac procedures. The first reported use of ECMO for extended periods in a pediatric heart patient was supplied by Soeter et al. who described the successful use of ECMO to support a 4-year-old girl with severe hypoxemia after repair of tetralogy of Fallot.[4] The patient was weaned from support within 48 hours, extubated two days later, and discharged on post-operative day 13.

Other landmark studies in the development of ECMO for pediatric cardiac support include those by Bartlett and Hill.[5-7] Although these reports focused on patients with respiratory failure, they also included descriptions of the successful use of ECMO for post-operative support in children undergoing congenital heart defect repairs. Important contributions provided by these early studies include the consideration of aspects of management which make ECMO for cardiac support unique. These issues include how best to handle anti-coagulation in post-operative cardiac surgical patients and the development of guidelines for appropriate patient selection. It is a testimony to the remarkable foresight of these pioneers that these same issues still retain central importance in the successful use of ECMO for pediatric cardiac support.

Current status of pediatric cardiac ECMO support

Examination of the ECLS Registry demonstrates that pediatric cardiac support (for patients ≤16 years) comprised ~29% of total ECMO cases for 2004 (Figure 1).[8] During the mid-1980s, a steady increase in pediatric cardiac cases compared to other patient groups was observed, which has leveled off during the past few years (Figure 2). This change reflects the greater use of ECMO to support circulatory failure in children as well as the decreased utilization of ECMO for respiratory failure due to the success of other respiratory support options such as inhaled nitric oxide (iNO) administration and high frequency ventilation (HFV). With these changes in ECMO utilization, a greater understanding of the practices that lead to successful support of pediatric cardiac patients has become increasingly important to ECMO centers.

Circuit-related and other technical aspects

Components of the circuit

The components of the ECMO circuit have been covered in Chapter 6. For children with cardiac disease, circuit components are similar to those utilized for the support of respiratory failure with some important differences. Most patients with cardiac disease require a venoarterial (VA) mode to provide circulatory as well as respiratory support; however, since substantial morbidity in congenital heart disease arises due to hypoxia, pulmonary hypertension, and right ventricular failure. Venovenous (VV) ECMO may currently be an under-utilized modality in pediatric cardiac patients.[9,10] While circulatory support is not achieved directly with VV ECMO, elimination of hypoxia along with decreased pulmonary vascular resistance may improve right ventricular function resulting in a substantial circulatory benefit. An interesting approach is the assistance respiratoire extra-corporelle (AREC) system which provides single-cannula VV ECMO using a non-occlusive rotary pump with tidal flow in the circuit provided by alternating clamps.[11] This system has been successfully used in pediatric cardiac patients

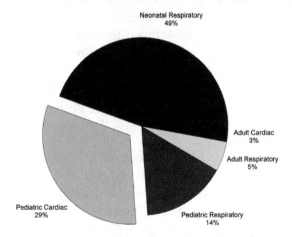

Figure 1. ELSO data for total number of patients requiring support by diagnostic group.

with hypoxia and pulmonary hypertension as the primary indication for ECMO support.[10,12]

Many centers utilize a standard ECMO circuit that employs a membrane oxygenator, a roller pump, and a heat exchanger. Membrane oxygenators are currently utilized by most centers; however, hollow-fiber oxygenators are also widely employed.[13-15] Hollow-fiber oxygenators combine highly efficient gas exchange with easy priming, especially important when ECMO is used for resuscitation tool cardiac arrest.[16] A significant limitation of hollow-fiber devices is plasma leakage across the oxygenator, which requires the device to be replaced frequently.[13] Although many centers continue to use roller pumps, centrifugal pumps, which maintain venous in-flow independent of gravity drainage, allow the patient to be maintained at any height relative to the pump and may even be clamped directly to the bed, substantially reducing tubing length. Centrifugal pumps may be especially useful in larger patients to maintain adequate venous return at higher flows.[17-20] An additional advantage of the centrifugal pump is that occlusion of arterial outflow from the pump

does not generate excessive arterial line pressure, reducing the risk of rupture of the arterial limb of the circuit. The chief disadvantage of the centrifugal pump is the high negative pressure that may be generated on the venous side of the circuit, potentially leading to cavitation and hemolysis.[21]

Anticoagulation

The whole-blood activated clotting time (ACT) is used to monitor anticoagulation. Achieving an ACT of 180-200 seconds with a continuous heparin infusion maintains the circuit with a minimal risk of significant thrombosis.[9,14,18,19,22-24] Platelets are maintained above 100,000/dl and, in patients requiring post-operative support where bleeding is a critical problem, above 150,000/dl. Clotting factors are supplied with infusions of fresh frozen plasma or cryoprecipitate to maintain fibrinogen levels above 100 mg/dl. Instituting the heparin infusion may be safely deferred for several hours until the ACT drifts downward in the bleeding post-operative patient.

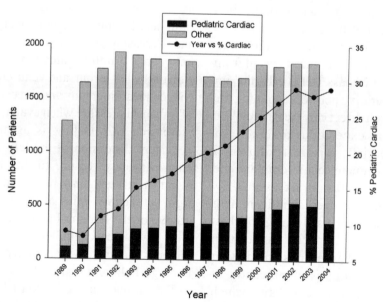

Figure 2. Comparison of ELSO data for annual number and percentage of total for pediatric cardiac support patients versus all other diagnostic categories.

Heparin-bonded hollow-fiber oxygenators and heparin-bonded tubing have been utilized in an attempt to decrease the amount of systemic heparin that is required.[13] Epsilon amino caproic acid (Amicar; Lederle Parenterals, Carolina, Puerto Rico) may be used to diminish the risk of post-operative hemorrhage.[9,25,26] Amicar is usually administered as an initial bolus, followed by a continuous IV infusion for 48 hours, and then discontinued. Maintaining the infusion for longer periods is usually unnecessary, as post-surgical bleeding subsides while circuit thrombosis resulting from prolonged administration becomes a greater concern. A recent review of nearly 300 patients treated with Amicar during ECMO failed to demonstrate decreased rates of intracranial hemorrhage; however, surgical site bleeding was reduced, particularly in cardiac surgical patients.[27]

Cannulation and left ventricular decompression

The approach to cannulation should be flexible and based on the underlying need for ECMO. Transthoracic cannulation of the right atrial appendage and the ascending aorta is most appropriate for cases that require intra-operative support due to failure to wean from cardiopulmonary bypass (CPB). In the immediate post-operative period, reopening the sternal wound with direct cardiac cannulation provides the most expeditious route to institute support, especially in patients who suffer cardiac arrest. Adequate venous drainage and excellent arterial perfusion are assured by chest cannulation; however, significant hemorrhage remains a major disadvantage of chest cannulation, making peripheral cannulation preferable in most other settings. In addition, the risk of mediastinitis is significantly increased with transthoracic cannulation which may make cardiac transplantation impossible if cardiac recovery does not occur.

Cannulation of the right internal jugular vein and the common carotid artery provides excellent venous drainage and perfusion and is the preferred cannulation site in neonates and children below ~15 kg. Cannulation of the femoral vessels provides adequate venous drainage and perfusion for larger children. A second venous drainage cannula placed in the right internal jugular vein may be added if venous drainage through the femoral route alone is inadequate. Risk of ischemia in the lower extremities is high with femoral arterial cannulation; however, this risk may be partially mitigated by placing a perfusion cannula in the distal femoral artery.[9,23] Venous congestion of the lower extremity may be prevented by placement of a "saphenous sump" catheter at the time of femoral venous cannulation.[17] The axillary artery and iliac vessels may be utilized for additional cannulation sites in difficult access cases.

Inadequate decompression of the left-sided cardiac chambers during ECMO support is common in cases of profound cardiac dysfunction. Steps should be taken to prevent pulmonary edema and further distension injury of the left ventricle. Left-sided distension is usually managed by increasing ECMO flow to empty the right heart, minimizing pulmonary blood flow, and decreasing pulmonary venous return to the left heart.[28] Careful evaluation to detect distension of the left atrium and ventricle is achieved with echocardiography and direct measurement of left atrial pressure when available. Although increasing ECMO flow is usually effective, persistent distension of the left-sided cardiac chambers may require further intervention: a left atrial vent may be introduced via the right pulmonary veins at the atrioventricular groove or the left atrial appendage in patients who have been cannulated transthoracically. Patients cannulated by peripheral routes may undergo balloon atrial septostomy performed in the cardiac catheterization laboratory or at the patient's bedside under echocardiographic guidance.[29,30]

Other management points

ECMO flow rates are generally maintained between 80-150 cc/kg/min until patients are ready for weaning. Inotropic support during ECMO for cardiac patients is usually substantially decreased compared to pre-ECMO levels. These patients are routinely maintained on low-dose dopamine and vasodilator infusions. This combination is aimed at improving peripheral and renal perfusion as well as encouraging some degree of ventricular emptying in a further attempt to limit left-sided distension. It is important to maintain moderate levels of ventilatory support for the cardiac patient who requires ECMO. Coronary perfusion is primarily derived from the left ventricle during ECMO if there is any appreciable cardiac ejection.[31,32] Measures must be taken to ensure that blood returning from the pulmonary veins is fully saturated and to maintain adequate myocardial oxygenation, increasing the patient's chance of ventricular recovery. In the absence of severe pulmonary parenchymal disease, fully saturated pulmonary venous blood is provided by maintaining moderate levels of ventilatory support during ECMO. The majority of ECMO-supported cardiac patients are maintained on 30-40% oxygen, 16 breaths/min, 5 cm H_2O positive end expiratory pressure (PEEP), and a tidal volume of 10 cc/kg.

Weaning from support

Weaning is performed under echocardiographic guidance to assess ventricular filling and function. Pulmonary arterial catheters are not routinely placed for cardiac output measurement or the determination of pulmonary capillary wedge pressure except in borderline cases. At the time of weaning, flows are gradually turned down over several hours until flows of 25-40 cc/kg/min are reached. Ventilatory support and inotrope infusions are simultaneously increased to appropriate levels. The arterial and venous

lines are then clamped, full anticoagulation is maintained, and the cannulas are intermittently flashed (every 15-20 minutes) until the patient is known to be stable without ECMO. Borderline patients can be maintained off ECMO for 1-2 hours with intermittent flashing of the cannulas until support is no longer needed. However, we have not capped the cannulas for periods of 24 hours or more as some groups have described in respiratory failure patients. One useful strategy in cases of profound ventricular dysfunction is to extend the weaning period over 48-72 hours with gradual reduction in flows. Fragile patients who might have failed with more rapid weaning may benefit from this approach by gradually accommodating to lower flows.

Clinical aspects

Cardiac diagnoses

The diagnostic categories from a large, single-center study using ECMO and ventricular assist devices (VAD) for pediatric cardiac patients are presented in Table 1.[9] More than half these cases were patients with complex cyanotic heart disease possessing either increased (33%) or decreased (25%) pulmonary blood flow. Reports from other centers reveal this to be a representative make-up of patient diagnoses. In Walters' report of a series of pediatric patients who required post-cardiotomy support, complete atrioventricular canal (20%), complex single ventricle anatomy (17%), and tetralogy of Fallot (14%) were the most common diagnoses.[33] Meliones in his 1991 review of ELSO Registry data for pediatric cardiac patients found patients with left-to-right shunt (24%), cyanosis with decreased pulmonary blood flow (22%), and cyanosis with increased pulmonary blood flow (17%) to be the most common diagnostic groups.[34] A comparison of the two modalities shows ECMO to be superior to VAD for the support of most children with complex cyanotic lesions where hypoxia, pulmonary hypertension, or biventricular failure contributes significantly to the pathophysiology necessitating mechanical circulatory support.[9,35] Due to the presence of an oxygenator in the circuit, ECMO addresses the underlying pathophysiology more directly and provides greater flexibility than VAD in these cases.

Indications for support

A review of several large clinical studies confirms that indications for support differ when ECMO is required in the pre-operative vs. post-operative period. Studies summarizing the pre-operative use of ECMO demonstrate that hypoxia and pulmonary hypertension are the most common indications leading to ECMO.[10,36] Post-operative support is most commonly initiated for failure to wean from CPB, cardiogenic shock, or cardiac arrest occurring in the ICU after cardiac surgery.[17-20,22-24,28,33,37,38]

Combined results of pre-operative, post-operative, and non-surgical pediatric cardiac patients demonstrate that hypoxia (36%), cardiac arrest (24%), and failure to wean from CPB (14%) were the most common indications for ECMO (Table 2).[9] Although hypoxia was the largest indication for ECMO in this study,

innovative therapies such as iNO administration and HFV may decrease the need for ECMO support in the treatment of pediatric patients with cardiac disease and refractory respiratory failure.[39-41] Kocis et al. reported the use of high frequency jet ventilation (HFJV) to successfully treat 7 of 8 patients with respiratory failure who would have otherwise required ECMO.[41] Goldman et al. used iNO to treat 10 patients with severe pulmonary hypertension after surgery for congenital heart disease, including 5 who could not be weaned from CPB.[39] ECMO was avoided in 8 of these 10 patients, with 80% surviving to hospital discharge.

Several studies have shown that failure to wean from CPB has a negative impact on survival.[9,14,20,33] However, a number of other studies did not find inability to wean from bypass to be a risk factor.[23,28] These latter studies stress the importance of the early application of ECMO before prolonged periods of low cardiac output in the post-operative patient that result in end-organ damage. The importance of early ECMO support cannot be over emphasized; however, we have observed that patients who are unable to wean from CPB without ECMO fare poorly due to excessive mediastinal hemorrhage and often exhibit a greater degree of ventricular dysfunction.

Table 1. Diagnostic groups and survival.

Diagnosis	Survivors (%)	Non-survivors (%)	Total (% of all groups)
Left to right shunt	1 (14%)	6 (86%)	7 (11%)
Left-sided obstruction	5 (42%)	7 (58%)	12 (18%)
Right-sided obstruction	1 (100%)	0	1 (1.5%)
Cyanosis, ↑ pulmonary blood flow	8 (36%)	14 (64%)	22 (33%)
Cyanosis, ↓ pulmonary blood flow	7 (41%)	10 (59%)	17 (25%)
ALCAPA	1 (100%)	0	1 (1.5%)
Cardiomyopathy	3 (75%)	1 (25%)	4 (6.0%)
Other	1 (33%)	2 (67%)	3 (4%)
Total	**27 (40%)**	**40 (60%)**	**67**

ALCAPA = anomalous left coronary artery from pulmonary artery.

Contraindications

As the use of ECMO for cardiac patients has increased, clinical features considered to be contraindications have evolved. It is universally understood that certain conditions constitute absolute contraindications, including incurable malignancy, advanced multi-system organ failure, extreme prematurity, and severe central nervous system damage.[9,18,33,38] Various reports have stressed that residual cardiac lesions after cardiac surgery should be viewed as a contraindication due to the poor outcome of these patients.[14,17] Patients who are not transplant candidates should be considered for support only in carefully selected cases, as any patient placed on ECMO may ultimately require cardiac transplantation for recovery.[18]

However, a number of conditions previously thought to be irreparable or at high risk for further complications with ECMO support have recently been treated with ECMO and should, at most, represent relative contraindications. For example, 10 years ago, single ventricle physiology was considered to be a contraindication for ECMO, while the ability to provide mechanical circulatory support is now considered an important adjunct in the treatment of these patients (see special topics: Perioperative support for hypoplastic left heart syndrome and other single ventricle forms).[9,28,33,42-45] In general, rigid contraindications for mechanical support, other than those mentioned above, have not been developed. Instead, each case should be evaluated individually. In addition to what is now routine support of shunted single ventricle patients, other "high-risk" patients have been successfully supported, including patients with pre-support cardiac arrest, patients undergoing palliative cardiac operations, and cardiac patients with co-existing congenital diaphragmatic hernia (CDH).

Complications

Complications by organ system from Children's Hospital, Boston are listed in Table 3.[9] These same trends are reflected in reports from other centers with hemorrhagic complications occurring in 10-70% of all patients.[14,18-20,23,24,33,37,38] Cardiovascular complications include arrhythmia or on-going significant ventricular dysfunction. Neurologic complications represent a source of considerable morbidity in these patients. Intracranial hemorrhage, seizures and cerebral infarction were the 3 most common neurologic complications, comprising 36%, 23%, and 18%, respectively, of all central

Table 2. Indications for ECMO support and survival.

Indication	Survivors (%)	Non-survivors (%)	Total (% of all)
Hypoxia	11 (44%)	14 (56%)	25 (36%)
Pre-op cardiac failure	1 (100%)	0	1 (1.4%)
Post-op cardiac failure	2 (29%)	5 (71%)	7 (10%)
Cardiac arrest	7 (41%)	10 (59%)	17 (24%)
Bridge to transplant	2 (67%)	1 (33%)	3 (4.4%)
Failure to wean from CPB	1 (10%)	9 (90%)	10 (14%)
Pulmonary hypertension	1 (25%)	3 (75%)	4 (5.8%)
Cardiac failure, no oper.	2 (67%)	1 (33%)	3 (4.4%)
Total	**27 (39%)**	**43 (61%)**	**70**

Note: The total number of indications (70) in table 2 exceeds the total number of diagnoses (67) in Table 1 due to 2 ECMO runs that were performed in 3 patients. Each run is considered to have its own indication while there is a single diagnosis per patient.

nervous system complications. Mechanical complications, including tubing rupture, cannula dislodgment, and important thrombus formation in the circuit, occurred in 26% of all cases. Like other published reports, this data shows that mechanical complications did not represent a risk factor for death.[19,23,28,34] Renal failure occurred in 21% of patients and was a risk factor for death; as confirmed by several other reports.[23,33,34]

Outcome and risk factors for death

Variable survival statistics have been reported for pediatric cardiac ECMO. In 2000, cumulative survival for cardiac ECMO in the ELSO Registry was 42%;[46] 5 years later, the cumulative survival rate is 43%.[8] In our single-center experience published in 1999, 76% of patients placed on ECMO were successfully weaned from support, with 40% of the original patients surviving to hospital discharge.[8] Contemporaneous studies reported similar weaning and hospital survival rates.[14,17-20,22-24,28,33,37,38,47,48] Interestingly, studies published in the last 5 years demonstrate rates of weaning (60-70%) and survival to hospital discharge (40-50%) which remain similar to reports from earlier eras despite advances in management.[42,49-52]

Ongoing cardiac failure and multi-system organ failure were the most common causes of death for ECMO supported patients in our experience (Table 4).[9] Analysis of the ELSO Registry by Meliones et al. listed ongoing cardiac failure (37%) and major central nervous system damage (15%) as the most common

Table 3. Complication rates and survival.

Complication	Incidence	Survival
Hemorrhage	28/70 (40%)	10/28 (36%)
Cardiovascular	26/70 (37.1%)	10/26 (38%)
Central nervous system	22/70 (31.4%)	10/22 (45%)
Any severe infection	19/70 (27.1%)	7/19 (37%)
Mechanical	18/70 (25.7%)	5/18 (28%)
Gastrointestinal	17/70 (24.3%)	6/17 (35%)
Renal failure[†]	15/70 (21.4%)	2/15 (13%)*
Pulmonary	15/70 (21.4%)	8/15 (53%)

†Dialysis or serum creatinine $\geq$ 3.0
*P=0.03 for renal complications impact on survival.

Table 4. Causes of death.

Cause of Death	Incidence (%)
Ventricular failure	14 (35%)
Multiple system organ failure	12 (30%)
Respiratory failure	4 (10%)
Anoxic brain injury	2 (5%)
Intracranial hemorrhage	2 (5%)
Arrhythmia	2 (5%)
Inadequate flow rates due to poor drainage	2 (5%)
Aortic cannula dislodgment	1 (2.5%)
Hemorrhage (torn umbilical vein)	1 (2.5%)
Total	**40**

causes of mortality.[34] Cardiac failure and complications arising from low cardiac output are, likewise, the most commonly reported causes of death in numerous other reports.[19,28,47] Thus, attempts to improve results achieved with pediatric cardiac ECMO should address optimization of ventricular function and avoidance of extended periods of low cardiac output. Prompt institution of ECMO support achieves both of these goals by preserving myocardial, central nervous system, and visceral perfusion. Allowing patients to remain in a low cardiac output state on increasing dosages of vasoconstrictive agents prior to ECMO may lead to end-organ damage that may not be reversible after circulatory support has been established. Once ECMO is initiated, meticulous patient management is required to limit infectious complications which may progress to multi-system organ failure. For the salvage of continuing severe cardiac dysfunction, an early and aggressive approach to cardiac transplantation may be the only life-saving therapy available.

Lack of return of ventricular function within 48-72 hours in post-cardiotomy patients, confers a poor prognosis.[9] Return of ventricular function is defined as the return of a pulsatile waveform on the peripheral arterial trace on maximal levels of support (80% of normal cardiac output provided by the device). The return of a pulsatile waveform on the arterial line trace by 72 hours of support was seen in 24 of 25 non-transplanted ECMO survivors (96%). This data has been used as additional prognostic information as post-cardiotomy patients without return of ventricular function within 48-72 hours of support are currently considered for transplantation or termination of support when transplantation is contraindicated. Delaying this decision while awaiting return of ventricular function beyond the first 48-72 hours of support is not justified based on these results. Due to the scarcity of pediatric organ donors, early consideration for transplantation optimizes the chances of successful organ procurement. While return

of ventricular function occurs early or not at all for ECMO supported patients after cardiac surgery, patients with myocarditis may require prolonged periods of mechanical circulatory support with ultimate complete recovery of ventricular function.[53-59] Myocarditis patients may be better managed with implantable VAD systems for prolonged periods with the anticipation of ultimate bridging to myocardial recovery (see ECMO for the treatment of acute fulminant myocarditis).

Long-term follow-up of mechanical circulatory support in children

Data are available that describe the long-term outcome for children requiring ECMO for primary respiratory failure; however, little information is available regarding the long-term outlook and quality-of-life for children who have survived mechanical circulatory support for cardiac indications. The long-term follow-up of children with cardiac disease who required mechanical circulatory support during a decade of experience at a single-center was analyzed.[60] This study followed 37 children who survived mechanical circulatory support (26 ECMO and 11 VAD survivors) for an average of more than 4 years. Only 1 patient died in either group for an overall long-term survival of 95%. For patients in both groups, 80% were described as exhibiting good to excellent general health, 90% were in New York Heart Association (NYHA) classes I or II, and echocardiographic evaluation of ventricular function was normal in all of the ECMO-supported patients and in 90% of the VAD-supported patients.

Poor neurologic outcomes were more common in ECMO-supported than VAD-supported patients. More than 60% of the ECMO-supported patients demonstrated moderate to severe neurologic impairment, while only 20% of the VAD survivors demonstrated this degree of neurologic impairment. Adverse neurologic outcomes were associated with low weight at the time of initial support and duration of hypothermic circulatory arrest in the children that received cardiac operations. Adverse neurologic outcomes were not associated with pre-support cardiac arrest, carotid cannulation, or carotid reconstruction.

Children with heart disease who survive to hospital discharge after requiring ECMO or VAD support demonstrate favorable long-term survival, general health, and cardiac outcomes. The relatively higher rates of neurologic complications in the ECMO-supported group are of concern and appear to suggest an advantage for VAD-support, possibly due to the decreased requirement for anticoagulation with less risk of neurologic complications such as intracranial hemorrhage; however, these results must also be interpreted with the understanding that the ECMO-supported group in this study had a higher proportion of critically ill neonates with more complex underlying cardiac conditions. Nevertheless, the potential for greater neurologic risk in ECMO patients should be appreciated and excess anticoagulation should be cautiously avoided.

Special topics

Perioperative support for hypoplastic left heart syndrome and other single ventricle forms

Review of a large single-center experience with pediatric mechanical circulatory support through 1996 demonstrated that only 2% of all cases were children with hypoplastic left heart syndrome.[9] A subsequent report from 2001 demonstrated that 28% of all pediatric cardiac cases requiring ECMO were for perioperative support for the Norwood procedure.[42] This difference over a 5-year period is representative of trends seen at other institutions; while previously felt to be at least a relative contraindication, patients who possess hypoplastic left heart syndrome and other forms of single ventricle physiology are now ECMO candidates. In fact, several reports have emphasized the importance of having an active ECMO program at pediatric cardiac centers in the event that such support is required in the perioperative care of these patients.[42-44] At least part of the difficulty in managing patients with shunted single ventricle physiology on ECMO arises from the difficulty of achieving balance between the pulmonary and systemic circulation in these patients during support. Increasing ECMO flow to higher than normal levels is almost always successful in maintaining adequate systemic perfusion and eliminating the effects of significant pulmonary "steal" of blood flow from the systemic circulation through the shunt. Occasionally, blood flow through the shunt must be physically limited to maintain adequate systemic perfusion and to avoid excessive pulmonary blood flow. This can be achieved by placing a metallic clip to partially constrict the shunt. This procedure can be performed at the patient's bedside. However, it is rarely necessary and great care must be taken to limit shunt flow without completely occluding the shunt resulting in extensive pulmonary infarction.[28]

While single ventricle physiology remains a risk factor for death in some reports,[50] a number of recent studies have reported success using ECMO to support these patients. Pizarro and Aharon described survival rates of 50% and 64%, respectively, for infants who required mechanical circulatory support after the Norwood procedure.[42,44] Interestingly, the report by Aharon noted higher survival for children with single ventricle physiology than for children with two ventricles who required ECMO. While conventional ECMO may be used in these patients, Darling et al. reported 80% survival utilizing a circuit configured without an oxygenator (no membrane oxygenator VAD [NOMO-VAD]) to support patients after a Norwood procedure.[43]

Transplantation experience

ECMO support may be used as a bridge to transplantation, as perioperative support (especially in children with elevated pulmonary vascular resistance after transplantation), and during rejection episodes. The use of ECMO as a bridge to pediatric cardiac transplant is well summarized by a number of recently published reports.[54,61-65] Reddy et al. reported that survival to transplantation for children who required mechanical bridging with either ECMO or VAD (82% survival to transplant) was no different than for patients who were medically managed (85% survival to transplant) even though the ECMO/VAD group was substantially more ill.[65] Del Nido et al. reported that at the University of Pittsburgh, 9 of 14 patients (64%) were successfully bridged to transplant after an average of 109 hours on ECMO support, with 6 of these patients (43%) surviving to hospital discharge.[61] Frazier et al. reviewed the experience at Arkansas Children's Hospital utilizing ECMO as a bridge to cardiac transplantation in 17 patients.[54] In this study, 15 of the 17 patients were either successfully bridged to transplantation (12) or recovered spontaneously (3), while 2 patients died awaiting transplantation on ECMO support. The duration of ECMO support was often quite prolonged, with a median duration of 269 hours (range 35-1078). In this experience, meticulous management led to very low infection rates despite prolonged periods of support, with only 1 patient developing significant infection that required removal from the transplant list. These studies emphasize the need for aggressive treatment for left ventricular distension, which these patients are prone to develop due to severe ventricular dysfunction. Other management techniques utilized by these successful programs include rigorous patient selection before bridging is initiated, consideration of donors over a broad size range to increase the donor pool, and measures to avoid infectious complications.

The utilization of ECMO for post-operative support at the time of cardiac transplantation in children is most often for treatment of pulmonary hypertension with right ventricular failure

or for support of graft dysfunction in the early post-operative period. Galantowicz and Stolar reported a multi-center analysis with a 40% survival rate in children who required ECMO in the immediate post-operative period after cardiac transplantation.[66] Other reports have demonstrated similar results.[9,67] Severe, acute rejection episodes after cardiac transplantation may be characterized by rapid deterioration, with ECMO providing temporary life-saving support until anti-rejection therapy becomes effective.[66,67]

Use of rapid resuscitation ECMO in the treatment of cardiorespiratory arrest

Cardiac arrest is a common indication for ECMO, comprising nearly 25% of all indications for ECMO in pediatric cardiac patients.[9] In addition, the survival of these patients is surprisingly high (~40%, equivalent to the rate of survival for all other indications) in a group that might be predicted to do poorly. Although pediatric cardiac patients that suffer cardiac arrest represent the most critically ill subset of an already challenging patient population, these observations suggest that this is a salvageable group that may do better with an aggressive approach. Several groups have developed systems that allow the expeditious institution of ECMO for children with cardiac disease who suffer cardiac arrest refractory to conventional cardiopulmonary resuscitation.[68-70]

One such system utilizes a modified ECMO circuit, an organized team of personnel to perform cannulation and a streamlined priming process.[69] This "rapid resuscitation" ECMO circuit is maintained vacuum- and CO_2-primed in the ICU. It is portable and battery-powered, allowing it to be used at any location in the hospital. If standard CPR is unsuccessful within 10 minutes of cardiac arrest, the circuit is moved to the patient's bedside and crystalloid priming is initiated while cannulation is proceeding. If cannulation is completed prior to the availability of blood products, ECMO flow is initiated with a crystalloid-primed circuit and blood products are added when they become available. The excess crystalloid volume is removed as blood is added to the circuit using exchange transfusions by hand and performing ultrafiltration after the hemodynamics have stabilized. Establishing a normal cardiac output with ECMO is the most critical factor for successful resuscitation of these children, even if the hematocrit is low at the time support is initiated due to the use of a crystalloid-primed circuit.

Rapid resuscitation ECMO was used in 11 pediatric patients who had suffered cardiac arrest. 9 of these patients were post-operative cardiac surgical patients, 1 had suffered cardiac arrest prior to surgery, and 1 had suffered cardiac arrest in the cardiac catheterization laboratory.[69] All patients were undergoing CPR at the time of ECMO cannulation. The median duration of CPR for these 11 patients was 55 minutes (range 15-103) compared to a median duration of CPR of 90 minutes (range 45-200) for 7 historical controls resuscitated with conventional means prior to the utilization of the rapid resuscitation system. 10 of the 11 rapid resuscitation patients were able to be weaned from ECMO, with 7 (64%) surviving to hospital discharge, compared to 2 survivors (29%) from the 7 historical controls.

Jacobs et al. reported results for a particularly innovative rapid resuscitation system that utilizes a hollow-fiber oxygenator to facilitate priming.[70] The circuit employs a centrifugal pump, short lengths of ¼ inch tubing, and is heparin-bonded throughout. It is fully portable and requires a priming volume of 250 ml. The use of a centrifugal pump eliminates the need for gravity drainage, allowing shorter tubing lengths and greater portability. The simplicity of the circuit facilitates priming and minimizes trauma to blood elements while the heparin-bonding minimizes blood loss. The authors reported their results with this system in 23 pediatric cardiac patients, many post-opera-

tive. All patients had support instituted with a crystalloid-primed circuit. The simplicity of this system and avoidance of the blood priming step enabled set-up time to be as brief as 5 minutes. The duration of cardiopulmonary resuscitation was only 12 minutes for the 4 patients who suffered cardiac arrest prior to cannulation, all of whom survived to hospital discharge.

These reports support the concept that pediatric cardiac patients who suffer cardiac arrest are often salvageable and deserve an aggressive approach with prompt institution of ECMO if conventional resuscitative measures fail. Rapid institution of circulatory support with modified ECMO systems can be life-saving with preservation of end-organ function in these patients.

ECMO for the treatment of acute fulminant myocarditis

Indications for the institution of ECMO in patients with myocarditis should be based on the clinical response to ICU management. Most patients that are considered for ECMO support are receiving high dose inotrope infusions with endotracheal intubation and muscle paralysis. If evidence of low cardiac output persists—clinically manifested as oliguria, poor cutaneous perfusion, and hypotension—despite routine measures, ECMO should be strongly considered. The need for escalating inotrope doses accompanied by significant ventricular ectopy is an especially lethal combination that suggests that mechanical circulatory support will be required, due to the tendency of these patients to develop sudden, intractable ventricular fibrillation. After ECMO is instituted, these patients are especially likely to develop left-sided cardiac distension and pulmonary edema due to the profound nature of their ventricular dysfunction.

The survival rate for children who require mechanical circulatory support for myocarditis is relatively good.[17,54,58,59,61,71,72] The ELSO Registry reports that myocarditis has the highest survival of any diagnostic group requiring ECMO, with 57% of patients successfully weaned from support.[8] A recent multi-institutional review of 15 patients with viral myocarditis supported by ECMO (12) or VAD (3) demonstrated an overall survival rate of 80%.[53] In this review, 9 of 15 patients were weaned from support, with 7 survivors (78%); the remaining 6 were successfully bridged to transplantation, with 5 survivors (83%). An especially important finding was that all non-transplanted survivors are currently alive with normal ventricular function. Two recent reports further emphasize the likelihood of recovery for these patients with survival rates of 73% and 100%; none of the patients in these 2 series required transplantation, and all survivors currently demonstrate normal ventricular function.[73,74] Historically, it was believed that a significant percentage of children with acute myocarditis would be expected to develop dilated cardiomyopathy with the ultimate need for cardiac transplantation; however, these studies suggest that children with acute fulminant myocarditis have an overall favorable outcome and a significant degree of disease reversibility if successfully supported during the acute phase of illness.

The reasons for better long-term outcomes and a decreased incidence of progression to dilated cardiomyopathy in patients most severely affected with myocarditis remain unknown; however, mechanical circulatory support may contribute to the improved long-term outcomes in these children. In patients with dilated cardiomyopathy, prolonged mechanical circulatory support may result in ultimate recovery of ventricular function due to favorable influences on the neurohormonal cardiovascular milieu and unloading of the left ventricle resulting in normalization of ventricular geometry through "reverse remodeling".[75] The institution of mechanical circulatory support in patients with acute fulminant myocarditis favorably impacts these same factors, resulting in ventricular recovery over a much shorter time course—a

process we described as "rapid reverse remodeling".[53] In these most severe cases of myocarditis, mechanical circulatory support provides the ultimate form of physiologic rest, similar to the simple bed rest and oxygen used to support less severe cases. It is compelling to speculate that normalization of ventricular geometry and function by the early institution of support may help to prevent the development of dilated cardiomyopathy.

Based on these results, the optimal approach for children presenting with acute fulminant myocarditis may be to provide mechanical circulatory support, even if required for prolonged periods, in anticipation of eventual ventricular recovery. Previous reports have documented full return of ventricular function in young adults with myocarditis after weeks or months of mechanical support.[56,76] Pulsatile paracorporeal or implantable VAD systems which allow extended periods of support have been used successfully in pediatric patients in Europe and have demonstrated the feasibility of this approach.[77,78] Prolonged mechanical circulatory support in a larger number of pediatric patients with fulminant myocarditis may reveal that support of these children for weeks or months will allow the return of native ventricular function, thereby avoiding transplantation, in virtually all of these children.

ECMO for patient transport

While it was previously believed to be too complex to provide ECMO support during transport, the use of ECMO for the transport of critically ill patients is now routinely performed at some highly specialized centers. Foley et al. described the University of Michigan experience with 100 patients who were transported on ECMO.[79] This experience included both adult and pediatric patients, and involved patients who required support for pulmonary as well as cardiac disease. This report detailed the technical aspects of establishing a successful ECMO transport program. For example, the transport team was comprised of 2 flight nurses, 1 ECMO specialist, and 1 ECMO surgical fellow. Most cases could be transported via ground ambulance; however, specially configured helicopters or jet aircraft were also used. Complications were experienced in 17% of transported patients, most commonly related to power failure of the circuit; however, all patients survived transport and 78% survived to hospital discharge.

Summary

The approach for children with complex cardiac disease has required the development of innovative measures to help ensure successful outcomes. The utilization of ECMO for cardiac support was a logical progression in pediatric centers after its widespread and highly successful treatment of neonatal respiratory failure. The ability to provide cardiac as well as respiratory support has been an important adjunct in the development of pediatric cardiology and cardiac surgery. It would be no overstatement to claim that a consistently successful surgical or medical approach to many of these cardiac lesions requires the availability of ECMO. This chapter has attempted to highlight important clinical and technical aspects of ECMO used for circulatory support in children. The topics of current importance should be appreciated in terms of their impact on the future of our field—innovative approaches to mechanical circulatory support for children, including the use of miniaturized VAD systems and even artificial heart technology—will become a reality. The principles employed presently in the application of ECMO to support the failing circulation in children will serve as the foundation for developing innovative circulatory support techniques for the future.

References

1. Park SJ, Tector A, Piccioni W, et al. Left ventricular assist devices as destination therapy: A new look at survival. *J Thorac Cardiovasc Surg* 2005; 129:9-17.

2. Rose EA, Gelijns AC, Moskowitz AJ, et al. Long term mechanical left ventricular assistance for end-stage heart failure. *N Engl J Med* 2001; 345:1435-1443.

3. Baffes TG, Fridman JL, Bicoff JP, Whitehill JL. Extracorporeal circulation for support of palliative cardiac surgery in infants. *Ann Thorac Surg* 1970; 10:354-363.

4. Soeter JR, Mamiya RT, Sprague AY, McNamara JJ. Prolonged extracorporeal oxygenation for cardiorespiratory failure after tetralogy correction. *J Thorac Cardiovasc Surg* 1973; 66:214-218.

5. Bartlett RH, Gazzaniga AB, Fong SW, Burns NE. Prolonged extracorporeal cardiopulmonary support in man. *J Thorac Cardiovasc Surg* 1974; 68:918-932.

6. Bartlett RH, Gazzaniga AB, Fong SW, Jefferies MR, Roohk HV, Haiduc N. Extracorporeal membrane oxygenator support for cardiopulmonary failure. *J Thorac Cardiovasc Surg* 1977; 73:375-386.

7. Hill JD, de Leval MR, Fallat RJ, et al. Acute respiratory insufficiency treatment with prolonged extracorporeal oxygenation. *J Thorac Cardiovasc Surg* 1972; 64:551-562.

8. ELSO Registry. Ann Arbor, MI: Extracorporeal Life Support Organization; January, 2005.

9. Duncan BW, Hraska V, Jonas RA, et al. Mechanical circulatory support in children with cardiac disease. *J Thorac Cardiovasc Surg* 1999; 117:529-542.

10. Trittenwein G, Furst G, Golej J, et al. Preoperative ECMO in congenital cyanotic heart disease using the AREC system. *Ann Thorac Surg* 1997; 63:1298-1302.

11. Chevalier JY, Couprie C, Larroquet M, Re-nolleau S, Durandy Y, Costil J. Venovenous single lumen cannula extracorporeal lung support in neonates. *ASAIO J* 1993; 39: M654-658.

12. Trittenwein G, Golej J, Burda G, et al. Neonatal and pediatric extracorporeal membrane oxygenation using nonocclusive blood pumps: the Vienna experience. *Artif Organs* 2001; 25:994-999.

13. Del Nido PJ. Extracorporeal membrane oxygenation for cardiac support in children. *Ann Thorac Surg* 1996; 61:336-339.

14. Langley SM, Sheppard SB, Tsang VT, Mon-ro JL, Lamb RK. When is extracorporeal life support worthwhile following repair of congenital heart disease in children? *Euro J Cardiothorac Surg* 1998; 13:520-525.

15. Saito A, Miyamura H, Kanazawa H, Ohzeki H, Eguchi S. Extracorporeal membrane oxygenation for severe heart failure after Fontan operation. *Ann Thorac Surg* 1993; 55:153-155.

16. Willms DC, Atkins PJ, Dembitsky WP, Jaski BE, Gocka I. Analysis of clinical trends in a program of emergent ECLS for cardiovascular collapse. *ASAIO J* 1997; 43:65-68.

17. Black MD, Coles JG, Williams WG, et al. Determinants of success in pediatric cardiac patients undergoing extracorporeal membrane oxygenation. *Ann Thorac Surg* 1995; 60:133-138.

18. Dalton HJ, Siewers RD, Fuhrman BP, et al. Extracorporeal membrane oxygenation for cardiac rescue in children with severe myocardial dysfunction. *Crit Care Med* 1993; 21:1020-1028.

19. Kanter KR, Pennington DG, Weber TR, Zambie MA, Braun P, Martychenko V. Extracorporeal membrane oxygenation for postoperative cardiac support in children. *J Thorac Cardiovasc Surg* 1987; 93:27-35.

20. Klein MD, Shaheen KW, Whittlesey GC, Pinsky WW, Arciniegas E. Extracorporeal membrane oxygenation for the circulatory support of children after repair of congenital heart disease. *J Thorac Cardiovasc Surg* 1990; 100:498-505.

21. Hirschl RB. Devices. In: Zwischenberger JB, Bartlett RH, eds. ECMO: Extracorporeal cardiopulmonary support in critical care. 2 ed. Ann Arbor, Michigan: ELSO, 1995:150-190.

22. Anderson HL, Attori RJ, Custer JR, Chapman RA, Bartlett RH. Extracorporeal membrane oxygenation for pediatric cardiopulmonary failure. *J Thorac Cardiovasc Surg* 1990; 99:1011-1021.

23. Delius RE, Bove EL, Meliones JN, et al. Use of extracorporeal life support in patients with congenital heart disease. *Crit Care Med* 1992; 20:1216-1222.

24. Raithel RC, Pennington DG, Boegner E, Fiore A, Weber TR. Extracorporeal membrane oxygenation in children after cardiac surgery. *Circulation* 1992; 86:II-305-II310.

25. Wilson JM, Bower LK, Fackler JC, Beals DA, Berhus BO, Kevy SB. Aminocaproic acid decreases the incidence of intracranial hemorrhage and other hemorrhagic complications of ECMO. *J Pediatr Surg* 1993; 28:536-541.

26. Horwitz JR, Cofer BR, Warner BH, Cheu HW, Lally KP. A multi-center trial of 6-aminocaproic acid (Amicar) in the prevention of bleeding in infants on ECMO. *J Pediatr Surg* 1998; 33:1610-1613.

27. Downard CD, Betit P, Chang RW, Garza JJ, Arnold JH, Wilson JM. Impact of AMICAR on hemorrhagic complications of ECMO: a ten-year review. *J Pediatr Surg* 2003; 38:1212-1216.

28. Ziomek S, Harrell JE, Fasules JW, et al. Extracorporeal membrane oxygenation for cardiac failure after congenital heart operation. *Ann Thorac Surg* 1992; 54:861-868.

29. Koenig PR, Ralston MA, Kimball TR, Meyer RA, Daniels SR, Schwartz DC. Bal-

loon atrial septostomy for left ventricular decompression in patients receiving extracorporeal membrane oxygenation for myocardial failure. *J Pediatr* 1993; 122: S95-99.

30. O'Connor TA, Downing GJ, Ewing LL, Gowdamarajan R. Echocardiographically guided balloon atrial septostomy during extracorporeal membrane oxygenation (ECMO). *Pediatr Cardiol* 1993; 14:167-168.

31. Kinsella JP, Gerstmann DR, Rosenberg AA. The effect of extracorporeal membrane oxygenation on coronary perfusion and regional blood flow distribution. *Pediatr Res* 1992; 31:80-84.

32. Secker-Walker JS, Edmonds JF, Spratt EH, Conn AW. The source of coronary perfusion during partial bypass for extracorporeal membrane oxygenation (ECMO). *Ann Thorac Surg* 1976; 21:138-143.

33. Walters HL, Hakimi M, Rice MD, Lyons JM, Whittlesey GC, Klein MD. Pediatric cardiac surgical ECMO: Multivariate analysis of risk factors for hospital death. *Ann Thorac Surg* 1995; 60:329-337.

34. Meliones JN, Custer JR, Snedecor S, Moler FW, O'Rourke PP, Delius RE. Extracorporeal life support for cardiac assist in pediatric patients. *Circulation* 1991; 84 :168-172.

35. Duncan BW. Mechanical circulatory support for infants and children with cardiac disease. *Ann Thorac Surg* 2002; 73:1670-1677.

36. Hunkeler NM, Canter CE, Donze A, Spray TL. Extracorporeal life support in cyanotic congenital heart disease before cardiovascular operation. *Am J Cardiol* 1992; 69:790-793.

37. Rogers AJ, Trento A, Siewers RD, et al. Extracorporeal membrane oxygenation for postcardiotomy cardiogenic shock in children. *Ann Thorac Surg* 1989; 47:903-906.

38. Weinhaus L, Canter C, Noetzel M, McAlister W, Spray TL. Extracorporeal membrane oxygenation for circulatory support after repair of congenital heart defects. *Ann Thorac Surg* 1989; 48:206-212.

39. Goldman AP, Delius RE, Deanfield JE, de Leval MR, Sigston PE, Macrae DJ. Nitric oxide might reduce the need for extracorporeal support in children with critical postoperative pulmonary hypertension. *Ann Thorac Surg* 1996; 62:750-755.

40. Journois D, Pouard P, Mauriat P, Malhere T, Vouhe P, Safran D. Inhaled nitric oxide as a therapy for pulmonary hypertension after operations for congenital heart defects. *J Thorac Cardiovasc Surg* 1994; 107:1129-1135.

41. Kocis KC, Meliones JN, Dekeon MK, Callow LB, Lupinetti JM, Bove EL. High-frequency jet ventilation for respiratory failure after congenital heart surgery. *Circulation* 1992; 86:II127-132.

42. Aharon AS, Drinkwater DC, Jr., Churchwell KB, et al. Extracorporeal membrane oxygenation in children after repair of congenital cardiac lesions. *Ann Thorac Surg* 2001; 72:2095-101.

43. Darling EM, Kaemmer D, Lawson DS, Jaggers JJ, Ungerleider RM. Use of ECMO without the oxygenator to provide ventricular support after Norwood Stage I procedures. *Ann Thorac Surg* 2001; 71:735-736.

44. Pizarro C, Davis DA, Healy RM, Kerins PJ, Norwood WI. Is there a role for extracorporeal life support after stage I Norwood? *Euro J Cardiothorac Surg* 2001; 19:294-301.

45. Booth KL, Roth SJ, Thiagarajan RR, Almodovar MC, del Nido PJ, Laussen PC. Extracorporeal membrane oxygenation support of the Fontan and bidirectional Glenn circulations. *Ann Thorac Surg* 2004; 77:1341-1348.

46. Duncan BW. Mechanical circulatory support in infants and children with cardiac disease. In: Zwischenberger JB, Bartlett RH, eds. ECMO Extracorporeal Cardio-

pulmonary Support in Critical Care. Ann Arbor, Michigan: ELSO, 2000.

47. Ferrazzi P, Glauber M, DiDomenico A, et al. Assisted circulation for myocardial recovery after repair of congenital heart disease. *Euro J Cardiothorac Surg* 1991; 5:419-424.

48. Trento A, Thompson A, Siewers RD, et al. Extracorporeal membrane oxygenation in children. *J Thorac Cardiovasc Surg* 1988; 96:542-547.

49. Johnson TR, Schamberger MS, Hart JC, Turrentine MW, Brown JW. After repair, atrioventricular valve regurgitation during cardiac extracorporeal membrane oxygenation predicts survival. *Ann Thorac Surg* 2003; 76:848-852.

50. Kolovos NS, Bratton SL, Moler FW, et al. Outcome of pediatric patients treated with extracorporeal life support after cardiac surgery. *Ann Thorac Surg* 2003; 76:1435-1441.

51. Morris MC, Ittenbach RF, Godinez RI, et al. Risk factors for mortality in 137 pediatric cardiac intensive care unit patients managed with extracorporeal membrane oxygenation. *Crit Care Med* 2004; 32:1061-1069.

52. Undar A, McKenzie ED, McGarry MC, et al. Outcomes of congenital heart surgery patients after extracorporeal life support at Texas Children's Hospital. *Artif Organs* 2004; 28:963-966.

53. Duncan BW, Bohn DJ, Atz AM, French JW, Laussen PC, Wessel DL. Mechanical circulatory support for the treatment of children with acute fulminant myocarditis. *J Thorac Cardiovasc Surg* 2001; 122:440-448.

54. Frazier EA, Faulkner SC, Seib PM, Harrell JE, Van Devanter SH, Fasules JW. Prolonged extracorporeal life support for bridging to transplant. *Perfusion* 1997; 12:93-98.

55. Helman DN, Addonizio LJ, Morales DLS, et al. Implantable left ventricular assist devices can successfully bridge adolescent patients to transplant. *J Heart Lung Transplant* 2000; 19:121-126.

56. Holman WL, Bourge RC, Kirklin JK. Circulatory support for seventy days with resolution of acute heart failure. *J Thorac Cardiovasc Surg* 1991; 102:932-934.

57. Kato S, Marimoto S, Hiramitsu S, Nomura M, Ito T, Hishida H. Use of percutaneous cardiopulmonary support of patients with fulminant myocarditis and cardiogenic shock for improving prognosis. *Am J Cardiol* 1999; 85:623-625.

58. Kawahito K, Murata S, Yasu T, et al. Usefulness of extracorporeal membrane oxygenation for treatment of fulminant myocarditis and circulatory collapse. *Am J Cardiol* 1998; 82:910-911.

59. Martin J, Sarai K, Schindler M, Van de Loo A, Yoshitake M, Beyersdorf F. Medos HIA-VAD biventricular assist device for bridge to recovery in fulminant myocarditis. *Ann Thorac Surg* 1997; 63:1145-1146.

60. Ibrahim AE, Duncan BW, Blume ED, Jonas RA. Long term follow-up of pediatric cardiac patients requiring mechanical circulatory support. *Ann Thorac Surg* 2000; 69:186-192.

61. del Nido PJ, Armitage JM, Fricker FJ, et al. Extracorporeal membrane oxygenation support as a bridge to pediatric heart transplantation. *Circulation* 1994; 90:II66-69.

62. Fiser WP, Yetman AT, Gunselman RJ, et al. Pediatric arteriovenous extracorporeal membrane oxygenation (ECMO) as a bridge to cardiac transplantation. *J Heart Lung Transplant* 2003; 22:770-777.

63. Gajarski RJ, Mosca RS, Ohye RG, et al. Use of extracorporeal life support as a bridge to pediatric cardiac transplantation. *J Heart Lung Transplant* 2003; 22:28-34.

64. Levi D, Marelli D, Plunkett M, et al. Use of assist devices and ECMO to bridge pediatric patients with cardiomyopathy to transplantation. *J Heart Lung Transplant* 2002; 21:760-770.

65. Reddy SL, Hasan A, Hamilton LR, et al. Mechanical versus medical bridge to transplantation in children. What is the best timing for mechanical bridge? *Eur J Cardiothorac Surg* 2004; 25:605-609.

66. Galantowicz ME, Stolar CJH. Extracorporeal membrane oxygenation for perioperative support in pediatric heart transplantation. *J Thorac Cardiovasc Surg* 1991; 102:148-152.

67. Delius RE, Zwischenberger JB, Cilley R, et al. Prolonged extracorporeal life support of pediatric and adolescent cardiac transplant patients. *Ann Thorac Surg* 1990; 50:791-795.

68. del Nido PJ, Dalton HJ, Thompson AE, Siewers RD. Extracorporeal membrane oxygenator rescue in children during cardiac arrest after cardiac surgery. *Circulation* 1992; 86:II300-304.

69. Duncan BW, Ibrahim AE, Hraska V, et al. Use of rapid-deployment extracorporeal membrane oxygenation for the resuscitation of pediatric patients with heart disease after cardiac arrest. *J Thorac Cardiovasc Surg* 1998; 116:305-311.

70. Jacobs JP, Ojito JW, McConaghey TW, et al. Rapid cardiopulmonary support for children with complex congenital heart disease. *Ann Thorac Surg* 2000; 70:742-750.

71. Cofer BR, Warner BW, Stallion A, Ryckman FC. Extracorporeal membrane oxygenation in the management of cardiac failure secondary to myocarditis. *J Pediatr Surg* 1993; 28:669-672.

72. Grundl PD, Miller SA, del Nido PJ, Beerman LB, Fuhrman BP. Successful treatment of acute myocarditis using extracorporeal membrane oxygenation. *Crit Care Med* 1993; 21:302-304.

73. Chen YS, Yu HY, Huang SC, et al. Experience and result of extracorporeal membrane oxygenation in treating fulminant myocarditis with shock: What mechanical support should be considered first? *J Heart Lung Transplant* 2005; 24:81-87.

74. Grinda JM, Chevalier P, D'Attellis N, et al. Fulminant myocarditis in adults and children: bi-ventricular assist device for recovery. *Eur J Cardiothorac Surg* 2004; 26:1169-1173.

75. Levin GR, Oz MC, Chen JM, Packer M, Rose EA, Burkhoff D. Reversal of chronic ventricular dilation in patients with end-stage cardiomyopathy by prolonged mechanical unloading. *Circulation* 1995; 91:2717-2720.

76. Levin HR, Oz MC, Catanese KA, Rose EA, Burkhoff D. Transient normalization of systolic and diastolic function after support with a left ventricular assist device in a patient with dilated cardiomyopathy. *J Heart Lung Transplant* 1996; 15:840-842.

77. Konertz W, Hotz H, Schneider M, Redlin M, Reul H. Clinical experience with the MEDOS HIA-VAD system in infants and children. *Ann Thorac Surg* 1997; 63:1138-1144.

78. Stiller B, Dahnert I, Weng Y, Hennig E, Hetzer R, Lange PE. Children may survive severe myocarditis with prolonged use of biventricular assist devices. *Heart* 1999; 82:237-240.

79. Foley DS, Pranikoff T, Younger JG, et al. A review of 100 patients transported on extracorporeal life support. *ASAIO J* 2002; 48:612-619.

29

Venoarterial Perfusion for Resuscitation and Cardiac Procedures: Cardiopulmonary Support

Susan P. Tourner, M.D. and Stephen J. Roth, M.D., M.P.H.

Introduction

Cardiopulmonary support (CPS), which is designated alternatively as extracorporeal cardiopulmonary resuscitation (eCPR), is an extracorporeal life support system for the short-term treatment of life-threatening cardiorespiratory emergencies. In pediatric applications, it is also referred to as rapid-deployment or rapid response ECLS. As a resuscitative technique, CPS relies on portability, rapid deployment, and percutaneous vessel cannulation to restore adequate tissue perfusion and oxygen delivery emergently after cardiovascular collapse. Deployment in hospital settings outside of the ICU, such as the emergency department, has proven to be feasible in resuscitations of adults in cardiogenic shock.[1] The portability of CPS systems allows for safer and easier patient transports for diagnostic testing, interventions in the OR or catheterization laboratory, and for inter-hospital transport.

The principal components of a CPS system are a centrifugal blood pump and hollow-fiber oxygenator. Together these can support both right and left heart function as well as gas exchange. CPS differs from other forms of extracorporeal support including cardiopulmonary bypass (CPB) and ECMO. CPB is a more complex pump and membrane oxygenator system used in the OR that can provide complete

cardiorespiratory support during cardiothoracic procedures. CPS is similar to venoarterial (VA) ECMO in that both are comprised of a pump and oxygenator system adapted for bedside use, but an ECMO circuit is larger, is often fitted with a roller instead of a centrifugal pump, and is designed to support patients for longer periods because the membrane oxygenator can function effectively for days versus only 6-24 hours for a hollow-fiber oxygenator.

Because a typical ECMO circuit contains more tubing and larger components than a CPS system, it may take up to 45 minutes for an experienced operator to assemble the circuit and prime it with fluid. To reduce this set-up time, some institutions have developed and maintained crystalloid-primed ECMO circuits for rapid-deployment that are stored in the ICU. For smaller pediatric patients, blood priming is often preferred to avoid marked hemodilution when circuit flow is initiated. Depending on the availability of blood products, blood priming may delay the initiation of support. In contrast, CPS circuits are designed for an asanguinous prime. Assembling and priming the circuit can take as little as 5 minutes, so the initiation of flow is possible within 5-15 minutes if the cannulas are in position.[2,3]

CPS is used in adults as a resuscitative tool for cardiac arrest refractory to standard advanced cardiac life support measures, as a short-term therapy for cardiogenic shock, as short-term support to allow myocardial recovery following cardiotomy, and as a temporary bridge to cardiac transplantation. CPS has also emerged as an elective mechanical support strategy during procedures that are likely to precipitate hemodynamic instability in patients with compromised myocardial function. In pediatrics, the use of CPS and rapid-deployment ECMO have increased significantly over the past 10 years, especially for cardiac patients. Many pediatric centers with significant experience in mechanical circulatory support have developed rapid-deployment ECMO as opposed to CPS for cardiopulmonary resuscitation.[4]

Equipment

The equipment for adult CPS is organized on a mobile cart that includes a centrifugal pump, hollow-fiber oxygenator, heat exchanger, back-up battery, ⅜-inch venous quick prime tubing, arterial tubing, and percutaneous arterial and venous cannulas. The entire circuit may be heparin-coated. Pre-packaged systems are available commercially. Alternatively, some institutions have elected to assemble their circuits from individual components.

When the decision is made to perform CPS, the components are assembled on the mobile cart. The oxygenator and tubing are first vacuum- and CO_2-primed to prevent bubble formation, and subsequently crystalloid-primed with a balanced electrolyte solution, calcium chloride, and human albumin. The oxygen delivery tubing is then connected, and the prime solution recirculated through the arteriovenous bridge. Ideally, red blood cells (RBCs), fresh frozen plasma (FFP) avoid additional delay in initiating flow, a circuit primed only with crystalloid may be used; colloid and other blood products are added when available. Excess fluid volume related to the prime can be removed from the patient either by exchange transfusion or by ultrafiltration once hemodynamic stability is

achieved.[5] When the arterial and venous cannulas are in place, the circuit is connected to the patient by stopping the pump, closing the arteriovenous bridge, and connecting the appropriate ends of the circuit tubing to the venous and arterial cannulas using sterile technique.

The centrifugal pump aspirates venous blood through a short length of tubing, generating flows up to 5 l/min in ideal conditions. Because the pump places continuous suction on the venous cannula, it may induce hemolysis. The blood is then pumped through the heat exchanger and the hollow-fiber oxygenator. When fully primed, these oxygenators tend to leak plasma, resulting in less effective gas exchange and limiting the circuit's effective function to 6-24 hours. Oxygenated blood is delivered back to the patient via the arterial cannula.

Vascular access

Vascular access is most often performed simultaneously with circuit assembly and priming. Because a circuit can be readied in 5-15 minutes, inserting the cannulas frequently becomes the rate-limiting step in initiating CPS. In cardiothoracic surgery patients who have undergone a recent sternotomy, the sternum can be reopened and the right atrium and aorta cannulated directly. In other patients, vascular access is achieved percutaneously using the modified-Seldinger technique. If a central venous and/or arterial catheter already exists, the catheter can be exchanged over a guide wire for a CPS cannula. If percutaneous methods are unsuccessful, a surgical cutdown can be performed.

Percutaneous access to the right atrium is obtained through a large vein, typically the internal jugular or femoral vein, with a CPS cannula varying between 17-23F in size. A femoral venous cannula passes through the inferior vena cava (IVC) and an internal jugular cannula traverses the superior vena cava (SVC) so that the tip of the cannula resides in the right atrium.

A transesophageal or transthoracic echocardiogram can be used to verify cannula tip location. Alternatively, the cannulas can be positioned utilizing fluoroscopy. Percutaneous access to a major artery such as the femoral artery or right common carotid artery is obtained using a 15-19F CPS cannula. The preferred location for the tip of a femoral artery cannula is the common iliac artery, whereas the target for a right common carotid artery cannula is the bifurcation of the right common carotid artery and aortic arch, with flow directed toward the descending aorta. Femoral artery cannulation can compromise limb perfusion distal to the cannula insertion site, resulting in significant leg ischemia. To prevent this complication, an additional 5F arterial catheter can be placed distally in the femoral artery to perfuse the leg.[5,6]

Because approximately half of adults who undergo CPS require conversion to longer-term mechanical support, some institutions insert ECMO cannulas in an effort to avoid the additional time and expense, as well as morbidities such as infection and bleeding, associated with repeat cannula placement.[7]

Patient management

Pump flow rate is selected to achieve adequate systemic perfusion. Mean arterial blood pressure (MAP), urine output, mixed venous O_2 saturation (SvO_2), and lactate levels are monitored to determine optimal circuit flow rates. An SvO_2 of at least 60% suggests adequate tissue oxygen delivery. A MAP of 50-80 mm Hg in adults and a MAP that is appropriate for age and size in pediatric patients is maintained using intravascular volume infusions and vasopressor and/or vasodilator agents, as needed. Both an arterial catheter and a central venous catheter are required to perform adequate bedside hemodynamic monitoring.

The waveform from an arterial catheter is monitored to assess left ventricular contractility. A stunned left ventricle may be unable to produce sufficient force to overcome the pressure generated by the pump and eject blood through the aortic valve. A poorly-contractile left ventricle may become progressively distended over time, resulting in myocardial ischemia, pulmonary venous hypertension and pulmonary edema, and an increased risk of ventricular thrombus. To restore pulsatility, volume expansion is indicated when central venous pressure (CVP) is low, and inotropic support is appropriate if the CVP is normal or elevated. If pulsatility cannot be restored and the aortic valve does not open, percutaneous balloon atrial septostomy should be performed by an interventional cardiologist to relieve left heart distension.[2,8] This problem can potentially be avoided by implanting an intra-aortic balloon pump (IABP) prior to CPS cannulation.[9]

Adequate mechanical ventilatory support to maintain a normal pulmonary venous oxygen level is important to preserve adequate coronary and cerebral oxygen delivery. A ventilatory strategy with high positive end expiratory pressure (PEEP) is commonly employed to minimize pulmonary edema and atelectasis, which can delay weaning and separation from the circuit. Typical mechanical ventilator settings are: peak inspiratory pressure (PIP) of 30 cm H_2O, a PEEP of 10 cm H_2O, rate of 6 breaths/minute, and FiO_2 of 0.5.

Systemic anticoagulation is required to prevent thrombus formation in non-heparin-bonded circuits, and heparin is the most common anticoagulant used. The standard test for monitoring the degree of anticoagulation produced by heparin is the activated clotting time (ACT). During cannulation, an IV heparin bolus of ~100 units/kg is administered to achieve an ACT of ~300 seconds. After the patient is connected to the circuit, a heparin infusion is initiated and adjusted to maintain an ACT of 180-220 seconds. If hemorrhage occurs, a lower ACT range of 160-200 seconds is targeted. If hemorrhage persists, as it may immediately after a surgical procedure, epsilon-aminocaproic acid (Amicar,

Xanodyne Pharmaceuticals, Florence, KY) can be administered. Heparin must be continued during treatment with epsilon-aminocaproic acid to prevent thrombosis. Also, as circuit flow is decreased, the target ACT range should be increased, since lower flow rates are associated with an increased risk of thrombosis.

During resuscitation, patients may sustain significant end-organ injury from ischemia. Therefore, after initiating CPS, it is important to assess the function of the kidneys, liver, and brain. Serum creatinine and urine output can reflect the degree of any renal injury; however, oliguria is common after initiation of CPS, even in those patients who subsequently regain normal kidney function. Liver enzymes, bilirubin, and coagulation parameters can reflect the extent of liver injury, but abnormal values may not develop in the immediate post-resuscitation period. It is also important whenever possible to avoid the use of neuromuscular blockade agents so that a neurologic examination can be performed. Serial electroencephalograms (EEGs) may be helpful in assessing for brain injury, but if hemorrhage or infarct is suspected, computed tomography (CT) or magnetic resonance imaging (MRI) may be required.

For patients who can be stabilized and are candidates to separate from CPS support in <24 hours, a strategy for weaning circuit flow and decannulation must be developed. Intravascular volume status and inotropic support should be optimized to achieve the best combination of preload, afterload, and contractility. A transesophageal or transthoracic echocardiogram is performed to determine the status of ventricular filling and systolic function. Mechanical ventilatory support is adjusted to achieve adequate oxygenation and ventilation. If a stable rhythm, systemic cardiac output, and gas exchange with an appropriate arterial blood pressure and SvO_2 on low-to-moderate doses of vasoactive medications and ventilator settings can be maintained as pump flow is reduced, then the patient is likely to separate successfully from CPS.[2]

If adequate recovery of cardiorespiratory function is not apparent within 6-24 hours, and particularly if the function of the hollow-fiber oxygenator is suspect, conversion to longer-term mechanical support should be considered. The possible need for and appropriateness of cardiac transplantation should also be considered at this time. In patients who have significant residual deficits in ventilation or oxygenation, VA ECMO may be required. If gas exchange is adequate and continued cardiac dysfunction is the primary problem, a ventricular assist device (VAD) or intra-aortic balloon pump (IABP) is appropriate.

Indications

CPS has been used successfully to resuscitate adults with cardiac arrest or cardiogenic shock due to acute myocardial infarction (MI) and subsequent ventricular septal or papillary muscle rupture, cardiotomy, transplant rejection, dysrhythmia, ruptured coronary artery graft, pericardial tamponade, cardiac trauma, and myocarditis. It has also been effective in patients with secondary cardiac failure due to respiratory insufficiency, hypothermic arrest from cold-water submersion, and drug overdose. The indications for CPS in cardiopulmonary resuscitation are summarized in Table 1.

Patient selection is the most important prognostic indicator.[5] The optimal adult patient is younger in age, has no major chronic illnesses, has experienced a witnessed decompensation or arrest, has curable disease, and is either in or close by the hospital. As a group, patients with cardiac disease caused by a condition that can be repaired or reversed and who have no, or minimal, co-morbidity have attained the best results. In patients who have the potential to recover, valid indications to perform CPS are the failure to achieve adequate ventilation or oxygenation with mechanical ventilatory support, correction of hypothermia, hypovolemic or cardiogenic shock, and to sustain a stable, perfusing cardiac rhythm.

Although some relative contraindications to CPS in adults have been proposed, there are few generally accepted absolute contraindications. Unwitnessed cardiac arrest, aortic valve insufficiency, aortic dissection, and terminal illness are considered by most to be contraindications (Table 2). Mortality after unwitnessed cardiac arrest is nearly 100% and has not been altered by the use of CPS.[3] Early and effective CPR can allow for neurologically-intact survivors, but this is less likely to occur in an unwitnessed arrest.[10,11] Aortic insufficiency accompanied by left ventricular dysfunction produces ventricular distension. Adverse effects of distension on subendocardial blood flow can result in additional myocardial dysfunction and the inability to separate from CPS.[2] Irreversible organ dysfunction such as portal hypertension with cirrhosis or pulmonary vascular obstructive disease are contraindications because CPS will not improve the underlying pathology and thus alter the patient's ultimate outcome.[3,5]

Table 1. Indications for Adult CPS.

Indications
Resuscitation
Cardiac arrest
Cardiogenic shock
Cardiac trauma
Respiratory insufficiency
Status asthmaticus
Smoke inhalation
Drug overdose
Pulmonary edema
Massive pulmonary embolism
Hypothermia
Procedural support
Angioplasty
Arrhythmia ablation
Pulmonary embolectomy
Coronary artery bypass grafting
Cerebral arteriovenous malformation resection
Donor heart preservation
Abdominal aortic graft replacement
Tracheal reconstruction
Ventricular assist device placement

Renal failure, hepatic failure, and significant neurologic disease are relative contraindications, depending on the existence of other therapeutic options and the degree of dysfunction. A recent cerebrovascular accident, major head trauma, and active bleeding were previously considered absolute contraindications to CPS due to the need for systemic anticoagulation. However, with the development of heparin-bonded circuits that allow for less systemic anticoagulation, CPS may be contemplated.[3]

Cardiac arrest and shock

Cardiac arrest and shock are the most common indications for CPS in adults. Outcomes of conventional cardiopulmonary resuscitation (CPR), including defibrillation and external cardiac massage, are poor with mortality approaching 100%.[3] Survival with meaningful neurologic function is <5% if cardiac arrest occurs outside the hospital and 5-15% inside the hospital.[8,12] In addition, patients who undergo CPR for >30 minutes have decreased hospital survival compared to those with <30 minutes of CPR[10,12,13] (Table 3). Early implementation of CPS can improve the survival rate to as much as 30-40%, as described in multiple published series (Table 4) and the ELSO Registry (Table 5).

Survival is impacted by the ability to quickly correct the pathology leading to cardiac arrest or shock. CPS can be therapeutic by providing adequate cardio-respiratory support to the body

Table 2. Contraindications for Adult CPS.

Contraindications
Unwitnessed cardiac arrest
Aortic insufficiency
Aortic dissection
Cardiac arrest >30 minutes
No correctable anatomic defect
Terminal illness
Diabetes mellitus
Peripheral vascular disease
Recent cerebrovascular accident

Table 3. Survival from cardiac arrest following CPR for ≤ 30 minutes vs. >30 minutes in adults.

Author	CPR ≤30 min Total	CPR ≤30 min Survivors	CPR >30 min Total	CPR >30 min Survivors	Unwitnessed Total	Unwitnessed Survivors
Hill[10] (1992)	54	14 (26%)	56	8 (15%)	10	0 (0%)
Willms[12] (1997)	44	15 (34%)	21	1 (5%)	–	–
Chen[13] (2003)	2	2 (100%)	55	16 (29%)	–	–

Table 4. Survivors of cardiac arrest and cardiac shock resuscitated with ECLS.

Author	Cardiac arrest Total N	Died on CPS	Died after CPS	Survival n	Survival (%)	Cardiac shock Total N	Died on CPS	Died after CPS	Survival n	Survival (%)
Younger[8] (1999)	21	8	4	9	(42.9)					
Hill[10] (1992)	125	100	6	17	(13.6)	44	25	0	17	(38.6)
von Segesser[32] (1999)	386	–	–	142	(36.8)	328	–	–	132	(40.2)
Potapov[7] (2003)						12	5	1	6	(50)
Willms[12] (1997)	68	–	–	17	(25)	13	–	–	3	(23.1)
Schwarz[5] (2003)	17	8	6	3	(17.6)	24	5	8	10	(41.7)
Aiba[14] (2001)						26	17	4	5	(19.2)
Sunami[18] (2003)	2	0	0	2	(100)					
Martin[1] (1998)	10	3	7	0	(0)					
Aliabadi[17] (1996)	2	0	0	2	(100)					
Mair[6] (1996)	3	0	1	2	(66.7)	2	1	0	1	(50)
Grambow[26] (1994)	7	7	0	0	(0)	23	10	7	6	(26.1)
Kitamura[23] (1999)						64	23	16	25	(39.1)
Rousou[24] (1994)	16	–	–	9	(56.3)					
Kawahito[25] (1994)	13	3	5	5	(38.5)					
Orime[9] (1998)						20	13	0	7	(35)
Noon[46] (1999)						141	64	46	31	(22)
Chen[13] (2003)	57	19	19	18	(31.6)					
Massetti[47] (2005)	40	23	9	8	(20)					
Total	**767**	**171**	**57**	**234**	**30.5**	**697**	**163**	**82**	**243**	**34.9**

Table 5. Adult CPS and pediatric eCPR survival as reported in ELSO Registry (1994-July 2005).

Year	Adult Total patients (>16 years)	Adult Survival n	Adult Survival (%)	Pediatric Total patients (≤16 years)	Pediatric Survival n	Pediatric Survival (%)
1994	0	0	(0)	1	1	(100)
1995	1	0	(0)	6	2	(33.3)
1996	2	1	(50)	3	2	(66.7)
1997	1	0	(0)	4	1	(25)
1998	12	5	(41.7)	27	8	(29.6)
1999	14	1	(7.1)	50	20	(66.7)
2000	35	11	(31.4)	70	29	(41.4)
2001	17	9	(26.9)	77	23	(29.9)
2002	26	7	(26.9)	87	39	(44.8)
2003	32	16	(5)	113	50	(44.2)
2004	34	7	(20.6)	119	51	(42.9)
2005 (Jan-Jul)	3	0	(0)	46	13	(28.3)
Total	**177**	**57**	**(32.2)**	**603**	**239**	**(39.6)**

during a limited period of time when the heart and lungs are improving from insults such as significant hypothermia, acute lung injury, or a severe metabolic disorder. CPS also improves survival in patients who experience cardiac arrest related to an anatomic lesion that can be corrected or palliated by an intervention. In one series, survival in patients who arrested because of non-anatomic disease was only 13.9% compared with 35.6% when a therapeutic intervention could be performed.[10]

Acute myocardial infarction

Cardiogenic shock is the leading cause of death in adult patients hospitalized for acute MI. Compared with IABP, CPS is a superior resuscitation technique, however, mortality remains high. The severity of shock associated with MI is the most important factor that predicts prognosis. Scoring systems for shock severity based upon systolic blood pressure, heart rate, hourly urine output, base excess, and mental status have been developed and used to classify shock as either mild, moderate, or severe.[14,15] Survival in moderate shock has been reported to be 5% when IABP is used for resuscitation compared to 38% with CPS; however, mortality in severe shock was 100% for both interventions.[14] CPS alone has a limited effect on outcome, but when combined with emergency coronary revascularization by angioplasty, it may improve survival. The hemodynamic impact of CPS is potentially limited in this setting because coronary perfusion may continue to be impaired. Blood returning to the right atrium bypasses the pulmonary circulation and returns instead to a peripheral artery, thereby increasing afterload on the myocardium without improving coronary blood flow. The diastolic pressure generated is likely to be insufficient to perfuse the myocardium adequately. This may explain why the concomitant use of IABP with CPS improves survival in patients with cardiogenic shock.[14]

Each year in the U.S., 25,000 deaths are attributed to post-infarction mechanical disruption of the myocardium, including the ventricular free wall, septum, and papillary muscles. After acute MI, 2% of patients develop ventricular septal rupture and 1% develop papillary muscle rupture with mortality approaching 80%.[16] CPS can be an effective bridge to more definitive treatment. In one case, a large apical ventricular septal defect was detected during percutaneous transluminal coronary angioplasty (PTCA) to open an occluded right coronary artery.[17] The patient developed pulseless ventricular tachycardia and received CPR for 5 minutes prior to the institution of CPS. Surgical repair in the OR resulted in full recovery.

Ventricular fibrillation

Intraoperative cardiac arrest victims are excellent candidates for CPS because the arrest is witnessed and CPR can be immediate. CPS can provide effective support during transient, unstable dysrhythmias refractory to conventional CPR techniques including antiarrhythmic medications and defibrillation. A report of 2 patients demonstrated the utility of CPS in ventricular fibrillation (VF) during general anesthesia for non-cardiac procedures.[18] Both patients had pre-existing cardiac disease and developed refractory VF in the OR. CPR was administered for 30-35 minutes until CPS could be initiated, and both patients had successful resuscitations with intact survival.

Drug overdose

CPS can be a beneficial temporizing measure in massive drug overdose.[11,19] Adequate tissue perfusion and oxygen delivery can be maintained until the drug is metabolized or eliminated, allowing for effective resuscitation. A case report of a successful resuscitation in a patient who intentionally ingested verapamil is an example of this application of CPS.[11] The patient developed refractory electromechanical dissociation (EMD) in an emergency department and underwent CPR for 2.5 hours until CPS could be initiated. After >6 hours on the circuit, a spontaneous circulation returned and the patient was successfully weaned off CPS within several hours. Full recovery of cardiac function occurred, and remarkably, without apparent neurologic deficit.

Cold water submersion

One exception to the contraindication of CPS in unwitnessed cardiac arrest is cold-water submersion with hypothermia. Hypothermia has a neuroprotective effect if it precedes hypoxia, so delay to initiation of CPR can still result in survival with a good neurologic outcome.[20] Severe hypothermia with core temperature <28°C results in cardiac arrest in 90% of cases.[21] During rewarming the most common cause of death is circulatory collapse and ventricular dysrhythmia. Passive rewarming is associated with profound hypotension due to decreased systemic vascular resistance and cardiac dysfunction; rewarming shock has mortality rates of 30-80%.[22] CPS can stabilize the cerebral and peripheral vasculature and enable controlled, active rewarming. The optimal rate of rewarming is unknown, but rates of 1°C every 10-30 minutes have been used. Because this injury is often unwitnessed, a heparin-coated CPS system should be used, if available, to avoid systemic anticoagulation in these patients because of the risk of associated trauma.

Post-cardiotomy myocardial failure

The incidence of post-cardiotomy myocardial failure is 2-6% in adult cardiac surgical patients.[7] Delays in the initiation of CPS have been associated with increased morbidity and mortality. For example, delay to onset of CPS has been reported to increase the incidence of biventricular vs. univentricular failure. If cardiac arrest followed, survival was reduced nearly 7-fold from 47% to 7%.[2,7] Although longer-term support is often required in post-cardiotomy myocardial failure, CPS is often the most expedient support strategy for preserving brain, kidney, and other major end-organ function. Conversion to a longer-term support system, which requires more preparation time, can be performed after stabilization with CPS.[23]

Post-operative VF and EMD are uniformly fatal when a stable rhythm and blood pressure are not restored with conventional CPR. Rousou et al. reported that 56% of a group of 16 patients survived ongoing post-operative VF or EMD when CPS was employed.[24] Similarly, 77% of a group of 13 patients described by Kawahito et al. successfully weaned off CPS after circulatory collapse from VF or EMD that was refractory to inotropic agents, IABP, and CPR.[25] These patients were managed using heparin-coated circuits plus low-dose systemic heparin while on CPS. This strategy may reduce mortality related to post-operative hemorrhage following a period of full anticoagulation on CPB.

Procedural support in the cardiac catheterization laboratory or OR

CPS has been utilized in the cardiac catheterization laboratory for resuscitation during sudden cardiovascular collapse and in both the catheterization laboratory and the OR to provide temporary support for interventional procedures. In a small, retrospective study by Grambow et al., rapid initiation of CPS (within 20 minutes) resulted in the rescue of patients in cardiogenic shock, but all patients who experienced cardiac arrest died despite CPS and further interventions.[26] Of those in shock who were initially salvaged with CPS, approximately 50% survived for 24 hours but only 25% to hospital discharge. Mortality after 24 hours was attributed to sepsis, multi-system organ dysfunction, or congestive heart failure.

Patients requiring coronary revascularization by angioplasty or surgery who have either severe left ventricular dysfunction or target vessels supplying greater than 50% of the myocardium are candidates for elective CPS. During catheterization, the contralateral femoral artery and vein are cannulated, and circuit flow is maintained either at 2 l/min or to maintain a MAP >50 mm Hg or to generate a pulmonary capillary wedge pressure >10 mm Hg while the intervention is performed.[26]

Aortic arch procedures

A CPS circuit can be used to support patients undergoing surgical interventions on the aortic arch or descending thoracic aorta. The left atrial appendage or the pulmonary vein at the left atrial junction is cannulated for "venous" access, and flow is returned either to the femoral artery or to the thoracic aorta distal to the surgical site.[27] A separate perfusion cannula to the left carotid artery can be inserted, if needed. Alternatively, vascular access can be achieved percutaneously though the femoral artery and vein, and the aorta can be exposed through a left posterolateral thoracotomy. The potential advantages proposed for a CPS-based approach compared to CPB include minimal aortic dissection, elimination of proximal and sequential aortic clamping, a bloodless field, better access to the proximal aortic arch and ascending aorta, and reduced blood loss.[28]

Complications

Bleeding and hemolysis, multi-system organ dysfunction, infection, and equipment failure are the common complications that contribute to morbidity and mortality associated with CPS in adults. The complications that have been reported to the ELSO Registry in adult patients treated with CPS are listed in Table 6, and data on complications and events reported in the ELSO Registry are shown in Table 7.

The most common complication associated with the use of CPS is bleeding from cannulation sites, with typical rates ranging from 4-14%.[3] Excessive bleeding is caused by multiple factors. Hepatic congestion and failure, malnutrition, multiple cannulation sites, low-dose anticoagulation with heparin, decreased platelet function, activation of the coagulation cascade secondary to hemolysis, and hyperfibrinolysis from contact with prosthetic surfaces all may contribute to increased bleeding. The use of heparin-coated circuits in addition to the serine protease inhibitor aprotinin and vitamin K therapies have contributed to lower bleeding rates.[2,3,26] Vena cava tears or rupture with retroperitoneal bleeding, and arterial or aortic injury

Table 6. Complications associated with ECLS.

Complications
Cannula-related
Perforated femoral or iliac artery
Retroperitoneal bleed
Aortic dissection
Limb ischemia
Poor venous drainage
Failure to cannulate
Hemorrhagic
Bleeding at cannulation site
Bleeding at surgical site
Pulmonary hemorrhage
Gastrointestinal bleeding
Cerbrovascular accident
Thromboembolic
Limb ischemia
Pulmonary infarction
Cerebrovascular accident
Insufficient perfusion
Ischemic brain injury
Renal failure
Hepatic failure
Mulit-system organ dysfunction
Technical
Equipment failure
Hemolysis
Infection
Insufficient ventricular unloading
Ventricular distension and pulmonary edema

Table 7. Complications reported to the ELSO Registry (1994-July 2005).

Complications	Pediatric n	Pediatric (%)	Adult n	Adult (%)
Mechanical				
Air in circuit	21	(3.5)	4	(2.2)
Cannula problems	68	(11.3)	13	(7.2)
Clots: Bladder	31	(5.1)		
Bridge	19	(3.2)	2	(1.1)
Hemofilter	28	(4.6)	7	(3.9)
Oxygenator	60	(10)	13	(7.2)
Other	50	(8.3)	10	(5.5)
Cracks in pigtail connectors	5	(0.8)	5	(2.8)
Heat exchanger malfunction	1	(0.2)		
Other tubing rupture	4	(0.7)	2	(1.1)
Oxygenator failure	52	(8.6)	39	(21.6)
Pump malfunction	6	(1)	1	(0.6)
Raceway rupture	3	(0.5)		
Metabolic				
Glucose <40	14	(2.3)	1	(0.6)
Glucose >240	83	(13.8)	75	(41.4)
Hyperbilirubinemia (>2 direct or >15 total)	30	(5)	14	(7.7)
pH <7.20	77	(12.8)	41	(22.7)
pH >7.60	25	(4.2)	14	(7.7)
Neurologic				
Brain death clinically determined	70	(11.6)	27	(14.9)
CNS hemorrhage by US/CT	42	(7)	1	(0.6)
CNS infarction by US/CT	43	(7.1)	24	(13.3)
Seizures				
Clinically determined	69	(11.4)	7	(3.9)
EEG determined	32	(5.3)	1	(0.6)
Pulmonary				
Pneumothorax requiring treatment	15	(2.5)	7	(3.9)
Pulmonary hemorrhage	55	(9.1)	11	(6.1)
Renal				
CAVHD required	41	(6.8)	39	(21.6)
Hemofiltration required	170	(28.2)	22	(12.1)

Table 7. Complications reported to the ELSO Registry (1994-July 2005). (Cont.)

Complications	Pediatric		Adult	
	n	(%)	n	(%)
Cardiovascular				
Cardiac arrhythmia	110	(17.3)	44	(24.3)
CPR required	48	(8)	12	(6.6)
Hypertension requiring vasodilators	74	(12.3)	13	(7.2)
Inotropes on ECLS	414	(68.7)	152	(84)
Myocardial stun by ECHO	38	(6.3)	4	(2.2)
PDA: Bidirectional	2	(0.3)		
L->R	2	(0.3)		
R->L	2	(0.3)		
Tamponade: Blood	35	(5.8)	21	(11.6)
Serous	2	(0.3)		
Hemorrhagic				
Cannulation site bleeding	105	(17.4)	40	(22.1)
Disseminated intravascular coagulation	37	(6.1)	5	(2.8)
GI hemorrhage	19	(3.2)	7	(3.9)
Hemolysis (Hgb >50 mg/dl)	75	(12.4)	28	(15.5)
Surgical site bleeding	101	(16.8)	53	(29.3)
Infectious				
Culture-proven infection	54	(9)	28	(15.5)
WBC <1,500	6	(1)		

CAVHD = continuous arteriovenous hemodialysis, CNS = central nervous system, CPR = cardiopulmonary resuscitation, CT = computed tomography, ECHO = echocardiography, EEG = electroencephalogram, GI = gastrointestinal, Hgb = hemoglobin, L = left, PDA = patent ductus arteriosus, R = right, US = ultrasound, WBC = white blood cell

including dissection and perforation that required surgical exploration and reconstruction have occurred.[4,6] Other non-cannula-related bleeding complications include pulmonary and gastrointestinal hemorrhage.[4]

Ischemic injury to the brain, kidneys, liver, and other end organs has been attributed to prolonged resuscitation as well as inadequate pump flow. Recovery from a moderate hypoxic-ischemic insult is possible for most organs; however, neurologic recovery is frequently limited. Emergency CPS and early coronary re-perfusion using PTCA can result in good myo-cardial recovery. By using mild hypothermia in conjunction with CPS during PTCA, a 2- to 5-fold increase in the rate of good neurologic recovery was achieved in a series reported by Nagao et al.[29]

Overall infection rates in temporary mechanical circulatory support have been reported to be as high as 30-40%.[2] Immobilization, poor nutritional status, and indwelling catheters and tubes are all likely to contribute to the high incidence of infection.

Although infrequent now, severe leg ischemia leading to limb amputation has occurred with femoral artery cannulation. Perfusion in the cannulated leg should be monitored closely for evidence of ischemia. Placement of a smaller, additional femoral artery cannula to perfuse the leg distal to the CPS cannula has reduced the risk of this complication. Limb complications were reported to occur in as many as 25% of patients prior to the use of the distal cannulation technique.[2,5]

Pediatric experience

The use of extracorporeal support for circulatory failure in the pediatric population has expanded significantly since the mid-1990s. This support is commonly referred to as eCPR or rapid deployment ECLS. Annual pediatric (<16 years old) cardiac runs reported in the ELSO Registry have increased more than 50% between 1994-2004, from 296 to 467 runs.[30] Compared with adult outcomes, pediatric survival rates have been superior, and pediatric applications of CPS and rapid-deployment ECMO have also grown (Table 5). Overall survival to hospital discharge, however, has remained steady at approximately 40% among pediatric patients in the ELSO Registry (Tables 5 and 8). Survival without significant neurologic impairment following a witnessed cardiac arrest is approximately 20% in children, and early implementation of eCPR can improve the proportion of survivors to ~50%.[2,5,8,32]

Equipment, vascular access, and patient management

In many pediatric centers, rapid-deployment ECMO is utilized rather than a CPS system because the time required to prepare the circuit and cannulate during a resuscitation is comparable.[4] A vacuum- and crystalloid-primed ECMO circuit can be constructed and maintained in the ICU for emergencies.

Whether flow is initiated with a circuit containing crystalloid only or blood, such pre-primed circuits can often be readied in less than 15-20 minutes and usually before cannulation is complete. The use of ECMO eliminates the requirement for a circuit change if mechanical support is necessary beyond the typical 6-24 hour lifespan of a hollow-fiber oxygenator. Pediatric patients frequently do require >24 hours of mechanical support: the average length of eCPR runs from 1994 through July 2005 was approximately 120 hours, with a maximum of 900 hours.[30]

The CPS and rapid-deployment ECMO equipment for pediatric patients is miniaturized to accomodate for the smaller vessels and lower circuit flow requirements of younger patients. A range of cannula, tubing, and membrane oxygenator sizes are available for ECMO to accommodate the diverse requirements of children ranging in age from birth to the late teenage years.[33]

Obtaining vascular access in children often becomes the rate-limiting step when preparing to initiate mechanical support in an emergency situation. The technical challenges of vascular access in pediatric patients are due to multiple factors including small vessel size, complex circulations in patients with congenital heart disease, and the higher prevalence of prior vascular injury (e.g., from vascular catheter placement in cardiac patients). In infants and small children, the neck vessels are the preferred site for access due to the relatively smaller size of the femoral vessels. Typically, the right carotid artery and right internal jugular vein are utilized.

Table 8. eCPR cases and survival by age reported to ELSO Registry (1994-July 2005).

Age group	Patients N	Survival n	(%)
0-30 days	210	83	(39.5)
31 days-<1 year	192	86	(44.8)
1 year-≤16 years	201	70	(34.8)
Adult (>16 years)	177	57	(32.2)
Total	**780**	**296**	**(37.9)**

Of note, neck vessel cannulation has not been shown to be a risk factor for major neurologic complications.[34] Early after sternotomy, vascular access can be obtained within the chest in post-operative cardiac patients by reopening the sternal wound. In cardiac patients who have had the sternum intentionally left open to promote cardiorespiratory stability in the early post-operative period, the chest vessels can be accessed for cannulation without an incision.[35,36] These patients are cannulated directly through the right atrium and aorta. Cardiac patients who are more likely to require ECMO support in the post-operative period (e.g., those with severe myocardial dysfunction before CPB surgery) are good candidates for delayed sternal closure.

Pediatric patients with complex congenital heart disease who have undergone surgery to create cavopulmonary connections (e.g., a Fontan operation or a bidirectional Glenn shunt) present additional challenges for vascular access.[37] Cannulation in patients with a Fontan circulation can be achieved using any combination of the femoral, neck, or chest vessels. The distal tip of the venous cannula should be positioned in the Fontan baffle between the SVC and IVC to optimize venous return, because maximal circuit flow is often limited by venous inflow. Patients with a bidirectional Glenn shunt can also be cannulated using any combination of the femoral, neck, and chest vessels. Due to the separation of the systemic venous return to the heart, with SVC blood directed into the lungs and IVC blood mixing with pulmonary venous blood before being pumped into the aorta, at least 2 venous cannulas are typically required to generate adequate circuit flow and systemic cardiac output. If a patient with a bidirectional Glenn shunt has significant systemic hypotension or is undergoing cardiac massage, the upper body should be cannulated before the lower body to reduce the SVC pressure. Elevated SVC pressure in combination with low systemic arterial blood pressure places these patients at

risk for inadequate cerebral perfusion, which likely contributes to the high incidence of major neurologic injury in those who are placed on ECMO during or following cardiac arrest.[37]

Previous cannulation of the large central vessels, especially in patients weighing <10 kg, predisposes patients to vessel occlusion from thrombosis and scarring.[38] This may result in fewer options for vascular access, thereby increasing the risk of cannulation failure. Therefore, it is important to determine, whenever possible, the patency of the large vessels in patients with a history of central venous and femoral arterial catheter placement(s) so that time is not expended attempting to cannulate occluded vessels. Ultrasonography is a reliable, non-invasive technique for evaluating the patency of deep vessels.[39]

Following cannulation and the initiation of circuit flow, an echocardiogram should be performed to verify cannula tip position, determine the degree of ventricular distension, and assess for mechanical distortion of the cardiac valves (e.g., tricuspid valve or aortic valve insufficiency). If the cause of a patient's decompensation is uncertain from the clinical course and non-invasive imaging, and especially in post-operative cardiac patients, then cardiac catheterization to evaluate the possibility of residual anatomic defects should be considered. Cardiac catheterization during mechanical circulatory support can be useful both for diagnostic and interventional purposes, and it can be performed safely and effectively despite the logistical challenges required for patient transport to the catheterization laboratory and the technical limitations associated with indwelling cannulas.[31] In patients with 2-ventricle physiology and no intracardiac shunts (e.g., myocarditis or cardiomyopathy), cardiac catheterization may be necessary to decompress the left heart to avoid left ventricular distention and pulmonary edema from left atrial hypertension. Left heart decompression can be achieved either by placement of a left atrial venting catheter, atrial septostomy or atrial septal stent placement.[31]

Indications for eCPR

CPS and rapid-deployment ECMO have been used to resuscitate pediatric patients in cardiac arrest or shock, to facilitate separation from CPB after cardiac surgery, and to rescue cardiac patients with severe, unremitting cyanosis or life-threatening dysrhythmias unresponsive to medical therapies. For patients in cardiac arrest who require initiation of mechanical circulatory support during resuscitation, the best candidates are those with a witnessed, in-hospital arrest who receive rapid and effective CPR for a reversible problem in the setting of single-organ dysfunction. Patients with irreversible cardiac dysfunction (e.g., severe dilated cardiomyopathy) who acutely deteriorate can also be suitable candidates provided that mechanical support can serve as a bridge to cardiac transplantation. For these patients, conversion to a VAD for longer-term support should be considered. Patients with multi-system organ dysfunction and those who are not candidates for transplantation have tended to have poor outcomes.[40,41]

Elective mechanical support for procedures has also been accomplished in pediatric patients. The types of patients anticipated to benefit from such a strategy have problems similar to those noted in adults, including poor ventricular function and a high likelihood of hemodynamic decompensation during the procedure or intervention. An example of elective procedural support was published by Carmichael et al.[42] A neonate with severe Ebstein's anomaly of the tricuspid valve failed antiarrythmic therapy for life-threatening episodes of accessory pathway-mediated supraventricular tachycardia. Because inducing tachycardia would be required to map the accessory pathway for radiofrequency ablation, the patient was electively placed on VA ECMO before transfer to the catheterization laboratory. ECMO support maintained hemo-dynamic stability during pathway mapping and ablation, and decannulation was successfully completed in the ICU.

Outcomes

Hospital survival after in-hospital cardiac arrest in the pediatric population has been >30% when eCPR (CPS or rapid-deployment ECMO) is employed as part of the resuscitation.[30,40,41] In a series of 64 children reported by Morris, et. al., survival following eCPR was comparable to survival following conventional CPR, even though all the eCPR patients initially failed conventional CPR.[41] Neither age, duration of CPR prior to initiation of ECMO support, nor duration of ECMO predicted survival in this series. Because hospital survival has not appeared to be related to the duration of chest compressions, cardiac massage for >30-60 minutes has not been a contraindication to the initiation of eCPR.[40,41] Although the number of patients is small, survival with intact neurologic function following 60-90 minutes of chest compressions prior to the initiation of eCPR has been reported, demonstrating that aggressive conventional resuscitation prior to the initiation of eCPR can provide adequate cerebral perfusion.[40,41,43] The results of eCPR in pediatric patients in the ELSO Registry are shown in Tables 5 and 8.

Pediatric cardiac patients with single-ventricle anatomy who have cavopulmonary connections have lower survival rates with mechanical circulatory support than other congenital heart disease patients.[37] ECMO supports the Fontan circulation better than the Glenn circulation, and patients with a Glenn shunt have both a higher risk of mortality and significant brain injury. The successful resuscitation of patients with passive pulmonary blood flow in a cavopulmonary circuit using conventional CPR is difficult because the baseline elevation of systemic venous pressure predisposes the end organs, and especially the brain, to inadequate perfusion. In the face of elevated intrathoracic pressures generated during conventional CPR, the systemic venous pressure is further increased, compromising cerebral as well as other end organ blood flow. Patients with Fontan and Glenn physiology are better managed if consideration for mechanical circulatory support is addressed prior to cardiac arrest.[37]

The potential for neurologic injury is significant whenever a child is placed on mechanical circulatory support, and the risk of injury is increased among those exposed to eCPR. In addition to the potential for intracranial hemorrhage from anticoagulation plus thromboemboli from the circuit, patients who require eCPR can suffer from ischemia, hypoxemia, and air or thrombotic emboli during conventional CPR. Cardiac patients also are susceptible to neurologic injury from intraoperative support techniques such as circulatory arrest.[44] A broad spectrum of neurologic sequelae in survivors of cardiopulmonary arrest and resuscitation with eCPR have been reported, including seizures, movement disorders, motor weakness, increased muscle tone, tremors, coordination problems, and global impairment.[43,44,45]

The most common causes of death after initiating eCPR in pediatric patients include unrecoverable cardiac dysfunction or inadequate cardiac output, multi-system organ dysfunction, uncontrollable hemorrhage, sepsis, and withdrawal of support.

Complications

Complications in the pediatric population are similar to those reported for adults (Table 7). The most common non-cardiac complications in patients in the ELSO Registry include cannulation and surgical site bleeding, hemolysis, equipment failure, and end organ dysfunction (primarily brain and kidneys). Compared to adults, oxygenator failure occurred less frequently (8.6 vs. 21.6%), but cannula problems were more frequent (11.3 vs. 7.2%). Culture-

proven infection was less common in pediatric patients compared to adults (9 vs. 15.5%). The proportion of patients determined to be clinically brain dead was similar (11.6% pediatric vs. 14.9% adult), and in both age groups, >30% underwent some form of renal replacement therapy.

Conclusions

The use of CPS as the most advanced component of cardiopulmonary resuscitation and as a cardiorespiratory support technique during high-risk procedures has increased and evolved in both adults and children during the past 10 years. Patient selection continues to be a key determinant impacting outcomes. One of the greatest growth areas in applications of ECLS has been in pediatric patients, especially those with cardiac disease. Many institutions with large pediatric cardiac surgical programs have developed rapid-deployment ECMO as their primary strategy for ECLS and use it as a resuscitative tool in post-operative patients. In both adults and children who undergo ECLS, neurologic complications and outcomes continue to be a significant concern. While certain risk factors for neurologic injury have been well defined, neurologic outcomes generally remain difficult to predict and to attribute to ECLS versus other associated risks (e.g., CPB surgery in neonates with cyanotic congenital heart disease). In programs with well-organized, multi-disciplinary teams that can prepare ECLS circuits in minutes, the rate-limiting step to initiating circuit flow is frequently vascular access. This limitation is particularly challenging to those managing pediatric patients, and improvements in vascular access techniques have the potential to improve survival and reduce morbidity.

References

1. Martin GB, Rivers EP, Paradis NA, Goetting MG, Morris DC, Nowak RM. Emergency department cardiopulmonary bypass in the treatment of human cardiac arrest. *Chest* 1998; 113:743-751.

2. Patel H, Pagani FD. Extracorporeal mechanical circulatory assist. *Cardiol Clin* 2003; 21:29-41.

3. Kurusz M, Zwischenberger JB. Percutaneous cardiopulmonary bypass for cardiac emergencies. *Perfusion* 2002; 17:269-277.

4. Duncan BW, Ibrahim AE, Hraska V, et al. Use of rapid-deployment extracorporeal membrane oxygenation for the resuscitation of pediatric patients with heart disease after cardiac arrest. *J Thorac Cardiovasc Surg* 1998; 116:305-311.

5. Schwarz B, Mair P, Margreiter J. Experience with percutaneous venoarterial cardiopulmonary bypass for emergency circulatory support. *Crit Care Med* 2003; 31:758-764.

6. Mair P, Hoermann C, Moertl M, Bonatti J, Falbesoner C, Balogh D. Percutaneous venoarterial extracorporeal membrane oxygenation for emergency mechanical circulatory support. *Resuscitation* 1996; 33:29-34.

7. Potapov EV, Weng Y, Hausmann H, Kopitz M, Pasic M, Hetzer R. New approach in treatment of acute cardiogenic shock requiring mechanical circulatory support. *Ann Thorac Surg* 2003; 76:2112-2114.

8. Younger JG, Schreiner RJ, Swaniker F, Hirschl RB, Chapman RA, Bartlett RH. Extracorporeal resuscitation of cardiac arrest. *Acad Emerg Med* 1999; 6:700-707.

9. Orime Y, Shiono M, Hata H, et al. Clinical experiences of percutaneous support: its effectiveness and limit. *Artif Organs* 1998; 22:498-501.

10. Hill JG, Bruhn PS, Cohen SE, et al. Emergent applications of cardiopulmonary support: a multi-institutional experience. *Ann Thorac Surg* 1992; 54:699-704.

11. Holzer M, Sterz F, Schoerkhuber W, et al. Successful resuscitation of a verapamil-intoxicated patient with percutaneous cardiopulmonary bypass. *Crit Care Med* 1999; 27:2818-2823.

12. Willms DC, Atkins PJ, Dembitsky WP, Jaski BE, Gocka I. Analysis of clinical trends in a program of emergent ECLS for cardiovascular collapse. *ASAIO J* 1997; 43:65-68.

13. Chen YS, Chao A, Yu HY, et al. Analysis and results of prolonged resuscitation in cardiac arrest patients rescued by extracorporeal membrane oxygenation. *J Am Coll Cardiol* 2003; 41:197-203.

14. Aiba T, Nonogi H, Itoh T, et al. Appropriate indications for the use of a percutaneous cardiopulmonary support system in cases with cardiogenic shock complicating acute myocardial infarction. *Jpn Circ J* 2001; 65:145-149.

15. Ogawa R, Fujita T. A scoring system for a quantitative evaluation of shock. *Jpn J Surg* 1982; 12:122-125.

16. Yip HK, Wu CJ, Chang HW, et al. Cardiac rupture complicating acute myocardial infarction in the direct percutaneous coronary intervention reperfusion era. *Chest* 2003; 124:565-571.

17. Aliabadi D, Roldan CA, Pett S, Follis F, Holland M. Percutaneous cardiopulmonary support for the management of catastrophic mechanical complications of acute myocardial infarction. *Cathet Cardiovasc Diagn* 1996; 37:223-226.

18. Sunami H, Fujita Y, Okada T, et al. Successful resuscitation from prolonged ventricular fibrillation using a portable percutaneous cardiopulmonary support system. *Anesthesiology* 2003; 99:1227-1229.

19. Behringer W, Sterz F, Domanovits H, et al. Percutaneous cardiopulmonary bypass for therapy resistant cardiac arrest from digoxin overdose. *Resuscitation* 1998; 37:47-50.

20. Kornberger E, Mair P. Important aspects in the treatment of severe accidental hypothermia: the Innsbruck experience. *J Neurosurg Anesthesiol* 1996; 8:83-87.

21. Vretenar DF, Urschel JD, Parrott JC, Unruh HW. Cardiopulmonary bypass resuscitation for accidental hypothermia. *Ann Thorac Surg* 1994; 58:895-898.

22. Wollenek G, Honarwar N, Golej J, Marx M. Cold water submersion and cardiac arrest in treatment of severe hypothermia with cardiopulmonary bypass. *Resuscitation* 2002; 52:255-263.

23. Kitamura M, Aomi S, Hachida M, Nishida H, Endo M, Koyanagi H. Current strategy of temporary circulatory support for severe cardiac failure after operation. *Ann Thorac Surg* 1999; 68:662-665.

24. Rousou JA, Engelman RM, Flack JE 3rd Deaton DW, Owen SG. Emergency cardiopulmonary bypass in the cardiac surgical unit can be a lifesaving measure in postoperative cardiac arrest. *Circulation* 1994; 90:1280-1284.

25. Kawahito K, Ino T, Adachi H, Ide H, Mizuhara A, Yamaguci A. Heparin coated percutaneous cardiopulmonary support for the treatment of circulatory collapse after cardiac surgery. *ASAIO J* 1994; 40:972-976.

26. Grambow DW, Deeb GM, Pavlides GS, Margulis A, O'Neill WW, Bates ER. Emergent percutaneous cardiopulmonary bypass in patients having cardiovascular collapse in the cardiac catheterization laboratory. *Am J Cardiol* 1994; 73:872-875.

27. Curtis JJ, Walls JT, Wagner-Mann CC, et al. Centrifugal pumps: description of devices and surgical techniques. *Ann Thorac Surg* 1999; 68:666-671.

28. Kouchoukos NT, Masetti P, Murphy SF. Hypothermic cardiopulmonary bypass and circulatory arrest for operations on the descending thoracic and thoracoabdominal aorta. *Ann Thorac Surg* 2002; 74:S1885-S1887.

29. Nagao K, Hayashi N, Kanmatsuse K, et al. Cardiopulmonary cerebral resuscitation using emergency cardiopulmonary bypass, coronary reperfusion therapy and mild hypothermia in patients with cardiac arrest outside the hospital. *J Am Coll Cardiol* 2000; 36:776-783.

30. Extracorporeal Life Support Organization. ECLS Registry report of the Extracorporeal Life Support Organization (ELSO). Ann Arbor, MI: University of Michigan: July 2005.

31. Booth KL, Roth SJ, Perry SB, del Nido PJ, Wessel DL, Laussen PC. Cardiac catheterization of patients supported by extracorporeal membrane oxygenation. *J Am Coll Cardiol* 2002; 40:1681-1686.

32. von Segesser LK. Cardiopulmonary support and extracorporeal membrane oxygenation for cardiac assist. *Ann Thorac Surg* 1999; 68:672-677.

33. Laussen PC, Roth SJ. Surgical approaches, cardiopulmonary bypass, and mechanical circulatory support in children. Mechanical circulatory support. In: Selke FW, del Nido PJ, Swanson SJ, eds. *Sabiston & Spencer Surgery of the Chest. 7th Edition.* Philadelphia, PA: Elsevier Saunders, 2005:1851-1862.

34. Stockwell JA, Goldstein RF, Ungerleider RM, Kern FH, Meliones JN, Greeley WJ. Cerebral blood flow and carbon dioxide reactivity in neonates during venoarterial extracorporeal life support. *Crit Care Med* 1996; 24:155-162.

35. Tabbutt S, Duncan BW, McLaughlin D, Wessel DL, Jonas RA, Laussen PC. Delayed sternal closure after cardiac operations in pediatric population. *J Thorac Cardiovasc Surg* 1997; 113:886-893.

36. McElhinney DB, Reddy VM, Parry AJ, Johnson L, Fineman JR, Hanley FL. Management

and outcomes of delayed sternal closure after cardiac surgery in neonates and infants. *Crit Care Med* 2000; 28:1180-1184.

37. Booth KL, Roth SJ, Thiagarajan RR, Almodovar MC, del Nido PJ, Laussen PC. Extracorporeal membrane oxygenation support of the Fontan and bidirectional Glenn circulations. *Ann Thorac Surg* 2004; 77:1341-1348.

38. Vitiello R, McCrindle BW, Nykanen D, Freedom RM, Benson LN. Complications associated with pediatric cardiac catheterization. *J Am Coll Cardiol* 1998; 32:1433-1440.

39. Kearon C, Ginsberg JS, Hirsh J. The role of venous ultrasonography in the diagnosis of suspected deep venous thrombosis and pulmonary edema. *Ann Intern Med* 1998; 129:1044-1049.

40. Morris MC, Ittenbach RF, Godinez RI, et. al. Risk factors for mortality in 137 pediatric cardiac intensive care unit patients managed with extracorporeal membrane oxygenation. *Crit Care Med* 2004; 32:1061-1069.

41. Morris MC, Wernovsky G, Nadkarni V. Survival outcomes after extracorporeal cardiopulmonary resuscitation instituted during active chest compressions following refractory in-hospital pediatric cardiac arrest. *Pediatr Crit Care Med* 2004; 5:440-446.

42. Carmichael TB, Walsh EP, Roth SJ. Anticipatory use of venoarterial extracorporeal membrane oxygenation for high-risk interventional cardiac procedure. *Respir Care* 2002; 47:1002-1006.

43. Parra DA, Totapally BR, Zahn E, et al. Outcome of cardiopulmonary resuscitation in a pediatric cardiac intensive care unit. *Crit Care Med* 2000; 28:3296-3300.

44. Ibrahim AE, Duncan BW, Blume ED, Jonas RA. Long-term follow-up of pediatric cardiac patients requiring mechanical circulatory support. *Ann Thorac Surg* 2000; 69:186-192.

45. Hamrick SE, Gremmels DB, Keet CA, et al. Neurodevelopmental outcome of infants supported with extracorporeal membrane oxygenation after cardiac surgery. *Pediatrics* 2003; 111:e671-675.

46. Noon GP, Lafuente JA, Irwin S. Acute and temporary ventricular support with BioMedicus centrifugal pump. *Ann Thorac Surg* 1999; 68:650-654.

47. Massetti M, Tasle M, Le Page O, et al. Back from irreversibility: extracorporeal life support for prolonged cardiac arrest. *Ann Thorac Surg* 2005; 79:178-183.

30

Adult Cardiac Failure: Management and Use of ECLS

Babak Sarani, M.D. and Robert L. Kormos, M.D.

Introduction

Adult cardiac failure is an increasingly prevalent disorder with approximately 550,000 new cases diagnosed annually in the U.S.[1] As such, the number of patients requiring some form of mechanical cardiac support is growing. Most often, this involves use of an intra-aortic balloon pump (IABP), but implantable ventricular assist devices (VADs) and ECMO have become standard tools in many tertiary care centers. Post-cardiotomy cardiac failure is the most common indication for ECMO in adult patients, but other indications include acute myocardial infarction (MI), cardiac arrest, primary graft dysfunction after cardiac transplant, fulminant myocarditis, and post-partum cardiomyopathy (PPCM). Use of ECMO for emergent support after cardiac arrest is addressed in Chapter 29. Table 1 lists the generally accepted indications for extracorporeal support, although many physicians liberalize these indications for ECMO because of its ease of cannulation and lower cost relative to VAD therapy.[2,3] ECMO is particularly useful when secondary organ complications or the abruptness of clinical presentation make the use of VADs less desirable.

Overall, there are no large, prospective trials on the utility of ECMO for adult cardiac failure. Consequently, the guidelines in this chapter are based mainly on small trials and case reports. A suggested algorithm for the role of ECMO in the management of adult cardiac failure is included (Figure 1).

Table 1. Indications for extracorporeal support after cardiac surgery.*[2,3]

Cardiac index <1.8 lpm/m^2 in conjunction with the following conditions:

- Left atrial or pulmonary capillary wedge pressure >20 mm Hg
- Systolic blood pressure <90 mm Hg
- Mean arterial blood pressure <60 mm Hg
- Urine output <20 cc/hr (adult with previously normal renal function)
- Metabolic acidosis
- Systemic vascular resistance >2,100 dynes/sec/cm^3

---

*With adequate preload, maximal pressor and IABP support, and inability to tolerate pharmacologic afterload reduction.

Post-cardiotomy cardiac failure

Post-cardiotomy cardiac failure is increasingly prevalent as patients who are referred for cardiopulmonary bypass (CPB) surgery are increasingly older and have impaired ventricular function pre-operatively. It is estimated that 1% of patients undergoing CPB surgery will not be able to wean from CPB despite pharmacologic and IABP support and thus will require extracorporeal mechanical support.[4]

Stunned myocardium, presumably from ischemia-reperfusion, is the most common cause of post-cardiotomy heart failure.[5] It is not possible to distinguish stunned myocardium from irreversible infarction in the immediate post-operative period.[6] Smedira et al. reported on 97 adult patients who required ECMO after cardiac surgery and found that factors associated with inability to wean from CPB included age >60 years, reoperation, emergent operation, left main coronary disease, history of cardiomyopathy or MI, renal failure, hepatic failure, or a neurologic event while on CPB.[7] Smedira suggested that patients with these risk factors receive 48-72 hours of ECMO support post-operatively, if needed, with conversion to VAD if the patient is a candidate for transplantation and weaning from ECMO is not possible.

Reports of outcomes of ECMO for post-cardiotomy cardiac failure generally show weaning from ECMO in 30-77%, and survival to hospital discharge after coronary bypass surgery in 16-37%.[8-11] Magovern et al. found 80% survival in 14 high-risk patients who required ECMO after coronary bypass surgery.[12] It is not clear why their findings were so favorable. In a study of 202 post-cardiotomy adult patients, Smedira et al. found that patients who required ECMO, but were ultimately bridged to transplant or to left VAD (LVAD), had the same 5-year survival (44%) as those who were weaned from ECMO.[11] In this study, 41% of the patients were not salvageable and had care withdrawn. Most investigators agree that outcomes can be improved by early utilization of ECMO, use of heparin-coated Carmeda membrane oxygenators, and optimal patient selection to exclude older patients or those with multiple other comorbidities such as renal or hepatic failure, or refractory ventricular arrhythmias.

The advantages and disadvantages of ECMO in the adult patient are listed in Table 2. Early institution of ECMO in lieu of VAD therapy for post-cardiotomy heart failure offers several advantages including ease of cannulation and rapid priming of the circuit at the bedside, ease of decannulation in case of cardiac recovery, biventricular support, pulmonary support with improved systemic oxygenation, ability to

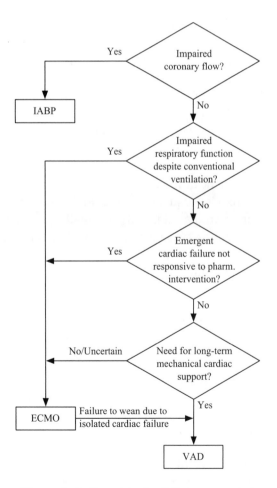

Figure 1. Left ventricular failure: suggested algorithm for the role of ECMO.

assess the patient off extracorporeal support temporarily with the addition of a bridge to the circuit, and lower cost. Thus, ECMO provides a much less expensive method to stabilize post-cardiotomy patients with refractory cardiogenic shock allowing time for possible cardiac recovery. If necessary, patients can be bridged to VAD or heart transplantation after ECMO. Mean duration of ECMO support for post-cardiotomy heart failure has been reported to be 25-120 hours.[6,9,12,13] In a study of 14 patients, Pagani et al. found that approximately 20% of patients with refractory cardiogenic shock and multi-organ system failure who were initially stabilized with ECMO were not candidates for heart transplantation or VAD therapy.[14] The authors concluded that the use of ECMO in place of VAD support is a cost-effective way to identify those patients most likely to benefit from continued aggressive care.

Initial experience with post-cardiotomy ECMO was poor largely because of excessive bleeding. This was often caused by lack of experience and the requirement for high-dose heparin to prolong circuit life. However, because of refinements in circuit design and heparin-coated Carmeda membrane oxygenators, these issues are not as problematic as they were in the past decade, and ECMO has become a promising treatment for post-cardiotomy heart failure.[6,15] Heparin-coated oxygenators have allowed activated clotting times to be maintained as low as 150-180 seconds. This has resulted in a marked diminution in the risk of bleeding, especially in the early post-operative period. Nevertheless, bleeding remains the most significant complication with ECMO, and the risk is highest in patients who require ECMO to separate from CPB in the OR.[6,16]

ECMO has several other disadvantages in comparison to VAD therapy. There are many reports of an increase in left ventricular systolic wall stress and oxygen consumption, as well as in afterload, both in laboratory models and patients.[6,17,18] This increase in afterload can be partially offset by increasing ECMO flow rates to decrease the volume of pulmonary venous blood returning to the left atrium, or by adding IABP support, but patients with impaired left ventricular ejection fraction may require left atrial venting via either atrial septostomy or diversion of blood flow from the left atrium to the venous limb of the ECMO circuit. Magovern et al. reported 100% mortality in 3 patients who required ECMO after mitral valve operation.[12] They reported that inability to offload the left ventricle and progressive left ventricular distention was the most likely cause of death in these patients. Thus, they conclude that the use of ECMO is a viable option in post-coronary bypass patients but should be avoided in patients in whom left ventricular venting may be required. Next, venoarterial (VA) ECMO has been shown to result in decreased pulmonary blood flow with a resultant need for prolonged mechanical ventilation after cardiac recovery.[6]

Table 2. Advantages and disadvantages of ECMO in comparison to VAD in the adult patient.

Advantages	Disadvantages
• Ability to cannulate and decannulate at bedside	• More bleeding potential in the immediate post-op period
• Biventricular support	• Increased left ventricular afterload
• Both cardiac and pulmonary support	• Potential for distal emboli or limb ischemia with VA ECMO
• Ability to assess patient off ECMO prior to decannulation	• Incomplete left ventricular decompression
• Less expense	

Lastly, VA ECMO carries the risk of distal emboli or extremity ischemia (with peripheral arterial cannulation).

The greatest potential of ECMO for post-cardiotomy support is as a bridge to other cardiac assist devices leading ultimately to cardiac transplantation or other long-term mechanical cardiac support. ECMO is used in this setting to support the patient long enough to establish viability for further long-term support. In particular, patients who present in cardiogenic shock with multi-organ failure often do not tolerate other forms of circulatory support because of severe pulmonary edema. In this scenario, LVADs fail to adequately support the circulation because of the concomitant right ventricular dysfunction that occurs with elevated pulmonary resistance. Indeed, even biventricular assist device support may fail if persistent hypoxemia and pulmonary edema occur.

Use of ECMO in heart/lung transplantation

Heart transplantation is the definitive treatment for end-stage cardiomyopathy. Mortality after heart transplant is highest in the first month following the procedure.[19] The most common causes for this high mortality include primary graft failure, acute rejection, bleeding, and infection.[20] Of these, primary graft failure and acute rejection are potentially treatable conditions but require time for therapy to take effect. Mechanical cardiac support may be needed in some cases to stabilize the patient and assess for response to therapy.

Primary graft failure in the absence of rejection is the most common cause of death in the first month after heart transplant. It occurs in 5-25% of all patients undergoing transplant, and accounts for 25-50% of all deaths in the early post-operative period.[20-22] Heart failure is caused by myocardial stunning which usually manifests as prolonged ventricular dysfunction. Myocardial stunning is affected by ischemic time, preservation injury, denervation, surgical manipulation, and vasoactive substances released during CPB.[23] Right ventricular failure is more common than left due to pre-existing pulmonary hypertension in most heart transplant recipients. Right ventricular failure is exacerbated by excess intravascular volume and/or increased pulmonary vascular resistance. Pulmonary hypertension is worsened by hypoxia and prolonged CPB at the time of transplant and is a proven predictor of mortality in this patient population. Isolated left ventricular failure is often secondary to preservation injury.

Acute rejection is the leading cause of death between 1-12 months after heart transplant.[22] It is estimated that 18% of patients are hospitalized within 1 year of transplantation for an episode of rejection.[24] Acute rejection is most often cellular-mediated and amenable to treatment using augmented immunosuppression. Patients with acute rejection rarely require mechanical cardiac support. However, those who do require such support take longer to recover than those with primary graft dysfunction caused by the pathophysiology of the underlying illness. ECMO also provides a support mechanism for combined aggressive immunosuppressive therapy and plasmapheresis in patients with presumed antibody-mediated rejection.

In their commentary, Fiser et al. note that ECMO may be necessary after heart transplantation for one of two reasons.[8] The first is severe pulmonary hypertension with right heart failure. Previous studies have shown that severe pulmonary hypertension can take as long as 2 weeks to resolve after transplant.[25,26] Second, as previously noted, primary graft failure is also a common indication for ECMO in this patient population.

Mechanical cardiac support is indicated once patients reach maximal medical therapy. Such support can include VADs or ECMO. IABP therapy is often not helpful as it can provide limited support to the left ventricle only. There are no large, prospective trials comparing the use of ECMO with VAD therapy for primary graft dysfunction; however, there are many case reports and small case series showing equal mortality outcomes using either modality in the short-term.[22,27] As with post-operative cardiomyopathy, ECMO provides many advantages over VAD support. Advantages specific to the heart or heart/lung transplant patient include the ability to provide both pulmonary and circulatory support and the ability to offload the right ventricle, although this may be offset by the increase in left ventricular afterload caused by ECMO. As with the post-cardiotomy patient, left ventricular overload can initially be treated with medication, increasing ECMO flow rates, and/or an IABP, but direct decompression of the left heart via atrial septostomy or left atrial cannulation with diversion of flow to the venous limb of the ECMO circuit may be necessary.[20,22,28] Again, as in standard post-cardiotomy ECMO support, the biggest advantage of ECMO is in supporting patients who develop multi-organ dysfunction caused by hyperacute or antibody-mediated rejection as part of the overall inflammatory response. Another significant advantage of ECMO is the ability to use the circuit to perform plasmapheresis to remove high levels of antibodies to histocompatability antigens as well as other inflammatory mediators.

As with other patient populations, the two most common complications of ECMO in the post-transplant patient are bleeding and neurologic injury.[29] Not surprisingly, the risk of bleeding is highest in the patients who require ECMO to separate from CPB in the OR, as these patients are fully anticoagulated and prone to platelet dysfunction following bypass.

In a retrospective study of 10 patients requiring ECMO after heart or heart/lung transplant, Whyte et al. found that adults had poorer outcomes relative to children less than 2 years of age, but no difference in ability to wean from ECMO between older patients and young adults.[29] Those >28 years of age had higher in-hospital mortality. Furthermore, the duration of ECMO had a negative correlation with survival, although the retrospective nature of the study did not allow the authors to establish whether the patients who required longer ECMO support died because of the underlying illness or from an ECMO complication. Finally, the authors found that the indication for ECMO in the post-transplant patient did not correlate with survival or ability to wean off ECMO. In reviewing the literature, Miniati et al. found other factors that are predictive of poor outcome: need for ECMO to separate from CPB in the OR, prolonged intubation, renal failure, mediastinal bleeding, and cardiac arrest before or during the initiation of ECMO.[22]

In comparing post-cardiotomy non-transplant patients requiring ECMO with post-heart or heart/lung transplant patients, Fiser et al. found that patients older than 65 years of age in either group were less likely to wean from ECMO and were less likely to survive.[8] Patients with an ejection fraction less than 30% 2 days after the initiation of ECMO were also less likely to wean or survive. There were no differences in cross-clamp time or cardiac bypass time between patients who were successfully weaned and those who were not, or those that survived and those that did not. Overall, post-transplant patients required longer ECMO times than non-transplant patients because of the underlying mechanism of cardiac failure.

Based on these and other similar studies, it is recommended that patients who require more than 2-3 days of ECMO support after non-transplant cardiotomy have a VAD placed and be considered for transplantation, if appropriate. Patients with post-transplant cardiac failure should be allowed 5-7 days of ECMO before being considered for VAD placement or re-transplant.[8,29] Mechanical cardiac support should be used sparingly in those >65 years of age as these patients rarely survive to hospital discharge.

ECMO for fulminant myocarditis or post-partum cardiomyopathy

There are only isolated case reports regarding the use of ECMO for acute myocarditis or PPCM with circulatory collapse. Both entities represent non-ischemic cardiomyopathies of uncertain etiology and have widely variable courses. Many have suggested that the underlying process involves an inappropriate activation of the immune system and/or inflammatory cascade.[30]

As with the treatment of primary graft dysfunction or acute rejection following transplant, extracorporeal circulatory support may be needed to stabilize the patient and provide time for medical therapy to be effective. Kawahito et al. and Chen et al. reported 15-20% mortality in patients with acute myocarditis requiring ECMO.[31,32] Those that survived to hospital discharge required 150-200 hours of ECMO support. Chen examined the surviving patients after 37 months and found that they had no clinical evidence of impaired ventricular function, although other investigators have reported various degrees of impaired cardiac ability especially in those with PPCM.[33,34]

Once patients with myocarditis or PPCM need mechanical cardiac support, they usually need either ECMO or VAD. IABP is not effective as these patients often have severely depressed ventricular function. In this setting, ECMO provides the same advantages as those noted above. Interestingly, neither Kawahito nor Chen reported high rates of complications related to their prolonged use of ECMO.[31,32] Therefore, patients with PPCM or acute myocarditis may be supported for longer periods of time with ECMO prior to implantation of a VAD or consideration for transplant, as many may ultimately recover and be weaned from support.

Combination of LVAD with ECMO

One of the most common complications of the use of an LVAD is right ventricular dysfunc-tion which mandates the use of a secondary right VAD (RVAD). Although the LVAD produces mild right ventricular dysfunction in all patients because of the leftward shift of the intraventricular septum, the reduction of pulmonary artery afterload produced by maximal left ventricular decompression allows the majority of patients to tolerate the right ventricular dysfunction. On the other hand, in the presence of severe pulmonary edema secondary to massive blood transfusion around the time of implant surgery, or inherent pre-operative pulmonary edema caused by congestive heart failure, the benefit of pulmonary afterload reduction is not seen, and patients can develop severe right heart failure. In these cases, the utilization of an ECMO circuit which drains the right ventricle and returns oxygenated blood to the left atrium provides time for restoration of pulmonary function and can usually be removed after 72 hours.

Weaning from ECMO

Once patients are on ECMO, the ventilator settings are rapidly weaned to low levels of ventilatory support to minimize ongoing pulmonary injury. Typically, the ventilator is set on volume control mode with fractional inspired oxygen less than 40%, respiratory rate of 8, tidal volume of 6 cc/kg, and positive end-expiratory pressure (PEEP) of 5 cm H_2O. Oxygen-carrying capacity is maximized by keeping the hematocrit between 35-40%. ECMO flow rates are maximized to generate 70-80 mm Hg negative pressure in the venous (outflow) limb. This usually generates a maximal flow rate of 7-8 liters per minute (lpm). Diuretics can be used to decrease endogenous cardiac output if the output is higher than the maximal flow rate which the ECMO circuit can support. Arterial blood gas and lactate levels are assayed regularly. A pulmonary artery catheter is inserted and continuous cardiac indices, including mixed venous oxygen saturation, are monitored. Vasopressors are used only as needed as they can further increase left ventricular afterload.

In the case of VA ECMO, weaning is performed under echocardiographic guidance with regular arterial blood gas and lactate measurements. ECMO flow rates are slowly weaned while pressor and ventilatory support are augmented after echocardiography confirms adequate ventricular filling and ejection. Blood gases and serum lactate levels are then assayed to confirm adequate gas exchange and oxygen delivery, respectively. Mixed venous oxygen saturation of 90% or greater is typical with full ECMO support; paradoxically, lower mixed venous oxygen saturation (60-70%) is indicative of cardiac recovery. As heart function improves, ECMO support is weaned and more blood is directed to the pulmonary circulation resulting in a low PO_2. Prior to decannulation, a bridge can be added to the circuit (if not already present) allowing a trial off ECMO. The patient can be thus monitored from hours to days as needed prior to decannulation.

Summary

In conclusion, adult cardiac failure is an increasingly common diagnosis. Most patients can be treated medically; however, 1% of patients undergoing cardiac bypass surgery and a similarly small percentage of patients undergoing cardiac transplant will require extracorporeal circulatory support. Such support can be provided using either ECMO or VADs. Previously noted bleeding diatheses associated with ECMO are now much less common as a result of the wide use of heparin-coated Carmeda membrane oxygenators and tubing, as well as improved anticoagulation management. ECMO is a better option for most of these patients as it is more readily reversible, can be urgently placed at the bedside, can provide both circulatory and pulmonary support, and is less expensive. VADs should be reserved for patients who cannot be weaned from ECMO or in those in whom it is known that an extended need for cardiac support will be necessary.

References

1. Rose EA, Gelijns AC, Moskowitz AJ, et al. Long-term mechanical left ventricular assistance for end-stage heart failure. *N Engl J Med* 2001; 345:1435-1443.

2. Fuhrman TM, Sturm JT, Holub DA, et al. Right and left ventricular hemodynamic indices as predictors of the need for and outcome of post-cardiotomy mechanical intraaortic balloon pump support. *Cardiovasc Dis* 1979; 6:350-358.

3. Normal JC, Cooley DA, Igo SR, et al. Prognostic indices for survival during postcardiotomy intra-aortic balloon pumping. Methods of scoring and classification, with implications for left ventricular assist device utilization. *J Thorac Cardiovasc Surg* 1977; 74:709-720.

4. Broderick T, Wechsler A. Ventricular Assist Devices and Artificial Hearts. In: Ayers S, ed. *Textbook of Critical Care.* 3rd ed. Philadelphia, PA: WB Saunders Co; 1995: 553-561.

5. Kloner RA, Przyklenk K, Kay GL. Clinical evidence for stunned myocardium after coronary artery bypass surgery. *J Card Surg* 1994; 9(3 Suppl):397-402.

6. Ko WJ, Lin CY, Chen RJ, Wang SS, Lin FY, Chen YS. Extracorporeal membrane oxygenation support for adult postcardiotomy cardiogenic shock. *Ann Thorac Surg* 2002; 73:538-545.

7. Smedira NG, Blackstone EH. Postcardiotomy mechanical support: risk factors and outcomes. *Ann Thorac Surg* 2001; 71(3 Suppl):S60-66; discussion S82-85.

8. Fiser SM, Tribble CG, Kaza AK, et al. When to discontinue extracorporeal membrane oxygenation for postcardiotomy support. *Ann Thorac Surg* 2001; 71:210-214.

9. Kawahito K, Ino T, Adachi H, Ide H, Mizuhara A, Yamaguci A. Heparin coated percutaneous cardiopulmonary support for the treatment of circulatory collapse after

cardiac surgery. *Asaio J* 1994; 40(4):972-976.

10. ELSO Data Registry Report: International Summary. University of Michigan, Ann Arbor, MI; 2001.

11. Smedira NG, Moazami N, Golding CM, et al. Clinical experience with 202 adults receiving extracorporeal membrane oxygenation for cardiac failure: survival at five years. *J Thorac Cardiovasc Surg* 2001; 122:92-102.

12. Magovern GJ Jr, Magovern JA, Benckart DH, et al. Extracorporeal membrane oxygenation: preliminary results in patients with postcardiotomy cardiogenic shock. *Ann Thorac Surg* 1994; 57:1462-1471

13. Muehrcke DD, McCarthy PM, Stewart RW, et al. Extracorporeal membrane oxygenation for postcardiotomy cardiogenic shock. *Ann Thorac Surg* 1996; 61:684-691.

14. Pagani FD, Lynch W, Swaniker F, et al. Extracorporeal life support to left ventricular assist device bridge to heart transplant: A strategy to optimize survival and resource utilization. *Circulation* 1999; 100(19 Suppl): II206-210.

15. Anderson H 3rd, Steimle C, Shapiro M, et al. Extracorporeal life support for adult cardiorespiratory failure. *Surgery* 1993; 114:161-172; discussion 72-73.

16. Lazzara RR, Magovern JA, Benckart DH, Maher TD, Jr., Sakert T, Magovern GJ Jr. Extracorporeal membrane oxygenation for adult post cardiotomy cardiogenic shock using a heparin bonded system. *Asaio J* 1993; 39:M444-447.

17. Bavaria JE, Furukawa S, Kreiner G, Gupta KB, Streicher J, Edmunds LH Jr. Effect of circulatory assist devices on stunned myocardium. *Ann Thorac Surg* 1990; 49:123-128.

18. Magovern GJ Jr, Christlieb IY, Kao RL, et al. Recovery of the failing canine heart with biventricular support in a previously fatal experimental model. *J Thorac Cardiovasc Surg* 1987; 94:656-663.

19. De Maria R, Minoli L, Parolini M, et al. Prognostic determinants of six-month morbidity and mortality in heart transplant recipients. The Italian Study Group on Infection in Heart Transplantation. *J Heart Lung Transplant* 1996; 15:124-135.

20. Ko WJ, Chen YS, Chou NK, Hsu RB, Wang SS, Chu SH. Extracorporeal membrane oxygenation rescue after heart transplantation. *Transplant Proc* 2000; 32:2388-2391.

21. Hauptman PJ, Aranki S, Mudge GH Jr, Couper GS, Loh E. Early cardiac allograft failure after orthotopic heart transplantation. *Am Heart J* 1994; 127:179-186.

22. Miniati DN, Robbins RC. Mechanical support for acutely failed heart or lung grafts. *J Card Surg* 2000; 15:129-135.

23. Taghavi S, Ankersmit HJ, Wieselthaler G, et al. Extracorporeal membrane oxygenation for graft failure after heart transplantation: recent Vienna experience. *J Thorac Cardiovasc Surg* 2001; 122:819-820.

24. Hosenpud JD, Bennett LE, Keck BM, Fiol B, Boucek MM, Novick RJ. The Registry of the International Society for Heart and Lung Transplantation: fifteenth official report--1998. *J Heart Lung Transplant* 1998; 17:656-668.

25. Bhatia SJ, Kirshenbaum JM, Shemin RJ, et al. Time course of resolution of pulmonary hypertension and right ventricular remodeling after orthotopic cardiac transplantation. *Circulation* 1987;76:819-826.

26. Bourge RC, Kirklin JK, Naftel DC, White C, Mason DA, Epstein AE. Analysis and predictors of pulmonary vascular resistance after cardiac transplantation. *J Thorac Cardiovasc Surg* 1991; 101:432-444; discussion 44-45.

27. Taghavi S, Ankersmit J, Zuckermann A, et al. A retrospective analysis of extracorporel membrane oxygenation versus right ventricular assist device in acute great failure after heart transplantation. *Transplant Proc* 2003; 35:2805-2807.

28. Duncan B. Extracorporeal Membrane Oxygenation for Circulatory Support. In: Franco K, Verrier E, eds. *Advanced Therapy in Cardiac Surgery.* 2nd ed. Philadelphia, PA: B.C. Decker; 2003: 405-414.

29. Whyte RI, Deeb GM, McCurry KR, Anderson HL 3rd, Bolling SF, Bartlett RH. Extracorporeal life support after heart or lung transplantation. *Ann Thorac Surg* 1994; 58:754-758; discussion 8-9.

30. Fenoglio JJ Jr, Ursell PC, Kellogg CF, Drusin RE, Weiss MB. Diagnosis and classification of myocarditis by endomyocardial biopsy. *N Engl J Med* 1983; 308:12-18.

31. Chen YS, Wang MJ, Chou NK, et al. Rescue for acute myocarditis with shock by extracorporeal membrane oxygenation. *Ann Thorac Surg* 1999; 68:2220-2224.

32. Kawahito K, Murata S, Yasu T, et al. Usefulness of extracorporeal membrane oxygenation for treatment of fulminant myocarditis and circulatory collapse. *Am J Cardiol* 1998; 82:910-911.

33. Hadjimiltiades S, Panidis IP, Segal BL, Iskandrian AS. Recovery of left ventricular function in peripartum cardiomyopathy. *Am Heart J* 1986; 112:1097-1099.

34. Lampert MB, Lang RM. Peripartum cardiomyopathy. *Am Heart J* 1995; 130:860-870.

31

Heart-lung Transplantation and ECLS

Thomas L. Spray, M.D. and Andrew I.M. Campbell, M.D.

Introduction

With survival to discharge following extracorporeal life support (ECLS) ranging from 33 to 77% depending on patient age and the etiology of organ failure,[1] and a significant number of non-survivors requiring withdrawal of therapy due to failure of heart or lung recovery, a sub-population of ECLS patients may benefit from thoracic transplantation. Mechanical circulatory support has become a viable option because of the following reasons: the growing wait list for thoracic organs, the related increase in severity of illness in organ recipients, the use of marginal donors in some centers,[2] and the likelihood of irreversible organ failure in pre-transplant patients, and in severe, but transient organ failure following transplantation. This chapter will outline the experience in utilizing ECLS as a bridge to thoracic transplantation and as a means of post-operative support for the transplanted heart or lung. As 95% of ECLS patients fall within the pediatric age group while only 10% of all thoracic transplant recipients fall within the same range the majority of these data are derived from the pediatric clinical experience.[3]

Heart transplantation and ECLS

Bridge to transplant

Since the mid-1980s, thoracic organ transplantation has become successfully estab-lished in the pediatric patient population. With progressive improvement in ECLS for cardiac support, many cardiac centers came to the conclusion that long-term ECMO support might prove a viable method of supporting patients with irreversible cardiac failure until a suitable graft could be found. The first published record of ECLS support for patients awaiting transplant came from the University of Michigan (U of M) in 1990 and revealed a discouraging 100% mortality,[4] with all 3 patients being withdrawn from consideration for transplantation due to irreversible damage to other organs. Subsequent reviews of the ELSO registry in 1991[5] and a second center-specific study from U of M[6] confirmed very poor survival in the bridge-to-transplant group in both children and adults, with the second study concluding that poor organ donor availability made ECLS an unacceptable choice for mechanical bridge to transplantation. A marked deviation from this opinion was expressed in a 1997 study of 17 patients, including both adults and children, from Arkansas Children's Hospital (ACH),[7] with 12 patients undergoing transplantation and 10 (83%) surviving to hospital discharge. Even more encouraging was the finding that, with aggressive treatment of even fungal sepsis, ECLS patients could safely be immunosuppressed and not experience overwhelming infection in the post-transplant period. In fact, post-transplant survival did not seem to be affected by pre-transplant ECMO support, and similar incidences of infection and rejection were observed in the ECMO-treated patients as compared to those with uncomplicated heart transplants in the relatively short follow-up period.

More recent studies have showed similarly variable results. A retrospective review from the Children's Hospital of Philadelphia (CHOP) in 2002 identified a 39% survival to transplantation but with no significant difference between ECMO-treated and non-treated heart transplant recipients over the first year.[8] Dr. Laks from UCLA reported a 53% survival to discharge in 19 patients who underwent pre-transplant non-pulsatile mechanical support, and again noted very acceptable rates of complications.[9] However, the apparent differences in these outcomes are easily explained by looking at the underlying diagnoses of the patient populations involved; 55% of the patients in the CHOP study had undergone a cardiac surgical procedure and then required ECLS support, whereas none of the patients in the UCLA study had required surgery. This may have left those individuals in the CHOP study more vulnerable to neurologic injury, infection, or secondary organ damage during the initial resuscitation period. This was further confirmed by a report from ACH in which 16 of 47 (32%) patients were successfully bridged to transplant, but only 2 of the 8 pediatric patients (25%) with a diagnosis of congenital heart disease survived vs. 7 out of 8 (88%) with a diagnosis of cardiomyopathy.[10] Additional evidence is found in a more recent paper from Great Ormond Street (GOS) in which a retrospective review of end-stage cardiomyopathy patients requiring mechanical assistance revealed a 92% survival to discharge in those supported with pre-transplant ECMO.[11] Unfortunately, these outstanding results may not be applicable in many other countries where donor accessibility is not as high, since in the GOS review the median waiting time for an organ was 7.5 days, while, in the U.S., the

wait time was approximately 14 days. With a doubling of the wait time, it is not surprising that a significant number of patients experience complications while on ECMO that would exclude them from transplantation.

ABO-incompatible transplantation has been proposed as a potential method of decreasing recipient waiting times and associated waiting list mortality in the general cardiac recipient population and could therefore be especially beneficial in those patients waiting on ECLS. In the pediatric cardiac population, the transplantation of ABO-incompatible organs may be particularly useful, as neonates do not produce antibodies to T-cell-independent antigens, including the major blood-group antigens. However, with a much greater recipient requirement than available donor pool, application of this process might simply translate into shorter waiting times for those already on mechanical support (with a resulting decrease in mortality), but much longer waiting times for those who are in a more stable hemodynamic condition (with a potential increase in waiting-list mortality). In countries where a minority of the infant cardiac donor pool is used, ABO-incompatible transplantation could have a significant effect on minimizing waiting list-related deaths.[12] Unfortunately, the use of large amounts of blood products necessary on ECMO and the inability ability to maintain a low isohemagglutinin titer makes ABO-incompatible transplantation difficult.

The most recent assessment of ECLS as a bridge to transplant comes from Columbia University (CU),[13] where, between 1984 and 2003, three hundred patients were listed for cardiac transplantation. Of the 21 patients who required pre-operative support, 10 survived to transplantation and 6 to hospital discharge (29%), underscoring the minimal improvement that has occurred in this area of ECLS in the last 15 years. If pre-operative ECLS support is then of limited utility in the overall cardiac transplant population, it becomes even more important, from a resource utilization perspective, to identify those patients which may benefit from its application. As stated previously, patients with cardiomyopathies have better survival both to transplant and to discharge, and in particular those who have not undergone a cardiac arrest should be considered the best candidates for bridging.[13] Secondly, preservation of renal function with the avoidance of dialysis while on ECMO has been associated with a higher likelihood of survival both before and after heart transplant.[14] Therefore, patients who fulfill both of these criteria will likely benefit from immediate transplant listing and aggressive supportive therapy.

The final consideration should be how to best manage those patients who are listed while on ECLS. Naturally, contraindications to transplantation may develop during the ECMO run which would require either a temporary or permanent removal of the patient from the waiting list, including severe irreversible neurologic injury, intractable bacterial or fungal sepsis, or withdrawal of parental consent. However, it is also necessary to maintain a proactive approach during this time to optimize the overall patient condition and particularly pulmonary status. This often requires balloon or blade atrial septostomy to insure that the left atrium is well decompressed and that there is no source for potentially elevated pulmonary artery pressures remains. Infection surveillance should include routine culturing of wounds, blood, sputum, and urine with aggressive treatment of positive cultures, due to the potential of initiating immunosuppression should a donor organ become available.

Mechanical support

The advantages of assist devices in optimizing the hemodynamics and organ function in children awaiting transplantation makes the development of pediatric assist devices a high priority for our specialty. Currently, however, only limited types of assist devices are available for bridge to transplantation in pediatric patients.

The currently available devices are either paracorporeal or implantable and are limited in their duration of support. The most commonly used bridges to transplantation in pediatric patients in the U.S. are short-term assist devices such as ECMO and centrifugal ventricular assist device (VAD) pumps as noted above. Long-term devices, which have only been used for medium-term support in most centers, include the Berlin Heart (Berlin Heart AG, Berlin, Germany) and Medos VAD (Medos Medizintechnik AG, Stolberg, Germany) systems, which have until recently only been available in Europe but now have had increasing use under humanitarian device exemption in the U.S. The Heartmate implant and Thoratec adult pulsatile devices (both Thoratec Corp, Pleasanton, CA) have been available for use in larger children and adolescents (>40 kg), but are not applicable for very small children and certainly not infants or neonates (<10 kg). Currently, modifications of adult axial flow devices, such as the DeBakey Child Device (MicroMed Technology, Houston, TX) may be more useful for older children and adolescents (>15-20 kg).

The use of VADs as a bridge to transplant will hopefully result in more patients being available for transplantation. The experience at CHOP for VAD support includes 12 patients; 3 patients receiving the Heartmate device, 7 the Thoratec device, and 2 infants were bridged with the Berlin Heart. Of these 12, 7 (58%) were successfully bridged to transplant. One patient died after transplantation was performed. One patient was successfully bridged to recovery, one patient died prior to transplant, and 3 are currently awaiting donor hearts.

It is apparent that options for mechanical circulatory support in children, particularly infants, continue to be severely limited in the U.S. ECMO is the most versatile option that can be initiated rapidly in patients of any size; however, overall survival to hospital discharge is limited by complications related to anticoagulation. Newer VADs which can be used in very small patients may significantly improve our ability for successful bridge to transplantation in the pediatric population.

Post-transplant support

Improvements in donor and recipient selection and advances in both surgical techniques and immunosuppressive therapy have contributed to a significant decrease in 30-day mortality following cardiac transplantation.[15] However, a number of patients, either due to the effects of brain death on the explanted organ, inadequate cardiac protection during retrieval, or concomitant illness within the donor or the recipient, will develop primary graft dysfunction in the immediate post-operative period and may only respond to extracorporeal mechanical support. The first documentation of this method of therapy came from U of M where 2 of 3 children placed on ECLS for graft failure survived to discharge.[4] Most encouragingly, of the 3 patients supported, no major difficulty was observed in management of their immunosuppressive therapy while on mechanical support, and no insurmountable infections developed. However, in a later study from Kosair Children's Hospital, only 1 of 3 neonates supported post-transplant for hypoplastic left heart syndrome survived to discharge, and that child suffered significant neurologic injuries.[16] A more comprehensive review from Kirshbom et al. in Philadelphia[8] highlighted the differences in early and late outcomes for mechanical support after transplantation. In this paper, 9 patients required support within 7 days of transplant (5 immediately) and 3 after that time point, with only 22% of the early patients surviving to discharge compared to 67% in the late group. It is interesting that none of the late group of patients were subsequently retransplanted, while 2 of the early group were, and that such a marked discrepancy

in survival would persist. The difference can potentially be explained by aggressive graft rejection in the late group leading to transient organ dysfunction, which can be successfully managed with changes in immunosuppression, while the predominant reason for early support is primary graft failure, which may not be recoverable.

Further evidence that the indication for ECMO after transplantation determines the outcome was provided in a recent study from Fenton et al.[17] The investigators noted that 11.9% of their pediatric transplant patients required ECLS support in the perioperative period and proposed that this number was much higher than in the adult population due to the greater likelihood of mild pulmonary hypertension in the congenital heart disease/single ventricle population. This mild dysfunction would be significantly worsened by cardiopulmonary bypass (CPB) and would then create an unacceptable pressure load for the transplanted right ventricle. A 53% survival to discharge in the early ECLS group (less than 6 weeks post-transplant) and a 40% survival in the late group were reported, but, of those patients who were placed on support for pulmonary causes (failure of oxygenation, pulmonary hypertension, or sepsis), none were weaned off ECLS.

Lung transplantation and ECLS

Bridge to transplant

Very limited data exists on the use of ECLS for bridging to pulmonary or cardiopulmonary transplantation. Experience at CHOP shows poor survival in patients listed for lung or heart-lung transplantation requiring pre-transplant ECMO support. Of the 14 patients in this group, only 1 patient underwent transplantation (a heart-lung patient), and remains alive 13 months after transplantation. Of the remaining 13 patients, 1 child (listed for heart-lung transplant) was successfully weaned and discharged home.

This child, who had a previously-repaired atrio-ventricular canal defect, had cardiopulmonary dysfunction after left atrioventricular valve replacement, and remains alive 19 months after ECMO. The remaining 12 children, including all of those listed for lung transplantation, did not survive to transplant or discharge.

Given the small number of patients who received a transplant or survived to discharge, statistical comparisons are impossible. However, some interesting information can be gleaned. First, all patients who had pre-ECMO cardiac arrests also had documented pulmonary hypertension. Of the 10 patients in the lung/heart-lung transplant group with pulmonary hypertension, 4 (40%) had a pre-ECMO cardiac arrest. These 4 patients had an average ECMO duration of 106 hours, and they were all removed from ECMO support because of arrest-related neurologic injuries. The pulmonary hypertension patients (n=5) who did not have cardiac arrests and who did not receive transplants had an average ECMO duration of 482 hours. Interestingly, the only patient who received a transplant with pulmonary hypertension was cannulated electively and underwent transplantation 13 hours later. None of the 4 patients without pulmonary hypertension had a cardiac arrest, and they were maintained on ECMO for an average of 855 hours until they either recovered function (n=1) or had complications that precluded transplantation (n=3).

Post-transplant support

The literature concerning post-transplant ECMO support is essentially the reverse of the pre-transplant ECMO literature in that there are more reports of support after lung transplantation than after heart transplantation. In the CHOP study,[8] survival in patients requiring ECMO after lung transplant was 63% for the ECMO group vs. 33% for the heart-transplant patients. The time course of support requirements and outcomes are interesting in that the majority of post-heart transplant patients required support early after

transplantation (9/12, or 75%), with relatively poor outcomes in the group (2/9, or 22% survival). Only 3 patients required support in the late period after heart transplantation, with 2 of the 3 surviving to discharge. The lung/heart-lung transplant patients, on the other hand, were more evenly divided between the early and late groups (3 vs. 5), and the early group had better early outcomes (100% survival to discharge vs. 40%).

The difference in outcome of patients requiring ECMO early after heart transplantation compared with lung/heart-lung transplantation is interesting. There have been several reports in the literature[18-20] describing ECMO support after lung transplantation, primarily in adult patients. In these reports and the CHOP study, patients with early or immediate reperfusion injury or graft dysfunction typically improved after 1-5 days of ECMO support. Patients who present late after transplant, however, do not recover function as often, and therefore ECMO support is in effect an attempt to bridge to retransplant. Lung-containing grafts injured by infectious processes, particularly adenovirus,[21] often do not recover and commonly recipient survival requires retransplantation.

Discussion

The options available for mechanical cardiopulmonary support in pediatric patients are limited in most institutions because of the lack of size-appropriate VADs. Also, the frequency of biventricular dysfunction and pulmonary hypertension in the pediatric population often makes the use of VADs difficult even when they are available. Placement of bilateral VADs in small children can be difficult and introduces a variety of potential complications. Because of these problems and the widespread use of ECMO for support of children with respiratory failure, ECMO remains the most commonly used method of mechanical circulatory support in children.

There are several advantages and disadvantages to ECMO that must be considered. The most obvious advantage of ECMO is the familiarity of most programs with this method of support. ECMO circuits can be prepared for use quickly, and patients can be cannulated and support initiated in the ICU if necessary. VADs, on the other hand, require a thoracotomy or sternotomy and a trip to the OR. In emergency situations, ECMO support can be instituted in 15-20 minutes. Another advantage of ECMO is its versatility. Essentially all forms of cardiopulmonary failure and all cardiac anatomic diagnoses can be treated with ECMO, including biventricular failure, right-sided failure with pulmonary hypertension, and isolated left-sided failure, while VADs are best suited to isolated failure of one ventricle in a biventricular heart. Although dual ventricular support is possible and not uncommon in adults, space considerations make bi-VAD support problematic in small children. The most significant disadvantages of ECMO are the requirements for immobilization, intensive care monitoring, and anticoagulation. Unlike some patients receiving intracorporeal VAD support, children on ECMO cannot be extubated and mobilized.

For patients awaiting transplantation, the duration of ECMO support is generally determined by organ allocation policies rather than patient-specific characteristics. The CHOP experience with long-term pre-transplant ECMO support includes a patient who required 1126 hours of support before a heart became available. Although this patient clearly represents the extreme, 4 CHOP patients underwent transplantation after >500 hours of ECMO support, and, of the 8 patients listed for heart transplants who remained on ECMO for >250 hours, 7 received transplants. These experiences indicate that there should be no arbitrary cutoff point for duration of support, so long as complications precluding transplantation have not developed.

Several reports have discussed the use of ECMO as a bridge to cardiac transplantation in children. The largest series in the literature was that of del Nido et al,[22] which included 14 children placed on ECMO and listed for heart transplantation between 1981-1993. Several interesting points

become apparent when comparing their experience and that of CHOP. First, postcardiotomy patients had a worse outcome than non-cardiotomy patients in both studies, with 25% (2/8) of the postcardiotomy patients surviving to discharge compared with 83% (5/6) of the non-cardiotomy patients in the earlier study. Second, del Nido et al. received organs for 64% (9/14) of patients after an average ECMO duration of 102 hours, whereas in the CHOP study, only 39% (12/31) of patients listed for heart transplants received organs, despite an average ECMO duration of 359 hours. This difference reflects the increasing scarcity of donor organs in the interval between the 2 reports. However, despite increased organ scarcity and longer duration of ECMO support, there was no difference in short-term outcomes between the 2 studies; early survival for the group as a whole was 50% in the previous study, compared with 48% in the current report.

The decision of when to list postcardiotomy patients for heart transplantation can be difficult because it is challenging to predict which patients might recover function. In this group, the patients who were successfully weaned from ECMO had an average ECMO duration of 4.5 days with a range from 1.4 to 7.9 days. Therefore, in general, those patients who will be successfully weaned from ECMO will do so within 8 days. Mehta et al.[23] reported a similar ECMO duration of 3.4 days for their postcardiotomy patients who were successfully weaned from support. However, the 3 postcardiotomy patients who were bridged to transplant received organs after 3, 8, and 10 days on the waiting list, respectively. The decision of when to list postcardiotomy patients for transplantation must be individualized on the basis of the management team's assessment of the likelihood of recovery. Patients who are believed to be unlikely to recover cardiac function on the basis of anatomy and intra-operative evaluation are generally listed earlier than those who are believed to be more likely to recover function. In most circumstances, patients are listed as soon as transplant candidacy is confirmed so as to maximize the patient's chance of receiving an organ before complications develop.

Although it may seem counterintuitive that a pre-ECMO cardiac arrest does not significantly affect outcome for patients listed for heart transplantation, previous studies have reported survival in the 33- 53%[20] range, which is consistent with the current report. For those patients who were placed on ECMO after a cardiac arrest (n=15; 11 heart, 3 lung, and 1 heart-lung) and who were not previously listed for transplantation, the timing of listing is variable and depends on exclusion of significant neurologic or other end-organ injury after the arrest. On average, these patients were listed for transplantation 1.4 days after the arrest with a range from 0-8 days. At CHOP, donor-organ size and distance-acceptance criteria are not altered for this group of patients, but suboptimal organs are occasionally considered.

Perhaps the most important finding of this study is that the long-term outcome for patients who receive heart transplants after ECMO bridge to transplant is not discernibly different from that of patients who undergo transplantation without pretransplant ECMO. This result is markedly different from the findings of Dellgren et al.,[24] who reported significantly worse outcomes for post-ECMO transplant patients (2-year survival of approximately 48% vs. 88% for non-ECMO patients, P<0.01). Given the results, aggregate outcomes may be further improved if organ allocation protocols were modified so as to minimize waiting times for patients on ECMO or other mechanical support.

Unfortunately, the outcome for patients who required ECMO support while waiting for lung or heart-lung transplants was not as favorable as that of the heart-transplant patients. Only 1 patient of the pre-transplant ECMO group received a heart-lung transplant, and none of the 8 patients listed for lungs survived to transplant. Equally disappointing was the low rate of successful weaning from ECMO, with only 1 patient surviving to discharge after discontinuation of support. Unlike patients with viral myocarditis or postcardiotomy

myocardial dysfunction, whose cardiac function occasionally improves if given time on mechanical support, most children listed for lung transplantation did not improve. The majority of patients listed for lung or heart-lung transplantation who required ECMO had pulmonary hypertension, with or without underlying cardiac disease. The outcome for patients with pulmonary hypertension who had a cardiac arrest while waiting for transplantation was particularly poor; all of these patients had neurologic injuries that rendered them unsuitable candidates for transplant. Support for such patients should be selectively applied, with the understanding that support will be withdrawn early if neurologic or other end-organ injury precluding transplant is identified.

References

1. Conrad SA, Rycus PT, Dalton H. Extracorporeal Life Support Registry Report 2004. *ASAIO J*. 2005; 51:4-10.

2. Pierre AF, Sekine Y, Hutcheon MA, Waddell TK, Keshavjee SH. Marginal donor lungs: a reassessment. *J Thorac Cardiovasc Surg* 2002; 123:421-427.

3. Bennett LE, Keck BM, Hertz MI, Trulock EP, Taylor DO. Worldwide thoracic organ transplantation: a report from the UNOS/ISHLT international registry for thoracic organ transplantation. *Clin Transpl* 2001; 25-40.

4. Delius RE, Zwischenberger JB, Cilley R, et al. Prolonged extracorporeal life support of pediatric and adolescent cardiac transplant patients. *Ann Thorac Surg* 1990; 50:791-795.

5. Meliones JN, Custer JR, Snedecor S, Moler FW, O'Rourke PP, Delius RE. Extracorporeal life support for cardiac assist in pediatric patients. Review of ELSO Registry data. *Circulation* 1991; 84:III168-72.

6. Kolla S, Lee WA, Hirschl RB, Bartlett RH. Extracorporeal life support for cardiovascular support in adults. *ASAIO J* 1996; 42:M809-819.

7. Frazier EA, Faulkner SC, Seib PM, Harrell JE, Van Devanter SH, Fasules JW. Prolonged extracorporeal life support for bridging to transplant: technical and mechanical considerations. *Perfusion* 1997; 12:93-98.

8. Kirshbom PM, Bridges ND, Myung RJ, Gaynor JW, Clark BJ, Spray TL. Use of extracorporeal membrane oxygenation in pediatric thoracic organ transplantation. *J Thorac Cardiovasc Surg* 2002; 123:130-136.

9. Levi D, Marelli D, Plunkett M, et al. Use of assist devices and ECMO to bridge pediatric patients with cardiomyopathy to transplantation. *J Heart Lung Transplant* 2002; 21:760-770.

10. Fiser WP, Yetman AT, Gunselman RJ, et al. Pediatric arteriovenous extracorporeal membrane oxygenation (ECMO) as a bridge to cardiac transplantation. *J Heart Lung Transplant* 2003; 22:770-777.

11. Goldman AP, Cassidy J, de Leval M, et al. The waiting game: bridging to paediatric heart transplantation. *Lancet* 2003; 362:1967-1970.

12. West LJ, Pollock-Barziv SM, Dipchand AI, et al. ABO-incompatible heart transplantation in infants. *N Engl J Med* 2001; 344:793-800.

13. Bae JO, Frischer JS, Waich M, Addonizio LJ, Lazar EL, Stolar CJ. Extracorporeal membrane oxygenation in pediatric cardiac transplantation. *J Pediatr Surg* 2005; 40:1051-1056.

14. Gajarski RJ, Mosca RS, Ohye RG, et al. Use of extracorporeal life support as a bridge to pediatric cardiac transplantation. *J Heart Lung Transplant* 2003; 22:28-34.

15. Hosenpud JD, Bennett LE, Keck BM, Boucek MM, Novick RJ. The Registry of the International Society for Heart and Lung Transplantation: seventeenth official report-2000. *J Heart Lung Transplant* 2000; 19:909-931.

16. McKay VJ, Stewart DL, Robinson TW, Cook LN, Austin EH 3rd. Preoperative versus postoperative extracorporeal life support in neonatal cardiac patients. *Perfusion* 1997; 12:179-86.

17. Fenton KN, Webber SA, Danford DA, Gandhi SK, Periera J, Pigula FA. Long-term survival after pediatric cardiac transplantation and postoperative ECMO support. *Ann Thorac Surg* 2003; 76:843-6.

18. Pereszlenyi A, Lang G, Steltzer H, et al. Bilateral lung transplantation with intra- and postoperatively prolonged ECMO support in patients with pulmonary hypertension. *Eur J Cardiothoracic Surg* 2002; 21:858-863.

19. Dahlberg PS Prekker ME, Herrington CS, Hertz MI, Park SJ. Medium-term results of extracorporeal membrane oxygenation for severe acute lung injury after lung transplantation. *J Heart Lung Transplant* 2004; 23:979-984.

20. Oto T, Rosenfeldt F, Rowland M, et al. Extracorporeal membrane oxygenation after lung transplantation: evolving technique improves outcomes. *AM Thorac Surg* 2004; 78:1230-1235.

21. Bridges ND, Spray TL, Collins MH, Bowles NE, Towbin JA. Adenovirus infection in the lung results in graft failure after lung transplantation. *J Thorac Cardiovasc Surg* 1998; 116:617-23.

22. del Nido PJ, Armitage JM, Fricker FJ, et al. Extracorporeal membrane oxygenation support as a bridge to pediatric heart transplantation. *Circulation* 1994; 90:II66-9.

23. Mehta U, Laks H, Sadeghi A, et al. Extracorporeal membrane oxygenation for cardiac support in pediatric patients. *Am Surg* 2000; 66:879-86.

24. Dellgren G, Koirala B, Sakopoulus A, et al. Pediatric heart transplantation: improving results in high-risk patients. *J Thorac Cardiovasc Surg* 2001; 121:782-91.

32

ECLS and the Kidney

Timothy E. Bunchman, M.D.

Introduction

Various events cause electrolyte and fluid disturbances in patients on ECMO. These events are often exaggerated by the underlying illness that led to the use of ECMO and will also be affected by the length of treatment. These factors may have an additive negative effect on patients who are critically ill and may have underlying fluid and electrolyte disturbances prior to the initiation of ECMO. The purpose of this review is to give a nephrologist's perspective on fluid and electrolyte disturbances, management, and outcome in patients who develop renal impairment on ECLS.

Factors influencing electrolyte disturbance

ECMO can cause electrolyte disturbances in three ways. First, connection of the ECMO circuit results in an increase in circulatory volume – a doubling in the case of neonates – which can cause electrolyte imbalance. Second, ECMO causes a reduction in renal blood flow. Third, ECMO causes cytokine activation, resulting in leaky capillary syndrome.[1-5]

Silicone membrane oxygenators used for ECMO require a large priming volume which is disproportionate to the patient's intravascular blood volume, due to a lack of appropriately-sized equipment. The ECMO circuit also influ-ences drug binding and drug clearance as drugs adhere to the plastic circuit.[6] Further volume effects can be caused by the innate circuit compliance, which is less of a problem with poly-methyl pentene (PMP) oxygenators compared to silicone. Membrane oxygenators (silicone or PMP) are an additional source of insensible fluid loss, while micro-porous polypropylene oxygenators can result in plasma leakage. All of these factors contribute to fluid and electrolyte disturbances.[7]

The ECMO circuit is primed with blood (with the exception of eCPR). This blood prime can be associated with immediate electrolyte disturbances. Banked blood is acidotic, hypo-calcemic, and hyperkalemic; careful attention to the components of the prime is necessary to mitigate complications related to its use. Techniques vary from center to center, but the addition of calcium and buffer (either bicarbon-ate or THAM) to the prime blood is essential to offset the hyperkalemia of the banked blood. Another technique is to wash the prime using pre-ECMO hemofiltration to normalize the electrolytes prior to initiating bypass. This lat-ter technique is extremely effective but quite time-consuming, taking 1-2 hours. Correction of acidosis, hyperkalemia, and hypocalcemia has been shown to have an important influence on patients undergoing continuous renal replace-ment therapy (CRRT).[8]

Effect on renal blood flow

Data have shown a reduction in renal blood flow as VV ECMO is initiated.[2] The cause is speculated to be related to the compliance of the tubing as well as the "cytokine storm."[4,5] Data have not shown whether VV or VA ECMO is better for the preservation of renal function. Published work in both animal models and in patient experience with ECMO treatment of diaphragmatic hernia, cardiac failure, and respiratory failure has not shown a marked difference in outcome between VV and VA ECMO, including renal dysfunction.[9-12]

Other factors in addition to the electrolyte disturbances of the blood prime can cause volume and electrolyte imbalance. ECMO patients often have significant problems with vasodilation, whether they are on VV or VA ECMO.[13] This results in a significant need for colloid resuscitation in the first 24-36 hours. Colloid is usually given in the form of packed red blood cells, albumin, or fresh frozen plasma. Since each of these products binds calcium, they all introduce a risk for hypocalcemia. Therefore, attention to calcium values at the initiation of and during blood product infusions is important. Fredrikson et al. showed that 15-20% of ECMO patients have transient hypercalcemia.[14] This may be partially explained by volume depletion in the presence of high albumin.

Skogby demonstrated that the "cytokine storm" occurs in patients as blood interfaces with the membrane and tubing, resulting in an increase in capillary permeability, also called "leaky capillary syndrome."[4] It has been suggested that early intervention with CRRT may improve the "cytokine storm." This has been debated greatly in the non-ECMO CRRT literature, continues to be controversial, and is an ongoing area of investigation.[15]

In a review by Zwischenberger et al. of ELSO Registry data, 24% of 13,000 neonates treated with ECMO either had transient renal dysfunction or a need for CRRT. This appeared to be related directly to the severity of illness, as well as to the duration on ECMO.[13]

The ELSO Registry provides data on the incidence of CRRT on ECMO, which is a subset of the total number of ECMO patients with ARF. From 1998-2004, 7,264 neonates ($\leq$30 days) and 3,276 children (>30 days and $\leq$10 years) underwent ECMO. In the infant population, 5,263 received VA ECMO and 2,001 received VV ECMO. The incidence of CRRT was 2% and 0.6%, respectively. In the pediatric population, 2,735 received VA and 541 received VV ECMO. The CRRT incidence was 4.9% and 6%, respectively, higher than in the neonatal population. One cannot determine from these data whether the CRRT need is greater for children than infants; this difference may be due to variations in clinical practice. Further, the greater use of CRRT in the older group may be the result of a larger portion of this patient population having sepsis as their primary indication for ECMO.

Another complication of ECMO is hypertension. Heaggen et al. noted that hypertension is significant and difficult to control in patients on ECMO.[16] Among the reasons for hypertension are fluid retention, sedation, and microemboli to the kidney. The latter is not dissimilar to the transient hypertension seen in the neonatal population when umbilical artery catheters are removed. Long-term follow-up of neonates with umbilical artery catheters shows that less than 5% are hypertensive 1 year later. Follow-up of ECMO patients has shown the incidence of hypertension to be minimal, suggesting that hypertension during ECMO is a transient yet significant problem. Work by McBride et al. showed that the use of IV nicardipine can easily improve the hypertension seen in neonates on ECMO.[17] However, this work also indicated a need for nicardipine at higher doses than are generally recommended, probably due to drug binding to the circuit and to the larger volume distribution.[18]

Drug kinetics

Various authors have looked at the impact of large extracorporeal blood volumes on drug kinetics.[7] Drug kinetics appear to be influenced by the extracorporeal blood volume, adherence to the membrane and tubing, and protein binding of the drugs. In studies by Mulla et al., theophylline clearance and kinetics varied with the volume of distribution and the extracorporeal blood volume, as well as the dose and duration.[19] When compared to non-ECMO patients, not surprisingly, the distribution of volume was much higher. In contrast, drugs such as midazolam are highly protein-bound and therefore demonstrate a longer plasma half-life.[20]

A review by Buck et al.[7] confirmed the importance of increased volume of distribution and drug binding on the pharmacokinetics of drugs during ECMO. Further, hemofiltration or dialysis of any mode will dramatically increase drug clearance. Dialysis has a significant impact on the clearance of drugs that are mostly non-protein bound, but depending on the mode of dialysis and the type of membrane used, significant removal may be seen for highly protein-bound drugs such as vancomycin, which historically were retained in ARF. Therefore, drug kinetics may be modulated by changes in renal blood flow, volume of distribution, and hepatic function, as well as the addition of hemofiltration.[7]

Dialysis on ECMO

The technique of dialysis is based upon solute (e.g., potassium and urea) or ultrafiltration (water) across a semi-permeable membrane. Water will come across the membrane based upon a pressure variance (transmembrane pressure [TMP]); the greater the TMP, the greater the ultrafiltration rate. In the hemodialysis (HD) and hemofiltration (HF) systems, the TMP is controlled by a venous pressure return. The greater the venous pressure, the higher the TMP and the greater the ultrafiltration rate. The rate at which a solute comes across the membrane is measured by its Sieving coefficient (SC). A low molecular weight solute that does not bind to protein – urea, for example – will have an SC ~1, denoting that, at the distal end of the membrane, the concentration of urea in the filtered solution will be the same as the concentration in the wash solution. Larger solutes and those that bind to proteins have lower SCs, indicating that they will not move through the filtration membrane as readily. For example, for a solute with an SC of 0.6, only 60% of the concentration will equalize on a pass through the filtration membrane. Further, the solute clearance will vary directly with the amount of dialysate or replacement fluid exposed per unit of time.

When comparing HD, HF (CVVH or CVVHD), and peritoneal dialysis (PD), HD uses 30-40 l/hr of dialysate, while CVVH or CVVHD may use 2 l/hr and PD may use 1 l/hr. Thus, HD is highly efficient per unit of time as compared to HF or PD. The difficulty with HD is that it is classically used for 3-4 hours per day or even every other day. In this time period, the solute clearance can be easily obtained, but the amount of net ultrafiltration that needs to occur at the next HD session, 24-48 hours later, may have a negative impact on volume status and hemodynamics, making HD impractical in this setting.[1,15]

Since the early 1980s, studies have demonstrated the benefit of adding hemofiltration for ECMO patients.[21] A recent study by Hoover et al. noted that early intervention with CRRT improved fluid balance and caloric intake and reduced the need for diuretics.[22] Additionally, they suggest that early CRRT-treated patients tended towards higher survival when compared to patients not requiring dialysis. This contradicts historical data that suggested that the use of dialytic therapy or the indication of dialytic therapy was associated with lower survival. Historical data from Kolovos et al. also suggest that the need for CRRT in cardiac patients requiring ECMO had a negative impact on survival.[10] The cause may be historical bias at that institution or late onset of intervention. More recent experience by Hoover suggests that early intervention with CRRT leads to survival rates equal to patients that do not require CRRT.

Techniques for CRRT include either peritoneal dialysis, which is advocated by many programs, or continuous hemofiltration.[23-25] The techniques of hemofiltration have been well described by our group.[1,15] The hemofiltration circuit can be constructed as a free-flow circuit using the ECMO pump to circulate the patient's blood flow, or can utilize a commercially-available hemofiltration circuit, using the hemofiltration pump for blood flow. In the latter situation, the hemofiltration circuit can be set up in a standard convective or in a diffusive model of hemofiltration for ECMO patients.[26-28] The free-flow system uses a continuous arterio-venous hemofiltration (CAVH) equivalent system, forcing consideration of medications prescribed. For example, a 3 kg infant will require ECMO at a blood flow rate of 300 ml/min in order to maintain adequate flow either on VV or VA ECMO. Introduction of a hemofilter into the system may result in blood flows of 150-200 ml/min across that membrane, depending on the particular techniques used. This is in stark contrast to the standard CRRT prescription for the same size child with blood flow at 30 ml/min. This 5- to 10-fold increase in blood flow will cause a significant increase on clearance, compared to standard dialysis. In addition, the ECMO pump flow rate must be increased to offset the hemofilter flow. An ultrasonic flow meter is helpful for monitoring flow when using free-flow CRRT. In standard dialysis, clearance is mostly related to saturation of dialysate, and is less dependent on the blood flow rate. However, the blood flow and the turnover of blood is so rapid that clearance may be excessive. Therefore, either the convective or the diffusive solution rate may require down-regulation to offset the high clearance. The effluence from the hemofilter in the free-flow technique is often controlled by an IV pump. These pumps have been reported to be inaccurate in an ECMO setting, putting the child at risk of inadvertent volume depletion from excessive ultrafiltration.[1] This will negatively impact nutrition and drug clearance, and can result in excessive hemodynamic compromise.[7,28] Therefore, it is useful to measure the effluent using a burette or similar device hourly to detect excessive fluid loss.

The location of an HF circuit on an ECMO circuit is important and has been previously described.[1] If the HF circuit is set up in parallel to the oxygenator, then the circuit with lower resistance (i.e., the HF) will cause blood to be diverted from the oxygenator. Figure 1 demonstrates various locations that a HF circuit can be placed during ECMO.

There is no published information on the relationship between the choice of HF membrane and outcome in ECMO or non-ECMO treated patients. Comparison of a AN-69 membrane to polysulfone membranes in a septic animal model suggest that the AN-69 membrane is superior for hemodynamic stability when used in a convective (CVVH) mode.[29] The AN-69 membrane has been associated with a bradykinin reaction at the onset of HF, with risk of hemodynamic compromise.[8] Recent work by Hackbarth et al notes that both of the membranes have some influence on bradykinin production, but this effect is easily avoided by dialyzing the circuit prior to initiation of CRRT.[30]

In those patients who are on CRRT on VV ECMO, the use of standard hemodynamic monitoring, including blood pressure and heart rate, is needed to help determine the degree of ultrafiltration. In patients on VA ECMO, however, excessive ultrafiltration may occur without hemodynamic compromise due to the fact that the VA ECMO circuit provides cardiovascular support. The bedside ECMO clinician can usually determine if a patient is intravascularly depleted when the pump is alarming for decreased venous return. In those patients who are hypervolemic, the ECMO blood flow rate can easily exceed 100 ml/kg/min. However, in those patients who are dry or in those patients with inadequate venous cannula size, often the blood flow rate is limited. Therefore, the addition of hemofiltration may impact the overall blood flow of the ECMO circuit, particularly when hemofiltration is excessive.

Diuretic therapy

Diuretics are commonly used in patients on ECMO in order to potentiate solute as well as fluid clearance. Whether a clinician uses CRRT or diuretics is a matter of preference. There is a bias that fluid clearance, either by diuresis or CRRT, will reduce lung water and improve gas exchange and ventilation. This has been standard clinical practice in most ECMO units for many years, but has never been subjected to a prospective, randomized

trial. There may be a negative impact for patients on VA ECMO due to hemodynamic compromise. In the last five years, there have been conflicting data as to the benefit vs. risk of diuretics for avoiding or mitigating the use of CRRT. Mehta et al. suggested that the early use of diuretics to avoid CRRT is associated with lower survival, but recent investigations are contradictory.[31,32] Medications for diuresis include loop diuretics (e.g., furosemide or bumetanide) or thiazide-like diuretics (e.g., oral metolazone or IV diurel). These drugs can be used independently or in combination to help augment fluid removal, but may not affect solute clearance. Since urine volume does not correlate with solute clearance, the nutritional support of the patient must be adjusted in order to maintain adequate balance between nutrition and solute clearance. Amino acid delivery, amino acid losses through the CRRT circuit, or urea losses through the urine must be considered.

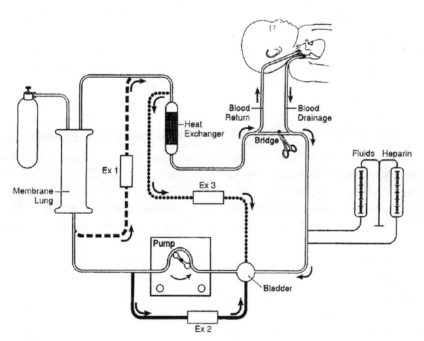

Figure 1. Schematic of a child on ECMO. The figure shows examples of the placement of a free-flow hemofilter or a hemofiltration pump "in-line" with the ECMO circuit. Example 1 bypasses the oxygenator and is less preferable. Example 2 and 3 both return to the bladder and are considered standard.

Outcome with CRRT

Two studies have looked at long-term renal function in patients who have been on ECMO and CRRT. Work by Golgej et al. examined 5 children who required hemofiltration on ECMO and were then converted over to peritoneal dialysis.[25] They found 4 of 5 patients came off dialysis within a short period after cessation of ECMO. Meyer et al. described 35 children requiring CRRT and hemofiltration.[33] Of those 35 patients, 20 patients were removed from ECMO and did not survive. Of the remaining 15, all patients were weaned off ECMO and required CRRT for varying period after discontinuation of ECMO. Of those 15 patients, 14 had full recovery of renal function within 3 months and had no long-term renal complications. The remaining patient had an ongoing need for end-stage renal disease therapy and ultimately received a kidney transplant for Wegener's Granulomatosis.

These data suggest that the use of CRRT may improve survival, and also refute historical data that CRRT was associated with lower survival. Patients who required CRRT during ECMO have a high likelihood of full recovery of renal function.

Conclusion

Electrolyte and fluid disturbances in patients on ECMO have several causes. Many are a result of the child's illness prior to initiation of ECMO, while others are attributable to ECMO itself. Many of these events are identifiable and preventable.

As with many disease processes, severity of illness continues to determine survival.[34,35] Extracorporeal devices are used to support the patient until specific therapy is provided or improvement occurs. Early intervention with CRRT may improve survival in children on ECMO, and in those who have ARF and need ECMO.

References

1. Smoyer WE, Maxvold NJ, Remenapp R, Bunchman TE. Renal replacement therapy. In: Farhman BP, Zimmerman JJ, eds. *Pediatric Critical Care.* 2nd ed. St. Louis, MO: Mosby; 1998.

2. Roy BJ, Cornish JD, Clark RH. Venovenous extracorporeal membrane oxygenation affects renal function. *Pediatrics* 1995; 95:573-578.

3. Ingyinn M, Rais-Bahrami K, Evangelista R, et al. Comparison of the effect of venovenous versus venoarterial extracorporeal membrane oxygenation on renal blood flow in newborn lambs. *Perfusion* 2004; 19:163-170.

4. Skogby M, Adrian K, Friberg LG, et al. Influence of hemofiltration on plasma cytokine levels and platelet activation during extra corporeal membrane oxygenation. *Scand Cardiovasc J* 2000; 34:315-320.

5. Golej J, Winter P, Schoffmann G, et al. Impact of extracorporeal membrane oxygenation modality on cytokine release during rescue from infant hypoxia. *Shock* 2003; 20:110-115.

6. Hewson M, Nawadra V, Oliver J, Odgers C, Plummer J, Simmer K. Insulin infusions in the neonatal unit: delivery variation due to adsorption. *J Paediatr Child Health* 2000; 36:216-20.

7. Buck ML. Pharmacokinetic changes during extracorporeal membrane oxygenation: implications for drug therapy of neonates. *Clin Pharmacokinet* 2003; 42:403-417.

8. Brophy PD, Mottes TA, Kudelka TL, et al. AN-69 membrane reactions are pH-dependent and preventable. *Am J Kidney Dis* 2001; 38:173-178.

9. Dimmitt RA, Moss RL, Rhine WD, Benitz WE, Henry MC, Vanmeurs KP. Venoarterial versus venovenous extra-

corporeal membrane oxygenation in congenital diaphragmatic hernia: the Extracorporeal Life Support Organization Registry, 1990-1999. *J Pediatr Surg* 2001; 36:1199-1204.

10. Kolovos NS, Bratton SL, Moler FW, et al. Outcome of pediatric patients treated with extracorporeal life support after cardiac surgery. *Ann Thorac Surg* 2003; 76:1435-1441.

11. Zahraa JN, Moler FW, Annich GM, Maxvold NJ, Bartlett RH, Custer JR. Venovenous versus venoarterial extracorporeal life support for pediatric respiratory failure: are there differences in survival and acute complications? *Crit Care Med* 2000; 28:521-525.

12. Hunter CJ, Blood AB, Bishai JM, et al. Cerebral blood flow and oxygenation during venoarterial and venovenous extracorporeal membrane oxygenation in the newborn lamb. *Pediatr Crit Care Med* 2004; 5:475-481.

13. Zwischenberger JB, Nguyen TT, Upp JR Jr, et al. Complications of neonatal extracorporeal membrane oxygenation. Collective experience from the Extracorporeal Life Support Organization. *J Thorac Cardiovasc Surg* 1994; 107:838-848.

14. Fridriksson JH, Helmrath MA, Wessel JJ, Warner BW. Hypercalcemia associated with extracorporeal life support in neonates. *J Pediatr Surg* 2001; 36:493-497.

15. Barletta GM, Bunchman TE. Acute renal failure in children and infants. *Curr Opin Crit Care* 2004; 10:499-504.

16. Heggen JA, Fortenberry JD, Tanner AJ, Reid CA, Mizzell DW, Pettignano R. Systemic hypertension associated with venovenous extracorporeal membrane oxygenation for pediatric respiratory failure. *J Pediatr Surg* 2004; 39:1626-1631.

17. McBride BF, White CM, Campbell M, Frey BM. Nicardipine to control neonatal hypertension during extracorporeal membrane oxygen support. *Ann Pharmacother* 2003; 37:667-670.

18. Flynn JT, Mottes TA, Brophy PD, Kershaw DB, Smoyer WE, Bunchman TE. Intravenous nicardipine for treatment of severe hypertension in children. *J Pediatr* 2001; 139:38-43.

19. Mulla H, Nabi F, Nichani S, Lawson G, Firmin RK, Upton DR. Population pharmacokinetics of theophylline during pediatric extracorporeal membrane oxygenation. *Br J Clin Pharmacol* 2003; 55:23-31.

20. Mulla H, McCormack P, Lawson, Firmin RK, Upton DR. Pharmacokinetics of midazolam in neonates undergoing extracorporeal membrane oxygenation. *Anesthesiology* 2003; 99:275-282.

21. Sell LL, Cullen ML, Whittlesey GC, Lerner GR, Klein MD. Experience with renal failure during extracorporeal membrane oxygenation: treatment with continuous hemofiltration. *J Pediatr Surg* 1987; 22:600-602.

22. Hoover N, Fortenberry J, Heard M, et al. Continuous venovenous hemofiltration (CVVH) use in pediatric respiratory failure patients on ECMO: a case-control study. Presented at: 3rd International Conference on Pediatric Renal Replacement Therapy; June 24-26, 2004; Orlando, FL.

23. Heiss KF, Pettit B, Hirschl RB, et al. Renal insufficiency and volume overload in neonatal ECMO managed by continuous ultrafiltration. *ASAIO Trans* 1987; 33:557-560.

24. Yap HJ, Chen YC, Fang JT, Huang CC. Combination of continuous renal replacement therapies (CRRT) and extracorporeal membrane oxygenation (ECMO) for advanced cardiac patients. *Ren Fail* 2003; 25:183-193.

25. Golej J, Boigner H, Burda G, Hermon M, Kitzmueller E, Trittenwein G. Peritoneal dialysis for continuing renal support

after cardiac ECMO and hemofiltration. *Wien Klin Wochenschr* 2002; 114:733-738.

26. Palevsky PM, Bunchman T, Tetta C. The Acute Dialysis Quality Initiative--part V: operational characteristics of CRRT. *Avd Ren Replace Ther* 2002; 9:268-272.

27. Maxvold NJ, Bunchman TE. Renal failure and replacement therapy. *Crit Care Clin* 2003; 19:563-575.

28. Maxvold NJ, Smoyer WE, Custer JR, Bunchman TE. Amino acid loss and nitrogen balance in critically ill children with acute renal failure: a prospective comparison between classic hemofiltration and hemofiltration with dialysis. *Crit Care Med* 2000; 28:1161-1165.

29. Rogiers P, Zhang H, Pauwels D, Vincent JL. Comparison of polyacrylonitril (AN69) and polysulphone membrane during hemofiltration in canine endotoxic shock. *Crit Care Med* 2003; 31:1219-1225.

30. Hackbarth RM, Eding D, Gianoli Smith C, Koch A, Sanfilippo DJ, Bunchman TE. Zero balance (A-BUF) in blood -primed CRRT circuits achieves electrolyte and acid-base homeostasis prior to patient connection. *Pediatr Nephrol* 2005; (Epub).

31. Mehta RL, Rasual MT, Soroko S, Chertow GM: PICARD Study Group. Diuretics, mortality, and nonrecovery of renal function in acute renal failure. *JAMA* 2002; 288:2547-2553.

32. Uchino S, Doig GS, Bellomo R, et al. Diuretics and mortality in acute renal failure. *Crit Care Med* 2004; 32:1669-1677.

33. Meyer RJ, Brophy PD, Bunchman TE, et al. Survival and renal function in pediatric patients following extracorporeal life support with hemofiltration. *Pediatr Crit Care Med* 2001; 2:238-242.

34. Swaniker F, Kolla S, Moler F, et al. Extracorporeal life support outcome for 128 pediatric patients with respiratory failure. *J Pediatric Surg* 2000; 35:197-202.

35. Bunchman TE, McBryde KD, Mottes TE, Gardner JJ, Maxvold NJ, Brophy PD. Pediatric acute renal failure: outcome by modality and disease. *Pediatr Nephrol* 2001; 16:1067-1071.

33

Nutritional Support of the ECMO Patient

Tom Jaksic, M.D., Ph.D.

Introduction

ECMO patients demonstrate a marked catabolic stress response that is qualitatively analogous to other forms of critical illness. Nutritional support is indicated and is predicated upon a clear understanding of the metabolism of ECMO patients, their metabolic reserves, and nutritional requirements.

Metabolism of patients on ECMO

It was once surmised that patients on ECMO were in a metabolic "rest state" secondary to the potentially beneficial effects of the ECMO circuit in decreasing both cardiac and pulmonary work. Quantitative stable isotopic studies, however, have not supported this concept. In fact, neonates on ECMO demonstrate some of the highest rates of protein catabolism reported.[1]

The hallmark of the catabolic response to critical illness is the accentuated breakdown of skeletal muscle protein that results in an enhanced movement of amino acids through the circulation. This provides amino acids needed for the rapid synthesis of proteins vital for the inflammatory response and tissue repair. Those amino acids not used for protein synthesis are channeled through the liver to create glucose from their carbon skeletons by a biochemical process termed gluconeongenesis. Hence, glucose requirements are effectively met. There is also a marked rise in the circulation of hepatically derived acute-phase proteins (e.g., C-reactive protein, fibrinogen, haptoglobin, alpha-1 antitripsin, and alpha-1 acid glycoprotein) and a concomitant decrease in hepatically derived nutrient transport proteins such as albumin and retinol binding protein. Depending upon their degree of illness, ECMO patients can manifest very high levels of acute phase proteins and the inflammatory mediator IL-6 that appears largely responsible for the acute phase response.[2]

The stereotypic metabolic response to illness is associated with a consistent hormonal and cytokine profile regardless of the specific disease process. There is a very transient decline in insulin concentrations followed by a persistent elevation. Despite higher insulin levels that, in theory, should promote anabolism, accelerated net protein breakdown remains. This may be explained, in part, by elevation of the catabolic hormones (glucagons, catecholamines, and cortisol) found during the acute phase of injury. Increased levels of cytokines released by activated macrophages also promote catabolism and are associated with increased mortality.[3] Although the hormonal and cytokine changes in the ECMO patient appear to ultimately follow this pattern, the extremely hormone-dilute circuit prime may also induce some further hemodynamic and metabolic instability.[4]

The catabolism of skeletal muscle to generate amino acids needed for tissue repair and to produce glucose for energy production is an excellent short-term adaptation; however, it is limited by the extent of the reserves. The progressive loss of skeletal muscle protein leads to respiratory compromise, cardiac dysfunction, increased susceptibility to infection, and increased mortality.[5] Survival is inversely proportional to the loss of lean body mass, and clinically, a 30% loss of lean body mass in adults is usually fatal.[6] It is interesting to note that a neonate on ECMO may lose approximately 15% of lean body mass in a 7-day treatment course.[1] Thus, the nutritional imperative is to quickly improve net protein balance and preserve lean body mass.

Metabolic reserves

One of the major differences in body composition between the adult and the child is the quantity of protein available. Adults have twice the protein stores of neonates. Adults also possess greater lipid stores, while carbohydrate reserves are constant across age groups. In addition to having reduced reserves, neonates and children have higher baseline requirements. The resting energy expenditure for neonates is up to 3-fold greater than that of adults, and the protein requirements may be 3.5 times the requirement for adults.[7] Thus, neonatal and pediatric ECMO patients are especially susceptible to the deleterious effects of protracted catabolic stress. The prompt institution of nutritional support, as soon as the patient has been adequately resuscitated, is prudent. In adults, the situation is somewhat less urgent, but early nutritional support is also recommended.

Nutritional requirements of the ECMO patient

Once a decision has been made to institute nutritional support, an individualized determi-

nation of nutrient requirements is needed. This assessment should include estimates of protein, total energy, carbohydrate, lipid, electrolyte, and micronutrient needs. An inability to precisely monitor growth, an active ongoing metabolic stress response, and clinical requirements for fluid restriction make adequate nutritional support in ECMO patients particularly challenging.

Protein requirements

Amino acids are the key building blocks for growth and tissue repair. The vast majority of amino acids make up protein molecules, and the remainder is in the free amino acid pool. Proteins are dynamic as they are continuously degraded and synthesized in a process termed "protein turnover". The reutilization of amino acids released from protein breakdown is extensive and, even under normal circumstances, provides the preponderance of amino acids used for the synthesis of new protein requirements. ECMO patients have accelerated protein turnover, and neonates on ECMO have a protein turnover that is twice that of healthy infants.[1] A salient advantage of high protein turnover is that it allows for the immediate synthesis of proteins needed for the inflammatory response and tissue repair. Acutely needed enzymes, serum proteins, and glucose (by way of gluconeogenesis) are, thus, synthesized. This process requires energy; hence, in critically ill children, there is a redistribution of the energy normally used for growth to fuel the metabolic stress response, while in adults, there is an increase in resting energy expenditure.[8] In patients on ECMO, the hallmarks of their altered protein metabolism are a marked increase in whole-body protein degradation as well as an increase in whole-body protein synthesis; however, it is the former that predominates causing these patients to manifest a negative net protein balance.[1] This catabolic tendency persists in critically ill neonates even 3 weeks after they are successfully weaned from the ECMO circuit, albeit to a reduced extent.[1]

The catabolism of skeletal muscle to generate glucose is a necessity as glucose is the preferred substrate for the brain, red blood cells, and renal medulla, and provides an energy source for injured tissues. Illness enhances gluconeogenesis in all patients; however, on a per kilogram body weight basis gluconeongenesis seems to be particularly elevated in neonates (presumably because of their relatively large brain to body weight ratio).[9] Interestingly, the provision of dietary glucose is relatively ineffective in quelling endogenous glucose production in a stressed state.[10]

Although skeletal muscle degradation is an excellent short-term adaptation in the ECMO patient, it is detrimental in the long-term. If the inciting stress for protein catabolism is not eliminated, the progressive loss of diaphragmatic and intercostal muscle as well as cardiac muscle perpetuates cardiopulmonary failure. Fortunately, amino acid nutritional supplementation improves protein balance, and protein synthesis appears to increase in ill patients, while protein degradation rates remain relatively unaffected.[11]

As neonates on ECMO have a 100% increase in protein breakdown the provision of dietary protein sufficient to optimize protein synthesis is the single most important nutritional intervention in the ECMO patient.[1] The quantities of protein (or amino acid solution) recommended for patients on ECMO are outlined in Table 1. Ultimately, the goal of protein provision in neonates and children on ECMO is not only to promote nitrogen balance but also to optimize growth and development. Excessive protein administration should be avoided, because toxicity can occur, particularly in patients with marginal renal or hepatic function. Even relatively healthy neonates fed protein allotments of 6 gm/kg/day have demonstrated azotemia, pyrexia, a higher incidence of strabismus, and a somewhat lower IQ.[12,13]

The use of enteral or parenteral glutamine supplementation (with and without other "immune enhancing" nutrients such as arginine, omega-3 fatty acids, and nucleotides) in an effort to limit septic complications in critically ill patients remains investigational, and larger studies are required before any cogent recommendation can be offered.

Hormonal manipulation of critically ill adults with the use of insulin has shown benefit.[14] The administration of insulin, through the use of a hyperinsulinemic euglycemic clamp in neonates on ECMO, results in a significant reduction in protein breakdown rates, but further investigation regarding insulin's effect upon protein synthesis in ECMO patients, as well as outcome analysis over a longer period, are required before any recommendations regarding the use of insulin may be made.[15]

Energy requirements

A careful appraisal of energy requirements in ECMO patients is necessary as both under- and over-estimates are associated with potentially harmful consequences. Inadequate caloric allotment will result in poor protein retention, especially if protein administration is marginal. In contrast, the provision of excess glucose calories in ECMO patients increases CO_2 production rates (exacerbating ventilatory failure) and even a paradoxical increase in net protein degradation.[2]

The severity of illness, persistence of illness, analgesia and anesthesia, and the properties of the ECMO circuit itself may affect

Table 1. Estimated protein requirements for neonates, children, and non-obese adolescents and adults on ECMO.

Age (years)	Estimated protein requirement (g/kg/day)
0 to 2	2.0-3.0
>2 to 13	1.5-2.0
14+	1.5

energy expenditure. Total energy requirements encompass resting energy expenditure, energy needed for physical activity, and diet-induced thermogenesis (a very small component). Resting energy expenditure in children includes the caloric requirement for growth. Although critically ill patients have increased energy requirements because of increased substrate (protein, carbohydrate, lipid) turnover, they also demonstrate growth arrest and decreased physical activity. Newborns undergoing major operations have only a transient 20% elevation in energy expenditure over baseline levels, and they return to normal within 12 hours.[16] Adequate anesthetic and analgesic management also play a significant role in muting the stress response, as evidenced by neonates undergoing patent ductus arteriosus ligation who do not manifest any discernable increase in resting energy expenditure post-operatively with fentanyl anesthesia and subsequent IV analgesia.[17]

The measurement of energy expenditure in ECMO patients is difficult; however, novel experimental assessments of energy needs have been made with the use of an adapted spirometry device and stable isotope technology.[1,2,18-21] Taken in aggregate, the data indicate that the mean total energy requirements of critically ill neonates on ECMO vs. age- and diet-matched controls are nearly identical, although the critically ill cohort does demonstrate a greater variability in energy expenditure. Further, a surfeit of calories in neonates on ECMO does not result in improved protein accretion.[2] Thus, for practical purposes, the recommended total dietary caloric intake for healthy subjects affords a reasonable estimate of caloric needs of patients on ECMO.[22] Table 2 outlines safe caloric provisions for patients on ECMO at various ages. It may be noted that these decrease with age on a per-kilogram basis. Predictive equations used in conjunction with arbitrary "stress factors" (to account for the degree of metabolic stress) have been shown to be inaccurate in determining individual energy expenditures in

ICU patients with respiratory failure and are not recommended.[23]

Once the patient has been weaned off ECMO and is in the convalescent phase, caloric provisions may be adjusted by measuring energy expenditure using an indirect calorimeter or by carefully monitoring growth on standardized growth charts. The need for the latter cannot be overstressed as caloric needs may actually increase as the patient assumes their own ventilation due to the increased work of breathing.[24] In practice, the clinician must often adjust diuretic management in conjunction with nutrient provision to obtain adequate growth without inducing respiratory compromise. Enterally fed patients, as a rule, require a further 10% increment in calories because of obligate malabsorption.

Once protein needs have been met, both carbohydrate and lipid energy sources have similar beneficial effects on net protein synthesis in ill patients.[25] The partitioning of energy-yielding substrates is based upon an understanding of carbohydrate and lipid utilization in the metabolic stressed state.

Carbohydrate requirements

Glucose production and availability is a priority in critical illness. Injured and septic adults have a 3-fold increase in glucose turnover, glucose oxidation, and an elevation in gluconeogenesis.[26,27] An important feature of the metabolic stress response is that the provision of dietary glucose does not halt gluconeongenesis,

Table 2. Estimated energy requirements for neonates, children, and non-obese adolescents and adults on ECMO.

Age (years)	Estimated energy requirement (kcal/kg/day)
0 to 3	90
>3 to 6	80
>6 to 8	70
>8 to 10	60
>10 to 12	50
>12 to 14	40
15+	30

and, consequently, the catabolism of proteins continues.[10] However, it is clear that a combination of glucose and amino acids effectively improves protein balance in illness primarily by augmenting protein synthesis.

In early nutritional support regimens for surgical patients, glucose and amino acid formulations with minimal lipids (only to obviate fatty acid deficiency) were often utilized, and energy allotments tended to be well above requirements. As may be predicted, the excess glucose was synthesized to fat, resulting in a net generation of carbon dioxide (CO_2). In contrast to glucose metabolism, excess lipids are merely stored as triglycerides and have no effect upon increasing CO_2 production. Administering high glucose, high caloric, and parenteral formulations in critically ill adults has been documented to result in a 30% increase in oxygen consumption, a 57% rise in CO_2 production, and a 71% increase in minute ventilation.[28] Thus, avoidance of overfeeding and the utilization of a mixed fuel system of nutrition employing both glucose and lipids to yield energy are of great utility in ECMO patients. Such an approach also tends to obviate hyperglycemia in the relatively insulin-resistant subject.

Lipid requirements

Lipid metabolism is similar to protein and carbohydrate turnover in generally being accelerated by illness proportionate to the degree of injury.[29,30] This process involves the recycling of free fatty acids and glycerol into (and hydrolysis from) triglycerides. Approximately 30-40% of released fatty acids are oxidized for energy and are, in fact, the prime source of energy in stressed patients. The glycerol portion of the triglyceride that is released may be converted to pyruvate and then, in turn, metabolized to glucose through gluconeogenesis. As with other catabolic processes caused by injury, the provision of dietary glucose does not decrease glycerol clearance or diminish lipid recycling.

It is also of interest to note that normal ketone body metabolism is impaired by the high levels of insulin present in the stressed metabolic state, making glucose the fundamental fuel for the brain.

As the energy needs of the critically ill patient are met largely by the mobilization and oxidation of free fatty acids, deficiency states can evolve. Additionally, neonates have limited stores of essential fatty acids; therefore, fatty acid deficiency may manifest in this group within 1 week.[31] In infants, linoleic and linolenic acid are considered essential, and arachidonic acid and docosahexaenoic acid may be essential as well. The clinical syndrome of fatty acid deficiency consists of susceptibility to bacterial infection, failure to thrive, thrombocytopenia, dermatitis, and alopecia.

The use of commercially available lipid solutions in ECMO obviates the risk of fatty acid deficiency, results in improved protein utilization, and does not significantly increase CO_2 production or metabolic rate. However, these advantages are balanced by potential risks of excess lipid administration—hypertriglyceridemia, increased infections, and decreased alveolar oxygen diffusion capacity.[32-34] Although the evidence is far from conclusive, the potential for adverse effects of lipid infusions have resulted in most ECMO centers starting lipid supplementation at 0.5 gm/kg/day, and advancing to 2-3 gm/kg/day while carefully monitoring triglyceride levels.[1,2] The precipitation of lipid emulsions in the ECMO membrane has not been a problem with this approach. Usually, lipid administration is restricted to a maximum of 30-40% of total calories during critical illness, although this practice has not been validated by clinical trials.

Electrolyte requirements

Electrolyte requirements (Na^+, K^+, Ca^{++}, Cl^-, HCO_3^-) must be frequently evaluated while providing nutritional support on ECMO. In addition to routine electrolyte monitoring, careful attention to phosphate and magnesium levels is needed as unsupplemented alimentation may lead to hypophosphatemia (resulting in thrombocytopenia and respiratory muscle dysfunction) and magnesium deficiency (resulting in cardiac arrhythmias). Renal failure tends to result in retention of phosphate and, thus, nutritional allotments must be reduced accordingly. Diuresis is frequently necessary on ECMO, and consequent Cl^- loss can result in metabolic alkalosis. Alkalosis tends to inhibit respiratory drive, drive K^+ intracellularly, and decrease ionized Ca^{++} by increasing the affinity of albumin for Ca^{++}. Increased Cl^- is administered through the parenteral nutrition formula to correct this problem. Severe metabolic acidosis caused by hypoperfusion or sepsis may also be addressed through the parenteral nutrition formulation. The provision of 1 mEq of excess acetate per kg administered over a 24-hour period is usually a safe adjunct to other measures which treat metabolic acidosis.

Vitamin and trace mineral requirements

The vitamin and trace mineral requirements of ECMO patients have not been studied. The fat-soluble vitamins A, D, E, and K, as well as the water-soluble vitamins ascorbic acid, thiamine, riboflavin, pyridoxin, niacin, pantothenate, biotin, folate, and vitamin B_{12} are all required and routinely administered. Since vitamins are not stoichiometrically consumed in biochemical reactions, but rather act as catalysts, the administration of large supplements of vitamins in ECMO is not logical from a nutritional standpoint.

The trace minerals that are required for normal development are zinc, iron, copper, selenium, manganese, iodide, molybdenum, and chromium. Trace minerals are used primarily in the synthesis of a ubiquitous and extraordinarily important class of enzymes called metalloenzymes. Metalloenzymes, along with vitamins,

act as catalysts. The vitamin and trace mineral requirements of humans are well defined in the literature, and little evidence exists that they are nutritionally inadequate in stressed states such as those found in ECMO patients.[22] In the event of severe hepatic failure, copper and manganese accumulation occurs, so parenteral trace mineral supplementation should be limited to once per week.

The pharmacologic use of vitamins and trace minerals in critical illness is controversial. Reviews of both vitamin and trace mineral toxicity clearly demonstrate that excessive dosage is a health risk.[35,36]

Route of nutrient provision

The standard form of initial nutritional support in ECMO patients is parenteral nutrition. This allows for the concentrated administration of nutrients and permits the attainment of nutritional goals without excessive fluid allotments.

Large scale studies of enteral nutrition in ECMO patients have not been performed. Generally, the use of enteral nutrition is preferable in critical illness provided that the GI tract is functional and there is no associated hypoperfusion. Continuous post-pyloric feeds minimize the risk of aspiration and appear to reduce complications and cost in treating critically ill children.[37] A series of 27 adult patients on venovenous (VV) ECMO receiving enteral feedings with or without parenteral supplementation has been reported without significant morbidity.[38] The vast majority was also treated with prokinetic agents. A series of 14 enterally fed pediatric patients on both venoarterial (VA) and VV ECMO, demonstrated no complications that could be attributed to the route of nutrient provision.[39] Vigilance is prudent in enterally fed ECMO patients because of the risks of necrotizing enterocolitis in neonates and small bowel necrosis in older patients.[39]

The passing of a post-pyloric feeding tube intra-operatively in patients undergoing congenital diaphragmatic (CDH) repair is a useful adjunct to later nutritional management.

Conclusion

The catabolism evident in patients on ECMO is severe and qualitatively resembles that of other critically ill states. Judicious administration of carbohydrates, lipids, vitamins, trace minerals, and particularly protein is needed to optimize lean body mass and reduce morbidity and mortality.

References

1. Keshen TH, Miller RG, Jahoor F, Jaksic T. Stable isotopic quantitation of energy expenditure and protein metabolism in neonates on and post extracorporeal life support (ECLS). *J Pediatr Surg* 1997; 32:958-962.
2. Shew SB, Keshen TH, Jahoor F, Jaksic T. The determinants of protein catabolism in neonates on extracorporeal membrane oxygenation. *J Pediatr Surg* 1999; 34:1086-1090.
3. Sullivan JS, Kilpatrick L, Costarino AT, et al. Correlation of plasma cytokine elevations with mortality rate in children with sepsis. *J Pediatr* 1992; 120:510-515.
4. Agus MS, Jaksic T. Critically low hormone and catecholamine concentrations in the primed extracorporeal life support circuit. *ASIAO J* 2004; 50:65-67.
5. Moyer E, Cerra F, Chenier R, et al. Multiple systems organ failure: VI. Death predictors in the trauma-septic state, the most critical determinants. *J Trauma* 1981; 21:862-869.
6. Gump FE, Kinney JM. Energy balance and weight loss in burned patients. *Arch Surg* 1971; 103:442-443.
7. Kashyap S, Schulze KF, Forsyth M, et al. Growth, nutrient retention, and metabolic response in low birth weight infants fed varying intakes of protein and energy. *J Pediatr* 1988; 113:713-721.
8. Jaksic T, Shew SB, Keshan TH, Dzakovic A, Jahoor F. Do critically ill surgical neonates have increased energy expenditure? *J Pediatr Surg* 2001; 36:63-67.
9. Keshen T, Miller RG, Jahoor F, et al. Glucose production and gluconeogenesis are negatively related to body weight in very-low birthweight neonates. *Pediatr Res* 1997; 41:132-138.
10. Long CL, Kinney JM, Geiger JW. Non-supressibility of gluconeongenesis by glucose in septic patients. *Metabolism* 1976; 25:193-201.
11. Duffy B, Pencharz P. The effects of surgery on the nitrogen metabolism of parenterally fed human neonates. *Pediatr Res* 1986; 20:32-35.
12. Goldman HI, Freudenthal R, Holland B, et al. Clinical effects of two different levels of protein intake on low birth weight infants. *J Pediatr* 1969; 74:881-889.
13. Goldman HI, Liebman OB, Freudenthal R, et al. Effects of early protein intake on low birth weight infants: evaluation at 3 years of age. *J Pediatr* 1971; 78:126-127.
14. van den Berghe G, Wouters P, Weekers F, et al. Intensive insulin therapy in the critically ill patients. *N Engl J Med* 2001; 345:1359-1367.
15. Agus MSD, Javid PJ, Dzakovic A, et al. Intravenous insulin improves protein breakdown in infants on extracorporeal membrane oxygenation. *J Pediatr Surg* 2004; 39:839-844.
16. Jones MO, Pierro A, Hammond P, Lloyd DA. The metabolic response to operative stress in infants. *J Pediatr* Surg 1999; 34:1086-1090.
17. Shew SB, Keshen TH, Glass NL, et al. Ligation of a patent ductus arteriosus under fentanyl anesthesia improves pro-

tein metabolism in premature neonates. *J Pediatr Surg* 2000; 35:1277-1281.

18. Cilley RE, Wesley JR, Zwischenberger JB, et al. Method of pulmonary and membrane lung gas exchange measurement during extracorporeal membrane oxygenation. *ASAIO J* 1986; 525-529.

19. Cilley RE, Wesley JR, Zwischenberger JB, et al. Metabolic rates of newborn infants with severe respiratory failure treated with extracorporeal membrane oxygenation. *Curr Surg* 1987; 44:48-51.

20. Cilley RE, Wesley JR, Zwischenberger JB, Bartlett RH. Gas exchange measurements in neonates treated with extracorporeal membrane oxygenation. *J Pediatr Surg* 1988; 23:306-311.

21. Shew SB, Beckett PR, Keshen TH, et al. Validation of a [13C] Bicarbonate tracer technique to measure neonatal energy expenditure. *Pediatr Res* 2000; 47:787-791.

22. National Academy of Sciences. *Recommended Dietary Allowances 10th ed.* Washington, DC; 1989.

23. Hunter D, Jaksic T, Lewis D, et al. Resting energy expenditure in the critically ill: estimations versus measurement. *Br J Surg* 1988; 75:875-878.

24. Muratore CS, Utter S, Jaksic T, Wilson JW. Nutritional Morbidity in survivors of congenital diaphragmatic hernia. *J Pediatr Surg* 2001; 36:1171-1176.

25. Jones MO, Pierro A, Garlick PJ, et al. Protein metabolism kinetics in neonates: effect of intravenous carbohydrate and fat. *J Pediatr Surg* 1995; 30:458-462.

26. Long CL, Spencer JL, Kinney JM, Geiger JW. Carbohydrate metabolism in normal man and effect of glucose infusion. *J Appl Physiol* 1971; 31:102-109.

27. Long CL, Spencer JL, Kinney JM, Geiger JW. Carbohydrate metabolism in normal man: effect of elective operations and major surgery. *J Appl Physiol* 1971; 31:110-116.

28. Askhanazi J, Rosenbaum SH, Hyman AI, et al. Respiratory changes induced by the the large glucose loads of total parenteral nutrition. *JAMA* 1980; 243:1444-1447.

29. Jeevanandam M, Youg DH, Schiller WR. Nutritional impact on energy cost of fat fuel mobilization in polytrauma victims. *J Trauma* 1990; 30:147-150.

30. Nordenstrom J, Carpetier YA, Askanazi J, et al. Metabolic utilization of intravenous fat emulsion during total parenteral nutrition. *Ann Surg* 1982; 196:221-231.

31. Friedman Z, Danon A, Stahlman MT, Oates JA. Rapid onset of essential fatty acid deficiency in the newborn. *Pediatrics* 1976; 58:640-649.

32. Cleary TG, Pickering LK. Mechanisms of intralipid effect on polymorphonuclear leukocytes. *J Clin Lab Immunol* 1983; 11:21-26.

33. Perriera GR, Fox WW, Stanley CA, et al. Decreased oxygenation and hyperlipidemia during intravenous fat infusions in premature infants. *Pediatrics* 1980; 66:26-30.

34. Freeman J, Goldmann DA, Smith NE, et al. Association of intravenous fat emulsion and coagulase-negative staphylococcal bacteremia in neonatal intensive units. *N Engl J Med* 1990; 323:301-308.

35. Marks J. The safety of vitamins: an overview. *Int J Vitam Nutr Res* 1989; 30:S12-20.

36. Foldin NW. Micronutrient supplements: toxicity and drug interactions. *Prog Food Nutr Sci* 1990; 14:277-331.

37. de Lucas C, Moreno M, Herce JL, et al. Transpyloric enteral nutrition reduces the complication rate and cost in the critically ill child. *J Pediat Gastroenterol Nutr* 2000; 30:175-180.

38. Scott LK, Boudreaux K, Thaljeh F, et al. Early enteral feeding in adults receiving veno-venous extracorporeal membrane oxygenation. *J Parenter Enteral Nutr* 2004; 28:295-300.

39. Pettignano R, Heard M, Davis R, et al. Total enteral nutrition versus total parenteral nutrition during pediatric extracorporeal membrane oxygenation. *Crit Care Med* 1998; 26:358-363.

40. Munshi IA, Steingrub JS, Wolpert L. Small bowel necrosis associated with early post post-operative jejunal feeding in a trauma patient. *J Trauma* 2000; 49:163-165.

34

Sedation and Management of Pain on ECLS

Björn Frenckner M.D., Ph.D. and Dick Tibboel M.D., Ph.D.

Introduction

Patients on mechanical ventilation in the ICU are generally heavily sedated. The purposes of sedation are to relieve pain, decrease anxiety, induce amnesia, decrease oxygen consumption and CO_2 production, prevent the patient from removing lines, and promote synchronous breathing with the ventilator. Sedation is achieved principally by continuous infusion of opiates, benzodiazepines, major tranquilizers, and anesthetic agents at adequate doses to promote a stuporous or comatose level of consciousness. Sedation policies have evolved during decades of progress in intensive care, but there is a lack of clinical studies on the effect of sedation on patient recovery. In fact, routine use of continuous heavy sedation has recently been questioned, and it has been pointed out that sedation does not come without a price.[1]

Sedation has been identified as an independent risk factor for ventilator-associated pneumonia in an observational study of 250 adult patients (median age 64) during the first 48 hours of mechanical ventilation.[2] Continuous sedation may prolong the duration of mechanical ventilation. In a study of 240 consecutive patients receiving mechanical ventilation, continuous sedation was associated with prolonged ventilation compared to patients receiving no IV sedation or only bolus administration.[3] Daily interruptions of sedative infusions have been shown to shorten the length of mechanical ventilation and to reduce complications.[4] Furthermore, minimal sedation or daily interruption enables the patient to undergo neurological assessment on a regular basis.

Suitable protocols for limited sedation are considered important in reducing the length of mechanical ventilation and the incidence of ventilator-associated pneumonia.[5] It is well known that ventilation of healthy lungs with low FiO_2 and low inspiratory pressures can be performed over long time periods without harmful effects on the lungs. This has been confirmed in studies of patients suffering from polio or victims of cervical spinal cord injuries.[6] On the other hand, ventilation with elevated airway pressures is directly injurious to the lung and results in lung injury now referred to as ventilator-induced lung injury (VILI).[7,8] It is important to emphasize that it is not solely the intrapulmonary pressure that is damaging, but rather the Tran pulmonary pressure difference, causing alveolar over distension. During coughing, extremely high intrapulmonary pressures can be obtained, but due to similar increase in intrathoracic extrapulmonary pressure, the transpulmonary pressure gradient is not affected. In positive pressure ventilation, however, the inspiratory pressure is directly transmitted to open air-filled alveoli and increases the transpulmonary pressure, as there is no counter pressure. The alveoli are thereby subjected to shear forces, which are believed to result in lung damage.

Pulmonary fluid balance is profoundly altered in acute respiratory distress syndrome (ARDS). In some experimental work, interest has, therefore, been focused upon lymph drainage from the lungs. Frostell et al. evaluated the effect of positive pressure ventilation and positive end expiratory pressure (PEEP) in healthy dogs and in dogs subjected to oleic acid lung damage.[9] There was a dramatic increase of thoracic lymph flow, mainly caused by drainage from the lungs after induction of lung damage. In both healthy lungs and lungs with induced injury, PEEP (10 cm H_2O) diminished the lymph flow by half. Spontaneous breathing significantly increased pulmonary lymph drainage when compared to positive pressure ventilation.

In the ARDS Network Study, ventilation of ARDS patients with lower tidal volumes (6 ml/kg) was associated with lower mortality when compared to ventilation with more traditional tidal volumes (12 ml/kg).[10] In another study, it was shown that a lung protective strategy of ventilation (i.e., with low tidal volumes) resulted in significantly lower levels of inflammatory mediators both in bronchoalveolar lavage and in plasma.[11]

ECLS alone does not cure the underlying disease of the patient, but helps to support cardiorespiratory function while the patient improves. When it is performed for respiratory indications, the primary goal is to recover lung function. The ventilation strategy is, therefore, of great importance, and the patient must not be subjected to any treatment that can cause further lung damage. As drugs for sedation and pain management influence and may potentially increase the requirements of mechanical ventilation, they may affect the chance for pulmonary recovery. Because of this, the mode of sedation and pain management is probably more critical in patients on ECLS for respiratory indications than for cardiac indications.

Current sedation strategy in ECLS

In order to understand the sedation policies currently employed in ECLS patients, a questionnaire was sent to all ELSO centers in November 2003. There were separate forms for neonatal, pediatric, and adult patient groups. The centers were asked if they routinely sedate the ECLS patient continuously, and if "yes", to provide the reasons for sedation. They were asked to give the top three most important reasons, choosing from the following alternatives: decrease anxiety, decrease pain, induce amnesia, facilitate synchronous breathing with the ventilator, prevent patients from removing lines, decrease oxygen consumption/CO_2 production, withdrawal, staff wishes, wishes of parents/relatives, or other. The centers were also asked which drugs were used, if routine muscle relaxation was used, if the sedation policy in cardiac patients differed from that in respiratory patients, and if the sedation policy had changed over the last years. The centers could briefly describe their general policy regarding sedation, how it was different for cardiac patients, and finally if and how their policy had changed over the last years. Replies were received from 51 neonatal, 37 pediatric, and 8 adult centers. These centers had together performed an annual average of 510 neonatal, 115 pediatric, and 59 adult cases for respiratory support and 240 neonatal, 160 pediatric, and 50 adult cases for cardiac support, which account for ~60% of cases reported to the ELSO Registry.

For respiratory indications, the vast majority of centers routinely sedated ECLS patients continuously (45/49 for neonates, 33/36 for pediatric, and 5/6 for adult patients). The main reasons for sedating the patients were to relieve pain and to relieve anxiety (Figure 1). Sedation was considered important in preventing the patients from removing lines and decreasing oxygen consumption and CO_2 production. Adults were also sedated in order to promote synchronous breathing with the ventilator and induce amnesia. Routine muscle relaxation was administered by 9 out of 49 neonatal centers (18%), by 13 out of 33 pediatric centers (39%), and by 1 out of 7 (14%) adult centers providing a response to this question.

About one-third of the centers (neonatal 33%, pediatric 24%, adult 40%) had a different policy regarding sedation in cardiac patients. There was not a consistent manner in which way the policy differed. Some were more liberal in the use of sedation in cardiac patients, as these patients were frequently post-operative, while other centers tried to use less, since most cardiac runs are shorter.

About one-third of the centers (neonatal 37%, pediatric 32%, adult 40%) indicated

their sedation policy had changed over the last years. The most frequent change was to use less sedation or muscle relaxation. However, one center used increased sedation because the nursing staff wanted to further decrease patient movement.

Pharmacology

The most frequently used drugs for sedation and pain management during ECLS are midazolam or other benzodiazepines, morphine, and fentanyl (Figure 2). Propofol is also frequently used in adults. The disposition of drugs is altered during ECLS due to:

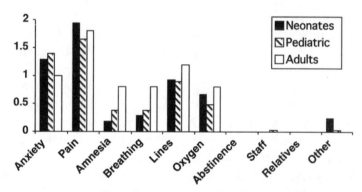

Figure 1. Diagrammatic representation of reasons for sedating patients. Each center responding to the questionnaire ranked the three most important reasons. The most important ranked three, the second ranked two and the third ranked one. The bars represent the total ranking divided by the numbers of centers answering.

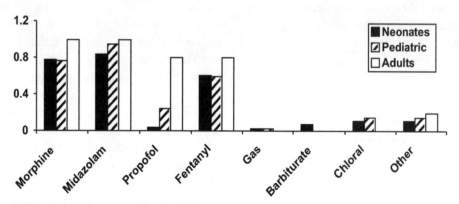

Figure 2. Diagrammatic representation of the most commonly used drugs for sedation. Each center indicated which drugs they routinely use. The bars indicate the total number of centers using the drug divided by the number of centers (i.e., the chance that a certain drug is used in a center).

- Expanded blood volume and increased volume of distribution
- Intrinsic increase in intra- and extra cellular volume
- Non-pulsatile blood flow
- Reduced plasma protein concentration, with resulting effects on pharmacokinetics and dynamics (PK/PD).

An overview of the effect of ECLS on pharmacokinetics of a number of analgesic and sedative drugs adapted from Buck is presented in Table 1.[12]

Morphine metabolism

A small fraction of morphine is excreted unchanged with the majority being metabolized into morphine-6-glucuronide (M6G) by the enzyme UDP-glucuronosyl transferase (UGT 2B7), and into morphine-3-glucuronide (M3G) by UGT2B7 and the enzyme-family GT1A. Physicians should be aware of M3G and M6G clearances because these metabolites contribute to both clinical effects and side effects. The M6G metabolite has pharmacological actions and side effects indistinguishable from those of morphine, while the potency of this metabolite is 47 to 650 times greater than that of morphine. M3G has little affinity for opioid receptors but contributes to neurotoxic symptoms such as hyperalgesia, allodynia, and myoclonus. Some investigators suggest that M3G antagonizes morphine-induced analgesia; others have refuted this finding.[13]

Table 1. Medication administered during neonatal ECLS.

Analgesics/sedatives	Altered pharmacokinetics
Morphine	+
Fentanyl	+
Midazolam	+
Diazepam	+
Lorazepam	+
Propofol	+
Pentobarbitol	unknown

Studies have demonstrated that ECLS affects drug metabolism,[12-15] but those investigating morphine pharmacokinetics during ECLS have concentrated only on the morphine rather than metabolite clearances.[15-17]

There is little literature published concerning the effects of age, size, concomitant medications, ECLS flow or duration, or disease processes on morphine pharmacokinetics, in contrast to other drugs.[13] Clinicians, therefore, must adjust morphine dose by extrapolating from data published on its use in post-operative neonates, and neonates on mechanical ventilation, and by clinical observations. It is imperative, therefore, to assess differences in morphine pharmacokinetics between neonates on ECLS and post-operative children.

In neonates on ECLS, metabolic clearance of morphine to M3G and M6G is increased; after 10 days this clearance is equal to the metabolic clearance in post-operative children.[13] This finding suggests that increased clearance will result in decreases in plasma concentrations during the first 10 days and that dose increases may be necessary.

Furthermore, studies in infants[16,19,20] and in adults[18] have shown that morphine clearance is significantly lower in patients requiring mechanical ventilator support, those with cardiac insufficiency, or those with history of hypoxia. Hypoxia prior to ECLS, due, for example, to meconium aspiration syndrome, may result in liver ischemia and lower activity of the liver enzymes responsible for morphine glucuronidation.

The alterations in M3G:M6G ratio changes during the first 2 weeks of life are unknown. Such changes seem likely as the M3G:M6G ratio is known to be low in early infancy but increases to reach adult values during the first six months of life.[19,21] This suggests that young infants may be less susceptible to M3G-related side effects than children or adults. The impact of ECLS-related factors or duration of morphine administration on morphine clearance, or on clearance of M3G and M6G is unknown.

Formation clearance to M3G and M6G is reduced during the first 10 days of ECLS, probably reflecting the severity of illness. Clearance of M3G and M6G is directly related to creatinine clearance, while ECLS flow has a small effect on metabolite clearance. Using the NONMEM software package (GloboMax, Hanover, MD) for population PK/PD data analysis, we found that higher flows were associated with decreased formation clearances, possibly reflecting illness severity.

Effect of co-medication

Apart from the absence of data on plasma levels, NONMEM analysis revealed that the concurrent use of furosemide, vecuronium, midazolam, and fentanyl had no effect on morphine formation clearance to M3G and M6G or the elimination clearance of M3G and M6G.

There is no documented effect of midazolam or fentanyl on morphine formation clearance to M3G and M6G or elimination clearance of these metabolites. The reason is that morphine is largely glucuronidated by uridine 5'-disphosphate glucuronosyltransferase UGT2B7 to M3G and M6G,[22] midazolam by the cytochrome P450 system (i.e., by CYP3A4, CYP3A5, and, to a much lesser extent, by CUP3A7),[22] and fentanyl by CYP3A4.[23]

Midazolam

Mulla et al.[14] reported that the volume of distribution of midazolam in ECLS-treated neonates was three to four times greater than in critically ill neonates not treated with ECLS. Clinicians should be aware that due to the increased volume of distribution, plasma concentrations will fall, especially during the first 10 days on ECLS.[13,16] Midazolam therapy should be guided by clinical monitoring, preferably by validated pain[25,26] or comfort scales,[27] as increased tolerance occurring with prolonged use will also further reduce the predictability of the drug effect.[12,24]

Minimal sedation

A policy and tradition of minimal sedation has evolved at the Karolinska Institute (Stockholm, Sweden) due to reasons outlined earlier in this chapter and from successful clinical experiences with this approach. It has been observed on several occasions that tidal volumes decrease substantially when patients on ECLS with spontaneously-triggered pressure-supported ventilation receive general anesthesia for a surgical procedure. In these cases it was necessary to increase the extracorporeal flow in order to achieve adequate oxygenation. An example of one such case follows.

Case report

A 7-year-old girl with pneumocystis carinii pneumonia following chemotherapy due to leukemia was successfully treated with venovenous (VV) ECLS. Pulmonary function recovered after 6 weeks, and she was ready for decannulation after a successful 12-hour trial-off period. She was fully awake and on pressure-supported spontaneous ventilation. Prior to decannulation, she received general anesthesia with muscle relaxation, after which it became impossible to maintain adequate oxygenation. The tidal volumes could not be maintained, gas flow to the oxygenator was re-initiated and ECLS flow was increased to prior levels. The patient was successfully decannulated 1 week later under ketamine anesthesia and spontaneous pressure-supported ventilation.[28] Her vital capacity was 38% of normal 5 weeks after decannulation and 64% of normal another 4 weeks later. Presently, she is a healthy 18-year-old.

Following initiation of ECLS, it is standard practice to heavily sedate and often paralyze all patients. The general policy at Karolinska University Hospital has been to withdraw muscle relaxation as soon as the patients are on bypass. The degree of sedation is then gradually decreased, and by the end of long runs most patients are only on a low dose morphine infusion. Clonidine has frequently been used to facilitate weaning of opiates. Common causes for anxiety should be sought and addressed. Hypoxemia is avoided by adjusting the ECLS flow. The sweep gas is adjusted to avoid hypercarbia and the anxiety caused as a result, but PCO_2 is maintained at levels that promote spontaneously triggered ventilation. Patients are mildly sedated when needed, mostly during nighttime with morphine, and propofol or midazolam, to facilitate sleeping. Special care is taken to maintain the normal 24-hour day. In short runs (i.e., <7 days) it is generally not possible to discontinue infusions of sedation, but with longer runs it has been possible to keep most patients awake during the daytime, allowing communication with the staff and family and other activities such as television viewing (Figure 3). Establishing a close relationship between staff and the patient is essential in decreasing the need for pharmacological sedation. Gentle patient care, friendly talking to the patient, and physical contact with the patient are potent sedatives. For children, it is important to have one of the parents at the

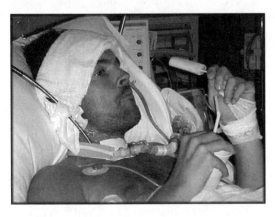

Figure 3. Adult patient at the end of a VV ECLS run. The neck cannula withdrawing blood from the right atrium, the tracheostoma, and the nasogastric tube are easily seen. The patient is fully awake and able to communicate. The picture illustrates the patient eating ice cream and drinking. (Published with permission from the patient).

bedside most of the time. Reading books and telling stories are highly effective in keeping children calm. Nursing care of ECLS patients is further outlined in Chapter 41.

Pain management during ECLS is adjusted on an individual basis. Treatment with ECLS is not painful in and of itself, but most patients on extracorporeal support have an underlying, often complicated illness. Some have been subjected to surgery, and some patients are on bypass post-trauma. Prior to minor procedures such as line or chest drain placement or other patient care, administration of analgesics should always be considered.

Decannulation after percutaneous venous cannulation is performed under mild sedation without anesthesia. Arterial cannulas or venous cannulas introduced during an open procedure are removed under local anesthesia with mild sedation, or in some cases under ketamine anesthesia.

In spite of a lower level of sedation, the doses have, in some cases, remained fairly high due to tachyphylaxis. It has not been possible to manage all patients successfully at the desired low level of sedation.

There are no controlled studies comparing high or low levels of sedation and the effect on ECLS outcome. The effects in terms of survival to hospital discharge in a cohort of patients treated with minimal sedation at Karolinska University Hospital have been comparable to results in the ELSO Registry. Out of 200 patients (104 neonates, 50 pediatric, and 46 adult patients) the survival rates were 80% vs. 77%, 54% vs. 54%, and 65% vs. 50%, for those treated with minimal sedation when compared to ELSO Registry survival rates, respectively.[29] It is not possible to compare differences in outcome between single centers and a common database, as many variables are different, including diagnose and condition at initiation of ECLS. The data demonstrates that a strategy of minimal sedation during ECLS treatment as outlined above can be used with good results.

In an early follow-up study, interviews were conducted with adult survivors. Half of the patients that were managed with low levels of sedation during ECLS could recall certain episodes that occurred during bypass. They were generally happy with the low level of sedation, and no adverse psychological effects were observed.[30]

Summary

The goals for sedating patients on ECLS are similar to those for sedating patients receiving conventional intensive care (e.g., to relieve pain and anxiety). However, sedation and pain management during ECLS have not been well studied. Different ECLS centers have varied policies, both in the choice of drugs, and the desired level of sedation. The policies have evolved from those used in conventional intensive care. There are no randomized studies comparing outcomes between groups treated with different levels of sedation. Certain facts should be considered when managing sedation and pain in ECLS patients. PK/PD are altered by factors such as the greater circulating blood volume. Monitoring the clinical effects of sedatives may, therefore, be more important in patients on ECLS compared to those receiving conventional intensive care.

The level of sedation may affect the need for and mode of mechanical ventilation required. In patients on ECLS for cardiac support, the mode of mechanical ventilation is probably of less importance, as the lungs are generally healthy with a normal compliance. For respiratory support, however, the mode of ventilation is more crucial as it may cause further pulmonary damage. Administration of sedatives and analgesics may be more crucial in this group.

As in conventional intensive care, intermittently lowering the level of sedation allows for neurological evaluation. Normal reaction of the patient when sedation is lowered can rule out severe central nervous system complication and

will decrease the demand for neuroradiological imaging.

The level of sedation also affects staffing demands. Managing an alert patient on ECLS may require increased staffing levels. It can be demanding for nursing staff when the patient expresses anxiety and there are difficulties with communication. This topic is further outlined in Chapter 41.

ECLS is not painful in itself, thus the need for pain control in most patients is limited. However, some patients on extracorporeal support have complicated illness. Some have been subjected to minor or major trauma or are on bypass post-operatively. Pain management in such patients must be adjusted on an individual basis. Administration of analgesics should always be considered.

References

1. Heffner JE. A wake-up call in the intensive care unit. *N Engl J Med* 2000; 342:1520-1522.

2. Rello J, Diaz E, Roque M, Vallés J. Risk factors for developing pneumonia within 48 hours of intubation. *Am J Respir Crit Care Med* 1999; 159:1742-1746.

3. Kollef MH, Levy NT, Ahrens TS, Schaiff R, Prentice D, Sherman G. The use of continuous i.v. sedation is associated with prolongation of mechanical ventilation. *Chest* 1998; 114:541-548.

4. Schweickert WD, Gehlbach BK, Pohlman AS, Hall JB, Kress JP. Daily interruption of sedative infusions and complications of critical illness in mechanically ventilated patients. *Crit Care Med* 2004; 32:1272-1276.

5. Kollef MH. Prevention of hospital-associated pneumonia and ventilator-associated pneumonia. *Crit Care Med* 2004; 32:1396-1405.

6. Adams AB, Whitman J, Marcy T. Surveys of long-term ventilatory support in

Minnesota: 1986 and 1992. *Chest* 1993; 103:1463-1469.

7. Adams AB, Simonson DA, Dries DJ. Ventilator-induced lung injury. *Respir Care Clin N Am* 2003; 9:343-362.

8. Ricard JD, Dreyfuss D, Saumon G. Ventilator-induced lung injury. *Eur Respir J Suppl* 2003; 42:2s-9s.

9. Frostell C, Blomqvist H, Hedenstierna G, Halbig I, Pieper R. Thoracic and abdominal lymph drainage in relation to mechanical ventilation and PEEP. *Acta Anaesthesiol Scand* 1987; 31:405-412.

10. ARDS-network. Ventilation with lower tidal volumes as compared with traditional tidal volumes for acute lung injury and the acute respiratory distress syndrome. *N Engl J Med* 2000; 342:1301-1307.

11. Ranieri VM, Suter PM, Tortorella C, et al. Effect of mechanical ventilation on inflammatory mediators in patients with acute respiratory distress syndrome: a randomized controlled trial. *JAMA* 1999; 282:54-61.

12. Buck ML. Pharmacokinetic changes during extracorporeal membrane oxygenation: implications for drug therapy of neonates. *Clin Pharmacokinet* 2003; 42:403-417.

13. Dagan O, Klein J, Bohn D, Koren G. Effects of extracorporeal membrane oxygenation on morphine pharmacokinetics in infants. *Crit Care Med* 1994; 22:1099-1101.

14. Mulla H, McCormack P, Lawson G, Firmin RK, Upton DR. Pharmacokinetics of midazolam in neonates undergoing extracorporeal membrane oxygenation. *Anesthesiology* 2003; 99:275-282.

15. Peters JW, Anderson BJ, Simons SH, Uges DR, Tibboel D. Morphine pharmacokinetics during venoarterial extracorporeal membrane oxygenation in neonates. *Intensive Care Med* 2005; 31:257-263.

16. Dagan O, Klein J, Bohn D, Barker G, Koren G. Morphine pharmacokinetics in children following cardiac surgery: effects of disease and inotropic support. *J Cardiothorac Vasc Anesth* 1993; 7:396-398.

17. Geiduschek JM, Lynn AM, Bratton SL, et al. Morphine pharmacokinetics during continuous infusion of morphine sulfate for infants receiving extracorporeal membrane oxygenation. *Crit Care Med* 1997; 25:360-364.

18. Berkenstadt H, Segal E, Mayan H, et al. The pharmacokinetics of morphine and lidocaine in critically ill patients. *Intensive Care Med* 1999; 25:110-112.

19. Lynn A, Nespeca MK, Bratton SL, Strauss SG, Shen DD. Clearance of morphine in post-operative infants during intravenous infusion: the influence of age and surgery. *Anesth Analg* 1998; 86:958-963.

20. Pokela ML, Olkkola KT, Seppälä T, Koivisto M. Age-related morphine kinetics in infants. *Dev Pharmacol Ther* 1993; 20:26-34.

21. McRorie TI, Lynn AM, Nespeca MK, Opheim KE, Slattery JT. The maturation of morphine clearance and metabolism. *Am J Dis Child* 1992; 146:972-976.

22. de Wildt SN, Kearns GL, Leeder JS, van den Anker JN. Glucuronidation in humans: pharmacogenetic and developmental aspects. *Clin Pharmacokinet* 1999; 36:439-452.

23. Phimmasone S, Kharasch ED. A pilot evaluation of alfentanil-induced miosis as a noninvasive probe for hepatic cytochrome P450 3A4 (CYP3A4) activity in humans. *Clin Pharmacol Ther* 2001; 70:505-517.

24. Mao J, Price DD, Mayer DJ. Mechanisms of hyperalgesia and morphine tolerance: a current view of their possible interactions. *Pain* 1995; 62:259-274.

25. Peters JW, Koot HM, Grunau RE, et al. Neonatal facial coding system for assessing post-operative pain in infants: item reduction is valid and feasible. *Clin J Pain* 2003; 19:353-363.

26. van Dijk M, de Boer JB, Koot HM, Tibboel D, Passchier J, Duivenvoorden HJ. The reliability and validity of the COMFORT scale as a post-operative pain instrument in 0 to 3-year-old infants. *Pain* 2000; 84:367-377.

27. Ambuel B, Hamlett KW, Marx CM, Blumer JL. Assessing distress in pediatric intensive care environments: the COMFORT scale. *J Pediatr Psychol* 1992; 17:95-109.

28 Linden V, Karlen J, Olsson M, et al. Successful extracorporeal membrane oxygenation in four children with malignant disease and severe pneumocystis carinii pneumonia. *Med Pediatr Oncol* 1999; 32:25-31.

29. Frenckner B, Frisén G, Palmér P, Lindén V. Swedish experiences with ECMO treatment with an artificial lung. *Lakartidningen* 2004; 101:1272-1275, 1278-1279.

30. Holstensson L, Lindén V, Palmér P, Frenckner B. Psycho-social follow-up of adult patinets surviving ECMO for ARDS. Presented at: 11th Annual ELSO Conference; 2000; New Orleans, LA.

35

Neurological Benefits of Mild Hypothermia

Denis Azzopardi, M.D.

Introduction

Brain injury is devastating for affected individuals as well as their families and is a major public health and social problem. Experimental and clinical studies have shown that cerebral insults lead to multiple complex pathophysiological processes, and these may be altered by timely interventions to lessen brain injury and improve outcome. Several neuroprotective interventions have been investigated in experimental studies, and mild hypothermia appears to be the most promising. This chapter will review the pathophysiological events that follow cerebral insults and the experimental and clinical evidence demonstrating neurological benefit by a modest reduction of body temperature.

Pathophysiological events associated with cerebral insults

Different cerebral insults may cause diverse patterns of injury but the pathophysiological processes that ensue are often similar.[1] Traumatic brain injury can cause compression of cerebral tissue, tearing of white and gray matter, and hemorrhage. These injuries can cause focal or diffuse histological abnormalities. Later, secondary injury caused by ischemia may occur due to alterations in cerebral blood flow.

Ischemic insults result from a severe reduction in cerebral blood flow because of occlusion of the cerebral or extracerebral circulation (or the in utero placental circulation in the fetus), cardiac arrest, or severe hypotension. Perinatal brain injury occurring in the term or near-term infant is primarily attributed to a combination of hypoxia and ischemia.

Reduction in oxygen and glucose delivery caused by severe hypoxia and/or ischemia rapidly results in cessation of cerebral oxidative metabolism, cerebral lactic acidosis, cell membrane ionic transport failure, and necrotic cell death.[2-4] Resuscitation following cessation of hypoxia-ischemia results in rapid recovery of cerebral energy metabolism. However, this is followed some hours later by a secondary fall in the concentration of cerebral high-energy phosphates accompanied by a rise in intracellular pH and the characteristic cerebral biochemical disturbance at this stage, lactic alkalosis.[4-7] In neonates, the severity of this secondary impairment in cerebral metabolism and persistent elevation of cerebral lactate and intracellular pH is associated with subsequent abnormal neurodevelopment and reduced head growth.[8-10] The secondary deterioration in cerebral metabolism that occurs some hours after the cerebral insult is presumably the result of a culmination of adverse biological events that ensue after restoration of oxygen supply and reperfusion of cerebral tissues. These processes result in accumulation of excitatory neurotransmitters, generation of reactive oxygen radicals, intracellular calcium accumulation, and mitochondrial dysfunction.[11-13]

Apart from the pathophysiological events that culminate in cellular energy failure and subsequent necrotic cell death, other mechanisms occur that lead to increased apoptosis.[14] While necrotic cell death is prominent in the immediate and acute phases of severe cerebral insults, apoptosis may be more important with less severe insults and may occur over a longer period.[15] Apoptosis occurs following the activation of pro-apoptotic proteins, the caspases, which cause characteristic damage to nuclear DNA that can be observed with gel electrophoresis (DNA laddering) or with a special staining technique, terminal deoxnucleotidyl nick end labeling (TUNEL). The initiation and progression of apoptosis is dependent on the balance between triggering events, such as oxidative stress and excessive glutamate stimulation, and the protective activity of anti-apoptotic proteins, such as BcL-2. Apoptosis appears to be a particularly important feature of delayed cell death following perinatal brain injury, perhaps because apoptosis is more prominent during development.[16]

In addition to biochemical and other processes, an inflammatory response also occurs following an acute cerebral insult. Disruption of the blood-brain barrier allows entry of leukocytes and macrophages that may phagocytose cells. Acute injury is also followed by the release of inflammatory molecules, such as cytokines, and activation of microglia, which take on the morphology of macrophages. Inflammation induced by lipopolysaccharide, a bacterial product, and pro-inflammatory cytokines such as cytokine IL-1 may play an important role in acute neuronal injury by enhancing the damaging effects of ischemia and the excitotoxicity due to accumulation of glutamate.[17-20] However, besides contributing to injurious processes, the inflammatory response may also have beneficial effects by isolating and removing damaged cells and by promoting repair and recovery. The balance between the detrimental and beneficial effects of inflammation may influence the severity of cerebral injury and determine outcome.[21]

As a result of the increased understanding of the pathophysiological processes that contribute to delayed secondary injury and the evidence suggesting that there may be a therapeutic window lasting several hours following cerebral injury, novel pharmaceutical products are being developed that may have neuroprotective properties. These products include calcium channel blockers, free radical scavengers, glutamate receptor blockers, anti-inflammatory and anti-apoptotic agents, and growth factors that promote repair. While many of these agents have shown benefit in experimental studies, the greatest benefit may result from therapies that target multiple pathophysiological mechanisms. Because temperature is critical to many aspects of cellular metabolism, there is active investigation regarding its effect on acute neurological injury.

Experimental studies of treatment with mild hypothermia following cerebral insults

There is substantial experimental data showing that a reduction of body temperature by about 3°C (mild hypothermia) during or following cerebral ischemia, hypoxia-ischemia, or trauma reduces brain damage. The beneficial effect of hypothermia is probably due to several mechanisms. First, mild hypothermia attenuates blood-brain barrier damage, reducing vasogenic edema, hemorrhage, and neutrophil infiltration.[22] Second, release of excitatory neurotransmitters is reduced, limiting intracellular calcium accumulation.[23,24] Third, free radical production is lessened, which protects cells and organelles from oxidative damage during reperfusion.[25]

Activation of the cytokine and coagulation cascades may contribute to the major organ dysfunction that occurs following acute insults and during cardiopulmonary bypass. Mild hypothermia may be protective in these situations by increasing interleukin-10 (IL-10, an anti-inflammatory cytokine) and reducing tumor necrosis factor alpha (TNF-α) concentrations through increased activation of suppressor signaling pathways, and by inhibiting release of platelet-activating factor.[26,27]

Perhaps, as a consequence of these multiple beneficial effects, as well as the decrease in the systemic metabolic rate that occurs with a reduction in body temperature, mild hypothermia has important positive effects on cerebral metabolism both during and following cerebral insults. Hypothermia decreases the cerebral metabolic rate for glucose and oxygen and reduces the loss of high energy phosphates during ischemia or hypoxia-ischemia.[28] Mild hypothermia also prevents or ameliorates secondary cerebral energy failure, which preserves cerebral high energy phosphates (nucleotide triphosphate [NTP] and exchangeable triphosphate pool [EPP]) and reduces cerebral lactic alkalosis.[29,30] In addition, it prevents the simultaneous increase in cytotoxic edema and loss of cerebral cortical activity that accompanies secondary energy failure (Figures 1 and 2).[31,32]

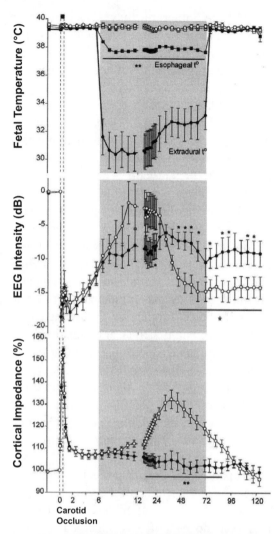

Figure 2. Time sequence of changes in fetal temperature and neurophysiologic variables. The 30-minute period of cerebral ischemia is shown by the dotted lines and solid bar, whereas cooling is shown by the gray highlighted area. The top panel shows changes in extradural (●) and esophageal (■) temperature in the hypothermia group and extradural (O) and esophageal (□) temperature in the sham-cooled group. The lower two panels show changes in EEG intensity, and cortical impedance (expressed as percentage of baseline) in the hypothermia (●) and sham-cooled (O) groups. The hypothermia group shows greater recovery of EEG intensity after resolution of delayed seizures, and complete suppression of the secondary rise in impedance. Mean ± SEM, *P <0.05, **P <0.001 hypothermia vs. sham-cooled fetuses, for individual time points or intervals (solid bars).[32]

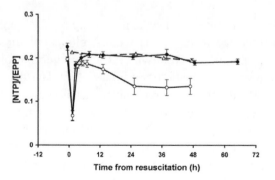

Figure 1. [NTP/EPP] in the 3 groups of piglets. ● = hypothermia (n=6), O =normothermia (n=12), and ∇=sham operated controls (n=6). Values are means and SEM.[31]
NTP: nucleotide triphosphate
EPP: exchangeable triphosphate pool

Mild hypothermia may also reduce the apoptosis which occurs after acute cerebral insults.[33] Experimental and clinical studies indicate that the number of apoptotic neurons (but not necrosis) is reduced, caspase activity is lessened, and cytochrome c translocation is diminished by mild hypothermia.[33-35] Hypothermia is thought to act early in the apoptotic pathways, perhaps by increasing the anti-apoptotic protein BcL-2 expression.[36]

The multiple beneficial biological effects of mild hypothermia observed in experimental studies are associated with a long-lasting reduction in cerebral tissue injury and improved cerebral function. Review of experimental studies of focal cerebral ischemia indicates that mild hypothermia is associated with a near 50% reduction of infarct size. Following global hypoxia, hypoxia-ischemia, or traumatic insults, mild hypothermia reduces damage in the cortex, thalamus, and hippocampus. Animals treated with mild hypothermia also demonstrate preserved neurological function. Although some of these benefits may diminish over time, long-term protection with hypothermia has also been demonstrated.[37,38]

Experimentally, neuroprotection has been observed even when mild hypothermia is initiated some hours after the cerebral insult. However, no benefit was observed in some studies when hypothermia was initiated very early, perhaps because recovery was hindered, secondary cerebral energy failure and epileptic activity had commenced, or inadequate sedation during hypothermia had resulted in an increased adrenergic stress response.[39-43] It has been suggested that mild hypothermia may increase the therapeutic window, thus allowing for other neuroprotective interventions.

Because of the diverse nature of the experimental models employed, ranging from cell culture studies to animals of different maturity, and because of the variation in mode of insult and application of hypothermia, uncertainty remains about clinical relevance. Despite un-certainty about which patients may benefit from hypothermia, when and for what duration, the method by which cooling should be applied, what the appropriate target temperature is, and the logistical problems of undertaking studies in comatose patients, the positive experimental results have prompted intensive clinical investigations of treatment with mild hypothermia following cerebral insults.

Clinical studies of treatment with mild hypothermia following cerebral insults

Early studies of treatment with hypothermia utilized profound hypothermia to protect the brain during operative procedures during which circulatory arrest was required. Following the introduction of heart-lung bypass procedures, profound hypothermia (18-20°C) became limited to specific situations, such as during the clipping of giant cerebral aneurysms and during certain cardiac operations where bypass cannot be continued throughout because the aortic arch and cerebral vessels are involved in the repair. Mild or moderate hypothermia has been investigated more recently in an effort to provide neuroprotection following traumatic brain injury, cerebral ischemia, or hypoxia-ischemia.

Traumatic brain injury

In the early 1990s, promising results were reported in preliminary small clinical studies of neuroprotection with mild hypothermia following traumatic brain injury. Pilot data from 80 patients in two randomized trials suggests a positive effect and no life threatening complications in patients treated with hypothermia.[44,45] Subsequently, a large, randomized multi-center study (the National Acute Brain Injury Study: Hypothermia) was initiated. The study was halted before completion because interim assessment suggested that treatment with mild hypothermia was futile.[46] The study enrolled 392 patients 16-65 years of age with coma from brain injury but without major multiple trauma. The target rectal temperature in the treated group of 33°C was achieved at 8.4 ±3 hours and was maintained for 48 hours. At 6 months after injury, no difference in the primary outcome of severe disability, vegetative state, or death was found between the two groups, but patients who were hypothermic on admission and were randomized to hypothermia had better Glasgow Coma scores at 6 months. Medical complications were increased in patients over 45 years of age who were treated with hypothermia. Some investigators have suggested that the negative result of this study was related to variations in clinical management, but this has been refuted by the study authors.[47]

In recent meta-analysis and systematic review of all clinical studies of neuroprotection with mild hypothermia following traumatic brain injury, there was no evidence of benefit with hypothermia, and there was a higher rate of sepsis in cooled patients.[48,49] A possible explanation for the failure to demonstrate benefit with mild hypothermia in these studies is the inclusion of patients with very severe traumatic injury who are unlikely to benefit from any intervention and delay in achieving the target body temperature.[50] These issues need to be addressed in future clinical studies.[51]

Stroke

Only a few feasibility studies have been carried out regarding treatment with mild hypothermia following ischemic stroke.[52-55] In these studies, the target core body temperature of 33°C was maintained for 24-72 hours by whole body surface cooling or by an intravascular cooling device, but initiation of cooling was delayed for several hours because of the need to perform neuroimaging and other procedures. Hypothermia appeared to be helpful in controlling intracranial pressure, but a rebound rise of intracranial pressure that necessitated further treatment was often noted during rewarming.[56]

There was a trend toward increased risk of sepsis, especially pneumonia, and there was no suggestion of improvement in neurological outcome or survival with hypothermic treatment. Overall, these preliminary studies do not support the use of hypothermia for neuroprotection following stroke. Future studies will need to overcome the logistical problems of achieving the target temperature within a few hours of initiation of stroke, minimizing complications, and maintaining cooling for longer periods of time.

Following cardiac arrest

In contrast to the predominantly negative studies of therapeutic hypothermia following traumatic brain injury and stroke, reports from two randomized, controlled studies published in 2002 suggest that mild hypothermia after cardiac arrest improves neurological outcome. The larger of the two studies, the multi-center "Hypothermia After Cardiac Arrest" study, enrolled 275 patients who were resuscitated after cardiac arrest caused by ventricular fibrillation.[57] In the group randomized to hypothermia, the target temperature of 32-34°C was achieved within 8 hours of restoration of spontaneous circulation and maintained for 24 hours using an external cooling device that delivered cold air over the entire body. The primary outcome was the achievement of good recovery or moderate disability on the Pittsburgh cerebral performance scale within 6 months; 55% of patients in the hypothermia group compared with 39% in the normothermia group achieved the primary outcome. Therefore, 6 patients would need to be treated with hypothermia to achieve good recovery or moderate disability, and the mortality was reduced by 14% (absolute risk reduction [ARR] = 14%, number needed to treat [NNT] to prevent one death = 7). Complications were similar in the two groups, but there was an increased incidence of sepsis in patients treated with hypothermia.

The other prospective controlled study was carried out in a single institution and enrolled 77 comatose survivors of out-of-hospital cardiac arrest.[58] Surface cooling with ice packs was commenced by paramedics following restoration of circulation, and the target temperature of 33°C was achieved within 2 hours and maintained for 12 hours. Within this group, 49% of patients treated with hypothermia had a good neurological outcome compared with 26% receiving normothermia (P=0.0046, ARR 23%, NNT 4.3). The improved outcome associated with cooling remained after adjustment for baseline differences in age and time from cardiac arrest to return of circulation, and there was no difference in the frequency of adverse events.

The benefits demonstrated by these studies, in contrast to the negative studies of hypothermia following traumatic brain injury or stroke, may be attributed to the early initiation of hypothermia and the exclusion of patients with the most severe anoxic insults (i.e., those with a delay of more than 60 minutes before restoration of spontaneous circulation). As a result of these two studies, hypothermia is now considered to be standard clinical practice for patients with cardiac arrest caused by ventricular fibrillation or tachycardia, but it is not known if hypothermia is helpful in patients after asystolic or pulseless electrical activity cardiac arrest. Also, the optimal temperature and duration of cooling remain uncertain.

Perinatal brain injury

Hypothermia was first reported as a method of resuscitation for asphyxiated newborns in the 1950s, but this practice was abandoned following the introduction of endotracheal intubation and mechanical ventilation. Perinatal asphyxia is an important cause of mortality and morbidity in the newborn. Studies of mild hypothermia for neuroprotection following perinatal asphyxia commenced after experimental studies in immature animals suggest that mild hypothermia applied soon after an asphyxial insult lessened pathophysiological abnormalities and improved functional outcome.

Two techniques of applied hypothermia were investigated. Gunn et al. introduced head cooling using a cap of coiled tubing filled with cooled fluid wrapped around the head to lessen the risk of potential complications associated with systemic hypothermia.[59] Excessive systemic cooling was prevented by use of an overhead heater and shielding of the head. With this technique, the rectal temperature was maintained at approximately 34.5°C, but the brain temperature achieved by this method was not measured. Studies employing newborn piglets (head size equivalent to a preterm infant) suggest that effective brain cooling may be achieved by this method, but computer modeling indicates that this may not be the case in a full term infant.[60,61] An alternative method has been to use whole body cooling with a target rectal temperature of 33.5°C using cooled air or a fluid-filled mattress.[62-64] Rectal temperature is usually used as a surrogate for brain temperature in these studies, because it is known to correlate closely with deep brain temperature.[65] This correlation is maintained following a cerebral insult and during whole body cooling, but it may be altered by medications such as pentobaribital.[65,66]

Since accidental hypothermia in premature infants is harmful, the primary aim of preliminary clinical studies following perinatal asphyxia was to assess the safety of induced, prolonged mild hypothermia. Cooling is associated with physiological changes in cardiovascular parameters. Blood pressure rises and heart rate falls linearly with decreases in the rectal temperature. These changes were also observed in clinical studies carried out in asphyxiated newborns (Figure 3), but no corrective intervention was required.[62,67] However, rectal temperature, blood pressure, and heart rate were less stable during hypothermia induced by head cooling, most likely because fluctuations in the power of the overhead heater altered peripheral vascular tone.[67] The Q-T interval has been reported to lengthen with cooling in newborns, but it has not been associated with arrhythmias, as has been observed in adults when the rectal temperature falls below 33°C.[68]

Apart from these cardiovascular effects, hypothermia may also alter clotting as well as biochemical and metabolic measurements. No significant differences in blood viscosity, thrombocytopenia, or acidosis were noted between cooled and normothermic infants; however, cooled infants had higher blood glucose and lower blood potassium levels, but these were not clinically significant.[62,69] Although increased sepsis rates have been observed in adults treated with cooling, this has not been reported in clinical studies of newborns.

The use of appropriate entry criteria is critical to the success of clinical studies involving novel treatments. In initial studies, it is necessary to select subjects who are most likely to

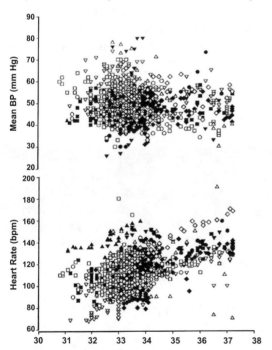

Figure 3. Relationships among mean blood pressure, heart rate, and rectal temperature in cooled infants. Different symbols represent data from individual infants.[62]

benefit from treatment in an effort to avoid unnecessary exposure of infants to potentially toxic effects when they are unlikely to benefit. It is also important to limit the size of the study to the minimum required for statistical significance. Some studies have used a combination of clinical features to identify infants at high risk of developing progressively severe asphyxial encephalopathy, but clinical assessment may not be sufficiently accurate immediately after birth. The amplitude-integrated EEG (aEEG), a simple form of single channel EEG monitoring, has been used as an additional criterion to identify and exclude those infants who are likely to have a normal prognosis.[62] The combination of an abnormal aEEG with abnormal early neurological examination increases the positive predictive value when compared with either one alone.[70]

After preliminary studies indicated that prolonged treatment with mild hypothermia soon after birth was feasible and could be applied safely, multi-center randomized studies commenced. Studies have been completed using either head cooling combined with mild body cooling (rectal temperature 34.5°C) or employing whole body cooling to 33-33.5°C, and others are ongoing.

The first study to report its findings was the "CoolCap Study".[71] Since this was the first large randomized study of treatment with hypothermia following perinatal asphyxia, the study's scientific committee decided to include infants with severe encephalographic changes, even though it was hypothesized that cooling was unlikely to be protective in these infants. In this study, 234 infants with moderate to severe encephalopathy and an abnormal aEEG were randomized to either head cooling for 72 hours starting within 6 hours of birth with rectal temperature maintained at 34.5°C, or to conventional care. Although there was no difference in the primary outcome of death or severe disability, results suggest a protective effect of hypothermia when controlling for severity of encephalopathy determined by pre-randomization aEEG (P=0.05, odds ratio [OR]: 0.57, 95% confidence intervals [CI]: 0.32-1.01). There was no effect of hypothermia in the 46 infants in the study with the most severe aEEG abnormalities. In the remaining 172 infants, the combined outcome measure (death or severe disability) was reduced from 65.9% in controls to 47.6% in cooled infants (P=0.01, OR:0.42, CI 0.22-0.8). In this less severe group, deaths were reduced from 38.6% to 28.6% and severe disability from 27.8% to 11.7%. However, these changes were not statistically significant. There were no clinically important complications associated with cooling. The inclusion of infants with very severe asphyxia may explain the lack of a neuroprotective effect of hypothermia in the total study population.

A similarly sized study employing whole body cooling to 33.5°C for 72 hours in infants selected by clinical assessment without an EEG has also been completed; its findings have been presented but not published.[72] In this study, 45 of 102 infants in the cooled group died or were disabled at 18 months compared with 64 of 106 control infants. The relative risk reduction (RR) was 0.72 (0.55-0.93) and 0.77 (0.6-0.98) after adjustment by center and severity of encephalopathy. A borderline significant reduction in deaths was observed in the cooled group (24/102 vs. 38/106, RR:0.66, CI:0.43-1.01), but not in disability.

A smaller study of whole body cooling in 65 asphyxiated newborns has also been reported.[73,74] In this study, infants randomized to hypothermia were cooled to 33°C for 48 hours and outcome was assessed at 12 months. Fewer cooled infants died (10/32 vs. 14/33) and fewer survivors treated with cooling had severely abnormal neurodevelopmental motor scores (4/17 vs. 7/11). However, perhaps because of the small study size, these differences were not statistically significant, but the difference in the combined outcome (death or severely abnormal neurodevelopmental motor scores) between cooled and control infants was significant (14/27 vs. 21/25, P=0.019).

The combined results of these three studies suggest that mild hypothermia is associated with a significant reduction in death and severe disability following perinatal asphyxia (Figure 4). However, there are major differences between

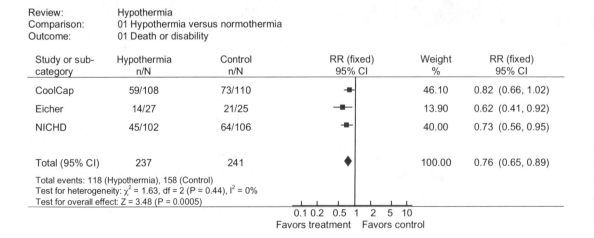

Review: Hypothermia
Comparison: 01 Hypothermia versus normothermia
Outcome: 01 Death or disability

Study or sub-category	Hypothermia n/N	Control n/N	RR (fixed) 95% CI	Weight %	RR (fixed) 95% CI
CoolCap	59/108	73/110		46.10	0.82 (0.66, 1.02)
Eicher	14/27	21/25		13.90	0.62 (0.41, 0.92)
NICHD	45/102	64/106		40.00	0.73 (0.56, 0.95)
Total (95% CI)	237	241		100.00	0.76 (0.65, 0.89)

Total events: 118 (Hypothermia), 158 (Control)
Test for heterogeneity: χ^2 = 1.63, df = 2 (P = 0.44), I^2 = 0%
Test for overall effect: Z = 3.48 (P = 0.0005)

0.1 0.2 0.5 1 2 5 10
Favors treatment   Favors control

Figure 4. Analysis of randomized controlled trials of mild hypothermia following perinatal asphyxia. A significant reduction in death or disability at 12-18 months is observed. Studies included are: Cool-Cap,[71] Shankaran,[72] and Eicher.[73-74]

these studies that might invalidate such meta-analysis. The studies had different methods of selection; variations in the cooling method and duration of therapy, most likely resulting in diverse brain temperatures in the cooled infants; and different evaluations of outcome. Pending full publication of these studies and the completion of ongoing studies it remains uncertain whether mild hypothermia is beneficial following perinatal asphyxia.

Neuroprotection with hypothermia has also been examined in infants undergoing ECMO for severe respiratory failure, a group of infants known to have a high incidence of neurological abnormalities. Brain injury in infants treated with ECMO may be caused by preceding events or may arise during ECMO. Respiratory failure from inhalation of meconium is a common indication for referral to ECMO. Meconium aspiration often occurs prior to delivery and may be associated with fetal hypoxia-ischemia. These infants are also severely ill and prolonged episodes of hypoxia are common prior to the initiation of ECMO. Cerebral injury may also occur as a result of the inflammatory and coagulation response to ECMO, which includes complement activation, activation of platelets and neutrophils, and release of cytokines and free radicals.[75] These effects may induce pulmonary inflammation and the clinical features associated with systemic inflammatory response syndrome, but it is not clear whether they contribute to neurological injury. Recently, the safety and feasibility of using mild hypothermia was tested in neonates receiving ECMO in a non-randomized pilot study of 25 infants divided into five groups with the core temperature maintained at 34-37°C. No major clinical or circuit problems were noted. There were no significant differences between groups in the molecular markers of coagulation, complement, cytokines, or platelet activation, but the group sizes were small.[76,77] This pilot study suggests that a multi-center, randomized, controlled trial would be feasible.

Challenges facing clinical studies of neuroprotection with hypothermia

Experimental data in the laboratory clearly demonstrate that mild hypothermia following diverse cerebral insults ameliorates molecular, biochemical, and metabolic abnormalities; reduces the extent of cerebral tissue injury; and improves neurological outcome. The challenge has been to demonstrate these benefits in a clinical trial. The initial promising results of pilot clinical studies have not always been confirmed in large, multi-center randomized studies. There are several reasons why experimental results may not be reproduced in clinical studies. Apart from the obvious reasons, such as species differences, uncertainty about timing, etiology, and severity of injury, there are difficult logistical problems in carrying out clinical studies of rapid therapeutic interventions in comatose patients. The initial resuscitative treatment and assessment, which may include neuroimaging and neurophysiological testing, may be prolonged which delays enrollment, and because some conditions, such as perinatal asphyxia are uncommon in countries with the resources necessary to undertake large studies, study recruitment may be drawn out and require many centers to participate, increasing the complexity and expense of the study. These logistical issues need to be recognized and addressed in the planning stages so that sufficient resources are assembled to ensure the success of the study.

Although the optimal time for induction of hypothermia following brain injury is uncertain, experimental data suggest that the opportunity for intervention is short and may vary with the type of insult and species studied. It is probably significant that in the large clinical trials showing benefit, cooling was induced very rapidly following resuscitation. This was achieved by enrollment at the site of presentation immediately after resuscitation and assessment were completed, involvement of paramedic staff when appropriate, and waiving the need to obtain consent from relatives prior to enrollment.[58]

Informed consent is required for most medical research studies, but may be waived in cases of comatose patients when urgent treatment is required. Institutional Review Boards are more likely to agree to waive or defer consent when the treatment window is short. In the two studies demonstrating benefit of mild hypothermia following cardiac arrest, consent was deferred until after randomization and was rarely refused.[57] The requirement for informed consent varied in the studies of traumatic brain injury. Patient enrollment was improved and time to enrollment was shorter when consent was waived. The requirement for informed consent is estimated to decrease patient enrollment by about 40% when consent must be obtained within 6 hours.[78] This requirement may also influence patient demographics. Enrollment of patients in minority groups increased after waiver of consent was allowed midway through the National Brain Injury Study. For the reasons outlined above, it has been suggested that it is impractical to perform studies without waiver of consent when the treatment window is less than 6 hours.

Current trials of hypothermia following perinatal asphyxia require written informed consent before randomization even though enrollment must be within 6 hours of birth. However, the validity of informed consent is questionable when it is required urgently.[79] When consent is required in such circumstances, a significant proportion of parents are later unable to recall whether they had been asked to consent to study enrollment.[80,81] The requirement of informed consent when there is insufficient time for deliberation hinders patient recruitment and weakens the scientific validity of the study. Deferred consent may be preferable when intervention is required soon after birth, provided there is minimal risk from the intervention and consent is sought as soon as practicably possible.[82]

Conclusion

The impressive benefits of mild hypothermia following cardiac arrest prove that neuroprotection following cerebral insult is possible. Inadequate selection procedures and logistical issues may explain why similar benefits have not been found in studies of hypothermia following traumatic brain injury or stroke. Similar difficulties are complicating current trials in neonates with perinatal asphyxia. The ethical and logistical issues identified in these studies need to be addressed in future studies of neuroprotection. Preliminary reports suggest that hypothermia may improve neurological outcome in infants with moderate but not severe perinatal asphyxia. Further studies are essential to determine optimal temperature, timing of hypothermia, and combination treatment with pharmacological agents.

References

1. Bramlett HM, Dietrich WD. Pathophysiology of cerebral ischemia and brain trauma: similarities and differences. *J Cereb Blood Flow Metab* 2004; 24:133-150.

2. Siesjo BK, Katsura K, Kristian T. The biochemical basis of cerebral ischemic damage. *J Neurosurg Anesthesiol* 1995; 7:47-52.

3. Siesjo BK. Cell damage in the brain: a speculative synthesis. *Acta Psychiatr Scand Suppl* 1984; 313:57-91.

4. Blumberg RM, Cady EB, Wigglesworth JS, McKenzie JE, Edwards AD. Relation between delayed impairment of cerebral energy metabolism and infarction following transient focal hypoxia-ischemia in the developing brain. *Exp Brain Res* 1997; 113:130-137.

5. Amess PN, Penrice J, Wylezinska M, et al. Early brain proton magnetic resonance spectroscopy and neonatal neurology related to neurodevelopmental outcome at 1 year in term infants after presumed

hypoxic-ischæmic brain injury. *Dev Med Child Neurol* 1999; 41:436-445.

6. Lorek A, Takei Y, Cady EB, et al. Delayed ("secondary") cerebral energy failure after acute hypoxia-ischemia in the newborn piglet: continuous 48-hour studies by phosphorus magnetic resonance spectroscopy. *Pediatr Res* 1994; 36:699-706.

7. Edwards AD, Azzopardi DV. Perinatal hypoxia-ischemia and brain injury. *Pediatr Res* 2000; 47:431-432.

8. Azzopardi D, Wyatt JS, Cady EB, et al. Prognosis of newborn infants with hypoxic-ischemic brain injury assessed by phosphorus magnetic resonance spectroscopy. *Pediatr Res* 1989; 25:445-451.

9. Robertson NJ, Cox IJ, Cowan FM, Counsell SJ, Azzopardi D, Edwards AD. Cerebral intracellular lactic alkalosis persisting months after neonatal encephalopathy measured by magnetic resonance spectroscopy. *Pediatr Res* 1999; 46:287-296.

10. Roth SC, Edwards AD, Cady EB, et al. Relation between cerebral oxidative metabolism following birth asphyxia, and neurodevelopmental outcome and brain growth at one year. *Dev Med Child Neurol* 1992; 34:285-295.

11. Siesjo BK, Elmer E, Janelidze S, et al. Role and mechanisms of secondary mitochondrial failure. *Acta Neurochir Suppl (Wien)* 1999; 73:7-13.

12. Siesjo BK, Katsura K, Zhao Q, et al. Mechanisms of secondary brain damage in global and focal ischemia: a speculative synthesis. *J Neurotrauma* 1995; 12:943-956.

13. Siesjo BK, Katsura K, Kristian T. The biochemical basis of cerebral ischemic damage. *J Neurosurg Anesthesiol* 1995; 7:47-52.

14. Taylor DL, Edwards AD, Mehmet H. Oxidative metabolism, apoptosis and perinatal brain injury. *Brain Pathol* 1999; 9:93-117.

15. Northington FJ, Ferriero DM, Graham EM, Traystman RJ, Martin LJ. Early neurodegeneration after hypoxia-ischemia in neonatal rat is necrosis while delayed neuronal death is apoptosis. *Neurobiol Dis* 2001; 8:207-219.

16. Edwards AD, Yue X, Cox P, et al. Apoptosis in the brains of infants suffering intrauterine cerebral injury. *Pediatr Res* 1997; 42:684-689.

17. Hagberg H, Peebles D, Mallard C. Models of white matter injury: comparison of infectious, hypoxic-ischemic, and excitotoxic insults. *Ment Retard Dev Disabil Res Rev* 2002; 8:30-38.

18. Mallard C, Welin AK, Peebles D, Hagberg H, Kjellmer I. White matter injury following systemic endotoxemia or asphyxia in the fetal sheep. *Neurochem Res* 2003; 28:215-223.

19. Allan SM, Rothwell NJ. Inflammation in central nervous system injury. *Philos Trans R Soc Lond B Biol Sci* 2003; 358:1669-1677.

20. Allan SM, Rothwell NJ. Cytokines and acute neurodegeneration. *Nat Rev Neurosci* 2001; 2:734-744.

21. Nguyen MD, Julien JP, Rivest S. Innate immunity: the missing link in neuroprotection and neurodegeneration? *Nat Rev Neurosci* 2002; 3:216-227.

22. Smith SL, Hall ED. Mild pre- and posttraumatic hypothermia attenuates blood-brain barrier damage following controlled cortical impact injury in the rat. *J Neurotrauma* 1996; 13:1-9.

23. Busto R, Globus MY, Dietrich WD, Martinez E, Valdes I, Ginsberg MD. Effect of mild hypothermia on ischemia-induced release of neurotransmitters and free fatty acids in rat brain. *Stroke* 1989; 20:904-910.

24. Nakashima K, Todd MM. Effects of hypothermia on the rate of excitatory amino acid release after ischemic depolarization. *Stroke* 1996; 27:913-918.

25. Globus MY, Alonso O, Dietrich WD, Busto R, Ginsberg MD. Glutamate release and

free radical production following brain injury: effects of posttraumatic hypothermia. *J Neurochem* 1995; 65:1704-1711.

26. Akisu M, Huseyinov A, Yalaz M, Cetin H, Kultursay N. Selective head cooling with hypothermia suppresses the generation of platelet-activating factor in cerebrospinal fluid of newborn infants with perinatal asphyxia. *Prostaglandins Leukot Essent Fatty Acids* 2003; 69:45-50.

27. Qing M, Nimmesgern A, Heinrich PC, et al. Intrahepatic synthesis of tumor necrosis factor-alpha related to cardiac surgery is inhibited by interleukin-10 via the Janus kinase (Jak)/signal transducers and activator of transcription (STAT) pathway. *Crit Care Med* 2003; 31:2769-2775.

28. Erecinska M, Thoresen M, Silver IA. Effects of hypothermia on energy metabolism in Mammalian central nervous system. *J Cereb Blood Flow Metab* 2003; 23:513-530.

29. Amess PN, Penrice J, Cady EB, et al. Mild hypothermia after severe transient hypoxia-ischemia reduces the delayed rise in cerebral lactate in the newborn piglet. *Pediatr Res* 1997; 41:803-808.

30. Bona E, Hagberg H, Loberg EM, Bagenholm R, Thoresen M. Protective effects of moderate hypothermia after neonatal hypoxia-ischemia: short- and long-term outcome. *Pediatr Res* 1998; 43:738-745.

31. Thoresen M, Penrice J, Lorek A, et al. Mild hypothermia after severe transient hypoxia-ischemia reduces the delayed rise in cerebral lactate in the newborn piglet. *Pediatr Res.* 1995; 37:667-70.

32. Gunn AJ, Gunn TR, Gunning MI, Williams CE, Gluckman PD. Neuroprotection with prolonged head cooling started before postischemic seizures in fetal sheep. *Pediatrics* 1998; 102:1098-1106.

33. Edwards AD, Yue X, Squier MV, et al. Specific inhibition of apoptosis after cerebral hypoxia-ischemia by moderate post-insult hypothermia. *Biochem Biophys Res Commun* 1995; 217:1193-1199.

34. Xu L, Yenari MA, Steinberg GK, Giffard RG. Mild hypothermia reduces apoptosis of mouse neurons in vitro early in the cascade. *J Cereb Blood Flow Metab* 2002; 22:21-28.

35. Zhu C, Wang X, Cheng X, et al. Post-ischemic hypothermia-induced tissue protection and diminished apoptosis after neonatal cerebral hypoxia-ischemia. *Brain Res* 2004; 996:67-75.

36. Zhang Z, Sobel RA, Cheng D, Steinberg GK, Yenari MA. Mild hypothermia increases BcL-2 protein expression following global cerebral ischemia. *Brain Res Mol Brain Res* 2001; 95:75-85.

37. Tomimatsu T, Fukuda H, Endoh M, et al. Long-term neuroprotective effects of hypothermia on neonatal hypoxic-ischemic brain injury in rats, assessed by auditory brainstem response. *Pediatr Res* 2003; 53:57-61.

38. Colbourne F, Corbett D, Zhao Z, Yang J, Buchan AM. Prolonged but delayed postischemic hypothermia: a long-term outcome study in the rat middle cerebral artery occlusion model. *J Cereb Blood Flow Metab* 2000; 20:1702-1708.

39. MacLellan CL, Girgis J, Colbourne F. Delayed onset of prolonged hypothermia improves outcome after intracerebral hemorrhage in rats. *J Cereb Blood Flow Metab* 2004; 24:432-440.

40. Taylor DL, Mehmet H, Cady EB, Edwards AD. Improved neuroprotection with hypothermia delayed by 6 hours following cerebral hypoxia-ischemia in the 14-day-old rat. *Pediatr Res* 2002; 51:13-19.

41. Tooley JR, Satas S, Porter H, Silver IA, Thoresen M. Head cooling with mild systemic hypothermia in anesthetized piglets is neuroprotective. *Ann Neurol* 2003; 53:65-72.

42. Gunn AJ, Bennet L, Gunning MI, Gluckman PD, Gunn TR. Cerebral hypothermia is not neuroprotective when started after postischemic seizures in fetal sheep. *Pediatr Res* 1999; 46:274-280.

43. Thoresen M, Satas S, Loberg EM, et al. Twenty-four hours of mild hypothermia in unsedated newborn pigs starting after a severe global hypoxic-ischemic insult is not neuro-protective. *Pediatr Res* 2001; 50:405-411.

44. Clifton GL, Allen S, Barrodale P, et al. A phase II study of moderate hypothermia in severe brain injury. *J Neurotrauma* 1993; 10:263-271.

45. Marion DW, Obrist WD, Carlier PM, Penrod LE, Darby JM. The use of moderate therapeutic hypothermia for patients with severe head injuries: a preliminary report. *J Neurosurg* 1993; 79:354-362.

46. Clifton GL, Miller ER, Choi SC, et al. Lack of effect of induction of hypothermia after acute brain injury. *N Engl J Med* 2001; 344:556-563.

47. Polderman KH, Girbes AR, Peerdeman SM, Vandertop WP. Hypothermia. *J Neurosurg* 2001; 94:853-858.

48. Henderson WR, Dhingra VK, Chittock DR, Fenwick JC, Ronco JJ. Hypothermia in the management of traumatic brain injury. A systematic review and meta-analysis. *Intensive Care Med* 2003; 29:1637-1644.

49. McIntyre LA, Fergusson DA, Hebert PC, Moher D, Hutchison JS. Prolonged therapeutic hypothermia after traumatic brain injury in adults: a systematic review. *JAMA* 2003; 289:2992-2999.

50. Polderman KH, van Zanten AR, Nipshagen MD, Girbes AR. Induced hypothermia in traumatic brain injury: effective if properly employed. *Crit Care Med* 2004; 32:313-314.

51. Marion DW. Moderate hypothermia in severe head injuries: the present and the future. *Curr Opin Crit Care* 2002; 8:111-114.

52. Schwab S, Georgiadis D, Berrouschot J, Schellinger PD, Graffagnino C, Mayer SA. Feasibility and safety of moderate hypothermia after massive hemispheric infarction. *Stroke* 2001; 32:2033-2035.

53. Schwab S, Schwarz S, Spranger M, Keller E, Bertram M, Hacke W. Moderate hypother-mia in the treatment of patients with severe middle cerebral artery infarction. *Stroke* 1998; 29:2461-2466.

54. Kammersgaard LP, Rasmussen BH, Jorgensen HS, Reith J, Weber U, Olsen TS. Feasibility and safety of inducing modest hypothermia in awake patients with acute stroke through surface cooling: a case-control study: the Copenhagen Stroke Study. *Stroke* 2000; 31:2251-2256.

55. Krieger DW, De Georgia MA, Abou-Chebl A, et al. Cooling for acute ischemic brain damage (cool aid): an open pilot study of induced hypothermia in acute ischemic stroke. *Stroke* 2001; 32:1847-1854.

56. Tokutomi T, Morimoto K, Miyagi T, Yamaguchi S, Ishikawa K, Shigemori M. Optimal temperature for the management of severe traumatic brain injury: effect of hypothermia on intracranial pressure, systemic and intracranial hemodynamics, and metabolism. *Neurosurgery* 2003; 52:102-111.

57. Mild therapeutic hypothermia to improve the neurologic outcome after cardiac arrest. *N Engl J Med* 2002; 346:549-556.

58. Bernard SA, Gray TW, Buist MD, et al. Treatment of comatose survivors of out-of-hospital cardiac arrest with induced hypothermia. *N Engl J Med* 2002; 346:557-563.

59. Gunn AJ, Gluckman PD, Gunn TR. Selective head cooling in newborn infants after perinatal asphyxia: a safety study. *Pediatrics* 1998; 102:885-892.

60. Van Leeuwen GM, Hand JW, Lagendijk JJ, Azzopardi DV, Edwards AD. Numerical modeling of temperature distributions within the neonatal head. *Pediatr Res* 2000; 48:351-356.

61. Tooley J, Satas S, Eagle R, Silver IA, Thoresen M. Significant selective head cooling can be maintained long-term after global hypoxia ischemia in newborn piglets. *Pediatrics* 2002; 109:643-649.

62. Azzopardi D, Robertson NJ, Cowan FM, Rutherford MA, Rampling M, Edwards AD.

Pilot study of treatment with whole body hypothermia for neonatal encephalopathy. *Pediatrics* 2000; 106:684-694.

63. Shankaran S, Laptook A, Wright LL, et al. Whole-body hypothermia for neonatal encephalopathy: animal observations as a basis for a randomized, controlled pilot study in term infants. *Pediatrics* 2002; 110:377-385.

64. Debillon T, Daoud P, Durand P, et al. Whole-body cooling after perinatal asphyxia: a pilot study in term neonates. *Dev Med Child Neurol* 2003; 45:17-23.

65. Mellergard P. Monitoring of rectal, epidural, and intraventricular temperature in neurosurgical patients. *Acta Neurochir Suppl (Wien)* 1994; 60:485-487.

66. Mellergard P. Changes in human intracerebral temperature in response to different methods of brain cooling. *Neurosurgery* 1992; 31:671-677.

67. Thoresen M, Whitelaw A. Cardiovascular changes during mild therapeutic hypothermia and rewarming in infants with hypoxic-ischemic encephalopathy. *Pediatrics* 2000; 106:92-99.

68. Gunn TR, Wilson NJ, Aftimos S, Gunn AJ. Brain hypothermia and Q-T interval. *Pediatrics* 1999; 103:1079.

69. Battin MR, Penrice J, Gunn TR, Gunn AJ. Treatment of term infants with head cooling and mild systemic hypothermia (35.0 degrees C and 34.5 degrees C) after perinatal asphyxia. *Pediatrics* 2003; 111:244-251.

70. Shalak LF, Laptook AR, Velaphi SC, Perlman JM. Amplitude-integrated electroencephalography coupled with an early neurologic examination enhances prediction of term infants at risk for persistent encephalopathy. *Pediatrics* 2003; 111:351-357.

71. Gluckman PD, Wyatt JS, Azzopardi D, Ballard R, et al. Selective head cooling with mild systemic hypothermia to improve neurodevelopmental outcome following neonatal encephalopathy: multicenter randomized trial. *Lancet* 2005; 365:663-70.

72. Shankaran S. Whole-body hypothermia for neonatal encephalopathy. Presented at: Hot Topics in Neonatology, December 12-14, 2004, Washington, D.C.

73. Eicher DJ, Wagner CL, Katikaneni LP, et al. Moderate hypothermia in neonatal encephalopathy: safety outcomes. *Pediatr Neurol* 2005; 32:18-24.

74. Eicher DJ, Wagner CL, Katikaneni LP, et al. Moderate hypothermia in neonatal encephalopathy: efficacy outcomes. *Pediatr Neurol* 2005; 32:11-17.

75. Peek GJ, Firmin RK. The inflammatory and coagulative response to prolonged extracorporeal membrane oxygenation. *ASAIO J* 1999; 45:250-263.

76. Ichiba S, Killer HM, Firmin RK, Kotecha S, Edwards AD, Field D. Pilot investigation of hypothermia in neonates receiving extracorporeal membrane oxygenation. *Arch Dis Child Fetal Neonatal Ed* 2003; 88:F128-F133.

77. Horan M, Ichiba S, Firmin RK, et al. A pilot investigation of mild hypothermia in neonates receiving extracorporeal membrane oxygenation (ECMO). *J Pediatr* 2004; 144:301-308.

78. Clifton GL, Knudson P, McDonald M. Waiver of consent in studies of acute brain injury. *J Neurotrauma* 2002; 19:1121-1126.

79. Allmark P, Mason S, Gill AB, Megone C. Obtaining consent for neonatal research. *Arch Dis Child Fetal Neonatal Ed* 2003; 88:F166-F167.

80. Ballard HO, Shook LA, Desai NS, Anand KJ. Neonatal research and the validity of informed consent obtained in the perinatal period. *J Perinatol* 2004; 24:409-415.

81. Stenson BJ, Becher JC, McIntosh N. Neonatal research: the parental perspective. *Arch Dis Child Fetal Neonatal Ed* 2004; 89:F321-F323.

82. Manning DJ. Presumed consent in emergency neonatal research. *J Med Ethics* 2000; 26:249-253.

36

Immunosuppressed Patients and ECLS

Heidi J. Dalton, M.D.

Introduction

The past few years have been distinguished by the expansion of extracorporeal support to patient groups who previously would have been excluded. Trauma, cardiac arrest, and septic shock were formally contraindications for ECLS as little as a few years ago.[1-8] However, patients with these conditions have recently been supported successfully with ECLS with acceptable survival rates. The experience gained from support of these complicated cases has advanced the field of ECLS. New equipment and techniques have also helped reduce the risk of bleeding, blood cell trauma, and mechanical complications. However, uncertainty remains as to the appropriateness of ECLS support for patients with underlying immune dysfunction.

In the past, immunosuppressed patients were considered inappropriate candidates for ECLS because of several concerns. One factor was the poor survival of immunosuppressed patients who require intensive care. Difficulties with infection, bleeding, and multi-organ failure, as well as the short life expectancy of many of these patients, has led to the often unspoken presumption that labor-intensive and invasive techniques such as ECLS are unsuitable. In fact, intensive care support has often been withdrawn in many of these patients due to perceived futility without consideration of the option of ECLS.

Another factor was the belief that the patient's abnormal immune function, coupled with the effects on the immune system of ECLS, would place the patient at great risk for lethal infection. Studies of immune function and white blood cell function during cardiopulmonary bypass (CPB) and ECMO have shown deleterious changes in immune system function, at least on a temporary basis.[9-11] Additionally, many immunocompromised patients have malignancy as a primary diagnosis. These patients often have the triad of severe neutropenia, thrombocytopenia, and anemia. The combination of poor immune function and increased risk of bleeding have excluded these patients from consideration for ECLS. Further, the long-term quality of life for such patients has been reported as poor, which has also discouraged the use of ECLS.

Traditionally, ECLS has been reserved for those patients with an acute, reversible disease expected to have a good quality of life should recovery occur. Concerns over whether ECLS in immunocompromised patients merely acts to delay the dying process have led to many thought-provoking discussions. It is difficult to establish specific criteria for ECLS use among previously healthy patients with more straight-forward diseases such as simple pneumonia or acute respiratory failure (ARF); determining whether a patient with a complicated immune disease should be considered for ECLS is even more challenging.

Little information is available to address whether ECLS should be used in the immuno-compromised patient. This chapter reviews the information at hand regarding the definition of immunosuppressed patients, the experience of such patients on ECLS, and possible future directions.

Immunocompromised patients

The category of primary immune dysfunction is typically defined as including those patients with underlying malignancy or an immune deficiency disorder. Patients with autoimmune diseases such as systemic lupus erythematosus, rheumatoid arthritis (juvenile rheumatoid arthritis in pediatric patients), Wegener's Granulomatosis, Goodpasture's syndrome, or other causes of vasculitis are among those placed in this category. Immune dysfunction also occurs in patients are receiving immunosuppressive medications or who become compromised during an acute illness from bone marrow depression. Although even common diseases such as asthma, allergies, or eczema which are treated with chronic medications such as corticosteroids can result in immunosuppression, this chapter focuses on patients with immune deficiency disorders or underlying malignancy, as well as post-transplant patients.

Case Report

One subgroup of patients with autoimmune disease in which the use of ECLS has been described are those with concomitant pulmonary hemorrhage.[12] While the systemic heparinization administered with ECMO, with its consequent risk of further bleeding, had led to reluctance to place such patients on ECLS, patients with Wegener's granulomatosis have been placed on ECLS.[13] A typical case report of such a patient follows.

A 16-year-old, previously healthy male presented with fever, cough, and chills. He had been treated as an outpatient for sinusitis. There was a history of mild asthma, with no other illness. There was no travel history or ill contacts. He had occasional epistaxis over a 3-week period. He was admitted to a community hospital due to continued cough and fever, and diagnosed with bilateral pneumonia and status asthmaticus. He was placed on antibiotics and inhaled steroids. By hospital day 5, his worsening respiratory status resulted in transfer to a tertiary pediatric ICU for worsening dyspnea and hypoxemia. On admission, the patient was febrile, tachypneic, and in respiratory distress. Initial use of a non-rebreather oxygen mask helped to relieve distress. Antibiotic coverage was broadened and repeat cultures were sent, as well as vasculitis labs. Bronchoscopy was planned for the next morning. During bronchoscopy preparation, the patient had an acute deterioration requiring intubation. Massive pulmonary hemorrhage was noted on intubation and 6 units of packed red blood cells (PRBCs) were required for stabilization. The patient was too unstable for bronchoscopy. Rapid escalation of ventilator settings occurred, and the patient was placed on high frequency ventilation (HFV) within 24 hours with a mean airway pressure (MAP) of 32 cm H_2O and FiO_2 60%. The patient was maintained on HFV with PaO_2 70-80 mm Hg, MAP 25, FiO_2 50%. Laboratory results noted an ANA <1.40, C3 114, C4 21, IgG 1551, IgA 150, IgM 71, pANCA <21, cANCA 138. A suspicious lesion in the nasal cavity was biopsied. The patient developed airleak syndrome over the next 24-48 hours requiring thoracostomy tubes. Pathologic examination of the nasal biopsy was consistent with We-

gener's granulomatosis. The patient was maintained on high dose corticosteroids without improvement and was started on Cytoxan. Worsening airleak syndrome and intermittent episodes of hypoxemia and hemodynamic instability occurred. Improvement in oxygenation was also intermittent and ventilator settings were able to be reduced but not sustained at lower levels consistently. Discussion was held regarding the utility of ECLS in this patient, and he was placed on venovenous (VV) ECMO percutaneously on hospital day 10 (Figure 1). During ECMO, plasmapheresis and continuous renal replacement were performed (Figure 2). No bleeding or other complications occurred. Following 6 days of ECMO support, the patient was successfully decannulated and was extubated 2 days later. The patient recovered completely and remained in remission from his underlying disease.

In a series of 8 patients with acute pulmonary hemorrhage treated with either venoarterial (VA) or VV ECMO, none had worsening hemorrhage and survival was 100%.[14] Neither recurrent hemorrhage nor infection were found

to be complications during ECMO. While the number of case reports is small and represents only a fraction of the types of primary immune disorders that are encountered, they nonetheless are encouraging as to the potential benefit of ECLS for this population.

Use of ECLS in malignancy

The use of ECLS in patients with malignancy or following transplant is controversial. As with other immune disorders, overall outcome in cancer and transplant patients requiring intensive care has been poor.[15,16] This fact, coupled with the assumption that children with cancer have a limited and poor quality-of-life, has led to the perception that aggressive ICU support for these patients may be unwarranted. A few years ago, it was not uncommon to hear the phrase, "Once they go into the ICU, they never come out," from families, nursing, and medical staff alike when a cancer patient required ICU therapy. For patients that did not experience prompt recovery, discussions by the medical team often focused on withdrawal or limitation of support rather than continued aggressive intensive care. This expectation of poor outcome discouraged studies of new therapies and techniques; cancer patients and those with

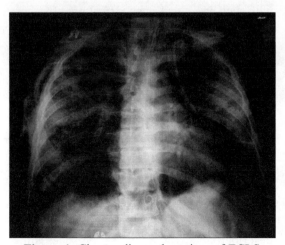

Figure 1. Chest radiograph at time of ECLS initiation.

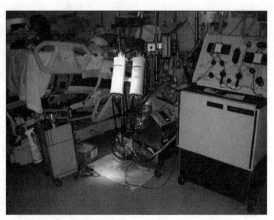

Figure 2. Concomitant use of ECMO and plasmapheresis.

transplantation are frequently excluded from studies so as not to skew results.[17] Cancer and transplant patients have been excluded not only from ECLS, but also from the use of inhaled nitric oxide (iNO), HFV, surfactant, and other therapies.[18-21] At the same time that outcome for cancer and transplant patients entering the ICU has been poor, the numbers of these patients entering the ICU has increased. Data from the Pediatric ICU Evaluations (PICUEs) project, a large database of >30,000 ICU patients from multiple ICUs, showed that although cancer patients comprised 1% of the ICU population in the period between 1996-98, this proportion had risen to 5% between 1998-2001.[16] Medical science has increased the availability of effective treatment regimens for these patients. The overall survival in pediatric cancer has increased to the point where disorders such as leukemia are now considered to be >90% curable.[22] The quality of life in cancer survivors has also improved, especially in children with uncomplicated treatment courses who may go on to live normal lives.

There are also some indications that the outcome of cancer patients in the ICU may be improving. In one evaluation of 1,000 pediatric cancer patients admitted to the pediatric ICU, again using the PICUEs database, overall survival to discharge among patients who did not require either mechanical ventilation or vasoactive medications was >90%.[16] Even in those patients presenting with acute illness requiring both mechanical ventilation and inotropic therapy, survival to discharge was 47%. This apparent improvement has triggered a reassessment of the use of aggressive therapies such as ECLS in patients who are non-responsive to conventional intensive care.

There are still few descriptions of use of ECLS in patients with malignancy, and what is available mainly represents single case reports. In one small published case series by Linden of 4 cancer patients who received ECLS for pneumocystis pneumonia and respiratory failure, survival was reported to be 75%.[23] All 3 patients with underlying hematologic malignancy survived. This report is probably the largest experience with blood cancer patients and ECLS which exists in the literature to date. There are multiple reports available now which outline use of ECLS following surgical treatment of solid tumors, in pediatric and adult patients.[24] ECLS has also been used as an adjunct during surgical resection of laryngotracheal masses to provide cardiopulmonary support.[25]

ECLS management concerns in cancer patients

In addition to concerns with reversibility and long-term outcome, other factors influence the risk-benefit ratio of ECLS for cancer patients. Consideration must be given when in the course of the disease to consider ECLS and how to manage chemotherapy during ECLS. While there remains hesitancy to apply ECLS in patients with neutropenia and thrombocytopenia, as discussed previously, experience has shown that successful use of ECLS in patients with low platelet counts (<50,000) or profound neutropenia is possible.[26,27] The fact that massive bleeding does not always occur or that overwhelming infection does not develop has emboldened ECLS clinicians to forge ahead when faced with such patients. Because treatment for these patients remains difficult and controversial, it is not uncommon for ECLS clinicians to consult each other when faced with specific patient care issues. This interaction is valuable for obtaining updates regarding patients being considered for ECLS, as well as for maintaining open dialogue about the ECLS management of these patients. A frequently discussed topic is how to manage chemotherapy while on ECLS. In the past, chemotherapy was discontinued due to concerns that its use would extend the duration of bone marrow suppression. Several case reports now describe patients who have been successfully induced or maintained on chemotherapy for cancer treatment while concomitantly receiving ECLS support. No pharmacokinetic studies of chemotherapeutic agents have been performed on ECLS but in the limited experience of caring for these patients, dose adjustments have not been routinely performed during ECLS. Patients with chronic granulomatous disease treated with WBC transfusions during ECLS in an attempt to clear Aspergillus infection have good recovery and function of transfused WBCs after they passed through the ECLS circuit.

Outcome of cancer patients treated with ECLS

The ELSO Registry reported that 90 children <21 years of age with neoplasms received ECMO,[28] 64 patients had hematologic disease, and 26 had solid tumors. Mean age was 7.5 years (range 0-21 years). ECMO was initiated for pulmonary support in 74 patients, for cardiac support in 11, and for rapid resuscitation (eCPR)

in 5. Mean duration of ECMO was 9.8 days (range 3 hours-59 days). Overall survival was 41% (37 of 90). The causes of death were irreversible organ failure (n=37), diagnosis incompatible with life (n=10), and hemorrhage (n=6). Risk factors associated with death included cardiac arrest prior to ECMO and development of renal or cardiopulmonary complications during the ECMO course. As an additional aspect of this report, a questionnaire was completed by 116 ELSO centers asking whether children with cancer should be offered ECMO, 110 (95%) responded that they would consider placing a child with cancer on ECMO. In a recent study of 333 children in the ELSO Registry who had received solid organ transplant, overall ECMO survival was not different from the overall pediatric population (54%), but survival to hospital discharge in post-transplant patients was significantly lower (40%, P=0.003).[29] Patients with combined heart-lung or liver transplant had worse survival (26% and 28% to discharge,

Table 1. Outcomes from pediatric ICU studies in BMT patients.

Author	BMT patients requiring CMV n (%)	Duration of mechanical ventilation (days)	Successful extubation n (%)	6-Month survival n (%)	Age (years)
Todd (1973-90)	54 (19%)	8 (1-52) Surv 3.5	6 (11%)	5 (9%)	10.2
Nichols (1978-88)	23 (7%)	–	–	2 (9%)	11-19
Warwick (1976-92)	196 (22.6%)	8 (1-102)	79 (40%)	33 (17%)	8.2
Rossi (1986-95)	39 (11%)	4 Surv 5.5 NS 3	17 (44%)	14 (36%)	6.5
Keenan (1983-96)	121 (11%)	Surv 6 NS 9	19 (16%)	8 (7%)	9.2
Diaz de Heredia (1991-95)	31 (18%)	2.5	12 (64%) Pneum 17%	6 (23%)	7.8
Hayes (1987-97)	33 (9%)	5	5 (15%)	4 (12%)	8.3
Total:	497 (14%)		138 (29%)	72 (15%)	

Surv: survivors, NS: non-survivors

respectively) than other groups. Use of ECLS in the pre- and post-transplantation of heart or lung has been associated with good outcomes and is considered standard care in some centers.[30]

ECMO for bone marrow transplant patients

There is little information on ECLS use in patients who have received bone marrow or other transplantation as part of their treatment regimen. The ELSO Registry reported on 11 patients between 1985-2002 with bone marrow transplant (BMT). Overall, 18% of these patients were able to be weaned off ECMO, but none survived to hospital discharge. Characteristics of these patients included the following: average age 107 $\pm$6.83 months, duration of intubation prior to ECMO 4 $\pm$4.5 days, oxygen index (OI) prior to ECMO 47 $\pm$12, PaO$_2$/FiO$_2$ 68 $\pm$44 and duration of ECMO 12 $\pm$16 days.[31] Based on these disappointing results, prior BMT has been a basis for exclusion at many ECMO centers. As more patients have received BMT and treatment regimens have been refined, new questions regarding this exclusionary practice have been raised. With the advent of stem cell transplant, where the immunosuppressive regimen is less severe and recipient recovery occurs more quickly than in traditional BMT patients, oncolo-gists are suggesting to ICU colleagues that highly aggressive care may be suitable for those patients who suffer acute illness following BMT.

The increase in patients receiving BMT over time is shown in Figures 3 and 4. With this increase, more BMT patients are entering the ICU environment. The highest risk for ICU admission is in the 3 month period following transplant and is associated with acute disease that occurs prior to or during early engraftment.[32] Patients who survive this initial risky period often have good long-term outcome if successful engraftment occurs. Dismal outcomes have been reported in BMT recipients requiring intensive care.[33-35] Outcomes from 7 pediatric ICU studies of BMT patients are shown in Table 1. Overall survival was 15%. It can be argued that mortality in these patients is so high that exposure to an invasive therapy such as ECLS, even with all the concerns discussed previously, is warranted and will not make the outcome any worse. Statistical impact on survival would be high if survival were achieved in only a few patients.

Mortality predictions

The ability to determine the appropriate timing and selection criteria for the use of ECLS is

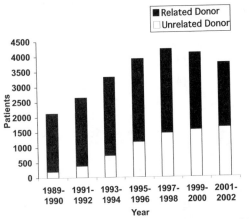

Figure 3. Allogenic transplants in patients ≤20 years registered with Center for International Blood and Marrow Transplant Research, 1989-2002, by donor type.

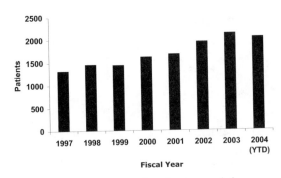

Figure 4. Number of patients receiving a transplant through National Marrow Donor Program (NMDP). Fiscal years 1997-2004 (Sept-Oct). 2004 data through July 2004.

crucial in this patient population. While no specific criteria have been developed, available data provide a reasonable foundation to help guide medical judgment. Development of respiratory failure or multi-organ dysfunction following BMT is uniformly associated with poor outcome. The duration and severity of organ failure has also been identified as a key feature. Rossi found that survival of BMT patients in the pediatric ICU was inversely correlated with the patients' worst OI (the OI was 11 in survivors vs. 30 in non-survivors).[34] In other reports, predictors of mortality have included the presence and duration of respiratory failure, number of total organ failures, severity of graft vs. host disease, and degree of hepatic dysfunction.[36] In an evaluation of 126 children with allogeneic BMT from St. Jude's Hospital[37] of whom 88 (70%) required mechanical ventilation for acute hypoxemic respiratory failure, 33% survived to ICU discharge, 16% were discharged from the hospital, and 9% were still alive 6 months after their intubation.[37] Survival in patients ventilated for <7 days compared to ≥7 days was 43% vs. 25% (P=0.08). This may suggest better outcome in patients receiving shorter courses of mechanical ventilation, although larger numbers of patients are needed to determine statistical significance. Other factors associated with survival included PaO_2/FiO_2 at

day 15 (patients with a PaO_2/FiO_2 <200 failed to survive), the presence of cardiac failure (55% in survivors vs. 76% in non-survivors, P=0.04), hepatic failure (17% in survivors vs. 39% in non-survivors, P=0.04), and neurologic injury (0% survival vs. 25% in non-survivors, P=0.001). In larger studies of adult BMT patients, the need for mechanical ventilation >4 days is almost universally fatal. Investigators at Duke University developed a scoring system based on severity of dysfunction and number of organs affected, which correlated with outcome in 39 pediatric BMT patients (Table 2).[38] A score >10 was associated with <5% survival in those patients requiring mechanical ventilation. Validation of such a score by a larger number of patients from multiple institutions is required to determine its utility for predicting outcome and, thus, for guiding therapy. Until definitive ECLS criteria are developed for patients with immune dysfunction, the clinician must rely on their best judgment and an assessment of the risks and benefits in the individual patient when deciding if ECLS should be initiated.

Case report

A patient case report follows to highlight these issues.

A 15-month-old boy with immune polyendocrine, X-linked syndrome (IPEX syndrome), who was status post second bone marrow transplant following failed engraftment, presented with respiratory distress 15 days after transplant. He was transferred to the pediatric ICU where he developed pulmonary hemorrhage and required immediate intubation. Within 12 hours, he was on HFV at a MAP of 35 cm H_2O and FiO_2 100%. His best arterial blood gas had a pH of 7.28, a $PaCO_2$ of 56 mm Hg and a PaO_2 of 46 mm Hg. He was given an epinephrine bolus for an acute bradycardic event and was started on vasoactive infusions. His WBC count

Table 2. Organ failure score (adapted from Gupta V et al. Crit Care Med 2003; 31:A136.)

Organ failure score	Probability of survival (odds ratio)	95% CI
0	0.67	0.42, 0.85
1	0.58	0.37, 0.77
2	0.49	0.32, 0.66
3	0.39	0.26, 0.55
4	0.31	0.19, 0.46
5	0.23	0.13, 0.39
6	0.17	0.08, 0.33
7	0.12	0.05, 0.29
8	0.09	0.03, 0.26
9	0.06	0.01, 0.23

was 0.1, platelet count was 76,000, and prothrombin time was 43 seconds. A discussion was held among ICU staff regarding the appropriateness of ECLS at an early time point in this patient. VA ECLS was instituted within 24 hours of intubation. The patient had no recurrence of pulmonary bleeding and bronchoscopy revealed no infection. Respiratory failure improved rapidly, and the patient was weaned from ECLS support after 48 hours. Extubation occurred 3 days later, and the patient returned to the ward by day 7.

While it can be argued that this patient may have recovered without ECLS, it is uncommon to see resolution of such severe respiratory disease requiring high levels of mechanical support, to the point where the patient can be extubated and discharged within such a short time span. The early use of ECLS, despite its risk for bleeding, may have limited lung injury and secondary organ damage, thus promoting rapid healing and recovery. Such case reports are countered by a multitude of other experiences in which multiple complications arose and outcome was poor. Given the poor outcome of BMT patients requiring intensive care in an environment that has included extraordinary therapies such as ECLS, it may be appropriate to develop a new algorithm of care that includes early consideration for ECLS. An example of an algorithm that includes other available support techniques is shown in Figure 5. While a randomized, controlled trial of ECLS vs. conventional therapy may be considered the optimal

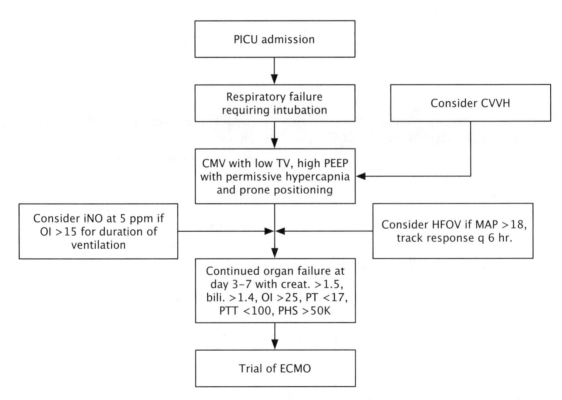

Figure 5. Sample treatment algorithm for pediatric respiratory failure in immunosuppressed patients.

manner to answer the question, the myriad of difficulties such as the small number of patients make it unlikely that this will occur. As a practical step, perhaps use of an algorithm for care such as that presented, combined with specific data collection and outcome evaluation, would provide improved information to help guide care. At the current time, it seems appropriate to consider use of ECLS in immunocompromised patients, especially those with cancer and BMT, in the same manner as the use of ECLS in cardiac arrest patients.

While acute cardiac arrest patients in the past were often excluded from ECLS support because of concerns of futility, bleeding complications, and a poor risk-benefit ratio, use of ECLS in cardiac arrest is now becoming commonplace with good survival.[39,40] This reversal of opinion has come about not due to randomized, controlled trials or landmark publications, but as a result of clinicians "pushing the envelope," followed by small case reports discussing patients and techniques and critical analysis of patient results. Once a larger experience with immunocompromised patients is analyzed, more rational decision-making regarding the overall utility of ECLS in these patients can be made.

Summary

Expansion of ECLS to patients with immune dysfunction is occurring. Development of care algorithms, specific data collection, and outcome evaluation from multiple centers are needed to help refine this effort. The willingness of clinicians to consider use of ECLS in patients with BMT and other complex diseases is needed to help determine if ECLS is a viable support mode or if such actions are misdirected in certain patient populations. Until medical science identifies an effective and less invasive therapy to support immune-deficient patients failing conventional treatment, ECLS should be considered and studied as a potential treatment modality.

References

1. Fortenberry JD, Meier AH, Pettignano R, Heard M, Chambliss CR, Wulkan M. Extracorporeal life support for posttraumatic acute respiratory distress syndrome at a children's medical center. *J Pediatr Surg* 2003; 38:1221-1226.

2. Dalton HJ, Siewers RD, Fuhrmana BP, et al. Extracorporeal membrane oxygenation for cardiac rescue in children with severe myocardial dysfunction. *Crit Care Med* 1993; 21: 1020-1028.

3. Szocik J. Rudich S, Csete M. ECMO resuscitation after massive pulmonary embolism during liver transplantation. *Anesthesiology* 2002; 97:763-764.

4. Sheridan RL, Schnitzer JJ. Management of the high risk pediatric burn patient. *J Pediatr Surg* 2001; 36:1308-1312.

5. Michaels AJ, Schreiner RJ, Kolla S, et al. Extracorporeal life support in pulmonary failure after trauma. *J Trauma* 1999; 46:638-645.

6. Goldman A, Kerr S, Butt W, et al. Extracorporeal support for intractable cardiorespiratory failure due to meningococcal disease. *Lancet* 1997; 349:466-469.

7. MacLaren G, Pellegrino V, Butt W, Preovolos A, Salamonsen R. Successful use of ECMO in adults with life-threatening infections. *Anaesth Intensive Care* 2004; 32:707-710.

8. Carcillo JA, Fields AI: American College of Critical Care Medicine Task Force Committee Members. Clinical practice parameters for hemodynamic support of pediatric and neonatal patients in septic shock. *Crit Care Med* 2002; 30:1365-1378.

9. Zavadil DP, Stammers AH, Willett LD, Deptula JJ, Christensen KA, Sydzyik RT. Hematological abnormalities in neonatal patients treated with extracorporeal membrane oxygenation (ECMO). *J Extra Corpor Technol* 1998; 30:83-90.

10. Brody JL, Pickering NJ, Fink GB, Behr ED. Altered lymphocyte subsets during cardiopulmonary bypass. *Am J Clin Pathol* 1987; 87:626-628.

11. Zach TL Steinhorn RH, Georgieff MK, Mills MM, Green TP. Leukopenia associated with extracorporeal membrane oxygenation in newborn infants. *J Pediatr* 1990; 116:440-444.

12. Daimon S, Umeda T, Michishita I, Wakasugi H, Genda A, Koni I. Goodpasture's-like syndrome and effect of extracorporeal membrane oxygenator support. *Intern Med* 1994; 33:569-573.

13. Hernandez ME, Lovrekovic G, Schears G, et al. Acute onset of Wegener's granulomatosis and diffuse alveolar hemorrhage treated successfully by extracorporeal membrane oxygenation. *Pediatr Crit Care Med* 2002; 3:63-69.

14. Kolovos NS, Scheurer DJ, Moler FW, et al. Extracorporeal life support for pulmonary hemorrhage in children: a case series. *Crit Care Med* 2002; 3:577-580.

15. Peters SG, Meadows JA, Gracey DR. Outcome of respiratory failure in hematologic malignancy. *Chest* 1988: 94:99-102.

16. Dalton HJ, Slonim AD, Pollack MM. MultiCenter outcome of pediatric oncology patients requiring intensive care. *Pediatr Hematol Oncol* 2003: 20:643-649.

17. Butt W, Barker G, Walker C, Gillis J, Kilham H, Stevens M. Outcome of children with hematologic malignancy who are admitted to an intensive care unit. *Crit Care Med* 1988; 16:761-764.

18. Dobyns EL, Cornfield DN, Anas NG, et al. Multicenter randomized controlled trial of the effects of inhaled nitric oxide therapy on gas exchange in children with acute hypoxemic respiratory failure. *J Pediatr* 1999; 134:406-412

19. Willson DF, Jiao JH, Bauman L, Zaritsky A, et al. Calf's lung surfactant extract in acute hypoxemic respiratory failure in children. *Crit Care Med* 1996; 24:1316-1322.

20. Herting E, Moller O, Schiffman JH, Robertson B. Surfactant improves oxygenation in infants and children with pneumonia and acute respiratory distress syndrome. *Acta Paediatr* 2002; 91:1174-1178.

21. Arnold JH, Hanson JH, Toro-Figuero LO, Gutierrez J, Berens RJ, Anglin DL. Prospective, randomized comparison of high-frequency oscillatory ventilation and conventional mechanical ventilation in pediatric respiratory failure. *Crit Care Med* 1994; 22:1530-1539.

22. Waskerwitz MJ, Ruccione K. An overview of cancer in children in the 1980s. *Nurs Clin North Am* 1985; 20:5-29.

23. Linden V, Karlen J, Olsson M, et al. Successful extracorporeal membrane oxygenation in four children with malignant disease and severe Pneumocystis carinii pneumonia. *Med Pediatr Oncol* 1999; 32:25-31.

24. Shiraishi T, Kawahara K, Shirakusa T, et al. Primary tracheal fibrosarcoma in a child: a case of tracheal resection under ECMO support. *Thorac Cardiovasc Surg* 1997; 45:252-254.

25. Hines MH, Hansell DR. Elective extracorporeal support for complex tracheal reconstruction in neonates. *Ann Thorac Surg* 2003; 76:175-178.

26. Dager WE, Gosselin RC, Yoshikawa R, Owings JT. Lepirudin in heparin-induced thrombocytopenia and extracorporeal membranous oxygenation. *Ann Pharmacother* 2004; 38:598-601.

27. Deitcher SR, Topoulos AP, Bartholomew JR, Kichuk-Chrisant MR. Lepirudin anticoagulation for heparin-induced thrombocytopenia. *J Pediatr* 2002; 140:264-266.

28. Gow KW, Heard ML, Heiss KF, Katzenstein HM, Wulkan ML, Fortenberry JD. ECMO in children with malignancies. In: *20th Annual CNMC Symposium on ECMO and*

Advanced Respiratory Therapies;, February 22-26, 2004; Keystone, CO. Abstract 23.

29. Naclerio AL, Gosnell R, Rycus P, DiGeronimo R. Peditric Extracorporeal Membrane Oxygenation in patients with immunocompromise. In: *20ᵗʰ Annual Children's National Medical Center Symposium for ECMO and Advanced Respiratory Diseases*; February 22-26, 2004; Keystone, CO. Abstract 43.

30. Oto T, Rosenfeldt F, Rowland M, et al. Extracorporeal membrane oxygenation after lung transplantation: evolving technique improves outcomes. *Ann Thorac Surg* 2004; 78:1230-1235.

31. ELSO Registry. Ann Arbor, MI: Extracorporeal Life Support Organization; 2004.

32. Nichols DG, Walker LK, Wingard JR, et al. Predictors of acute respiratory failure after bone marrow transplantation in children. *Crit Care Med* 1994; 22:1485-1491.

33. Wolfson RK, Kahana MD, Nachman JB, Lantos J. Extracorporeal membrane oxygenation after stem cell transplant: clinical decision-making in the absence of evidence. *Pediatr Crit Care Med* 2005; 6:200-203.

34. Rossi R, Shermie SD, Calderwood S. Prognosis of pediatric bone marrow transplant recipients requiring mechanical ventilation. *Crit Care Med* 1999; 27:1181-1186.

35. Rubenfield GD, Crawford SW. Withdrawing life support from mechanically ventilated recipients of bone marrow transplant: a case for evidence-based guidelines. *Ann Intern Med* 1996; 125:625-633.

36. Rossi R, Shernie SD, Calderwood S. Prognosis of pediatric bone marrow transplant recipients requiring mechanical ventilation. *Crit Care Med* 1999; 27:1181-1186.

37. Tamburro R, West N, Fiser RT, Sillos EM, Schmidt JE, Hale G. Outcome of acute hypoxemic respiratory failure in children receiving allogeneic bone marrow transplants. *Crit Care Med* 2002; 29(Suppl): A143.

38. Gupta V, Martin P, Craig D, Hagen S, Cheifetz I. Organ failure score as a predictor of mortality in pediatric BMT patients. *Crit Care Med* 2003; 31:A136.

39. Dalton HJ, Siewers RD, Fuhrmana BP, et al. Extracorporeal membrane oxygenation for cardiac rescue in children with severe myocardial dysfunction. *Crit Care Med* 1993; 21:1020-1028.

40. Morris MC, Wernovsky G, Nadkarni VM. Survival outcomes after extracorporeal cardiopulmonary resuscitation instituted during active chest compressions following refractory in-hospital pediatric cardiac arrest. *Pediatr Crit Care Med* 2004; 5:440-446.

37

Extracorporeal Organ Support in Liver Failure

Rajiv Jalan, M.B.B.S., M.D., F.R.C.P., F.R.C.P.E., Ph.D.

Introduction

Liver failure, whether acute with no pre-existing liver disease (acute liver failure [ALF]) or an acute episode of decompensation superimposed on a chronic liver disorder (acute-on-chronic liver failure [ACLF]), carries a high mortality. In ALF patients, the lack of detoxification, metabolic, and regulatory functions of the liver leads to life-threatening complications, including kidney failure, encephalopathy, cerebral edema, severe hypotension, and susceptibility to infections culminating in multi-organ failure.[1] The standard therapy for such patients is liver transplantation, but currently one-third of these patients die waiting for a transplant and organ shortage is increasing.[2] However, liver failure, of both types is potentially reversible and considerable research has been conducted over many years to develop effective liver support devices.

Development of these devices has followed two distinct approaches. The first, biological devices, aim to provide all the normal liver functions[3,4] and are based on the use of living liver cells with either human hepatic cells (e.g., extracorporeal liver assist device [ELAD])[5] or porcine hepatocytes (e.g., bio-artificial liver [BAL] device).[6] Other devices are under development in the Netherlands[7]

and Germany.[8] The second approach is based on detoxification functions using only membranes and adsorbents, which can remove the putative toxins associated with liver failure. Such entirely artificial devices are substantially less costly, about 10% the cost, than those based on living liver cell lines. The earliest of the artificial systems developed was based on perfusion of the blood through the adsorbent charcoal.[9,10] Although some of the toxins present in liver failure were shown to be adsorbed to the charcoal, other compounds tightly bound to proteins in the plasma were not removed.[9,10] Another system known as the BioLogic-DT (HemoCleanse Technologies, Lafayette, IN) is a combination of flat-membrane dialysis against adsorbent solution,[11] but several studies have shown only limited efficacy in removing protein-bound substances.[3,12] The molecular adsorbents recirculating system (MARS) is an extracorporeal device that is able to remove albumin bound substances from the plasma. This is achieved by dialyzing the plasma from the patient across a polysulfone membrane using human albumin as the dialyzate.[13-19] Additionally, there is a dialysis component for the removal of water-soluble toxins.

This chapter will define the goals of artificial liver support and provide a critical review of data from clinical studies on the MARS system for albumin dialysis.

Liver support devices

The ideal liver support system would provide many of the normal liver functions, it would be easy to use, have minimal complications, and be cost-efficient. From the pathophysiological perspective, it would have a significant biosynthetic capacity, the ability to detoxify, and the ability to bio-transform by altering the key processes which allow regeneration and healing. Although the biosynthetic function of the liver is important, it is possible to provide orally or IV many of the substances that the liver manufactures (e.g., glucose, albumin, trace elements and vitamins, clotting factors).[4] The ability of an artificial liver support system to mimic the detoxification functions of the liver is crucial to its success. Liver failure causes the accumulation of various toxic substances (e.g., ammonia, mediators of oxidative stress, bile acids, nitric oxide [NO], lactate, products of arachidonic acid metabolism, benzodiazepines, indoles, mercaptans)[16,17] which are important factors in the pathogenesis of end organ dysfunction, alteration in vascular function, abnormalities in acid-base balance, and may also impair liver regeneration.[18,19] The biological device for liver support is primarily designed to provide the synthetic functions, whereas the artificial device is primarily for detoxification function. If all these functions are to be achieved by a potential liver support system, then it is difficult to imagine that a purely biological device would fulfill these roles. On the other hand, removal of toxins alone may allow biotransformation and the recovery of biosynthetic and metabolic functions without additional synthetic activity. Although the primary aim of using a liver support device is to improve the transplant-free survival of patients with liver failure, alternative objectives may be to serve as an effective bridge to liver transplantation, to prevent the occurrence of liver failure in those that are predisposed to it, or to provide functional capacity to improve end organ function.

Technical aspects

Newer artificial liver systems, which use albumin as the transport medium for toxins and utilize a membrane with a small pore size, are substantially more selective with regards to their detoxifying capacity than the previous generation of devices based on charcoal hemoperfusion.[9,10] They are specific for albumin-bound substances, which form the majority of the toxins accumulating in liver failure,[16] while larger molecules (e.g., immunoglobulins, growth factors) that might be physiologically important are prevented from crossing over.

The system that has been developed over the last decade and is currently under extensive clinical investigation is the MARS machine (Gambro Hospal LTD, Huntingdon, U.K.) (Figure 1).[14,18] This uses a hollow-fiber dialysis module in which patient blood is dialyzed across

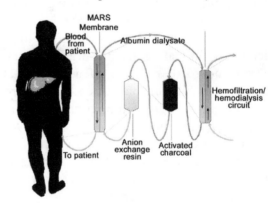

Figure 1. Schematic diagram of the MARS circuit, showing the direction of blood flow and the dialysate (20% albumin). The albumin-bound toxins from the blood pass on to the albumin in the dialysate, which is then cleansed sequentially by a hemodialysis/hemofiltration module (removing water-soluble substances), and adsorber columns containing activated charcoal and anion-exchange resin (removing most of the albumin-bound substances). The dialysate is thus regenerated, and once more capable of taking up more toxins.

an albumin-impregnated polysulfone membrane (with a cut-off of 50 kDa), while maintaining a constant flow of 600 ml of 20% albumin as dialysate in the extra-capillary compartment. In vitro studies has demonstrated that toxins bound to albumin in the blood will detach and bind to the membrane's binding sites[18] since albumin, when attached to polymers, have a higher affinity for albumin-bound toxins.[19] These pass on to the albumin in the dialysate, which is then cleansed sequentially by a hemodialysis/hemofiltration module (removing water-soluble substances), and adsorber columns containing activated charcoal and an ion-exchange resin (removing most of the albumin-bound substances). The dialyzate is thus regenerated and is once more capable of taking up toxins from the blood.

Another type of albumin dialysis that was introduced in 1999 is the fractionated plasma separation and adsorption (FPSA) method, using an albumin-permeable membrane with a cut-off of 250 kDa.[20] Albumin and the albumin-bound toxins cross the membrane and pass through special adsorbers (1-2 columns in series in the secondary circuit, containing a neutral resin adsorber and an anion exchanger) which remove the toxins. The cleansed albumin is returned to the plasma. In the newly introduced Prometheus system (Fresenius Medical Care AG, Bad Homburg, Germany) the FPSA method is combined with direct high-flux hemodialysis of the blood.[21] This approach differs from the MARS system, in which hemodialysis/filtration is performed in the albumin dialyzate.

Results from clinical studies

Molecular adsorbents recirculating system

Compared to the biological devices, MARS is easy to use and relatively inexpensive with a cost of ~£4,000-7000 (~$2,250-4,000) for full treatment.[22-32] Some of the important studies evaluating MARS are summarized in Table 1. In contrast to trials of the biological devices which have been tested in the context of ALF, most of the clinical studies with MARS have

Table 1. Summary of important studies evaluating the MARS device.

Study	Patient population	Study design	End-point	Outcome
Stange et al. (2000)[41]	ACLF with intrahepatic cholestasis (bilirubin >20 mg/dl) (n=26)	Prospective case series	In-hospital mortality	UNOS 2a status: 7/16 survived UNOS 2b status: 10/10 survived
Mitzner et al. (2000)[33]	Type-I hepatorenal syndrome (n=13)	Two-center randomized controlled	30-day mortality	Mortality: controls- 100% (day-7), MARS- 62.5% (day-7), and 75% (day-30) (P<0.01)
Heemann et al. (2002)[34]	ACLF (n=24)	Two-center randomized controlled	Primary: reduction of serum bilirubin Secondary: in-hospital mortality	Improvement of bilirubin, and 30-day survival with MARS (11/12 vs. 6/11 controls, P<0.05)
Jalan et al. (2003)[42]	ACLF due to acute alcoholic hepatitis (Maddrey's discriminant function >32) (n=8)	Prospective case series	In-hospital mortality	Improvement of 3-month predicted mortality (pre-MARS: 76%, post-MARS: 27%), 3-month survival: 4/8

been in ACLF patients with a survival benefit shown in 2 small, randomized, controlled trials.[33,34] This is an effective detoxification device which can remove substances bound to a variety of plasma proteins, and which have the potential to bind to albumin.[35] MARS therapy in patients with ACLF has a major beneficial effect on the circulating neurohormones, NO, free radicals production, and markers of oxidative stress.[36] The clinical effects of these changes are reflected in individual organ function with temporal improvement in cholestasis and liver function, renal function, encephalopathy, and in some patients in the mean arterial pressure (MAP).[37] The improvement in liver function may result from reduced hepatocyte cell death and an improved environment for regeneration. Alternatively, it may be the result of improved hepatic hemodynamics. The most marked and consistent effect of MARS is to decrease the severity of hepatic encephalopathy while not affecting the circulating ammonia levels,[36,38] suggesting that MARS may modify the blood-brain barrier characteristics, which determine the effects of hyperammonemia on the brain. Alternatively, it may exert this effect through reduction in oxidative stress and/or removal of unknown protein-bound factors that either act alone or with ammonia to produce encephalopathy. These data are supported by studies in animal models, of ALF, where MARS-treated animals were observed to have significantly lower intracranial pressure without any difference in arterial ammonia.

In the first randomized trial of MARS, 13 ACLF patients with type-I hepatorenal syndrome were allocated to treatment with MARS or standard medical therapy including hemodiafiltration.[33] The mortality rate at day 7 was 100% in the group receiving hemodiafiltration (n=5) compared with 62.5% in the MARS group at day 7 (n=8) and 75% at day 30 (P<0.01). Mean survival was 25.2 ±34.6 days in the MARS group and 4.6 ±1.8 days in the control group (P<0.05). In addition, a significant decrease in

serum bilirubin and creatinine, and an increase in serum sodium and prothrombin activity were observed in the MARS group, but not in the control group. MAP at the end of treatment was significantly higher in the MARS group. Although there was no statistically significant increase in urine volume in the MARS group, 4 of 8 MARS patients showed an increase in urine volume, compared with none in the control group.

The most recent and largest randomized, controlled trial performed in two centers, included 24 patients with ACLF and marked hyperbilirubinemia (serum bilirubin >20 mg/dl [340 μmol/l]) who were randomized to receive standard therapy alone (n=12) or standard therapy with MARS (n=12).[34] The primary endpoint of bilirubin <15 mg/dl for 3 consecutive days was reached in 5 of 12 patients in the MARS group and 2 of 12 patients in the control group. Compared to controls, bilirubin, bile acids, and creatinine decreased, and MAP and encephalopathy improved in the MARS group. Most importantly, albumin dialysis was associated with a significant improvement in 30-day survival (11/12 vs. 6/11 in controls). At present, a multi-center, randomized, controlled trial looking at the mortality of ACLF patients is being conducted in the U.K. and other European countries, while another, focused on short-term benefit in hepatic encephalopathy, is nearing completion in the U.S.

The safety of this device has been evaluated by its use in over 3,000 patients worldwide. The MARS Registry, which is maintained by the University of Rostock (Rostock, Germany), contains data on about 500 patients treated with this device.[38,39] In general, the treatment is well tolerated and the only consistent adverse finding with the use of MARS is thrombocytopenia. Critical analysis of the data in patients with ACLF suggests that its use is contraindicated for those with established disseminated intravascular coagulation (DIC) or in those patients with incipient DIC characterized by progressive thrombocytopenia and coagulopathy.

Prometheus

The results of Prometheus treatment in 11 patients with ACLF and accompanying renal failure will be published.[21] Improvement of serum levels of conjugated bilirubin, bile acids, ammonia, cholinesterase, creatinine, urea, and blood pH occurred. A drop of blood pressure in 2 patients and uncontrolled bleeding in 1 patient were the adverse events noted. Prospective, controlled trials are planned.

Clinical trials

The results of randomized clinical trials evaluating the various liver support systems are summarized in Figure 2. The results of trials using the biological liver-support devices

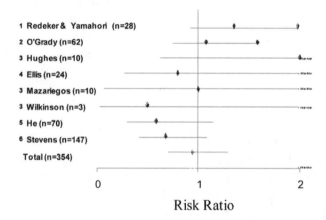

A

ACUTE LIVER FAILURE (ALF)

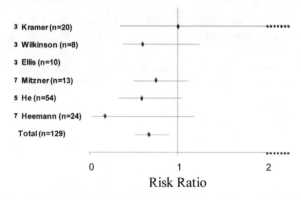

B

ACUTE-ON-CHRONIC LIVER FAILURE (ACLF)

Figure 2. Randomized, controlled trials with artificial and bio-artificial liver support devices, showing the effects on mortality in ALF (A) and ACLF (B).[40] 1: Whole blood exchange; 2: Charcoal hemoperfusion; 3: Biologic-DT; 4: ELAD; 5: Hemoperfusion; 6: BAL; 7: MARS. The only device to show significant effects on mortality is the MARS device, in the context of ACLF.

in ALF have been disappointing, with little evidence of significant benefits in terms of synthetic functions. This may be either because they are ineffective, or because the trials have not allowed the effects of these devices to be fully explored. Demetriou's study using the bioartificial liver device exemplifies the latter. Although this trial was intended to focus on patients with ALF,[25] patients with primary graft dysfunction were also included. Although the overall analysis indicated no significant differences in survival, a post hoc analysis revealed a near-survival benefit in the ALF group. The group of patients they assessed was a group for whom recovery of the native liver function, even with auxiliary liver transplant, can take up to a year (Table 2). In contrast to these results, the use of MARS has been shown to improve systemic hemodynamics, severity of hepatic encephalopathy, and renal function which has translated into improved survival in 2 small studies in patients with ACLF.[17,33,34,39] These 2 randomized clinical trials illustrate that if treatment is applied before organ failure is manifest, progression to full-blown ACLF may be prevented. In the study by Heeman et al.[34] mortality in the control group was ~45%, but in the study by Mitzner et al.[33] mortality of the control group was 100%. Intervention with MARS resulted in an increase in survival in the Heeman study to >90%, but survival in the MARS-treated patients in the Mitzner study was ~20%. The timing of intervention with liver

support is of critical importance in determining whether a device will improve outcome. By the time multi-organ failure manifests, the benefits of intervention with these devices is unlikely to be fully realized.

Current status of MARS

The use of MARS is supported by studies showing improvement in organ function with its use and early data showing improvement in survival in patients with ACLF. An important question with the MARS device is whether the clinical course of these patients is altered and survival of the patient improved. Based on critical evaluation of the results presented above, guidelines have been drawn up as to the use and contraindications, and these are being followed in the current multi-center trial in the U.K. and are strongly recommended to all those who use MARS (Table 3). It is particularly important for there to be a clear appreciation that the use of this device is contraindicated in cases of severe thrombocytopenia, progressive coagulopathy, and sepsis, which together may be indicative of incipient DIC.

Not surprisingly, MARS is also being used to treat ALF. The largest single-center experience from Helsinki suggests benefits in bridging patients to transplant; in addition , some patients experienced spontaneous recovery. However, controlled clinical trials will be needed before any firm recommendations can be made. Such

Table 2. Summary of the Demetriou study evaluating the bioartificial device (BAL) Hepat-Assist.

Study	Patient population	Study design	End-point	Outcome	Comments
Demetriou et al. (2001)[25]	ALF (n=147), primary graft non-function (n=24)	Multi-center randomized controlled	30-day mortality	30-day survival- *All patients:* BAL-71%, controls-62% *Subgroups:* All ALF: BAL-73%, controls-59% (P=0.1) ALF due to Parcetamol: BAL-70%, controls-37% (P<0.05)	Substantial impact of transplantation (54% of all patients) on outcome

a trial is being planned in France, but given the experience with trials of bioartificial devices in ALF, the timing of randomization may well determine the outcome of the study. Further difficulties in the design and analysis of such trials arises from the different timing of liver transpantation. In addition to uses for liver failure, MARS appears to have a clinical benefit in poisoning cases with protein-bound drugs or toxins. This is due to the ability of MARS to remove protein-bound drugs. In addition, early data show that MARS is effective in the treatment of pruritus in patients with cholestasis.

Summary

Clearly, the role of MARS in liver failure will only become clear when the results of current trials are available. However, the interest in MARS has resulted in further interest in the pathophysiology of ACLF. There is a growing realization that a large number of patients with liver failure have a high mortality rate and require considerable resources. With better understanding of the basis of acute decompensation, availability of emerging medical therapies such as MARS could bring about a considerable improvement in survival as well as reduction of hospital in-patient stay.

Table 3. Indications, contraindications, and monitoring for MARS therapy.

Indications
Acute on chronic liver failure (ACLF)
Severe alcoholic hepatitis
Severe pruritus due to cholestasis
Intoxication from protein-bound substances

Relative contraindications
Progressive coagulopathy indicative of DIC
Uncontrolled sepsis
Uncontrolled bleeding

Monitoring during therapy
Electrolytes including phosphates, magnesium, and calcium
Coagulation (check for DIC)
Drug levels (protein-bound drugs may be removed)

References

1. Stockmann HB, JN IJ. Prospects for the temporary treatment of acute liver failure. *Eur J Gastroenterol Hepatol* 2002; 14:195-203.

2. The Organ Procurement and Transplantation Network. Transplant and waiting list resourses. www.optn.org. Accessed July 22, 2005.

3. Allen JW, Hassanein T, Bhatia SN. Advances in bioartificial liver devices. *Hepatology* 2001; 34:447-455.

4. Strain AJ, Neuberger JM. A bioartificial liver--state of the art. *Science* 2002; 295:1005-1009.

5. Sussman NL, Chong MG, Koussayer T, et al. Reversal of fulminant hepatic failure using an extracorporeal liver assist device. *Hepatology* 1992; 16:60-65.

6. Rozga J, Williams F, Ro MS, et al. Development of a bioartificial liver: properties and function of a hollow-fiber module inoculated with liver cells. *Hepatology* 1993; 17:258-265.

7. Flendrig LM, la Soe JW, Jorning GG, et al. In vitro evaluation of a novel bioreactor based on an integral oxygenator and a spirally wound nonwoven polyester matrix for hepatocyte culture as small aggregates. *J Hepatol* 1997; 26:1379-1392.

8. Gerlach JC, Schnoy N, Encke J, Smith MD, Muller C, Neuhaus P. Improved hepatocyte in vitro maintenance in a culture model with woven multicompartment capillary systems: electron microscopy studies. *Hepatology* 1995; 22:546-552.

9. O'Grady JG, Gimson AE, O'Brien CJ, Pucknell A, Hughes RD, Williams R. Controlled trials of charcoal hemoperfusion and prognostic factors in fulminant hepatic failure. *Gastroenterology* 1988; 94:1186-1192.

10. McGuire BM, Sielaff TD, Nyberg SL, Hu MY, Cerra FB, Bloomer JR. Review of

support systems used in the management of fulminant hepatic failure. *Dig Dis* 1995; 13:379-388.

11. Ash SR, Blake DE, Carr DJ, Carter C, Howard T, Makowka L. Clinical effects of a sorbent suspension dialysis system in treatment of hepatic coma (the BioLogic-DT). *Int J Artif Organs* 1992; 15:151-161.

12. Hughes RD, Pucknell A, Routley D, Langley PG, Wendon JA, Williams R. Evaluation of the BioLogic-DT sorbent-suspension dialyser in patients with fulminant hepatic failure. *Int J Artif Organs* 1994; 17:657-662.

13. Mitzner S, Stange J, Freytag J, Lindemann S, Schmidt R. Role of transport proteins in bioartificial liver assist systems. *Int J Artif Organs* 1996; 19:49-52.

14. Stange J, Mitzner S. A carrier-mediated transport of toxins in a hybrid membrane. Safety barrier between a patients blood and a bioartificial liver. *Int J Artif Organs* 1996; 19:677-691.

15. Stange J, Mitzner S, Ramlow W, Gliesche T, Hickstein H, Schmidt R. A new procedure for the removal of protein bound drugs and toxins. *ASAIO J* 1993; 39:M621-625.

16. Mitzner SR, Stange J, Klammt S, Peszynski P, Schmidt R, Noldge-Schomburg G. Extracorporeal detoxification using the molecular adsorbent recirculating system for critically ill patients with liver failure. *J Am Soc Nephrol* 2001; 12 Suppl 17:S75-82.

17. Sen S, Jalan R, Williams R. Extracorporeal albumin dialysis in acute-on-chronic liver failure: will it stand the test of time? *Hepatology* 2002; 36:1014-1016.

18. Stange J, Ramlow W, Mitzner S, Schmidt R, Klinkmann H. Dialysis against a recycled albumin solution enables the removal of albumin-bound toxins. *Artif Organs* 1993; 17:809-813.

19. Hughes R, Ton HY, Langley P, et al. Albumin-coated Amberlite XAD-7 resin for hemoperfusion in acute liver failure. Part II: in vivo evaluation. *Artif Organs* 1979; 3:23-26.

20. Falkenhagen D, Strobl W, Vogt G, et al. Fractionated plasma separation and adsorption system: a novel system for blood purification to remove albumin bound substances. *Artif Organs* 1999; 23:81-86.

21. Rifai K, Ernst T, Kretschmer U, et al. Prometheus-a new extracorporeal system for the treatment of liver failure. *J Hepatol* 2003; 39:984-990.

22. Matsumura KN, Guevara GR, Huston H, et al. Hybrid bioartificial liver in hepatic failure: preliminary clinical report. *Surgery* 1987; 101:99-103.

23. Chen SC, Hewitt WR, Watanabe FD, et al. Clinical experience with a porcine hepatocyte-based liver support system. *Int J Artif Organs* 1996; 19:664-669.

24. Samuel D, Ichai P, Feray C, et al. Neurological improvement during bioartificial liver sessions in patients with acute liver failure awaiting transplantation. *Transplantation* 2002; 73:257-264.

25. Demetriou AA, Brown RS Jr, Busuttil RW, et al. Prospective, randomized, multicenter, controlled trial of a bioartificial liver in treating acute liver failure. *Ann Surg* 2004; 239:660-667.

26. Ellis AJ, Hughes RD, Wendon JA, et al. Pilot-controlled trial of the extracorporeal liver assist device in acute liver failure. *Hepatology* 1996; 24:1446-1451.

27. Millis JM, Kramer DJ, O'Grady J, et al. Results of phase I trial of the extracorporeal liver assist device for patients with fulminant hepatic failure. *Am J Transplantation* 2001;1:391.

28. van de Kerkhove MP, Di Florio E, Scuderi V, et al. Phase I clinical trial with the AMC-bioartificial liver. Academic Medical Center. *Int J Artif Organs* 2002; 25:950-959.

29. Sauer IM, Kardassis D, Zeillinger K, et al. Clinical extracorporeal hybrid liver support-phase I study with primary porcine liver

cells. *Xenotransplantation* 2003; 10:460-469.

30. Mitzner SR, Klammt S, Peszynski P, et al. Improvement of multiple organ functions in hepatorenal syndrome during albumin dialysis with the molecular adsorbent recirculating system. *Ther Apher* 2001; 5:417-422.

31. Sorkine P, Ben Abraham R, Szold O, et al. Role of the molecular adsorbent recycling system (MARS) in the treatment of patients with acute exacerbation of chronic liver failure. *Crit Care Med* 2001; 29:1332-1336.

32. Stange J, Mitzner SR, Risler T, et al. Molecular adsorbent recycling system (MARS): clinical results of a new membrane-based blood purification system for bioartificial liver support. *Artif Organs* 1999; 23:319-330.

33. Mitzner SR, Stange J, Klammt S, et al. Improvement of hepatorenal syndrome with extracorporeal albumin dialysis MARS: results of a prospective, randomized, controlled clinical trial. *Liver Transpl* 2000; 6:277-286.

34. Heemann U, Treichel U, Loock J, et al. Albumin dialysis in cirrhosis with superimposed acute liver injury: a prospective, controlled study. *Hepatology* 2002; 36:949-958.

35. Sen S, Rose C, Ytrebo LM, et al. Molecular Adsorbents Recirculating Systems (MARS): A potential model for removing midazolam, fentanyl and possibly other protein-bound drugs. *Hepatology* 2003; 38:238A.

36. Sen S, Davies NA, Mookerjee RP, et al. Pathophysiological basis of extracorporeal albumin dialysis with MARS in acute-on-chronic liver failure due to alcohol. *Hepatology* 2003; 38:239A.

37. Sen S, Jalan R, Williams R. Liver failure: basis of benefit of therapy with the molecular adsorbents recirculating system. *Int J Biochem Cell Biol* 2003; 35:1306-1311.

38. Steiner C, Zinggrebe A, Viertler A. Experiences with MARS therapy in liver disease: analysis of 385 patients of the International MARS Registry. *Hepatology* 2003; 38:239A.

39. Sen S, Steiner C, Williams R, Jalan R. Artificial liver support: Overview of Registry and controlled clinical trials. In: Arroyo V, Forns X, Garcia-Pagan JC, Rodes J, eds. Progress in the treatment of liver diseases. Barcelona, Spain: Ars Medica, 2003: 429-435.

40. Kjaergard LL, Liu J, Als-Nielsen B, Gluud C. Artificial and bioartificial support systems for acute and acute-on-chronic liver failure: a systematic review. *JAMA* 2003; 289:217-222.

41. Stange J, Mitzner SR, Klammt S, et al. Liver support by extracorporeal blood purification: a clinical observation. *Liver Transpl* 2000; 6:603-613.

42. Jalan R, Sen S, Steiner C, Kapoor D, Alisa A, Williams R. Extracorporeal liver support with molecular adsorbents recirculating system in patients with severe acute alcoholic hepatitis. *J Hepatol* 2003; 38:24-31.

38

Management of Bleeding During ECLS

Giles J. Peek, M.D., F.R.C.S., C.Th., Birgit Wittenstein, Dr. Med., Chris Harvey, M.B.B.S., F.R.C.S., and David Machin, B.Sc., A.C.P.

Introduction

Bleeding is one of the most feared complications of ECLS, dreaded by both physicians and surgeons alike. In the early days of ECLS, copious bleeding around cannulation sites contributed greatly to the morbidity and probably also to the high mortality seen in the first adult cases.[1] As experience with ECLS grew, iatrogenic bleeding was largely eliminated, less heparin was used, and cannulation techniques improved. Preventative strategies forbidding "unnecessary" invasive procedures during ECLS, and more recently, improvements in extracorporeal technology have lead to further reductions in ECLS patients' propensity for hemorrhage.

Unfortunately, however, patients can still experience severe and sometimes fatal hemorrhage during ECLS. In this chapter, we will discuss the management of these challenging cases.

Epidemiology and etiology

The ELSO Registry Report in 2005 documented surgical site bleeding in 31.4% of cardiac patients, 21.9% of adult respiratory patients, 15.3% of pediatric respiratory, and 6.1% of neonatal respiratory patients. Cannulation site bleeding occurs in 7.4%, 12.7%, 10.1%, and 6.3%, respectively. A small number of GI bleeds and cardiac tamponade from clots are also reported in all patient groups, the latter being most common in the cardiac group at 5.5%. It is readily apparent that bleeding is a common problem for ECMO patients.

Approach to the bleeding patient

Three basic principals that underlie the management of bleeding are optimization of coagulation, drug therapy, and surgical treatment. The clinician must initially assess the severity of the problem. What appears to be a minor amount of bleeding observed for a short time at bedside can develop into a life-threatening hemorrhage if allowed to persist for several days. Bleeding of 1 ml/min equates to nearly 1.5 l/day. Bleeding can usually be managed with a slight reduction in activated clotting time (ACT), local pressure, or a simple suture. Severe bleeding is usually obvious and mandates immediate surgery. Decision making for patients with moderate bleeding, who comprise the majority of patients, is more difficult. Not all patients require the entire clinical pathway, and the pathway should be adapted to match the severity of the patient's problem. In the next sections, the optimization of coagulation/heparinization and drug therapy, including anti-fibrinolytics, will be discussed followed by a discussion of surgical principles.

Optimization of coagulation

The optimization of the coagulation system may be all that is required to deal with diffuse hemorrhage (e.g., pulmonary hemorrhage). In patients with moderate bleeding when surgery is planned, or in elective surgery (e.g., CDH repair), the coagulation system should be optimized prior to surgery. In patients with life-threatening bleeding, transfusion and drug treatment will be accomplished in parallel with emergency surgery.

Coagulation cascade

Assays of the coagulation system should be near normal with the exception of evidence of limited heparinization. The level of heparin present during ECLS usually has little effect on the prothrombin time. Thus, any prolongation in the prothrombin time represents a coagulopathy and is an indication for transfusion of fresh frozen plasma (FFP). Aliquots of 10 ml/kg are given against the corrected weight of the patient until the prothrombin ratio or international normalized ratio (INR) falls to <1.5. The corrected weight is the weight the patient would be with a blood volume equivalent to the ECLS circuit plus their own blood volume (a 3 kg neonate with a 500 ml circuit volume would have a corrected weight of 3 + 500/80 = 9.25 kg). In adults, it is usually sufficient to give 4 units of FFP. If rapid correction is required or fluid balance is a problem, larger volumes can be given with the excess volume removed by hemofiltration.

The activated partial thromboplastin time (aPTT) and the thrombin time will naturally be prolonged by the presence of heparin and often by aprotinin, if used. These indices are, therefore, not helpful, other than demonstrating the presence of heparin.

The formation of a sound clot depends upon normalization of the intrinsic and extrinsic pathways and the presence of sufficient functional platelets and fibrinogen. It is standard clinical practice, therefore, to measure the fibrinogen concentration and to transfuse cryoprecipitate if the concentration is <200 mg/dl. Usually 1-2 units of cryoprecipitate are sufficient for a neonate and ~6 units for an adult. The needed dose is more a function of circuit size, as with FFP, than body weight.

Near-patient thromboelastography is becoming available for measuring platelet function in a clinically meaningful time frame. As of yet, we do not have experience with its use, so we are limited to estimating platelet function by their number. Experience has taught us that spontaneous bleeding is rare in a neonate on ECLS (with a silicone oxygenator) if the platelet count is >75-100,000/μl. The same experience has shown that, when surgery is performed, bleeding is more manageable if the platelet count is >150,000/μl. In a patient not on ECLS, it is standard practice to transfuse if the platelet count drops <30,000/μl. From this, we infer that only ~30% of the platelets are functioning when on ECLS with a silicone oxygenator. We believe that platelet function may be better preserved with the newer poly-methyl pentene oxygenators.[2] Generally, platelet count is maintained >150,000/μl in patients who are bleeding, undergoing surgery, or have had an operation in the last 3-4 days. The usual dose of platelets for a neonate is 1 single donor unit, and 4-6 units for an adult. It is likely that in the future we will use near-patient testing of platelet function to assist with our transfusion decisions.

Drug therapy

The most commonly used classes of drugs in bleeding ECLS patients are vitamin K and the anti-fibrinolytics; however, recombinant activated factor VII has recently become available and appears useful. A short discussion of its use will follow at the end of this section.

Vitamin K is often given IV to neonates who are bleeding on ECMO as an empirical treatment since it has been standard perinatal practice. It does not appear to cause any problems with thrombus promotion in the circuit; however, its efficacy in this setting is unproven.

One of the fundamental problems with ECLS is that the circuit acts as a continued thrombotic stimulus with the generation of thrombin despite the presence of heparin.[3] This, in turn, leads to continued up-regulation of the fibrinolytic system, which has the effect of lysing clots that have formed. It is common for a post-operative cardiac patient to be bleeding on post-op day 2-3 on ECLS. This phenomenon is a result of fibrinolysis. The use of anti-fibrinolytic agents is essential if clot stability is to be maintained and bleeding stopped definitively. The three anti-fibrinolytics in common use are tranexamic acid, epsilon amino-caproic acid, and aprotinin.

Tranexamic acid (Cyklopron)

Tranexamic acid is commonly used to both prevent and arrest bleeding after cardiopulmonary bypass (CPB) in adults and to a lesser extent in children.[4,5] It is inexpensive and easy to administer. Its effectiveness was shown in one small open-label study by reducing surgical bleeding from a mean of 390 ml to only 57 ml during congenital diaphragmatic hernia (CDH) repair on ECLS.[6] This translates into a reduced red cell transfusion requirement (1.13 vs. 2.95 ml/kg/hr). Unfortunately, 2 of the 19 neonates in the study developed severe thrombotic complications. Tranexamic acid is not in widespread use for hemorrhage control during ECLS, as there are better agents available, therefore, it generally is not recommended.

Epsilon-amino caproicacid (Amicar)

Amicar is probably the most widely used drug worldwide for hemorrhage control during ECLS. It is also commonly used for CPB-related bleeding.[7] Amicar is an amino acid which exerts its anti-fibrinolytic effect by saturating the lysine binding sites of plasminogen, thereby displacing plasminogen from fibrin and preventing fibrinolysis. There are many experienced teams using Amicar routinely both to prevent hemorrhage during elective surgery on ECLS and to control ongoing bleeding.[8,9] Experience has been very positive and many surgeons would be reluctant to operate on ECLS patients without Amicar. There is one small, randomized, controlled trial in the literature which examines the use of Amicar to prevent hemorrhage in neonates on ECLS, excluding babies with CDH.[10] In this study, Amicar was used in a dose of 100 mg/kg bolus, followed by an infusion at 25 mg/kg/hr for 72 hours. Twenty-nine patients were enrolled and were randomized to receive either Amicar or placebo; 13 received Amicar and 16 placebo. In the treatment group, 23% developed intracranial hemorrhage (ICH), compared with 12.5% in the control group. There was no statistically significant difference in the incidence of ICH, circuit complications, or transfusion requirements between the groups. Two patients, both in the control group, developed inferior vena cava thrombosis. The authors concluded that Amicar does not prevent ICH in neonates on ECLS. The negative findings of this small, but well conducted study do not, however, negate the use of Amicar to treat hemorrhage, or as an adjunct to surgery. Amicar is significantly more cost efficient than aprotinin and remains the mainstay of anti-fibrinolytic treatment in most ECLS programs. A typical dose regime for Amicar is a loading dose of 100 mg/kg, administered over 60 minutes; a maintenance dose range from 20-30 mg/kg/hr in 5% dextrose in water adjusted for renal failure (creatinine ≥ 2 and ≤ 0.5 cc/k/hr urine output) to 15-20 mg/kg/hr; and rebolus after exchange transfusion or circuit change. During Amicar infusion, the ACT must be maintained at "normal" ECMO levels; failure to do this can result in widespread thrombosis of the circuit.

Aprotinin

At Glenfield Hospital (Leicester, U.K.), aprotinin forms the mainstay of drug management for patients who are bleeding or undergoing surgery. The pharmacologic properties of aprotinin are complex and not completely understood.[3] It acts as an antifibrinolytic, preserves platelet function, has anti-inflammatory properties, and speeds up some parts of the coagulation cascade, while slowing down others.

Aprotinin has been shown to be effective in both preventing and treating bleeding after cardiac surgery in adults and children.[11,12] It is not associated with thrombotic complications.[13] It has been used during ECLS with good success.[14] Aprotinin is given as a loading dose of 10,000 u/kg over ½ hour followed by 10,000 u/kg/hr as an infusion. When surgery is planned, the infusion should be started before the incision. The aprotinin infusion is maintained for a prolonged period, usually 24-48 hours after bleeding has ceased. During aprotinin infusion, it is common for a slow clot build-up to occur in the ECMO circuit; it is unusual for rapid occlusion of the circuit to occur.

The ACT functions by saturating the blood sample with a negatively-charged particulate activator to ensure factor XII is converted to factor XIIa. The test initiates an enzymatic cascade from one clotting factor to another via the intrinsic pathway of the blood coagulation system.[15] Traditionally, the ACT tube for the low heparin concentrations used during ECMO is the P214 glass bead particulate-activated tubes (Hemochron, [ITC, Edison, NJ]). Another option is the MAX-ACT(Array Medical, Sommerville, NJ) tube which contains multiple activators (glass, kaolin, and celite) to ensure maximum activation of factor XII to achieve optimal activation.[16] MAX-ACT values are consistently around 20 seconds lower than those obtained by the P214 tubes and Hemochron 401 and 801 ACT devices. P214 readings should be increased by 20 seconds during aprotinin administration to prevent possible circuit thrombosis. The action of aprotinin resulting in prolongation of ACT with some activators is not fully understood, but may be caused by its anticoagulant properties. Just as aprotinin can prolong the ACT, the aPTT ratio can also be prolonged during aprotinin infusion even if the circuit is being run without any heparin; this has been attributed to the known anticoagulant properties of aprotinin.[19] The presence of a kaolin activator is thought to additionally act on factor XI.[17] Thus, the proposed inhibitory effect of aprotinin on factor XII will not affect MAX-ACT values, because activation of factor XI can still proceed. Conversely, kaolin may bind to aprotinin and so cannot inhibit intrinsic pathway activation within the ACT tube.[18] Recognition of the type of activator and type of ACT machine used is paramount when considering the clinical relevance of ACT values.

Recombinant Factor VIIa

Recombinant factor VIIa (rFVIIa) has been used successfully at pharmacological doses in non-hemophilia patients with profuse bleeding related to severe trauma or major surgery. Administration of rFVIIa enhances the rate of thrombin formation, thereby ensuring increased platelet activation as well as formation of a stable fibrin plug resistant to premature lysis.[20] No data have been published thus far on rFVIIa administration in ECMO patients. rFVIIa has been used for severe, refractory bleeding on ECMO in 4 patients at Great Ormond Street Hospital (GOSH) in London, U.K. Activated factor VIIa initiates hemostasis by the formation of a complex with tissue factor (TF), a transmembrane protein released as a result of blood vessel or tissue injury.[21] The FVIIa/TF complex activates factor X which then induces thrombin formation from prothombin. Thrombin generation is amplified by the interaction of platelets, factor V, VII, and IX with factor Xa. Thrombin is crucial for the formation of a stable fibrin plug resisitant to premature fibrinolysis.[20] In addition, rFVIIa promotes platelet function independent of TF activation.[22] The duration of rFVIIa hemostasis is dose-dependent. The measurable effect is a correction of INR, prothrombin time (PT) and partial thromboplastin time (PTT).[23] A few case reports describe the successful use of rFVIIa to achieve hemostasis in severe, refractory bleeding after cardiac surgery in adult and pediatric patients.[24,25] The main concern with any procoagulant therapy in ECMO patients is the concomitant risk of thrombus formation. Thromboembolic events in the extracorporeal circuit are potentially life-threatening. Factor VIIa, at pharmacologically-relevant concentrations, is not able to induce thrombin generation or clot formation alone. FVIIa/TF complex formation is required for a procoagulant effect. Recent experimental data suggest that factor VIIa efficacy in vivo requires the simultaneous presence of TF and platelet accumulation at the site of a vascular lesion.[26] This implies that FVIIa-induced hemostasis is restricted to the site of tissue injury and active bleeding. The risk of thromboembolic events, therefore, should be very low. However, circulation of blood through an extracorporeal circuit with synthetic, non-endothelial cell surfaces, shear stress, turbulence, and pump-induced mechanical injury to blood cells generates a multi-faceted response. Complement, coagulation, and kallikrein cascades are activated, and monocytes and endothelial cells express TF on their cell surface.[27,28] These events result in a hypercoagulable state. To date, there is no convincing evidence for thromboembolic complications in patients receiving rFVIIa after CPB. There is only a single report of an adult patient with a left ventricular assist device (VAD), receiving rFVIIa for 7 days. No thrombin or platelet aggregates were detected in the mechanical pump chamber.[29]

A total of 17 pediatric patients were supported with ECMO immediately following open heart surgery at GOSH. Treatment with rFVIIa for refractory bleeding on ECMO occurred in 4; 3 of the patients were neonates, and 1 patient was a 33-month-old. All 4 patients underwent corrective surgery for congenital cardiac lesions; 2 patients for transposition of the great arteries (TGA) with ventricular septal defect (VSD), one with double outlet right ventricle (DORV), and one with supravalvular aortic stenosis. Two patients were cannulated through the chest and 2 via the right neck vessels. Routine treatment to control bleeding was given to all 4 patients in the ICU. This treatment consisted of the administration of FFP, cryoprecipitate, platelet transfusion to achieve platelet levels of >100,000/μl and continuous IV aprotinin-infusion at a rate of 10,000 u/kg/hr. In addition, all patients received 1 dose of IV vitamin K. Anticoagulation on ECMO was maintained with a heparin infusion with a target ACT of 150-180 seconds. All patients underwent exploration of the chest and cannulation site within 5 hours after initiation of ECMO because of ongoing severe bleeding. No surgical cause of bleeding was identified in any of the children.

Despite the aforementioned measures to control bleeding prior to rFVIIa application, severe blood loss continued at an average of 47 ml/kg/hr (range 25-70). The patients received, on average, 36 ml/kg/hr (range 20-75) of packed red blood cells (RBCs) to maintain a stable hematocrit. An average of 10 ml/kg/hr (range 7-18) of fresh frozen plasma, 2.5 ml/kg/hr (range 1.8-3.0) of cryoprecipitate, and 7.4 ml/kg/hr (range 6-10) of platelets were given during the observation period prior to rFVIIa (Figure 1). The first dose of rFVIIa was given 4-7 hours post-ECMO (mean 5.5 hours). The dose used was 90-120 mcg/kg, administered as a bolus infusion over 20 minutes through a central venous line. A second identical dose was given 4 hours after the first bolus. After the first dose of rFVIIa, bleeding decreased dramatically in all 4 patients within 30 minutes. Blood loss was reduced to an average of 8 ml/kg/hr (range 3.4-15.0) in all patients. Transfusion requirements fell to 8 ml/kg/hr (range 3.4-15.0) of packed RBCs, 1 ml/

kg/hr (range 0-2.3) of FFP, 0.2 ml/kg/hr (range 0-0.8) of cryoprecipitate, and 1.5 ml/kg/hr (range 0-2.3) of platelets (Figure 1). The second dose of rFVIIa was given prophylactically to maintain stable hemostasis. During the patients' further course on ECMO, blood loss remained moderate to low, and no further doses of rFVIIa were given. No side effects were observed during or after rFVIIa application. Inspection of the ECMO circuit revealed no thrombus formation

or clinical signs of thromboembolism. During treatment with rFVIIa, a primed ECMO circuit was available as emergency back-up in case of significant circuit clotting.

In summary, experience with rFVIIa in 4 patients on ECMO showed prompt and sustained control of severe hemorrhage with a concomitant fall in transfusion requirements. This dramatic reduction of allogeneic blood product exposure may suggest that an earlier use of rFVIIa to manage bleeding complications on ECMO is indicated.

Fixed micro-dose heparin

A fixed dose of heparin at 10 u/kg/hr is occasionally used in patients who continue to bleed despite surgical exploration; correction of INR, fibrinogen, and/or platelet count; and infusion of aprotinin. The lower dose heparin is frequently effective in controlling hemorrhage without assuming the risks of stopping heparin.

Stopping the heparin

Ultimately, if the patient is bleeding despite the above measures, and surgical treatment is not possible or has failed, then it is occasionally necessary to stop the heparin infusion. Before doing this, it is important to carefully consider whether any other treatment is possible. If stopping the heparin becomes necessary, it is general practice to have a replacement circuit immediately available. Even without heparin bonding of the circuit, it is usually possible to continue heparin-free ECMO for 6-36 hours before a circuit change is required. This is often effective in stopping the bleeding.

Surgical treatment

It is clear from clinical experience that large amounts of blood and clots in a body cavity act as a potent stimulus of fibrinolysis. Thus, initial bleeding leads to additional bleeding, and a

A
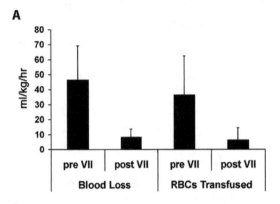

B
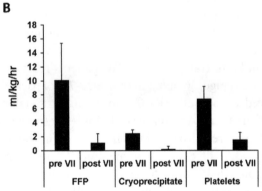

Figure 1. A: Blood loss and transfused packed RBCs before and after the first dose of recombinant factor VIIa. B: Clotting product requirement before and after the first dose of recombinant factor VIIa. The time interval "pre VII" is defined as the period between admission to CICU from the OR after ECMO cannulation until application of the first rFVIIa bolus. This interval was on average 5.5 hours (range 4-7). The time interval "post VII" is the observation period of 6 hours immediately following the first rFVIIa bolus. During this "post VII" period, all patients received a second rFVIIa bolus 4 hours after the first.

continuous bleeding cycle ensues. Timely and often repeated surgical exploration is the only way out of this downward spiral. Usually the best time to perform a surgical exploration is as soon as it is convenient following optimization of the coagulation parameters as detailed above. Obviously, bleeding causing intractable hypovolemia or tamponade mandates immediate surgery. Most explorations and elective CDH repair can be carried out in the ICU, but one should consider transferring the patient to the OR if direct visualization of the operative field is not possible. This is often the case with adult patients, as once the patient has been positioned close to the operating surgeon, the width of the patient's bed precludes all but the most basic involvement of the assistant surgeon. In the OR, with better lighting and a narrow operating table, exposure may be improved. However, moving a patient carries a significant risk of decannulation and circuit disruption. One must be certain that the benefit outweighs the risk.

Surgery should always be carried out by an experienced surgical specialist. These procedures are not suitable teaching cases for junior residents. A headlight is almost mandatory, especially when operating in the ICU, and should be supplemented by portable overhead lights, which are important so the assistant can see when the surgeon turns away from the field. Incisions should be generous to afford adequate exposure without tearing the tissue as can occur when a small incision is stretched open by retraction. Such tissue damage can lead to serious post-operative bleeding. All dissection should be carried out with electrocautery left in coagulation mode, as the cut mode does not stem capillary bleeding while on ECMO. Hemostasis of the incision should be painstaking with ligation of larger vessels; titanium ligaclips can save time. Blunt dissection should be avoided as much as possible. Bone wax can be used on the cut edges of the sternum or a cut rib. Bleeding points, when identified, are controlled by standard surgical techniques such as electrocautery, ligation, or suture. The use of autologous pericardial pledgets is particularly helpful when controlling bleeding from suture lines or cannulation sites on the heart. Bleeding will frequently occur around transthoracic cannulas, more often from the right atrial cannula rather than the aortic. This is because the right atrial tissue is much more fragile and the purse strings tend to tear over time. Placement of additional purse strings, ideally prolene on a round-bodied needle with multiple teflon pledgets, will usually control the bleeding for a time as the prolene suture slides through the tissue more easily than a braided suture. By placing pledgets on four sides of the purse string, the tissue can be bunched up around the cannula to stop the bleeding. Ultimately, the best way to control bleeding from the chest is to remove the cannulas and close the chest. It is usually fairly easy to place cannulas via the right side of the neck, allowing the aortic and venous cannulas to be removed from the chest. The use of moderate hypothermia (32°C) can make the transition between cannulas or circuits safer by reducing oxygen consumption. Venting the left heart via a septostomy rather than a left atrial cannula can allow removal of the cannula and closure of the chest. Neck cannulation has been correlated with higher survival in pediatric cardiac ECLS patients.[30]

Hypothermia has another important role as an adjunct to the use of surgical glue. Bleeding from needle holes along a suture line will often not stop and oversewing, even with pledgeted sutures, causes more bleeding from the needle holes. Glue can be useful in stopping this bleeding, but paradoxically, the glue will not work on actively bleeding tissue. However, reduction of blood pressure can stop the bleeding long enough for the glue (i.e., Tiseel or Bioglue) to be applied. In a patient on venoarterial (VA) ECMO, the arterial line is clamped, the venous line is left open, and blood is withdrawn from the bladder until the heart is empty and the blood pressure has dropped. In a neonate, this can be done by attaching two 60 ml syringes to the bladder ports, aspirating them in turn, and leaving them connected. The suture line is then sucked dry and the glue applied, taking care not to put so much glue into the chest that it causes distortion of other structures, particularly the coronary arteries following a switch operation. The circulation is kept empty in this manner until the glue is dry, the arterial line is unclamped, and, the volume re-infused. The whole procedure takes 1-2 minutes, which is well tolerated at 32°C. In a patient on venovenous (VV) ECMO, blood can be withdrawn in the same way, or inflow occlusion can be used, clamping and snaring the vena cava to prevent blood from entering the heart. Care must be taken not to damage the ECMO cannula during this procedure. On VV ECMO, it is probably safer to use 34°C and shorten the period of circulatory arrest to ≤2 minutes. Activated cellulose (Surgicel[Johnson and Johnson, New Brunswick, NJ]) is also useful either used alone or laid onto a suture line before glue is applied (Bioglue[Cryolife, Inc., Kennesaw, GA]), reminiscent of using fiberglass matting with epoxy resin. If circulatory arrest is not used, patients should be kept normothermic to encourage normal coagulation which is temperature-dependent. In general, suture lines constructed on ECMO should be glued, even if they are dry at the time. When performing a lung biopsy, the use of pericardial strips (peristrips) to buttress the staple line can prevent bleeding. Again, glue can be applied.

If bleeding cannot be controlled, the cavity should be packed with gauze swabs (soaking the swabs in aprotinin and wringing them out first has been helpful). In this case, repeated exploration will be required at least to remove the swabs, so it is common practice to just close the skin or sew a membrane into the skin edges. If the field looks dry, it is worth closing the wound formally. Most post-operative or iatrogenic bleeding will require 1-2 explorations; the actual closure of the wound probably helps

hemostasis by achieving tissue apposition. Formal closure is avoided in cases where multiple explorations are needed, as the repeated suturing will cause tissue damage and further bleeding. Large multiple chest drains should be placed.

Pulmonary hemorrhage

Most pulmonary hemorrhages will stop when ventilation is discontinued, and the patient is managed on continuous positive airway pressure (CPAP) of 10-15 cm H_2O. If the pulmonary hemorrhage is caused by left heart distension and high left atrial pressure, then it will not stop until the left atrium is decompressed, usually by atrial septostomy. In one of our adult respiratory patients on ECMO, this was not the case. Bleeding from an intra-parenchymal chest drain caused severe intrapleural bleeding. The chest was explored via a right thoracotomy, and the chest drain was seen transfixing the middle lobe and entering the right lower lobe. The wounds were oversewn, glue was applied, and the suture lines appeared dry. Two days later, the patient developed profuse bleeding via the endotracheal tube which did not stop with CPAP. The bleeding was life-threatening, originating from the right middle and lower lobes. Options such as embolization were discussed but discarded as impractical. Bilobectomy was also considered and discarded, as it would necessitate the removal of too much viable lung tissue. The patient was extubated under deep sedation while paralyzed, and the larynx was packed with wide ribbon gauze. The transfusion requirement decreased and eventually ceased over a 12-hour period, and the pack was left in situ for 3 days. Rigid bronchoscopy was performed which showed a cast filling the entire bronchial tree and protruding through the vocal cords. The clot was removed with biopsy forceps and suction down to the segmental bronchi. Lavage was initiated with perflurodecalin. This procedure was successful and the patient is a long-term survivor.

Glenfield experience

During 2004, Glenfield Hospital provided ECMO support for 19 adults, 23 neonates, and 20 pediatric patients (62 total). In all, 14 patients underwent a surgical procedure while on ECMO (4 adults, 2 neonates, and 8 children). Of these, 6 operations were for patients with bleeding post-median sternotomy (1 adult, 1 neonate, and 4 children). Four patients underwent a thoracotomy while on ECMO (1 patient had a bilateral thoracotomy, and 3 patients required re-exploration for bleeding). Other procedures included: fasciotomy, laparotomy, gastroscopy, and one video-assisted thoracoscopic exploration of the chest. All bleeding patients received aprotinin and aggressive correction of clotting abnor-malities. In 3 patients, bleeding was controlled by lowering the ACT to 140-160 seconds and hemostasis was achieved in another by dropping the ACT to 160-180 seconds. The heparin infusion rate was reduced to run at 10 units/hr in 7 patients with bleeding control achieved in 3. Heparin was totally discontinued in 5 patients with control of bleeding being achieved in 2. Two patients were taken off ECMO and 2 patients received factor VIIa. Three patients required a new circuit because of excessive clotting. Two patients died prior to gaining control of hemorrhage (1 from sudden cardiac arrest and 1 from elective withdrawal of treatment on the grounds of futility). The Glenfield algorithm for the bleeding patient is shown below (Figure 2).

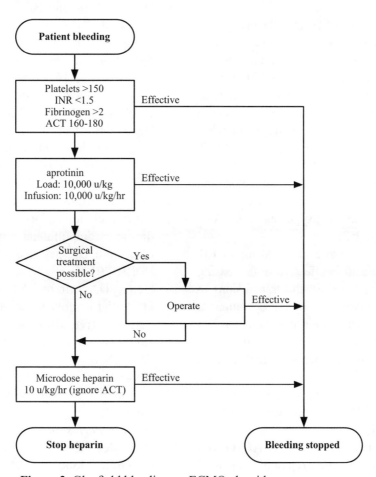

Figure 2. Glenfield bleeding on ECMO algorithm.

Conclusion

Bleeding complications are a major challenge to the skills of the ECMO team. Successful management requires an aggressive multi-modality approach in which surgery plays a central role. In ECMO programs which are not surgically led, it is essential to have prior discussion with appropriate surgeons about treatment protocols so that when bleeding does occur, it can be appropriately managed. Operations should be avoided which rely largely on natural hemostasis rather than surgical control. If at all possible, such procedures should be deferred until the patient has been decannulated from ECMO.

References

1. Zapol WM, Snider MT, Hill JD, et al. Extracorporeal membrane oxygenation in severe acute respiratory failure. A randomized prospective study. *JAMA* 1979; 242:2193-2196.
2. Peek GJ, Killer HM, Reeves R, Sosnowski AW, Firmin RK. Early experience with a polymethyl pentene oxygenator for adult extracorporeal life support. *ASAIO J* 2002; 48(5), 480-482.
3. Peek GJ, Firmin RK. The inflammatory and coagulative response to prolonged extracorporeal membrane oxygenation. *ASAIO J* 1999; 45:250-263.
4. Brown RS, Thwaites BK, Mongan PD. Tranexamic acid is effective in decreasing postoperative bleeding and transfusions in primary coronary artery bypass operations: a double-blind, randomized, placebo-controlled trial. *Anesth Analg* 1997; 85:963-70.
5. Zonis Z, Seear M, Reichert C, Sett S, Allen C. The effect of preoperative tranexamic acid on blood loss after cardiac operations in children. *J Thorac Cardiovasc Surg* 1996; 111:982-987.
6. van der Staak FH, De Haan AF, Geven WB, Festen C. Surgical repair of congenital diaphragmatic hernia during extracorporeal membrane oxygenation: hemorrhagic complications and the effect of tranexamic acid. *J Pediatr Surg* 1997; 32:594-599.
7. DelRossi AJ, Cernaianu AC, Botros S, Lemole GM, Moore R. Prophylactic treatment of postperfusion bleeding using EACA. *Chest* 1989; 96:27-30.
8. Wilson JM, Bower LK, Lund DP. Evolution of the technique of congenital diaphragmatic hernia repair on ECMO. *J Pediatr Surg* 1994; 29:1109-1112.
9. Wilson JM, Bower LK, Fackler JC, Beals DA, Bergus BO, Kevy SV. Aminocaproic acid decreases the incidence of intracranial hemorrhage and other hemorrhagic complications of ECMO. *J Pediatr Surg* 1993; 28:536-540; discussion 540-541.
10. Horwitz JR, Cofer BR, Warner BW, Cheu HW, Lally KP. A multicenter trial of 6-aminocaproic acid (Amicar) in the prevention of bleeding in infants on ECMO. *J Pediatr Surg* 1998; 33:1610-1613.
11. Jamieson WR, Dryden PJ, O'Connor JP, Sadeghi H, Ansley DM, Merrick PM. Beneficial effect of both tranexamic acid and aprotinin on blood loss reduction in reoperative valve replacement surgery. *Circulation* 1997; 96:II-96-100.
12. Codispoti M, Mankad PS. Management of anticoagulation and its reversal during paediatric cardiopulmonary bypass: a review of current UK practice. *Perfusion* 2000; 15:191-201.
13. Henry DA, Moxey AJ, Carless PA, et al. Anti-fibrinolytic use for minimising perioperative allogeneic blood transfusion. *Cochrane Database Syst Rev* 2001; CD001886.
14. Biswas AK, Lewis L, Sommerauer JF. Aprotinin in the management of life-threatening bleeding during extracorporeal life support. *Perfusion* 2000; 15:211-216.
15. Hattersley PG. Activated coagulation time of whole blood. *JAMA* 1966; 196:436-440.

16. Espana F, Ratnoff OD. Activation of Hageman factor (factor XII) by sulfatides and other agents in the absence of plasma proteases. *J Lab Clin Med* 1983; 102:31-45.
17. Heimark RL, Kurachi K, Fujikawa K, Davie EW. Surface activation of blood coagulation, fibrinolysis and kinin formation. *Nature* 1980; 286:456-460.
18. Dietrich W, Jochum M. Effect of celite and kaolin on activated clotting time in the presence of aprotinin: activated clotting time is reduced by binding of aprotinin to kaolin. *J Thorac Cardiovasc Surg* 1995; 109:177-178.
19. Landis RC, Haskard DO, Taylor KM. New antiinflammatory and platelet-preserving effects of aprotinin. *Ann Thorac Surg* 2001; 72:S1808-S1813.
20. Rapaport SI, Rao LV. Initiation and regulation of tissue factor-dependent blood coagulation. *Arterioscler Thromb* 1992; 12:1111-1121.
21. Mann KG. Biochemistry and physiology of blood coagulation. *Thromb Haemost* 1999; 82:165-174.
22. Monroe DM, Hoffman M, Oliver JA, Roberts HR. Platelet activity of high-dose factor VIIa is independent of tissue factor. *Br J Haematol* 1997; 99:542-547.
23. Erhardtsen E, Nony P, Dechavanne M, Ffrench P, Boissel JP, Hedner U. The effect of recombinant factor VIIa (NovoSeven) in healthy volunteers receiving acenocoumarol to an International Normalized Ratio above 2.0. *Blood Coagul Fibrinolysis* 1998; 9:741-748.
24. Hendriks HG, van der Maaten JM, de Wolf J, Waterbolk TW, Slooff MJ, van der MJ. An effective treatment of severe intractable bleeding after valve repair by one single dose of activated recombinant factor VII. *Anesth Analg* 2002; 93:287-289.
25. Egan JR, Lammi A, Schell DN, Gillis J, Nunn GR. Recombinant activated factor VII in paediatric cardiac surgery. *Intensive Care Med* 2004; 30:682-685.
26. Butenas S, Brummel KE, Paradis SG, Mann KG. Influence of factor VIIa and phospholipids on coagulation in "acquired" hemophilia. *Arterioscler Thromb Vasc Biol* 2003; 23:123-129.
27. Wachtfogel YT, Harpel PC, Edmunds LH, Jr, Colman RW. Formation of C1s-C1-inhibitor, kallikrein-C1-inhibitor, and plasmin-alpha 2-plasmin-inhibitor complexes during cardiopulmonary bypass. *Blood* 1989; 73:468-471.
28. Ernofsson M, Thelin S, Siegbahn A. Monocyte tissue factor expression, cell activation, and thrombin formation during cardiopulmonary bypass: a clinical study. *J Thorac Cardiovasc Surg* 1997; 113:576-584.
29. Zietkiewicz M, Garlicki M, Domagala J, et al. Successful use of activated recombinant factor VII to control bleeding abnormalities in a patient with a left ventricular assist device. *J Thorac Cardiovasc Surg* 2002; 123:384-385.
30. Balasubramanian S, Tiruvoipati R, Amin M, et al. Factors influencing the outcome of pediatric extracorporeal mechanical circulatory support. In: Abstract of the 15th Annual ELSO Conference; September 9-12, 2004; Ann Arbor, MI.

39

Plasmapheresis

Jeffrey B. Sussmane, M.D., F.C.C.M.

Introduction

Plasmapheresis is a treatment whose use and efficacy has grown exponentially since its introduction in the clinical setting in the 1960s.[1] Therapeutic plasma exchange (TPE) is the most frequent "pheresis" modality performed. Typically, a centrifuge or filter separates the components, and the replacement fluid is continuously returned to the patient during the filtration. The goal is to remove, replace, or deplete a unique circulating cell or substance responsible for the disease process. The term "plasmapheresis" are used to refer to the removal, exchange, modification, or filtration of the returning plasma component. Cytapheresis includes red cell pheresis or erythrocytapheresis, the removal of red blood cells (RBCs) and the return of predetermined replacement fluids, most commonly donor RBCs. Therapeutic leukodepletion is employed for the removal of white blood cells (WBCs), granulocytes or monocytes, thereby decreasing aggregates that interfere with blood flow, while leukapheresis refers to peripheral stem cell collection, performed to remove WBCs, specifically progenitor monocytes, from peripheral blood for storage and re-infusion at a later date.

TPE is used to treat infection, inflammatory, autoimmune, oncologic, metabolic, neurologic, or renal diseases.[2] In the past 10 years, many hospitals have developed programs for apheresis due to its growing success and the increase of therapeutic uses.[3] The technique has also gained widespread acceptance in Europe.[4] TPE is a supportive therapy used in conjunction with ongoing care and has been shown to increase the chance of recovery and survival in critically ill children and adults.[5-7]

Historical perspective

Apheresis stems from the Greek verb *aphairesis* meaning "to take away, withdraw, or separate". The original concept of removing circulating "toxins" or "humours" from the blood is centuries old and was once done routinely in an attempt to improve or restore health. Leeches and other bloodletting techniques were popular for many years. Historians continue to discuss the death of George Washington and his bloodletting for what was probably laryngotracheitis.[8] Modern TPE was introduced by Abel and Roundtree in 1914. They treated toxemia in an animal model by removing plasma and returning the cellular components, observing that an animal could survive the loss of large amounts of plasma if the "corpuscles" were returned along with a replacement solution. Extensive applications for plasma exchange were later focused on the removal of plasma to create and supply a donor pool of blood products during World War II. Improvements involved separating the components used for transfusion. Skoog and Adams in 1959, and Solomon and Fahey in 1963, first used plasma exchange in the treatment of hyperviscosity syndromes such as macroglobulinemia. Apheresis has since evolved from its primitive beginnings into a sophisticated, safe, and efficient therapy. Technological advances have allowed the customization of equipment and procedures to meet specific patient size and diagnostic needs, as well as to decrease adverse events.

Principles of operation

TPE for the clinically unstable patient is performed in the ICU at the bedside by registered nurses or technicians, under the supervision of a qualified physician. The patient's weight, sex, height, hematocrit, and procedure-specific information are manually entered into the device computer program to perform the patient appropriate separation. Two peripheral veins that accept 14 gauge catheters may provide adequate access for many procedures. Central venous access for children is often successful with a catheter as small as a double lumen 7F. Larger catheter sizes will facilitate all collections. A central, double lumen venous catheter provides the safest and most efficient means of withdrawing and returning continuous volumes of blood without interruption. Centrifugal separation occurs when a specific circuit is loaded into a centrifugal machine for each treatment. A filtration method of separating blood components is also available. The device is primed in a similar manner to the centrifugal systems. Anticoagulation and replacement fluids are also programmed to be returned to the patient after filtration and removal of the designated components. Once connected, the patient's blood is pumped into the machine along with an anticoagulant that is automatically added based on pre-programmed information. The centrifuge separates the blood into layers primarily based on molecular weight and density. RBCs are the densest and collect against the centrifuge wall,

followed by WBCs, platelets, and plasma. Optical sensors are used to detect the plasma cell interface to minimize contamination of cell and fluid layers by other components during centrifugal TPE. The desired components/layers are automatically removed to collection bags, and the remaining blood components, along with appropriate replacement fluids, are returned to the patient.

Rotary peristaltic pumps control the flow of all fluids throughout the entire procedure. They are programmed to regulate; the rate amount of whole blood initially removed from the patient, the rate of infusion of anticoagulation into the system, the rate and amount of each component separated from the centrifuge, the rate and amount of fluid sent to collection bags, and the rate and amount of returned blood components and replacement fluids returned to the patient. Warmers can be added to the circuit to heat replacement fluid, preventing hypothermia caused by infusion of fluids that are cold or at room temperature. Most apheresis machines have the ability to select the percentage of fluids removed to be automatically re-infused. These alarms are preset to insure that there is no significant change in the volume of fluid removed or added to the patient. They also alert the operator to any changes in the rate at which fluids are removed or added.

TPE may also be performed using a filtration technique. An anticoagulated extracorporeal circuit passes the blood through a filter; separation of the plasma is achieved, followed by reinfusion of the cellular components. This technique performs well for specific plasma filtration scenarios but is reliant upon the filter pore size. TPE using filtration has been studied in a number of clinical conditions.[9-12]

Types of therapeutic apheresis treatments

Therapeutic plasma exchange

TPE removes specified plasma volumes and returns predetermined replacement fluids, most commonly plasma and/or albumin. The manipulation of returning plasma initiates an immune response which can be seen in the elevation of all major circulating immune complexes within 1-3 hours of treatment. Complement levels of C3a, C4a, C5a, in some patients, become elevated towards the end of the first treatment, but most commonly increase after the first and during the second treatment. Immunoglobulins are decreased after all procedures and often require replacement. Granulocytes and macrophages also increase with complement after and during the second treatment due to this apparent inflammatory immunomodulation. Lymphocytes increase in treatment three, and the T helper/suppressor ratio increases in treatment four. Pediatric indications for TPE include sepsis, hemolytic uremic syndrome, Kawasaki syndrome, toxic shock, meningococcemia, transplant incompatibilities, and circulating immune disorders including Guillian-Barre Syndrome, systemic lupus erythematosus, rheumatoid arthritis, multiple sclerosis, myasthenia gravis, Goodpasture disease, Steven Johnson syndrome, and coagulopathies such as those associated with acute hepatic failure.[13,14] In adults, TPE is used in the treatment of thrombotic thrombocytopenic purpura, myasthenia gravis, chronic inflammatory demyelinating polyneuropathy, macrobulinemia,[15] and toxicology emergencies.[16-18] TPE involves cycling 100% of the patient's total blood volume, thereby removing putative pathologic material in the patient's plasma. The efficacy of treatment may be measured by a reduction in concentration of pathologic and toxic substances such as the cytokines previously mentioned.[19] The aggressive use of immunoglobulin G (IgG) concomitant with plasmapheresis has been widely reported for pre-transplant patients and for blood group incompatibilities incurred with transplantation and rejection.[20-23]

TPE is currently used in sepsis to decrease the amount of circulating inflammatory mediators. In 1980, Vain[24] demonstrated that the use of exchange transfusion in neonates with severe septicemia improves survival. Busund[25] in 1991 reported that plasma exchange with albumin replacement significantly reduced plasma tumor necrosis factor, endotoxin, and IL-1 activity during septic shock. This reduction in cytokine activity was associated with an increased survival and improved cardiovascular performance relative to control patients. In a prospective study, Garlund and Sjolin[26] found that the mortality of a group with primary septic shock that received plasmapheresis was lower than the group that did not. They concluded that TPE may be a therapeutic option in the early stages of septic shock. Fatalities occurred in the patients for whom TPE was delayed >12 hours. TPE administered in conjunction with conventional intensive care treatment of septic shock may improve survival.[27] However, case reports and retrospective control studies have shown mixed results with response to plasmapheresis in sepsis.[28] In a prospective, randomized trial of septic shock, the relative risk for 28-day mortality in the plasmapheresis group was 0.61 with the number needed to treat of 4.9.[29]

TPE may also be applied to diseases that are primarily immunologically mediated. Goodpasture Disease, an anti-glomerular basement membrane disease, is the first humorally-mediated condition to be treated effectively with plasmapheresis.[30] Dyck in 1986,[31] conducted a prospective, randomized, double-blind trial of plasma exchange and sham exchange for chronic inflammatory demyelinating polyradiculoneuropathy, demonstrating that plasma exchange had a beneficial effect. He also explored the use of plasma exchange in polyneuropathy associated with monoclonal gammopathy, finding that plasma exchange prevented worsening of the neuropathic deficit and even ameliorated it. There was an additional benefit to muscle strength and muscle action potentials.

Jansen observed that patients receiving plasmapheresis for Guillian-Barre experienced a decrease in time spent on mechanical ventilation and overall costs, and were quicker to regain motor function.[32] Plasmapheresis influenced the duration of mechanical ventilation, the time to regain the ability to walk independently, and the chance to regain full strength after 1 year. The use of plasmapheresis in Guillian-Barre has improved the management of this disease, when severe, from a supportive to an active treatment. Plasmapheresis has also been successfully utilized in the treatment of other acute inflammatory demyelinating polyneuropathies. Plasmapheresis has been utilized in acute episodes of fulminant central nervous system (CNS) inflammatory demyelination and fulminant vasculitis as well as polyneuritis and neuropathies.[33] Superior results in the treatment of thrombotic thrombocytopenic pupura or hemolytic uremic syndrome (HUS) and other thrombotic conditions have also been documented with plasma exchange.[34-36]

Circulating inflammatory mediators are widely recognized to contribute to the morbidity and mortality of certain clinical conditions. The direct filtration of these mediators had not been possible until the recent improvement in biocompatibility of membranes. An immunoadsorption column with protein A covalently bound to a microprocessed silicone filter (Prosorba [Fresenius HemoCare, Redmond, WA]) has been widely utilized and may be added to the circuit, in combination with therapeutic plasmapheresis. This greatly amplifies the immunomodulation of the extracorporeal circuit. The Prosorba column may be indicated for patients with chronic or idiopathic thrombocytopenic purpura (ITP), increased IgG, and associated circulating immune complexes. The Prosorba column has also proven to be effective in treating patients with rheumatoid arthritis who are intolerant of, or who failed treatment with, disease-modifying anti-rheumatic drugs.[37] The Prosorba column has been utilized to prevent graft vs. host reactions in organ recipients based on the rationale that removal and modulation of circulating immune complexes decreases the possibility of rejection. A polymixin-B-immobilized fiber has been shown to significantly decrease circulating

levels of endotoxin after plasmapheresis,[38] but no study has shown a benefit to these absorptive therapies.

Therapeutic cytapheresis

Therapeutic cytapheresis is the removal of cellular components (WBCs, RBCs, or platelets). Cytapheresis can be further subdivided into three categories: erythrocytapheresis, leukapheresis, and plateletpheresis.

Erythrocytapheresis, also known as red blood cell exchange (RBCX), is indicated in illnesses such as sickle cell disease (for anemia, acute chest syndrome, priapism, and stroke), cyanotic congestive heart disease (for hyperviscosity syndrome), neonatal hemolytic anemia, and thalassemia. RBCX is most frequently employed in patients who require rapid RBCX transfusions (e.g. sickle cell disease or malaria). The treatment involves the depletion of RBCs and replacement with leukocyte-poor donor RBCs. RBCX has been shown to improve tissue oxygenation, correct anemia and polycythemia, and correct blood viscosity, as well as improve pulmonary compliance. Benefits of RBCX over manual exchange transfusions include the decreased risk of complications such as iron overload, stroke, hypoxia, allo-antibody formation, and exposure to anticoagulants.[39]

Leukapheresis (WBCX) may be subdivided into 2 procedures: peripheral hematopoetic stem cell collection (PBSC) and leukodepletion. PBSCs are done to harvest undifferentiated, pluripotential monocytes. Ideally, this is achieved from the patient (autologous) decreasing the chances of graft vs. host disease post-transplant. An additional option is to retrieve stem cells from a sibling (allogenic), identical twin (syngenetic), or an unrelated donor (allogenic). The cells are processed, cryopreserved, and stored until needed for re-transfusion at a later date to rescue or reconstitute bone marrow in patients who have received high-dose chemotherapy and/or radiation.

First introduced in 1986, PBSC has become an accepted clinical procedure for many oncology patients.[40] Candidates for stem cell collection include patients with leukemia, neuroblastoma, relapsed lymphoma, and renal cancer. Stem cells are progenitor monocytes produced in the bone marrow that can differentiate into specific mature cells. PBSCs target the collection of mononuclear cell lymphocytes, specifically the CD 34+ monocytes, which are also phagocytic antagonists of certain microorganisms and are involved in immune modification. Depending on the institutional protocol, the stem cell donor may undergo a 7-10 day regimen of bone marrow stimulation with a hematopoietic cytokine, granulocyte colony stimulating factor (gCSF), before the collection.[41] gCSF mobilizes stem cells into the peripheral bloodstream and may increase their number up to 100-fold; in addition, it allows for rapid recovery of the bone marrow. Each treatment takes between 4-6 hours for 3-5 days and entails processing 3-6 times the donor's blood volume. The objective is to collect 10^7 CD34$^+$ cells in order to increase the chances of a successful transplant. Since there is currently no laboratory method to directly quantify stem cells, a surrogate marker, the CD34$^+$ cell antigen, is utilized to estimate the number of stem cells collected. In the experience at Miami Children's Hospital, a pre-collection value >2.0 x 10^5/mm^3 WBCs in the peripheral blood has been shown to improve collection success. The collection is preserved and stored in a blood bank until the patient is deemed ready to receive it as a bone marrow transplant post-ablative chemotherapy. In comparison to a bone marrow harvest, peripheral stem cell collection allows for frequent collection, decreases the risk of tumor cell contamination, and avoids general anesthesia. Future applications for cardiac, neurologic, and metabolic diseases are now being studied.

Leukodepletion is employed to reduce the number of circulating WBCs to decrease patient morbidity and mortality as a result of leukostasis.[42,43] In pediatric patients, leukodepletion is used as a first-line adjunct therapy to chemotherapy for acute lymphocytic leukemia or acute myelocytic leukemia in which the WBC count is >2.0 x 10 ^{5}/mm^3 to decrease the WBC load and thus, the risk of leukostasis, stroke, and tumor lysis syndrome. Leukopheresis may be performed by collecting the buffy coat layer; this typically drops the WBC count by 50-75% post-procedure. Patients receiving leukodepletion may experience fewer electrolyte abnormalities during induction chemotherapy.

Therapeutic plateletpheresis

Therapeutic plateletpheresis is indicated in patients with symptomatic thrombocytosis. The goal is to decrease the platelet count by 30-50%; this may dramatically reverse the signs and symptoms related to cerebral and myocardial ischemia, pulmonary embolism, and gastrointestinal bleeding. Therapeutic plateletpheresis is also useful for reducing the platelet count in severe thrombocytosis with or without vasculitis.[44] It should be noted that spleen size plays an important role in determining the efficacy of this treatment, since mobilization of platelets from the spleen occurs during plateletpheresis.

Physiologic considerations

The clinical application of TPE begins with the consideration of patient age and determination of intravascular volume. Double lumen catheters (7F or larger) are optimal for establishing adequate blood flow to maintain circuit integrity. Smaller children may tolerate the insertion of a 5F catheter for exchange via the femoral vein. TPE catheters can be placed using a sterile field at bedside, eliminating the need for the OR. These non-tunneled catheters are designed for short-term use only and can be used immediately after placement. Bilateral antecubital peripheral access, with 14 gauge catheters in small children, may be insufficient to maintain adequate blood flow due to recurrent obstruction, patient movement and discomfort. The type of priming fluid for the circuit is dependent on the patient age. The typical centrifuge circuit requires 350 cc for priming and has a circuit volume of ~150 cc. The 18 kg child will have ~12% dilution from the circuit, and the circuit may be primed with blood to minimize the dilutional effects of priming. Packed RBCs (PRBCs) will prevent dilution of the hematocrit with anemia or, in some cases, hypovolemia.[45] Smaller children are at greater risk, while larger children (>20 kg) may tolerate priming with colloid. The choice of replacement fluids also varies depending on the diagnosis, indication, and/or institutional protocol. The decision to utilize fresh frozen plasma (FFP) or fractionated human albumin should be made clinically, based on the immunologic, protein, pulmonary, and cardiovascular condition of the child. Crystalloid solutions (e.g., normal saline) and colloid solutions (e.g., albumin or FFP) may be utilized alone or in combination. The risk of transfusion and physiologic complications increases with the use of foreign protein and plasma, but children with unstable or suboptimal physiology often benefit from the use of a combination of FFP and fractionated human albumin. FFP is the replacement of choice if coagulation factors are depleted; however, administration requires immunologic compatibility and carries an increased risk of exposure to foreign protein.

TPE treatments usually take from 1-3 hours once a day or every other day for a period of 3-10 days. The number of treatments is dependent upon patient response and can usually be established by the completion of the first two treatments, as reflected by improved laboratory values and clinical status. Repeated therapies should be cycled with days without TPE to minimize the depletion of healthy circulating cofactors. Coagulation cofactor replacements may be carried out utilizing FFP. Many centers also measure IgG levels and replace accordingly. Careful monitoring of coagulation profiles will document both improvement and depletion of coagulation cofactors.

It is important to calculate the plasma volume to exchange. One blood volume plasma exchange will exchange 63% of the circulating blood volume or toxin. A two blood volume plasma exchange will remove 86%. Single volume exchanges are typically chosen as they are well tolerated and more successful when repeated after an intervening period. Repeated exchanges follow daily and every-other-day profiles. The typical course is 4-7 treatments for sepsis and related immunologic disorders as plasma- and protein-bound substances are readily removed during TPE.

Cardiorespiratory

Acute decreases in preload, changes in peripheral vascular resistance, and alteration of right ventricular compliance may occur both from the exposure to the extracorporeal circuit and volume shifts. The initiation of any extracorporeal circuit must take into consideration the underlying right and left ventricular lusitropic (myocardial relaxation) and inotropic condition, as well as the peripheral vascular resistance. Ventilated patients who are marginally preload-dependent may suffer a decrease in pulmonary blood flow and left ventricular pressure. Patients who exhibit acute intravascular depletion often respond to a decrease in the rate of removal of whole blood, and therapeutic volume boluses. Intravascular depletion often leads to clinical instability in smaller patients. Colloid solutions are routinely given during plasmapheresis. Inotropic support is rarely required, except in septic patients, or those with cardiomyopathies and other conditions with cardiovascular decompensation. Warming of the replacement fluids can help prevent complications such as hypothermia and sickling in susceptible patients. While there is no evidence for a change in pulmonary compliance or gas exchange, sudden changes in peripheral vascular resistance from exposure to foreign surfaces may be seen and are usually amenable to volume infusion. Improvement in left ventricular function[46] has been reported after therapy, with the reduction of circulating mediators, seen more commonly in patients with gram negative sepsis.[47]

Metabolic

The most frequently encountered electrolyte disturbances result from abnormalities in soluble calcium. Hypocalcemia is most frequently seen in patients with severe liver dysfunction, those receiving citrated FFP, or during procedures with a high citrate to blood ratio.[48] The use of relatively large volumes of unwashed blood in small children may precipitate episodes of hyperkalemia, especially with frequent and closely spaced procedures. Depletion of plasma proteins, especially coagulation factors, and immunologic factors may occur if repeated procedures are performed. Prevention and management of hypocalcemia includes administration of oral supplemental calcium or IV calcium (gluconate or chloride). Prolonged manipulation of intravascular volume with plasmapheresis will alter serum pH primarily due to the citrate exposure. Serum proteins will also be reduced unless adequately replaced during or after each procedure. Abnormal liver function with rising liver enzymes may be caused by the primary disease, the procedure, or exposure to citrate. Thus, it is important to monitor pH and serum protein and to follow the reduction of all circulating enzymes during a prolonged course of plasmapheresis.

Hematological

High blood flow rates may create hemolysis if a catheter is too small, twisted, or kinked. Significant hemolysis may precipitate disseminated intravascular coagulation (DIC) or mimic a transfusion reaction. Two examples of commonly used double lumen devices that may maintain high-flow rates during apheresis are the Bard catheter and the 8F Perm-cath (Quinton catheter) hemodialysis catheter. Hemolysis may be detected by monitoring the plasma color.

Monitoring of hemoglobin, hematocrit, platelet count, and coagulation factors such as prothrombin time (PT)/partial thromboplastin time (PTT), fibrinogen, and D-dimer are also essential for evaluation of the hematological status. A decrease in circulating immunoglobulins or coagulation cofactors may be addressed by the infusion of FFP, IgG, fibrinogen, or Factor VII. The importance of maintaining a properly functioning catheter cannot be overstated.

Circuit priming

The fluid status of the patient needs to be carefully evaluated prior to performing plasmapheresis. Typically the goal is to leave the patient in a fluid balance range of no more than 75-125% of calculated baseline. The COBE Spectra Apheresis System (Gambro BCT, Lakewood, CO) default volume level is 100% baseline (no net increase or decrease). Normal saline is commonly utilized for the initial circuit prime. Blood prime may be ordered by the physician. Children <20 kg often require one unit of donor-compatible CMV negative, irradiated, leukodepleted blood to prime the apheresis circuit. The methods of blood priming will be dependent on the physician's evaluation. Blood priming with reconstituted blood is often chosen when the hematocrit is normal or high. Anemic, volume overloaded, or volume-intolerant patients may require PRBCs when priming. Clinically stable children will tolerate either reconstituted blood or PRBCs.

The total volume required to prime a COBE Spectra Apheresis System circuit is 345 cc. The internal continuously circulating volume in the actual circuit is 150 cc. The "rinse-back" volume that is automatically delivered, if requested, is 195 cc. If the operator requests to leave the patient at "100% balance" then the patient will not have a net gain or loss of volume. If a "rinse-back" is requested, the patient will receive a 195 cc bolus after the machine registers the balance programmed, even if "100% balance" has been selected. This will leave the patient 195 cc positive. One should not rinse-back at the end of a procedure unless there is a need to increase the patient's volume. The recorded values can be subtracted from final run values to measure total volume given (Figure 1).

When blood priming with PRBCs, the machine should be programmed with the hematocrit (Hct) of the PRBCs in the banked blood bag. In small children it may be important to maintain the child's blood count. The blood inlet line should be monitored, and when the blood reaches the return saline manifold, the "volume-processed" values are recorded for; anticoagulant, inlet volume, and plasma. This total volume recorded will represent the total blood removed from the child and may be replaced in addition to other calculations if clinically applicable. This value recorded during priming may also be added to the target value of total blood products to be processed to achieve the desired results (Figure 1).

Anticoagulation

Anticoagulation is utilized to minimize clotting of the blood as it travels through the circuit. The most frequently used anticoagulant is citrate. The most commonly used form is acid-citrate-dextrose (ACD-A). Most ACD-A is processed from the circuit when exposed to the calcium in the circuit collection. Each 100 ml of ACD-A contains 2.2 grams sodium citrate hydrous, 730 mg citric acid anhydrous, and 2.45 grams dextrose anhydrous. The infusion rate for anticoagulation is dependent on the total blood volume and type of replacement fluid (ml of anticoagulation/min/l of total blood volume). This flow rate is designed by the Spectra control program to minimize overexposure to citrate. Citrate reactions are primarily related

to acute hypocalcemia but may also include primary acidosis and liver dysfunction. The clinical condition may alternatively require the use of heparin. Heparin binds antithrombin III and blocks the clotting factor activity of VII, IX, X, XI, and XII. The use of heparin requires the monitoring of clotting times. A convenient bedside determination of in vivo clotting is the measurement of an activated clotting time (ACT). An accepted range for ACTs utilizing the I-stat technique is 130-150 seconds. This may be within the "normal" range for blood clotting, as heparin is infused directly into the circuit, performing regional anticoagulation of the circuit and minimizing systemic anticoagulation and its associated complications.

Nursing care of apheresis patients

The patient's and/or family's understanding of the procedure is essential prior to the beginning of apheresis. Providing the patient and family with written materials about the purpose and benefits of the apheresis procedure and allowing time to answer any questions is optimal. Informed consent for the line placement, blood products, and the apheresis procedure is obtained.

Orders to be checked and verified include the type of procedure, type of catheter, site of catheter, type of replacement fluid, volume to be processed, and ending fluid balance. The patient's height, weight, and gender are programmed into the machine. The baseline laboratory tests include a complete blood count, ionized calcium, electrolytes, magnesium, phosphorus, and PT/PTT (if multiple runs are to be performed). Vital signs include EKG, temperature, blood pressure and pulse oximetry. A detailed medication history is required. Patients are monitored during the procedure with continuous cardiac monitoring and pulse oximetry. Blood pressure and heart rate are recorded at least every 15 minutes. Some patients require pre-medication with Solu-Medrol, Benadryl, or sedation. Sedation and pain medication are required for the line placement.

During the treatment the patient must be monitored for signs of hypocalcemia, hypotension, hypothermia, and transfusion reaction. The ionized calcium is repeated 1 hour after starting or midway into the procedure. After the procedure, ionized calcium, CBC, magnesium, and phosphorus are measured. If the patient requires multiple runs, the albumin, total protein, IgG, IgA, coagulation factors and PT/PTT are measured. Plasma- and protein-bound medications may also be removed during apheresis.

A clinical assessment of the patient is performed at the start of every procedure and includes vital signs, neurological status, perfusion,

and catheter site. The date and time of initiation and termination of treatment must be recorded. The effluent, including color or texture, and any mechanical problems during treatment are recorded. Documentation should also include fluid replacement used, any change in patient status during treatment, any intervention, and patient tolerance to treatment. A sample checklist for apheresis is shown (Table 1).

Complications

The Apheresis Program at Miami Children's Hospital began in 1994 and has provided care to more than 180 patients with almost 800 procedures. Complications that required interven-

---

A.

$$\text{Fluid balance} = \frac{(\text{Replacement rate} + \text{AC rate}) \times 100}{\text{Plasma flow rate}}$$

B.

$$\text{Volume of RBC post-dilution} = \frac{(\text{Hct RBC from banked blood bag}) \times (\text{vol. RBC bag})}{\text{Desired Hct for prime}}$$

C.

Volume of diluent to add to PRBC bag = (Total vol. RBC after dilution) - (Initial vol. PRBC bag)

D.

RBCs after dilution = Vol. of diluent − Vol. of initial PRBCs

---

Example:

RBC Hct = 70%
RBC vol. = 220 ml
Desired Hct for prime = 30%

Volume of RBC unit after dilution = (0.70) x (220 ml) = 513 ml
Volume of diluent = (513 ml) - (220 ml) = 293 ml

Add 293 cc fluid to the original unit of PRBCs to achieve desired Hct of 30%

Figure 1. Plasmapheresis calculations. A. Formula to calculate fluid balance; B. Formula for blood priming with reconstituted whole blood to a desired hematocrit; C. Formula for volume of diluent to add to PRBC bag; D. Formula for volume of RBCs after dilution. Note: The diluent may be a combination of FFP, 5% Albumin or Normal Saline. AC = anticoagulant, Hct = hematocrit, PRBC = packed red blood cells, RBC = red blood cells.

tion occurred in 47% of our treatments with one fatality. A summary of the complications encountered is shown in Table 2.

Hypocalcemia is the most frequent complication. The contributing factor is citrate in PRBC, FFP, and ACD-A. The patient may complain of tingling/numbness of lips, fingers or toes, and, at times, they may also feel light-headed or dizzy. In cases of severe hypocalcemia, the patient can develop dysrhythmias. The calcium in the blood binds to ACD, causing gradual depletion of circulating calcium. Electrolytes are monitored before, during, and after each procedure with special emphasis on magnesium, ionized calcium, and potassium levels. For procedures >1 hour, the calcium levels must be monitored every hour until the end of the procedure. The management of hypocalcemia includes slowing down the inlet flow (20 cc/min), sending a stat ionized calcium, and giving calcium replacements such as calcium chloride 10% (20-25 mg/kg/dose) and calcium gluconate (100-500 mg/kg/day continuous drip in 4 divided doses). Calcium gluconate drips can be used for lengthy treatments. For emergent arrhythmias, the procedure is stopped and IV calcium chloride is administered. If the calcium level is within normal limits, the procedure can be resumed with ongoing calcium monitoring. Pre-treatment with oral calcium supplements has decreased the incidence of hypocalcemia.

The etiology of coagulation abnormalities is due first to depletion of coagulation factors removed during TPE, and second to replacement fluids, such as albumin, which do not contain coagulation factors and result in a dilutional effect. Recovery of coagulation factors is characterized by a rapid 4-hour increase and a slow rise in circulating cofactors during the next 24 hours after a single exchange. When multiple treatments are performed over a short period (≥3 treatments/week), the depletion in clotting factors is more pronounced and may require several days for spontaneous recovery.[48] By using FFP as a replacement fluid, the risks of iatrogenic hemodilution of circulating coagulation cofactors can be minimized. There is an increased risk associated with using blood products that should always be considered.[49]

Transfusion reaction

Contributing factors include ABO mismatch (not following blood bank protocol) and multiple transfusions. Prevention includes administration of leukodepleted blood product and pre-medication of sensitive patients. Patients that receive multiple transfusions may be given an antihistamine prior to treatment. When a transfusion reaction occurs, the procedure is discontinued and institutional transfusion reaction protocols are followed. Perfusion should be maintained by giving crystalloids and osmotic diuretics and checking urine for hemolysis.

Thrombocytopenia

This can result from loss of platelets in the discarded plasma during dilution, or via filter thrombosis. There is a greater loss of platelets using the centrifugal method than by membrane plasma separation. Wood and Jacobs[50] have also shown decreases in the hematocrit of 10% after each plasmapheresis treatment in the absence of any extracorporeal losses or hemolysis.

Hypothermia

Contributing factors include the extracorporeal circuit, the use of cool replacement fluids, and patient size. The rapid loss of circulating volume may also cause patients to experience chills or shivering. Preventive measures include using warmed replacement fluids. Slowing down the inlet flow may also improve hypothermia. Comfort measures vary from providing blankets, to use of external warming units. It may also help to warm the infusing replacement fluid using the circuit warmer.

Table 1. Plasmapheresis procedure checklist.

Apheresis Check List

Date: _____   Reviewed by Medical Director:

Patient Name: _____   _____

Account #: _____   *Signature*

                                Date

Apheresis Specialist: _____

Date/Notes	Done	Procedure

		1. Pheresis consult obtained.
		  a. Attending notified.
		  b. Insurance information forwarded to Admitting for approval by referring source.

		2. Appropriate staff notified.
		  a. Fellow on call.
		  b. Nurse Manager/CNS.

		3. Family provided with apheresis brochure.

		4. Pre-apheresis criteria met:
		  a. Informed consent/blood transfusion consent obtained.
		  b. Appropriate labs reviewed and parameters met.
		  c. CBC with diff. (platelets >50,000, Hgb >8, hematocrit >24).
		  d. PT, PTT (<13, ≤35)
		  e. Ionized calcium (≥1.0)
		  f. If patient is <18 kg, complete type and cross match and send to blood bank (request hematocrit on bag).
		  g. EMLA cream applied to catheter site (femoral area).
		  h. Appropriate Quinton catheter ordered.

		5. Insurance verification confirmed by pheresis coordinator.
		6. Labs reviewed by critical care fellow and apheresis specialist (H/H, PT, PTT, ICA). Corrective action taken.

		7. Patient arrives to apheresis treatment area.
		  a) Fellow evaluates patient, (including height [cm], weight [kg], and temperature).
		  b) History/physical assessment done.
		  c) Administer calcium carbonate tablets (Tums 1000 mg).
		  d) Patient/family teaching reinforced. Consent reviewed. Documented in medical record.
		  e) Patient sedated per protocol for procedures.
		  f) Catheter inserted.
		  g) Machine primed and ready for use

		8. Patient's pre-pheresis condition reviewed and documented. Pheresis started.

		9. Notify:
		  a) Community blood center
		  b) Cell Laboratory
		    • Validate packing materials received for integrity, leaks, damage, and breakage.

		10. Reassessment/document (mid-procedure) by fellow and R.N.:
		  a. Sedation status
		  b. Neuro status
		  c. Vital signs
		  d. Treatment yield
		  e. Tolerance to procedure
		  f. Document signs or symptoms of hypocalcemia (tingling, lips quivering, tetany)
		  g. Hemoglobin and hematocrit if RBC exchange

		11. Obtain CD34 with differential.
		12. Product hand-delivered by pheresis specialist to lab.

		13. Patient condition reviewed and documented post-procedure including:
		  a. Sedation status
		  b. Neuro status
		  c. Vital signs
		  d. Treatment yield (amount)
		  e. How patient tolerated procedure

		14. **2 hours post-completion, obtain CBC and ionized CA^+**
		15. Fellow writes transfer orders including approximate time for subsequent treatment and criteria for transfusions if indicated. • Patient kept on bed rest.

Hypotension

Hypotension is often seen at the beginning of the procedure, especially if the patient's blood volume is suddenly depleted or the patient condition is unstable. There may also be a clinically relevant change in the intravascular compliance of some patients at the time that extracorporeal flow is initiated. This may manifest as a decrease in peripheral vascular resistance. Patients on inotropic support are at higher risk. Reducing the inlet flow will decrease the rate of volume depletion and may correct the problem. Fluid and inotropic boluses may also be given to the patient through the circuit, and the rate of inotropic infusion increased.

Apheresis specialist training and competencies

We recommend that individuals be certified as apheresis specialists upon successful completion of the following:

Didactic: The apheresis specialist will attend 32 hours of didactic lectures. Upon completion, a written test will be given and a passing score of 85% must be achieved.

Water Labs: The apheresis specialist will complete 8 hours of supervised water lab training plus a final test on emergency drills. This does not include individual practice sessions, which are required in order to pass the final test. These practice hours will vary according to the individual's skill level but will not be less than 4 hours.

Clinical Orientation: The apheresis specialist will complete a minimum of 36 hours of clinical orientation. Upon completion of these hours, the skills checklists will be reviewed by the nurse manager and ECMO Coordinator. If any skill requirements have not been met, further bedside orientation may be warranted.

Re-certification: Emergency water lab check-off is required four times annually. Didactic and/or practical continuing education in the form of lectures, workshops, or animal laboratory experience will consist of not less than 8 hours per year.

Family-centered care

Family-centered care is an integrated system of resources designed to meet patient and family needs and promote involvement of the family in the patient's hospitalization. A brief orientation to answer questions and set realistic goals and expectations is scheduled during the pre-treatment phase. The focus is on the family's individual needs, providing clinical information, supplemental teaching, and support while the patient is receiving treatment. Family members are encouraged to get involved and actively participate in the patient care.

The staff, in collaboration with the child life service, provides distractions and entertains the pediatric patient during treatment or painful procedures. Board games, television viewing, and reading materials are available. The healthcare team in the ICU and apheresis program provides reassurance and comfort, as well as reinforcing the treatment regimen and protocols to the family and patient.

Planned maintenance, calibration testing, and procedures for equipment failure

The performance of all medical equipment is tested according to standards set by the clinical engineering department. A planned maintenance

Table 2. Plasmapheresis complications requiring treatment.

Complications	Patients treated (%)
Hypotension	5.6%
Hypertension	3.5%
Hypocalcemia	11%
Nausea, vomiting, tachycardia,	6.2%
Other (e.g., hematoma, pneumo-/hemothorax, retroperitoneal bleed, infection, thrombosis)	<1%

program including calibration testing that assures the precision and longevity of the system must be established by the clinical engineering department in collaboration with the apheresis section. All calibration and maintenance testing is based on the recommendation of the manufacturer.

Summary

The intuitive concept of separating blood and providing therapeutic adjustments to benefit the patient has been explored throughout medical history. Diagnostic and technical advances in overall care are now focusing on plasmapheresis and the subsequently manipulation of patients who have some pathologic alteration in their immune system or immune response. This chapter primarily reviews the application and technique of pediatric plasmapheresis with an overview of the full spectrum of apheresis techniques and applications.

References

1. Kambic HE, Nose Y. Historical perspective on plasmapheresis. *Ther Apher* 1997; 1:83-108.
2. Friday J, Kaplan A. Indications for therapeutic plasma exchange. Available at www.uptodateonline.com. Accessed January 13, 2005.
3. Madore F. Plasmapheresis: technical aspects and indications. *Crit Care Clin* 2002; 8:375-392.
4. Pisani E. Regulatory framework for plasmapheresis in the European Union: industry's viewpoint. *Hematol Cell Ther* 1996, 38 Suppl 1:S35-38.
5. Clark WF, Rock GA, Buskard N, et al. Therapeutic plasma exchange: An update from the Canadian Apheresis Group. *Ann Int Med* 1999; 131:453-462.
6. Linenberger ML, Price TH. Use of cellular and plasma apheresis in the critically-ill patient: Part 1: technical and physiological considerations. *J Int Care Med* 2005; 20:18-27.
7. Kellum JA, Venkataraman R. Blood purification in sepsis: an idea whose time has come. *Crit Care Med* 2002; **30**:1387–1388.
8. The sudden death of Patsy Dustis, or George Washington on sudden unexplained death in epilepsy. *Epilepsy Behav* 2004; 5:598-600.
9. Malchesky PS, Sueoka A, Matsubara S, et al. Membrane plasma separation. 1983. *Therapeutic Apheresis* 2000; 4:47-53.
10. Yeh JH, Chen WH, Chiu HC. Complications of double-filtration plasmapheresis. *Transfusion* 2004; 44:1621-1625.
11. Unger JK, Haltern C, Dohmen B, et al. Maximal flow rates and sieving coefficients in different plasmafilters: effects of increased membrane surfaces and effective length under standardized in vitro conditions. *J Clin Apheresis* 2002; 17:190-198.
12. Gurland HJ, Lysaght MJ, Samtleben W, et al. A comparison of centrifugal and membrane-based apheresis formats. *Int J Artif Org* 1984; 7:35-38.
13. DePalo T, Giordano M, Bellantuono, et al. Therapeutic apheresis in children. *Int J Artif Org* 2000; 23:834-839.
14. Singer Al, Olthoff KM, Kim H. Role of plasmapheresis on the management of acute hepatic failure in children. *Ann Surg* 2001; 234:418-424.
15. Kawaguchi N, Kuwabara S, Nemoto Y, et al. The Study Group for Myasthenia Gravis in Japan. Treatment and outcome of myasthenia gravis: retrospective multicenter analysis of 470 Japanese patients, 1999-2000. *J Neurol Sci* 2004; 224:43-47.
16. Rock G, Buskard NA. Therapeutic plasmapheresis. *Curr Opin Hematol* 1996; 3:504-510.
17. Nenov VD, Marinov P, Sabeva J. Current applications of plasmapheresis in clinical

toxicology. *Nephrol Dial Transp* 2003; 18 Suppl 5:56-58.

18. Pond SM. Extracorporeal techniques in the treatment of poisoned patients. *Med J Aust* 1991; 155:62-63.

19. Motohashi K, Yamane S. The effect of apheresis on adhesion molecules. *Ther Apher Dial* 2003; 7:425-430.

20. Pisani BA, Mullen GM, Malinowska K, et al. Plasmapheresis with intravenous immunoglobulin G is effective in patients with elevated panel reactive antibody prior to cardiac transplantation. *J Heart Lung Transplant* 1999; 18:701-706.

21. Warren DS, Zachary AA, Sonnenday CJ, et al. Successful renal transplantation across simultaneous ABO incompatible and positive crossmatch barriers. *Am J Transp* 2004; 4:561-568.

22. Abraham KA, Brown C, Conlon PJ, et al. Plasmapheresis as rescue therapy in accelerated acute humoral rejection. *J Clin Apheresis* 2003; 18:103-110.

23. Debray D, Furlan V, Baudoouin V, et al. Therapy for acute rejection in pediatric organ transplant recipients. *Pediatr Drugs* 2003; 5:81-93.

24. Vain NE, Maziumian JR, Swarner W, Cha CC. Role of exchange transfusion in the treatment of severe septicemia. *Pediatrics* 1980; 66:693-697.

25. Busund R, Lindsetmo RO, Rasmussen LT, Rokke O, Rekvig OP, Revhaug A. Tumor necrosis factor and interleukin 1 appearance in experimental gram-negative septic shock. The effects of plasma exchange with albumin and plasma infusion. *Arch Surg* 1991; 126:591-597.

26. Gardlund B, Sjolin J, Nilsson A, et al. Plasma levels of cytokines in primary septic shock in humans: correlation with disease severity. *J Inf Dis* 1995; 172:296–301.

27. Stegmayr B. Plasmapheresis in severe sepsis or septic shock. Blood Purif 1996; 14:94–101.

28. McMaster P, Shann F. The use of extracorporeal techniques to remove humoral factors in sepsis. *Ped Crit Care Med* 2003; 4:2-7.

29. Busund R, Koukline V, Utrobin U, et al. E Plasmapheresis in severe sepsis and septic shock: a prospective, randomised, controlled trial. *Int Care Med* 2002; 28:1434-1439.

30. Klemmer PJ, Chalermskulrat W, Reif MS, et al. Plasmapheresis therapy for diffuse alveolar hemorrhage in patients with small-vessel vasculitis. *Am J Kid Dis* 2003; 42:1149-1153.

31. Dyck PJ, Daube J, O'Brien P, et al. Plasma exchange in chronic inflammatory demyelinating polyradiculoneuropathy. *N Engl J Med* 1986; 314:461-465.

32. Jansen PW, Perkin RM, Ashwal S. Guillian-Barre syndrome in childhood: natural course and efficacy of plasmapheresis. *Ped Neurol* 1993; 9:16-20.

33. Toyka KV, Hartung HP. Chronic Inflammatory polyneuritis and neuropathies. *Curr Opin Neurol* 1996; 9:240-250.

34. Rock GA, Shumak KH, Buskard NA, et al. Comparison of plasma exchange with plasma infusion in the treatment of thrombotic thrombocytopenia purpura. *N Engl J Med*, 1991; 325:393-397.

35. Nguyen TC, Stegmayr B, Busund R, et al. Plasma therapies in thrombotic syndromes. *Int J Artif Organs* 2005; 28:459-465.

36. Madore F. Plasmapheresis. Technical aspects and indications. *Crit Care Clinics* 2002; 18:375-392.

37. Felson DT, LaValley MP, Baldassare AR, et al. The Prosorba column for the treatment of refractory rheumatoid arthritis: a randomized double-blind, sham-controlled trial. *Arthritis Rheum* 1999; 42:2153-2159.

38. Aoki H, Kodama M, Tani T, et al. Treatment of sepsis by extracorporeal elimination of endotoxin using polymyxin B-immobilized fiber. *Am J Surg* 1994; 167:412–417.

39. Valbonesi M, Bruni R. Clinical application of therapeutic erythrocytapheresis (TEA). *Transfusion Science* 2000; 22:183-194.

40. Kessinger A, Armitage JO, Landmark JD, et al. Reconstitution of human hematopoietic function with autologous cryopreserved circulating stem cells. *Exp Hematol* 1986; 14:192-196.

41. Gorlin JB. Therapeutic plasma exchange and cytapheresis in pediatric patients. *Transfus Sci* 1999; 21:21-39.

42. Urbaniak SJ. Therapeutic plasma and cellular apheresis. *Clin Haematol* 1984; 13:217-251.

43. Grima KM. Therapeutic apheresis in hematological and oncological diseases. *J Clin Apheresis* 2000; 15:28-52.

44. Hamblin T, Oscier D. Polyarteritis presenting with thrombocytosis and palliated by plasma exchange. *Postgrad Med J* 1978; 54:615-617.

45. Kliman A, Carbone PP, Gaydos LA, et al. Effects of intensive plasmapheresis on normal blood donors. *Blood* 1964; 23:647-656.

46. Pahl E, Crawford SE, Cohn RA, et al. Reversal of severe late left ventricular failure after pediatric heart transplantation and possible role of Plasmapheresis. *Am J Cardiol* 2000; 85:735-739.

47. Berlot G, Tomasini A, Silvestri L, et al. Plasmapheresis in the critically ill patient. *Kidney Int Suppl* 1998; 66:S178-181.

48. Baldini GM, Silvestri MG. Quality assurance in hemapheresis: quality of fresh frozen plasma. *Int J Artif Organs* 1993; 16 Suppl 5:226-228.

49. Strauss RG. Apheresis donor safety--changes in humoral and cellular immunity. *J Clin Apheresis* 1984; 2:68-80.

50. Wood L, Jacobs P. The effect of serial therapeutic plasma pheresis on platelet count, coagulation factors, plasma immunoglobulin, and complement levels. *J Clin Apher* 1986; 3:124-128.

40

Carbon Dioxide Removal Devices; Intracorporeal Membrane Oxygenation and Artificial Lungs

James E. Lynch, R.R.T., Thomas D. Black, B.S., Brittany B. DeBerry, M.D., Scott K. Alpard, M.S., and Joseph B. Zwischenberger M.D.

Introduction

The primary goal of respiratory support is to minimize the requirement for high tidal volumes and airway pressures, and provide "lung rest". ECMO provides near total gas exchange (for both oxygen and CO_2) in infants and adults;[1-3] however, application of this technology involves significant blood-surface interactions that may exacerbate lung injury.[3,4] In addition, ECMO is extremely labor-intensive, time-limited, and costly, requiring expensive equipment and a highly trained team. In this chapter, we will discuss the functional properties and management techniques of CO_2 removal and intracorporeal membrane oxygenation, as well as look into the future of long-term gas exchange devices.

AVCO$_2$R

Recent trends in ventilator management limit inflation pressures and tidal volume (TV) often at the cost of increasing systemic arterial CO_2 levels. This technique, often called permissive hypercapnia, has been shown to reduce the baro/volutrauma and the need for high airway pressures and ultimately to improve survival in acute respiratory distress syndrome (ARDS).[5-10] Unfortunately, permissive hypercapnia is accompanied by respiratory acidosis causing substantial changes in hemodynamics and organ blood flow unless the arterial pH is controlled.[6,11]

Investigations into extracorporeal CO_2 removal (ECCO$_2$R) began in the late 1970s. Kolobow and Gattinoni introduced ECCO$_2$R using a modified form of ECMO with venovenous (VV) perfusion.[12-14] Their focus was CO_2 removal, allowing for a reduction in ventilatory support. Oxygenation was maintained by simple diffusion across the patient's alveoli, called apneic oxygenation, using low-frequency positive pressure ventilation. Unfortunately, the ECCO$_2$R system required all of the components of a standard ECMO circuit. Studies in animals[12,13] and humans[15-17] demonstrated the effectiveness of ECCO$_2$R in reducing ventilatory requirements. Despite the early success with ECCO$_2$R, a small, randomized study conducted at a single center comparing ECCO$_2$R with mechanical ventilation showed no difference in mortality.[18] While the results of this study were disappointing, other investigators began to look for simple CO_2 removal devices that would offer the benefits of gentle ventilation without all of the risks of ECMO or ECCO$_2$R.

The use of a simple arteriovenous (AV) shunt for extracorporeal gas exchange significantly reduces the complexity of conventional ECMO, yet allows sufficient gas exchange to achieve near total CO_2 removal. By reducing and eliminating circuit length and complexity, a number of complications associated with conventional ECMO are eliminated.[19] The use of an AV shunt with fewer circuit components allows for less monitoring, avoidance of the extracorporeal pump, substantially lower cost, and improves safety when compared to conventional ECMO. Barthelemy et al.[20] in a sheep model used a pumpless AV extracorporeal system in combination with apneic oxygenation to satisfy all the gas exchange requirements for up to 24 hours using a 2 m² hollow fiber oxygenator. Subsequently, Awad et al.[21] placed membrane oxygenators designed for CPB in an AV shunt in healthy dogs and sheep for up to 7 days. The animals tolerated the shunt with no alteration in hemodynamics. Extracorporeal was stable throughout the study. Young et al.[22] used a large membrane oxygenator with a surface area of 5 m² in an AV shunt in healthy sheep to achieve CO_2 removal. The resistance from the tubing and the oxygenator was the limiting factor for the gas exchange, although significant CO_2 removal was seen even at low blood flow. In all the studies described, AV flow rates were limited by circuit resistance. The mean arterial pressure (MAP) was between 120-130 mm Hg, and the pressure gradient across the device was >30 mm Hg.

The group at Galveston developed a technique of simplified extracorporeal AV CO_2 removal ($AVCO_2R$) with a new generation commercially available, low-resistance, hollow fiber gas exchanger to provide lung rest in the setting of severe respiratory failure.[23] The extremely low resistance of the $AVCO_2R$ gas exchange device (<10 mm Hg pressure difference) allows blood flow of as much as 25% of the animal's cardiac output (>1,300 ml/min). The cannulas used determined flow rates and are small in comparison to that which would be required for a typical adult ECMO patient (12F arterial, 16F venous). Groin access to the common femoral artery and femoral vein are the preferred routes of vascular access using $AVCO_2R$. Commercially available kits allow for percutaneous insertion of these small cannulas. The priming volume of the circuit is only 200 ml and given this volume crystalloid priming is performed, avoiding the need for the blood priming.

In adult sheep (~35 kg), as shunt blood flow (Qb) was increased with sweep gas flow (Qg) held constant at 3 l/min, a proportional increase in CO2 extraction was seen until Qb reached 1,000 ml/min. At this point CO2 removal plateaued at 112 ±3 ml/min (Figure 1). Similarly, CO2 removal increased proportionally with increasing Qg flow when Qb was held constant (Figure 2). The maximum Qg/Qb ratio was 2:1, and the pressure gradient across the device was <10 mm Hg throughout the experiment. Minute ventilation (MV) could be gradually decreased as Qb was increased. At maximal Qb (1417 +26 ml/min), MV was reduced from 6.9 ±0.8 l/min to 1.3 ±0.5 l/min (16% baseline) while maintaining normocapnia. At this maximal reduction in ventilator support, changes in PaCO2 were monitored while Qb was incrementally diminished. Hypercapnia was observed only at a flow rate of <500 ml/min (Figure 3). AVCO2R

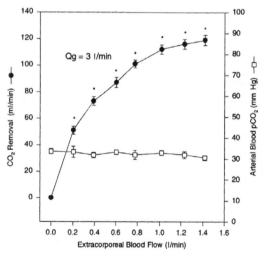

Figure 1. Proportional increase in CO_2 removal as $AVCO_2R$ flow increases from 0 ml/min at baseline to 1,417 ±26 ml/min. Sweep gas flow held constant at 3,000 ml/min. Normocapnia is maintained with PaCO₂ <40 mm Hg (P<0.01 vs. baseline).

proved to be capable of removing as much as 96% of total CO2 production. Reduction of ventilator support to 16% of baseline MV was possible while maintaining normal PaCO2. At flows of <500 ml/min, moderate hypercapnia (40-70 mmHg) occurred, but it was well tolerated without adverse hemodynamic effects.24

To compare pressure/flow characteristics of commercially available percutaneous vascular cannulas, different sizes of percutaneous cannulas used clinically were evaluated to allow adequate flow (800-1,100 ml/min) yet minimize vessel damage, especially to the femoral artery. The evaluation yielded a family of curves which allow size matching to achieve the desired flow for a targeted CO_2 removal. The blood flow during $AVCO_2R$ depends on three variables: 1) device resistance, 2) the pressure gradient between the arterial and venous systems, and 3) cannula resistance. The effect of venous resistance was minimized by using venous cannulas that were four F sizes larger than their paired arterial cannula. Percutaneous arterial cannulas that are ≥12F allow sufficient flow for maintaining normocapnia in adults.[25] Small adults and children tolerate proportionately smaller cannula. Ultrasound imaging can estimate the size of cannula the vessel can safely accommodate. A cannula with a transverse diameter ≤½-inch the size of the native vessel is recommended. Using this technique and systemic heparinization, distal limb ischemia has not been seen.[24]

To evaluate the effect of $AVCO_2R$ on ventilator requirements during ARDS, an ovine model of severe respiratory failure was created to reliably produce a LD 50 smoke inhalation injury.[19] This acute, 6-hour study attempted to determine the support possible using the $AVCO_2R$ device. No significant changes in hemodynamic variables were observed following shunt installation even with Qb through the $AVCO_2R$ device varying between 25-29% of cardiac output. As MV was reduced hourly during the study to achieve lung rest, CO_2 removal gradually increased to a maximum of 111 ±4 ml/min, accounting for 96% of total CO_2 production (121 ±9 ml/min). This allowed for significant reductions in ventilator support. These changes

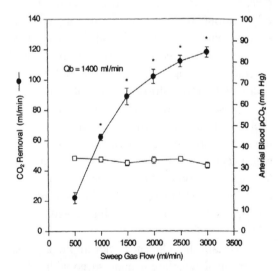

Figure 2. Proportional increase in CO_2 removal as sweep gas flow increases from 500-3,000 ml/min. $AVCO_2R$ flow held constant at 1.4 l/min. Normocapnia is maintained with $PaCO_2$ <40 mm Hg (P<0.01 vs. baseline).

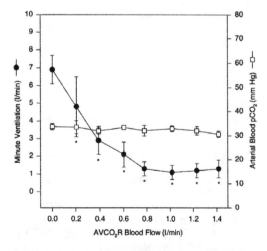

Figure 3. Reduction in MV during $AVCO_2R$. MV reduced from 6.9 ±0.8 l/min to 1.3 ±0.5 l/min as $AVCO_2R$ flow increased from 0 l/min at baseline to 1,417 ±26 l/min at maximal unimpeded flow while maintaining normocapnia (P<0.05 vs. baseline).

are shown in Figure 4. MV was decreased by 95% and peak inspiratory pressure (PIP) decreased by 52%, while $PaCO_2$ remains normal. Based on these short-term studies, $AVCO_2R$ appeared to be simple and effective in achieving lung rest.

Patients with ARDS are often hemodynamically unstable with a tendency toward a hypodynamic or hyperdynamic state.[26,27] To investigate the effect of long-term $AVCO_2R$ on hemodynamic variables in an ARDS model, adult sheep were subjected to a severe smoke inhalation injury.[28] $AVCO_2R$ was used to provide total CO_2 removal to evaluate the effects of sustained $AVCO_2R$ flow on critical

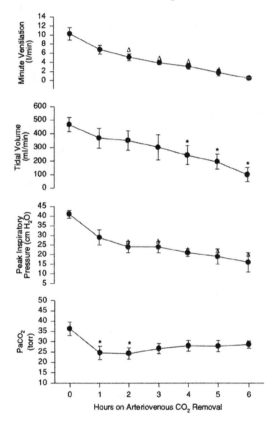

Figure 4. Reduction in MV, TV, and PIP during $AVCO_2R$. MV reduced from 10.3 ±1.4 l/min to 0.5 ±0 L/min at 6 hr. on $AVCO_2R$ while maintaining normocapnia; similarly, TV significantly reduced from 467 ±53 ml/min at baseline to 102 ±52 ml/min. With reductions in MV and TV, PIP was significantly reduced from 40.8 ±2.1 cm H_2O at baseline to 19.7 ±7.5 cm H_2O at 6 hr. on $AVCO_2R$ (P<0.05 and ΔP<0.01 vs. baseline).

hemodynamic variables over a 7 day period. This study confirmed that there was no hemodynamic instability; heart rate (HR), cardiac output (CO), MAP, pulmonary artery pressure (PAP), or Qb despite a 20-26% cardiac shunt through the $AVCO_2R$ circuit for 7 days remained stable.

However, $AVCO_2R$ does not provide substantial oxygen transfer when the arterial PaO_2 level is adequate because inflow to the device is already saturated (>90%) with a close to maximal oxygen carrying capacity. There is a small amount of oxygen transfer (<10%) and some benefit related to the increased oxygen content of the mixed venous blood reaching the pulmonary precapillary bed, which may alter the normal vasoconstrictive response to local hypoxia with reduction in the pulmonary shunt.[28]

Redistribution of blood flow, with decreased blood flow to muscles and skin, and preserved blood flow to the brain and heart has been observed in a high-shunt, high-output cardiac failure model in conscious rats.[29] Colored microspheres were used in a conscious sheep model to evaluate the effect of $AVCO_2R$ on regional organ/tissue perfusion at varying levels of shunt flow.[30] Overall, there was no evidence of adverse hemodynamic effect throughout the study despite a ≤25% AV shunt. Even though organ blood flow, expressed as a percent of the baseline measurement, showed no statistically significant differences, a modest alteration in flow distribution was noted. The vital organs, especially the brain, renal cortex, gut, and skeletal muscle sustained a mild reduction in end organ perfusion. In this study, the conscious animal, with intact autoregulatory mechanisms, was able to maintain blood flow to all critical organs (brain, heart, kidney, and mesentery) within 20% of baseline perfusion, despite an AV shunt equal to 25% of the resting CO.

To establish a clinically relevant model of severe respiratory failure in adult sheep with a 40% total body surface area (TBSA) full thickness cutaneous flame burn, and smoke inhalation injury, we developed a model of predictable severity based on the number (dose) of smoke breaths administered

(Figure 5).[31] Using the combined smoke inhalation injury and cutaneous burn model of severe respiratory failure, we evaluated percutaneous $AVCO_2R$ and its effect on ventilator-dependent days and survival. When animals met entry criteria for ARDS with PaO_2/FiO_2 <200 within 40-48 hours of injury, they were randomized to either $AVCO_2R$ or control. With percutaneous $AVCO_2R$ removing 90% of the CO_2 produced, significant reductions were possible in MV (13-1.6 l/min), TV (450-270 ml), PIP (25-14 cm H_2O), respiratory rate (RR) (25-16 breaths/min), and FiO_2 (0.86-0.34) while normocapnia was maintained. Along with the decreased ventilatory requirements associated with $AVCO_2R$, there was also a concomitant improvement in arterial oxygenation (Figure 6). The PaO_2/FiO_2 ratio improved to >300 by 72 hours. $AVCO_2R$ animals were weaned from mechanical ventilation three times earlier than control survivors (2.4 days of mechanical ventilation vs. 6.2 days, respec-

tively). All animals receiving $AVCO_2R$ and only 3 in the control group survived the 7-day study (Figure 7).

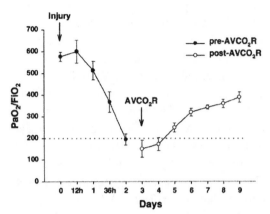

Figure 6. PaO_2/FiO_2 ratio (P/F) following smoke inhalation and cutaneous flame burn injury following placement of $AVCO_2R$. Entry criteria (P/F <200) were met at 48 hr. (194.8 ±25.9). At the time $AVCO_2R$ was initiated P/F was 151.5 ±40.0. After 36 hr., P/F had improved to >200 and after 72 hr. P/F was >300 (320.0 ±17.8).

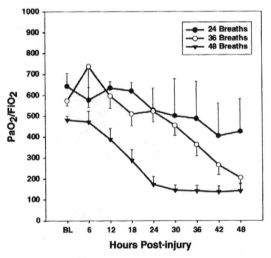

Figure 5. PaO_2/FiO_2 ratio (P/F) in sheep following smoke inhalation and cutaneous flame burn injury. Severe respiratory failure (SRF) = P/F <200. No animal in the 24 breath/40% TBSA III° cutaneous flame burn group met clinical criteria for SRF (P/F <200). All the animals in the 36 breath/40% TBSA III° cutaneous flame burn group met clinical criteria for SRF (P/F <200) within 48 hr. following injury. All the animals in the 48 breath/40% TBSA III° cutaneous flame burn group developed SRF within 24-36 hr.

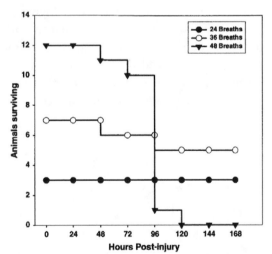

Figure 7. Kaplan-Meier curve depicting the number of sheep surviving the 7-day (168 hr.) study. All the sheep in the 24 breath/40% TBSA III° cutaneous flame burn group survived to 7 days. 5 of 7 sheep (71.4%) in the 36 breath/40% TBSA III° cutaneous flame burn group survived to 7 days (LD30). None of the sheep in the 48 breath/40% TBSA III° cutaneous flame burn group survived to 7 days. Only 1 sheep receiving 48 breaths of cotton smoke survived to day 4.

Clinical trials

In our initial clinical experience with AVCO$_2$R,[32] 5 patients were treated for ARDS and CO$_2$ retention at the University of Texas Medical Branch (UTMB) and the Louisiana State University Medical Center (LSUMC). Feasibility and safety of AVCO$_2$R placed by percutaneous femoral cannulation (10-12F arterial and 12-15F venous) was evaluated in a 72-hour trial. Mean AVCO$_2$R flow at 24, 48, and 72 hours was 837.4 $\pm$73.9 ml/min, 873 $\pm$83.6 ml/min, and 750 $\pm$104.5 ml/min, respectively. There were no vascular complications or significant change in HR or MAP. AVCO$_2$R proved capable of removing a maximum of 208 ml/min of CO$_2$ at a Qb of 1086 ml/min. This allowed a decrease in MV from 7.2 $\pm$2.3 l/min, at baseline, to 3.4 $\pm$0.8 l/min at 24 hours. PaCO$_2$ at baseline was 93.6 $\pm$9.0 mm Hg and upon initiation of AVCO$_2$R decreased to 69.0 $\pm$10.0 mm Hg. AVCO$_2$R removed ~70% of total CO$_2$ production over the 72 hours of the study (Figure 8). Oxygenation was successfully managed with gentle ventilation and near-apneic oxygenation. All patients survived the procedure without adverse sequelae and only minor complications. This initial study demonstrated that percutaneous AVCO$_2$R can support ~70% CO$_2$ removal in adults with ARDS and CO$_2$ retention without hemodynamic compromise or instability.

The success of these early studies has led to a steady increase in the number of AVCO$_2$R cases, termed pumpless extracorporeal lung assist (PECLA) in Europe. The European experience with PECLA includes well over 500 patients, and while the early data seems promising with >70% survival[33] no large, randomized trials have been performed. The PECLA circuit utilizes a hollow fiber gas exchanger (Novalung, Jostra, Hirrlingen, Germany) with excellent gas exchange and performance characteristics which is not yet Food and Drug Administration (FDA) approved (Figure 9).

Intravenacaval oxygenation and CO$_2$ removal with the intravascular oxygenator

The concept of an intravenacaval (intravascular) oxygenation (IVOX) and CO$_2$ removal device was originally conceived by Mortensen as an intracorporeal gas exchange device in

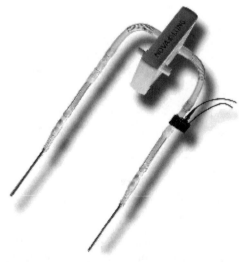

Figure 9. The symmetrical lung assist device is shown with 2 low resistance cannulas attached. The system's low pressure gradient allows use without a mechanical blood pump in an AV shunt created between the femoral artery and vein. (From: Matheis G, *Perfusion* 2003, 18:245-251, with permission.)

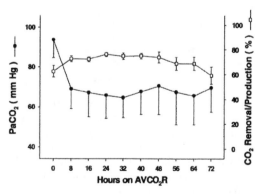

Figure 8. CO$_2$ removal with AVCO$_2$R. At baseline, PaCO$_2$ was 93.6 $\pm$9.0 mm Hg and decreased 69.0 $\pm$10.0 mm Hg on initiation of AVCO$_2$R. AVCO$_2$R removed approximately 70% of total CO$_2$ production throughout the 72-hour study.

patients with ARDS.[34,35] The IVOX consisted of multiple hollow fibers placed within the vena cava to provide oxygenation and CO_2 removal without the need for extracorporeal circulation (Figure 10). The fibers were joined together in a potted manifold that communicated with the dual lumen gas conduit at both its proximal and distal ends. The fibers were silicone-coated (Siloxone, Applied Membrane Technology Inc., Minnetonka, MN) and heparin-bonded to create a thin, "true" membrane on the previously porous hollow fibers.

The group at Galveston initially tested the IVOX for safety and efficacy and reported its experimental and clinical use.[36-39] The IVOX was initially tested in an ovine model to describe the design features and to delineate the experimental and potential clinical use. Implantation of the device did not adversely affect hemodynamic function, nor was there evidence of significant hemolysis, thromboembolism, blood foaming, catheter migration, or venacaval intimal injury. The significant reduction in foreign surface area as compared to ECMO resulted in fewer blood surface interactions as evidenced by reduced pulmonary leukosequestration and complement activation.[37] In the initial design, IVOX was capable of removing up to 30% of CO_2 production in an ovine model of severe smoke inhalation injury. The average CO_2 exchange was approximately 40 ml/min for size 7 IVOX and ranged from 30-55 ml/min. This represented ~30% of the CO_2 production of an adult sheep (150-180 ml/min).

Prior to implantation of the IVOX in humans, the vascular access site is evaluated for size and patency with Doppler ultrasound. The IVOX is passed into the vena cava over a guide wire utilizing fluoroscopy to ensure proper position. Prior to insertion, the patient is bolused with heparin followed by a continuous infusion to maintain the activated clotting time (ACT) at 200-250 seconds or partial thromboplastin (PT) time at 80-90 seconds. A vacuum pump draws 100% oxygen into the device and the exhaust gas is analyzed for CO_2 concentration by a capnometer using the formula:

$$CO_2 \text{ removal (ml/min)} = Q \times [CO_2],$$

where Q is the gas flow through the IVOX (ml/min) and $[CO_2]$ is the CO_2 concentration in the exhaust gas (%).

Estimation of oxygen transfer utilizing the exhaust gas required sophisticated techniques such as mass spectrometry, and results were highly variable. In clinical practice, oxygen transfer was estimated by measuring the changes in mixed venous oxygen saturation with the IVOX on vs. a brief period with the IVOX off:

$$O_2 \text{ transfer (ml/min)} = 0.134 \times Hgb \times CO \times SvO_2 \text{ (IVOXon} - \text{IVOXoff)} \times 10$$

where Hgb is hemoglobin concentration, CO is cardiac output, and SvO_2 is mixed venous oxygen saturation. Although easy to use, this method generated somewhat inaccurate results. Any minor change in CO, blood shunting in the superior or inferior vena cava, shunting through the natural lungs, instability in metabolism, or respiration compensation led to errors. These errors were caused by changes in blood oxygen and CO_2 concentrations between the time

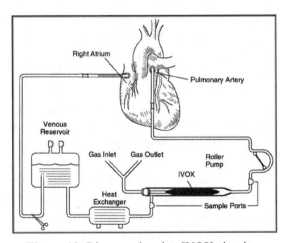

Figure 10. Diagram showing IVOX circuit.

points of IVOXon and IVOXoff.[40] A more precisely controlled bypass circuit would have been required for quantitative analysis of such an intravenacaval device.[41,42]

The performance of the IVOX was limited in comparison to native pulmonary function.[36] The IVOX in animal and human studies demonstrated an average of 40 ml/min of CO_2 and oxygen exchange, ~25-30% of the metabolic demand of the patients receiving the implanted device.[37,38] Therefore, IVOX could not be used as a substitute for ECMO to provide total support for patients with acute respiratory failure (ARF).

An international, multi-center phase I-II clinical trial of IVOX was conducted in major critical care centers in the U.S. and Europe.[43] Between 1990-93, 164 IVOX devices were utilized in 160 patients for temporary augmentation of gas exchange. These patients had developed severe but potentially reversible ARF. Basic entry criteria for the study in the U.S. and Europe were similar: mechanical ventilation for >24 hours; $PO_2 \leq 60$ mm Hg on $FiO_2 \geq 0.5$ with $PEEP \geq 10$ cm H_2O, and $pCO_2 > 40$ mm Hg with $MV \geq 150$ ml/kg/min.

All patients were adults and selected for IVOX implantation for ARF due to a variety of causes including pneumonia, trauma, sepsis, and ARDS. The right femoral or right jugular vein was used as a site for insertion. Oxygen and CO_2 exchange by IVOX was calculated by the formula previously described. The amount of oxygen transfer and CO_2 removal varied

Table 1. IVOX gas exchange in patients with ARDS.

Size (mm)	Surface area (m^2)	Fibers (no.)	O_2 Transfer*	CO_2 Removal*
7	0.21	589	40.3	43.8
8	0.32	703	45.6	60.2
9	0.41	894	54.2	60.1
10	0.52	1,107	72.5	71.0

*Average gas exchange of IVOX (ml/min) during severe respiratory failure in the controlled international multi-center trial.

from ~40-70 ml/min depending on the size of the implanted device (Table 1). Use of IVOX resulted in immediate blood gas improvement in the majority of patients, which allowed ventilator settings to be reduced. FiO_2, PEEP, mean or peak airway pressure, and MV were decreased by >10% in >60% of patients and by >25% in >40% of patients. Although overall survival of reported patients receiving IVOX was only 30%, survival was directly related to the severity of lung injury and patient selection. Patients with an increasing severity of lung injury or pulmonary malfunction, as indicated by Murray score, oxygenation index (OI), or intrapulmonary shunt had a lower survival. Unfortunately, there was no control arm to this study to evaluate effect of IVOX on survival. Complications or adverse events included mechanical and/or performance problems, patient complications (bleeding, thrombosis, infection, venous occlusion, arrhythmia), and user errors. Seven severe adverse events occurred in 4 patients and may have contributed to their death. These complications reflected the learning curve seen with new invasive devices.

Several publications resulted from investigators participating in the IVOX collective trial. Gentilello et al.[44] treated 9 adult patients with ARF for a mean duration of 5.6 days. Mean CO_2 removal by IVOX (sizes 7-10) was 40-51 ml/min. Although application of IVOX was associated with an increase in PaO_2 and decrease in $PaCO_2$, the quantity of gas transfer was not sufficient to allow a reduction in PEEP, FiO_2, or MV. In 5 patients with ARDS, High et al.[45] showed that IVOX could only achieve a maximum of 29% of total gas exchange allowing small reductions in ventilatory support. Jurmann et al.[46] implanted IVOX in 3 patients with severe respiratory failure and demonstrated partial gas exchange support and a moderate reduction in ventilator settings. In their experience with 8 patients, Kallis et al.[46] achieved an average of 58 (40-106) ml/min of CO_2 removal and 85 (68-140) ml/min of oxygen transfer in 8 patients. Conrad et al.[48] treated 2 patients with size 9 and 10 IVOX which transferred 43-92 ml/min of oxygen and 33-86 ml/min of CO_2 and achieved a significant reduction in FiO_2 and MV in both patients. In an adult patient with extended use of IVOX, von Segesser et al.[49] showed an increased PaO_2 that allowed a reduction in PEEP and FiO_2 together with improved hemodynamic function.

Based on the worldwide experience to date, IVOX demonstrated feasibility as a "booster" lung in patients with ARF. IVOX gas exchange is able to support 30% of the metabolic demands of the patient and allows a measurable reduction in ventilator settings. However, improvements in design and engineering are needed in order for IVOX to become a more clinically applicable device.

Lessons learned from the IVOX

Mathematical modeling of IVOX

A detailed mathematical model was developed to analyze the factors limiting oxygen and CO_2 exchange by IVOX and to explore possible ways to enhance performance.[50] Analysis showed that, countercurrent flow of blood and gas resulted in higher rates of CO_2 removal. Higher gas flow rates result in reduced back pressure of CO_2 in the gas phase, thereby augmenting CO_2 removal. Additionally, as the $PaCO_2$ of blood arriving at the device is allowed to rise, there is a near linear increase in the rate of CO_2 removal by the device due to increased concentration gradient for CO_2 diffusion.

Additional results using this model indicate that most of the mass transfer resistance to oxygen uptake and CO_2 removal is in the blood phase and could be diminished by enhanced mixing of blood in the vena cava. While an increase in fiber surface area could significantly enhance gas transfer, it could also result in increased resistance to venous return. Newer generations of IVOX designed to increase

blood/fiber mixing could significantly enhance the efficiency of gas exchange.

Functional performance of IVOX using an ex vivo VV bypass circuit

To allow precise measurement of gas exchange characteristics, better define the factors affecting the performance of IVOX, and evaluate engineering improvements in IVOX design, an ex vivo VV bypass circuit modeling the adult vena cava was used by Tonz et al.[42] and later modified by the group at Galveston.[41] The bypass circuit was flow-controlled and temperature-maintained, allowing accurate quantification of the gas exchange by IVOX at varying blood flow, hemoglobin concentration, and blood PCO_2 levels. Results obtained with the ex vivo circuit were similar to those predicted by the mathematical model. Total oxygen transfer for size 7 IVOX (589 fibers with 0.31 m^2 surface area) varied with blood flow up to 41 ml/min. CO_2 removal gradually increased from 17-42 ml/min as blood flow increased from 1.0-3.0 l/min, but higher blood flow did not further increase CO_2 removal. Hemoglobin concentration >8.0 g/dl did not result in proportional increase in oxygen transfer. These results demonstrated that IVOX is a diffusion-limited, perfusion-dependent device in which gas exchange performance needs further improvement. In addition, increases of blood pCO_2 from 45-90 results in linear increases in the pressure gradient across the IVOX membrane, doubling CO_2 removal from 41-81 ml/min.

Further studies using the ex vivo circuit also highlighted the potential improvement in gas exchange by active mixing of the blood in contact with IVOX device. As predicted by the mathematical model and previous investigation, IVOX is a diffusion-limited device with most of the mass transfer resistance occurring in the boundary layer of the blood phase. The efficiency of the IVOX can be enhanced by increased mixing of the blood in the vena cava. To further test this hypothesis, size 9 IVOX devices (894 fibers with 0.41 m² surface area) incorporated into the bypass circuit were studied.[50] Blood flow was controlled by a roller pump ranging from 1.0-4.0 l/min. An intra-aortic balloon (IABP) was placed near the shaft of the IVOX and pulsated at the rate adjusted to best improve the CO_2 removal (100-120 beats/min). Oxygen transfer and CO_2 removal were measured with and without balloon pulsation and varying flow rates. Blood mixing by balloon caused a 25-49% increase in oxygen transfer by IVOX, and this increase remained relatively constant throughout the full flow range. CO_2 removal was also increased up to 35%, but at flows between 3.5-4.0 l/min the effect of mixing was diminished (Figure 11). In summary, reduction in the mass transfer resistance by blood mixing improves gas exchange. Because O_2 is more diffusion-limited, it is more dependent on mixing of blood for gas exchange than CO_2. These results suggest that further design improvements to incorporate active mixing may enhance the gas exchange performance of IVOX.

Intravascular lung assist device

Vaslef et al.[52] developed an intravascular lung assist device (ILAD) by potting the membrane fibers into sub-units of rosette-like layers, increasing the membrane surface area up to 0.4–0.6 m² with blood flow perpendicular to the fibers without increasing the overall size of the device for intravascular placement. Similar to IVOX, ILAD gas exchange efficiency increases with blood flow and gas pressure gradient across its membrane. In addition, the fiber arrangement allowed cross-flow and significantly increased gas exchange. Although the device could achieve up to 100 ml/min of both oxygen and CO_2 exchange within the space of the vena cava in their in vitro studies, the blood pressure gradient needed to overcome the resistance of the device and achieve this gas exchange was very high (23-105 mm Hg). Further attempts were made by the same group to arrange the fibers in a helical or screw-like form.[53] Unlike conventional devices which depend on passive bulk blood flow around

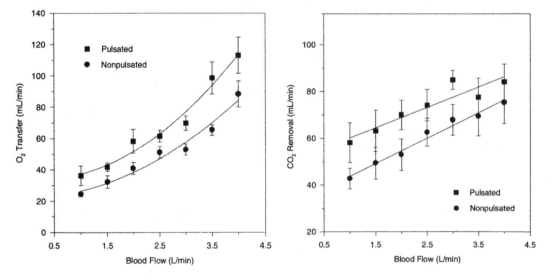

Figure 11. Increase in O_2 transfer (A) and CO_2 removal (b) of IVOX with trans-radial mixing of blood in the ex vivo bypass circuit.

them, this "pumping" ILAD causes an active mixing of for the blood when rotated, improving gas exchange.

Hattler respiratory assist catheter

Building on the lessons learned from the in vitro testing of the IVOX, the Hattler catheter incorporates a small pulsating balloon into the middle of a hollow fiber bundle (Figure 12). The balloon allows for convective mixing of the blood which increases the gas exchange capabilities of the device. In a recent report Hattler et al.[54] characterized in vivo and in vitro characteristics of their device. By testing a variety of balloon sizes and pulsation rates, it was determined that larger balloon volumes and higher pulsation rates increased both oxygen loading and CO_2 removal in a linear fashion (Figure 11). The in vivo models in healthy calves demonstrated much less consistent results between balloon sizes. Clinical trials are underway in Mexico and China; however, no data have been published to date.

Artificial lungs

Long-term support for the failing lung has lagged behind that of the heart and kidney. Dialysis allows for years of support for those awaiting transplant and new, modern ventricular assist devices (VAD) allow for bridge-to-transplant in heart patients, allowing for months of support. No such device yet exists for the lungs. ECMO allows a temporary bridge for ~1 month; however, currently there are no commercially available IVOX devices available. CO_2 removal devices such as arterial venous CO_2 removal (AVCO$_2$R) are also time-limited and have not demonstrated long-term durability or safety. Clearly, the need exists for a long-term bridge to lung transplantation, as 30% of candidates die awaiting a suitable donor. However, many obstacles must be overcome for the artificial lung to move from the bench-to-bedside.

Controversy remains as to what the proper configuration of an artificial lung should be. Current configurations being evaluated include pulmonary artery to left atrium (PA-LA), which

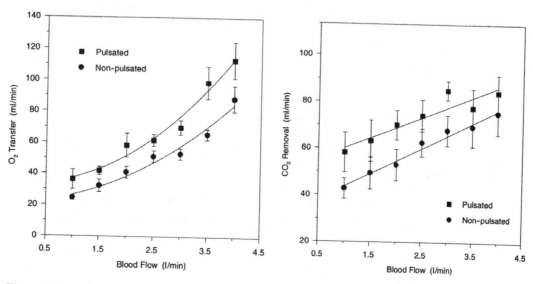

Figure 12. Schematic of the Hattler catheter tested in the acute implants. HE. Helium. (From: Golob JF, et al., *ASAIO J* 2001; 47:432-437, with permission.)

allows for partial support utilizing a pumpless artificial lung. The pressure gradient between the pulmonary artery and the left atrium provides flow through the device. Drawbacks to this configuration include unpredictability of flow through a device that depends on pulmonary vascular resistance, which can change dramatically over a short period of time, and loss of the lung vascular bed as a filter for clots. Additionally, device malfunction or need for change-out would involve considerable risk of systemic embolus or stroke.

A pulmonary artery to pulmonary artery (PA-PA) configuration uses the right heart as a pump, with the device receiving the total right ventricular output. Unfortunately, this configuration creates an excessive amount of right heart strain, resulting in a 50% incidence of right heart failure in an animal mode.[55] To combat the right heart strain, an inflow compliance chamber was added to the low resistance MC3 prototype.[56] The PA-PA configuration allows the artificial lung to be utilized in patients with elevated right heart pressures. Technically, the modified compliance chamber achieved significant augmentation, however, the pulsatile third wave introduced into the delicate pulmonary artery caused severe hemorrhage. This configuration would require a difficult surgery in humans for implantation. Sheep have very long main pulmonary arteries (6 centimeters), which enables easy proximal and distal-end to-side anastomosis. The relatively short human pulmonary artery (2.5-3 centimeters) would require either dividing the main pulmonary artery, with return of the blood post-oxygenator to the transected main pulmonary artery, or utilizing a graft to the side of the main pulmonary artery and diverting all blood flow to the device and back to the right pulmonary artery. Unfortunately, both of these techniques would require cardiopulmonary bypass (CPB) support and neither are attractive long-term options.[57]

A third configuration being explored is the right atrium to pulmonary artery (RA-PA) configuration. This configuration would require either integration or the coupling of the artificial lung to a pump. Functioning in a similar fashion to a right VAD, blood would flow from the right atrium to the device and be pumped into the main pulmonary artery. No CPB would be required for implantation and removal, and temporary use of the native circulation would be possible to allow for device change-out. Two distinct approaches to this configuration have emerged. In one strategy, the pump and artificial lung become one. Through the use of centrifugal pumps with membrane fibers incorporated into the spinning disk, these all-in-one devices provide forward flow and gas exchange simultaneously. Devices such as these remain at the animal testing stage.

Another option for this configuration involves the use of separate components with a blood pump and oxygenator placed in series. Utilizing a pulseless axial or centrifugal pump connected to an artificial lung, pump function and gas exchange function can be individually controlled based on the needs of the patient. Drawbacks to this system include the increased complexity of having two independent devices, as well as the added bulk that would come with adding a pump to an artificial lung.

Blood surface compatibility in the artificial lung provides a unique set of challenges. With the increased surface area of an artificial lung relative to a VAD, anticoagulation becomes more difficult. The length of time necessary for a device to be considered a bridge-to-transplant (≥ 6 months) presents anticoagulation challenges for the artificial lung that are not found in short-term support devices such as ECMO. Various events inevitable with long-term support present problems, including development of pulmonary hypertension from the constant barrage of small emboli to the lung bed, the constant need for anticoagulation, and low-level stimulation and complement activation.

Table 2. Comparison of ECMO, CPB, low-flow positive pressure ventilation with $ECCO_2R$, IVOX/Intravenous Membrane Oxygenator (IMO), $AVCO_2R$, and total artificial lung.

	ECMO	CPB	$ECCO_2R$	IVOX/IMO	$AVCO_2R$	Total artificial lung
Setting	Respiratory and/or cardiac failure	Cardiac surgery	Respiratory failure	Respiratory failure (investigational)	Respiratory failure (investigational)	Respiratory failure (experimental)
Location	Extrathoracic	Intrathoracic	Extrathoracic	Intravenacaval	Extrathoracic	Extrathoracic
Type of support	VA (cardiac) VV (respiratory)	VA (total bypass)	VV (respiratory) (CO_2)	Partial respiratory (O_2 & CO_2)	AV (respiratory) (CO_2)	PA-PA or PA-LA
Cannulation	VA: neck VV: neck and groin 2 cannulas (surgical or percutaneous) 1 cannula (VVDL)	Direct cardiac 2 cannulas (surgical)	Neck and groin 2 cannulas (surgical or percutaneous) 1 cannula (VVDL)	Groin (femoral vein insertion)	Groin 2 cannulas (percutaneous)	Transthoracic to major vessels
Blood flow	High (70-80% CO)	Total (100% CO)	Med (30% CO)	Passive (IVC/SVC/RA flow external to membrane)	Low (10-15% CO)	Total (100%)
Ventilatory support	Pressure-controlled ± High PEEP 10-12 breaths/min	None (anesthesia)	High PEEP 2-4 Breaths/min High FiO_2	4-6 Breaths/min ± High PEEP FiO_2 for PaO_2 >60	4-6 Breaths/min ± High PEEP FiO_2 for PaO_2>60	None necessary
Blood reservoir	Small (50 cc)	Yes (>1 liter)	Small (50 cc)	No	No	No
Arterial filter	No	Yes	No	No	No	No
Blood pump	Roller or centrifugal	Roller or centrifugal	Roller or centrifugal	None (pulsed fibers may gas exchange)	None	None
Heparinization	ACT 200-260	ACT >400	ACT 200-260	ACT 200-260	ACT 200-260	ACT 200-260
Average length of extracorporeal support	Days to weeks	Hours	Days to weeks	Days	Days to weeks	Days
Unique complications	Arterial emboli Bleeding	Arterial emboli Bleeding	Bleeding	Insertion and positioning Bleeding	Vascular access Bleeding	Thoracotomy Bleeding
Unique causes of death	Air embolism Circuit failure	Air embolism Circuit failure	Inadequate support	Inadequate support	Inadequate support	Right heart failure

Summary

Palliation of end-stage lung disease patients with total or partial gas exchange devices still remains a challenge. Short-term support can currently be accomplished with new generation hollow fiber oxygenation devices for up to 3 weeks. A bridge-to-transplant gas exchanger still remains in the animal testing phase. Implantable artificial lungs likely remain years away (Table 2).[57]

Many of the issues that have limited the application of extracorporeal devices for respiratory assistance or replacement have still remained unanswered. Although our understanding of blood surface interaction, extracorporeal gas exchange, and the hemodynamic effects of such devices has improved, we still are missing several key pieces to the puzzles. As anticoagulation and fiber technology improve, and devices become smaller with less surface area, a new era of respiratory support will likely emerge. This promise gives hope to the many investigators who have tried to solve this puzzle for the last 20 years or longer and to the patients who suffer from severe lung disease.

References

1. Anderson H, 3rd, Steimle C, Shapiro M, et al. Extracorporeal life support for adult cardiorespiratory failure. *Surgery* 1993; 114:161-172.

2. Cornish JD, Heiss KF, Clark RH, Strieper MJ, Boecler B, Kesser K. Efficacy of venovenous extracorporeal membrane oxygenation for neonates with respiratory and circulatory compromise. *J Pediatr* 1993; 122:105-109.

3. Zwischenberger JB, Cox CS, Jr., Minifee PK, et al. Pathophysiology of ovine smoke inhalation injury treated with extracorporeal membrane oxygenation. *Chest* 1993; 103:1582-1586.

4. Bartlett RH. Extracorporeal life support for cardiopulmonary failure. *Curr Probl Surg* 1990; 27:621-705.

5. Amato MB, Barbas CS, Medeiros DM, et al. Effect of a protective-ventilation strategy on mortality in the acute respiratory distress syndrome. *N Engl J Med* 1998; 338:347-354.

6. Bidani A, Tzouanakis AE, Cardenas VJ, Jr., Zwischenberger JB. Permissive hypercapnia in acute respiratory failure. *JAMA* 1994; 272:957-962.

7. Hickling KG, Walsh J, Henderson S, Jackson R. Low mortality rate in adult respiratory distress syndrome using low-volume, pressure-limited ventilation with permissive hypercapnia: a prospective study. *Crit Care Med* 1994; 22:1568-1578.

8. Milberg JA, Davis DR, Steinberg KP, Hudson LD. Improved survival of patients with acute respiratory distress syndrome (ARDS): 1983-1993. *JAMA* 1995; 273:306-309.

9. Rappaport SH, Shpiner R, Yoshihara G, Wright J, Chang P, Abraham E. Randomized, prospective trial of pressure-limited versus volume-controlled ventilation in severe respiratory failure. *Crit Care Med* 1994; 22:22-32.

10. Willms D, Nield M, Gocka I. Adult respiratory distress syndrome: outcome in a community hospital. *Am J Crit Care* 1994; 3:337-341.

11. Cardenas VJ, Jr., Zwischenberger JB, Tao W, et al. Correction of blood pH attenuates changes in hemodynamics and organ blood flow during permissive hypercapnia. *Crit Care Med* 1996; 24:827-834.

12. Gattinoni L, Kolobow T, Tomlinson T, et al. Low-frequency positive pressure ventilation with extracorporeal carbon dioxide removal (LFPPV-ECCO2R): an experimental study. *Anesth Analg* 1978; 57:470-477.

13. Gattinoni L, Kolobow T, Tomlinson T, White D, Pierce J. Control of intermittent positive pressure breathing (IPPB) by ex-

tracorporeal removal of carbon dioxide. *Br J Anaesth* 1978; 50:753-758.

14. Kolobow T, Gattinoni L, Tomlinson T, Pierce JE. An alternative to breathing. *J Thorac Cardiovasc Surg* 1978; 75:261-266.

15. Brunet F, Belghith M, Mira JP, et al. Extracorporeal carbon dioxide removal and low-frequency positive-pressure ventilation. Improvement in arterial oxygenation with reduction of risk of pulmonary barotrauma in patients with adult respiratory distress syndrome. *Chest* 1993; 104:889-898.

16. Gattinoni L, Agostoni A, Pesenti A, et al. Treatment of acute respiratory failure with low-frequency positive-pressure ventilation and extracorporeal removal of CO_2. *Lancet* 1980; 2:292-294.

17. Gattinoni L, Kolobow T, Agostoni A, et al. Clinical application of low frequency positive pressure ventilation with extracorporeal CO_2 removal (LFPPV-ECCO2R) in treatment of adult respiratory distress syndrome (ARDS). *Int J Artif Organs* 1979; 2:282-283.

18. Morris AH, Wallace CJ, Menlove RL, et al. Randomized clinical trial of pressure-controlled inverse ratio ventilation and extracorporeal CO_2 removal for adult respiratory distress syndrome. *Am J Respir Crit Care Med* 1994; 149:295-305.

19. Tao W, Brunston RL, Jr., Bidani A, et al. Significant reduction in minute ventilation and peak inspiratory pressures with arteriovenous CO_2 removal during severe respiratory failure. *Crit Care Med* 1997; 25:689-695.

20. Barthelemy R, Galletti PM, Trudell LA, et al. Total extracorporeal CO_2 removal in a pumpless artery-to-vein shunt. *Trans Am Soc Artif Intern Organs* 1982; 28:354-358.

21. Awad JA, Deslauriers J, Major D, Guojin L, Martin L. Prolonged pumpless arteriovenous perfusion for carbon dioxide extraction. *Ann Thorac Surg* 1991; 51:534-540.

22. Young JD, Dorrington KL, Blake GJ, Ryder WA. Femoral arteriovenous extracorporeal carbon dioxide elimination using low blood flow. *Crit Care Med* 1992; 20:805-809.

23. Brunston RL, Jr., Zwischenberger JB, Tao W, Cardenas VJ, Jr., Traber DL, Bidani A. Total arteriovenous CO_2 removal: simplifying extracorporeal support for respiratory failure. *Ann Thorac Surg* 1997; 64:1599-1604.

24. Zwischenberger JB, Alpard SK, Conrad SA, Johnigan RH, Bidani A. Arteriovenous carbon dioxide removal: development and impact on ventilator management and survival during severe respiratory failure. *Perfusion* 1999; 14:299-310.

25. Brunston RL, Jr., Tao W, Bidani A, Cardenas VJ, Jr., Traber DL, Zwischenberger JB. Determination of low blood flow limits for arteriovenous carbon dioxide removal. *ASAIO J* 1996; 42:M845-849.

26. Meade P, Shoemaker WC, Donnelly TJ, et al. Temporal patterns of hemodynamics, oxygen transport, cytokine activity, and complement activity in the development of adult respiratory distress syndrome after severe injury. *J Trauma* 1994; 36:651-657.

27. Ronco JJ, Belzberg A, Phang PT, Walley KR, Dodek PM, Russell JA. No differences in hemodynamics, ventricular function, and oxygen delivery in septic and nonseptic patients with the adult respiratory distress syndrome. *Crit Care Med* 1994; 22:777-782.

28. Brunston RL, Jr., Tao W, Bidani A, Alpard SK, Traber DL, Zwischenberger JB. Prolonged hemodynamic stability during arteriovenous carbon dioxide removal for severe respiratory failure. *J Thorac Cardiovasc Surg* 1997; 114:1107-1114.

29. Flaim SF, Minteer WJ, Nellis SH, Clark DP. Chronic arteriovenous shunt: evaluation of a model for heart failure in rat. *Am J Physiol* 1979; 236:H698-704.

30. Brunston RL, Jr., Tao W, Bidani A, Traber DL, Zwischenberger JB. Organ blood flow during arteriovenous carbon dioxide removal. *ASAIO J* 1997; 43:M821-824.

31. Alpard SK, Zwischenberger JB, Tao W, Deyo DJ, Traber DL, Bidani A. New clinically relevant sheep model of severe respiratory failure secondary to combined smoke inhalation/cutaneous flame burn injury. *Crit Care Med* 2000; 28:1469-1476.

32. Zwischenberger JB, Conrad SA, Alpard SK, Grier LR, Bidani A. Percutaneous extracorporeal arteriovenous CO2 removal for severe respiratory failure. *Ann Thorac Surg* 1999; 68:181-187.

33. Personal communication Heiko Frerichs, April, 2005.

34. Mortensen JD. An intravenacaval blood gas exchange (IVCBGE) device. A preliminary report. *ASAIO Trans* 1987; 33:570-573.

35. Mortensen JD, Berry G. Conceptual and design features of a practical, clinically effective intravenous mechanical blood oxygen/carbon dioxide exchange device (IVOX). *Int J Artif Organs* 1989; 12:384-389.

36. Cox CS, Jr., Zwischenberger JB, Graves DF, Niranjan SC, Bidani A. Intracorporeal CO2 removal and permissive hypercapnia to reduce airway pressure in acute respiratory failure. The theoretical basis for permissive hypercapnia with IVOX. *ASAIO J* 1993; 39:97-102.

37. Cox CS, Jr., Zwischenberger JB, Traber LD, Traber DL, Herndon DN. Use of an intravascular oxygenator/carbon dioxide removal device in an ovine smoke inhalation injury model. *ASAIO Trans* 1991; 37:M411-413.

38. Zwischenberger JB, Cox CS, Jr. A new intravascular membrane oxygenator to augment blood gas transfer in patients with acute respiratory failure. *Tex Med* 1991; 87:60-63.

39. Zwischenberger JB, Cox CS, Graves D, Bidani A. Intravascular membrane oxygenation and carbon dioxide removal--a new application for permissive hypercapnia? *Thorac Cardiovasc Surg* 1992; 40:115-120.

40. Mortenson J. *Augmentation of blood gas transfer by means of an intravascular blood gas exchanger (IVOX).* 1 ed. Berlin, Germany: Springer-Verlag; 1991:318-346.

41. Tao W, Zwischenberger JB, Nguyen TT, et al. Performance of an intravenous gas exchanger (IVOX) in a venovenous bypass circuit. *Ann Thorac Surg* 1994; 57:1484-1490.

42. Tonz M, von Segesser LK, Leskosek B, Turina MI. Quantitative gas transfer of an intravascular oxygenator. *Ann Thorac Surg* 1994; 57:146-150.

43. Conrad SA, Bagley A, Bagley B, Schaap RN. Major findings from the clinical trials of the intravascular oxygenator. *Artif Organs* 1994; 18:846-863.

44. Gentilello LM, Jurkovich GJ, Gubler KD, Anardi DM, Heiskell R. The intravascular oxygenator (IVOX): preliminary results of a new means of performing extrapulmonary gas exchange. *J Trauma* 1993; 35:399-404.

45. High KM, Snider MT, Richard R, et al. Clinical trials of an intravenous oxygenator in patients with adult respiratory distress syndrome. *Anesthesiology* 1992; 77:856-863.

46. Jurmann MJ, Demertzis S, Schaefers HJ, Wahlers T, Haverich A. Intravascular oxygenation for advanced respiratory failure. *ASAIO J* 1992; 38:120-124.

47. Kallis P, al-Saady NM, Bennett ED, Treasure T. Early results of intravascular oxygenation. *Eur J Cardiothorac Surg* 1993; 7:206-210.

48. Conrad SA, Eggerstedt JM, Morris VF, Romero MD. Prolonged intracorporeal support of gas exchange with an intravenacaval oxygenator. *Chest* 1993; 103:158-161.

49. von Segesser LK, Schaffner A, Stocker R, et al. Extended (29 days) use of intravascular gas exchanger. *Lancet* 1992; 339:1536.

50. Zwischenberger JB, Cardenas VJ, Jr., Tao W, Niranjan SC, Clark JW, Bidani A. Intravascular membrane oxygenation and carbon dioxide removal with IVOX: can improved design and permissive hypercapnia achieve adequate respiratory support during severe respiratory failure? *Artif Organs* 1994; 18:833-839.

51. Tao W, Schroeder T, Bidani A, et al. Improved gas exchange performance of the intravascular oxygenator by active blood mixing. *ASAIO J* 1994; 40:M527-532.

52. Vaslef SN, Mockros LF, Anderson RW. Development of an intravascular lung assist device. *ASAIO Trans* 1989; 35:660-664.

53. Makarewicz AJ, Mockros LF, Anderson RW. A pumping intravascular artificial lung with active mixing. *ASAIO J* 1993; 39:M466-469.

54. Hattler BG, Lund LW, Golob J, et al. A respiratory gas exchange catheter: in vitro and in vivo tests in large animals. *J Thorac Cardiovasc Surg* 2002; 124:520-530.

55. Zwischenberger JB, Anderson CM, Cook KE, Lick SD, Mockros LF, Bartlett RH. Development of an implantable artificial lung: challenges and progress. *ASAIO J* 2001; 47:316-320.

56. Lick SD, Zwischenberger JB, Wang D, Deyo DJ, Alpard SK, Chambers SD. Improved right heart function with a compliant inflow artificial lung in series with the pulmonary circulation. *Ann Thorac Surg* 2001; 72:899-904.

57. Lick SD, Zwischenberger JB. Artificial lung: bench toward bedside. *ASAIO J* 2004; 50:2-5.

41

Nursing Care of the Patient on ECMO

Robert T. Remenapp, R.N., B.S.N., Anke WinklerPrins, B.A., R.N., B.S.N., and Inger Mossberg, C.R.N.A., I.C.C.R.N., B.Sc.

Introduction

When the first patients were placed on ECMO in the 1970s, there was no nursing care paradigm in place to guide the nursing management of these patients. The technology was new, uncharted, and technologically complex. No articles or texts addressed the nursing care of ECMO patients. Nurses had to adjust care at the bedside as the needs of this new set of patients became evident.

ECMO support, while often considered extraordinary, is now standard in major medical centers worldwide. Years of experience have helped nurses understand the unique needs of this patient population and have allowed the development of strategies for ECMO nursing care in all age groups. A number of articles have been published in nursing journals highlighting the ECMO technology.[1-5] Some address the issues specific to the nursing care of this group of patients.[6,7]

Nursing care of the ECLS patient requires a unique skill set as well as strong critical care nursing skills. Patient care needs will vary depending on the underlying disease state, the patient age, and the level of clinical stability. Daily bedside care can vary from routine in the stable ECMO patient to stressful and highly technical in the patient with ECMO-related complications. This chapter discusses various care models, with a focus on the overall goals of care. Included are representative experiences from both the University of Michigan

in Ann Arbor, Michigan and the Karolinska Institute in Stockholm, Sweden.

How is ECMO different?

There are several aspects that make the nursing care for the ECMO patient unique as compared to other ICU patients. First and foremost, patients are wholly reliant on the ECMO circuit for survival. Failure of the ECMO circuit can be life-threatening. This circumstance demands a level of nursing vigilance and technologic expertise greater than that needed for most other patient management situations. Second, the family is informed that ECMO is being instituted as a last resort. If ECMO is unsuccessful there are generally no other treatment options available. The nursing care needs of a family faced with this situation can be arduous and time-consuming. Lastly, patients on ECMO often do not have the outward appearance of someone as critically ill as they actually are. Family members, nurses, physicians, and ECMO specialists may find themselves unprepared for a poor outcome when the patient appears stable on ECMO support.

The nursing care delivery system

Care of the ECMO patient involves providing nursing care to the patient (and family) as well as management of the ECMO circuit. The professional that manages the ECMO circuit has been designated the ECMO specialist. Registered nurses, respiratory care practitioners, and perfusionists all may function in this role. In some institutions, the nursing role and the ECMO specialist role are integrated; in others they are distinct.

Many factors influence an institution's choice of who should fill the ECMO specialist role. These include the patient population served (adults, children, or newborns), the type of ICU where ECMO is performed, and the skill levels and the availability of professionals. In Europe, for example, there is no respiratory care practitioner role, so management of the ECMO circuit is a nursing care responsibility. There is no single optimal model for program design; what is most critical is that the program continually evaluates its structure and responds to the changing needs of the patients.

Coordinating care between the ECMO specialist and bedside nurse requires a team approach. It is helpful for the caregivers to verbalize patient care goals, such as maintaining cardiovascular stability, increasing diuresis, or controlling bleeding. Communication of goals promotes mutual understanding and collaboration, and prevents interventions that are incongruent with the goals.

The bedside nursing care of the patient on ECMO is not unlike critical care nursing of the non-ECMO patient. It should be goal-directed and holistic, taking into account how alterations in individual organ systems affect the patient as a whole. The following discussion presents a conceptual basis of care with examples of specific nursing interventions for distinct patient groups. It is not meant to be an exhaustive or all-inclusive list. Each institution must seek to creatively solve clinical problems and share experiences with other members of the ECMO community.

Goals of nursing care

At a very basic level, the goals of nursing care for ECMO patients can be summarized as provision of comfort and rest, prevention of complications, and support while the healing process occurs. Nursing assessment, planning, and interventions are guided by these goals.

Comfort and rest

Comfort, the verb, is defined as, *"To soothe in time of affliction or distress, to ease physically; relieve."*[8] Comfort as provided by nurses encompasses physical comfort, emotional support, education, and advocacy. In the family-centered care model, the nurse provides care to the patient and family as a single unit. Family-centered care recognizes the family as the primary caregiver with the nurse supporting this relationship rather than assuming the primary caregiver role.[9]

Physical comfort is continuously assessed in ECMO patients and various interventions are used to promote rest and comfort. Medication, position changes, touch, and a calming physical environment are examples. There exists a great deal of variability within the medical community in regard to the management of pain and anxiety. While there is general agreement that patients should not be uncomfortable, assessment of their discomfort is difficult, particularly in the cases of cognitively impaired patients, and assessment can vary from nurse to nurse.[10,11] Additionally, the outward signs of anxiety can be misinterpreted as pain. Cultural/language differences can also affect the pain assessment.[12] Physiologic measures are used to assess pain, and can be misinterpreted. For example, tachycardia can be a symptom of pain, even without other signs of discomfort,[13] but it can also be a sign of a physiologic instability, such as hypovolemia. Lastly, the use of neuromuscular blockade limits the ability to objectively assess patient comfort level. Many pharmacologically paralyzed patients are managed with deep sedation, additionally restricting the assessment.[10] A novel approach is to manage the patient when awake and responsive, so pain and anxiety can be assessed more accurately. This approach is limited as it is difficult to implement in small children or cognitively impaired adults.

Emotional support

Empathy, optimism, reassurance, and hope tempered with reality are all tools the nurse can use to support the emotional needs of both the patient and family. At the same time, this support strengthens the relationship between the nurse and family.[14] This relationship allows the nurse to assist families to develop coping strategies for stressful situations and difficult decisions.[15]

Education

Nurses educate patients and their families about the ICU routines, the function and mechanics of the ECMO circuit, the medical plan, and the condition of the patient. This allows the family to develop a level of understanding which enables them to actively participate in the patient's care. It also helps them develop strategies to cope with potential outcomes.[16]

Advocacy

Nurses function as patient advocates in many ways. They serve as intermediaries between the family and health care system, they ensure medical orders are congruent with the stated goals of care, they encourage the family to be involved in patient care, and they look out for the patient's and family's well-being, both physically and emotionally.

Complication prevention

The prevention of complications is the most critical of nursing goals when caring for an ECMO patient. Prior to the initiation of ECMO, most of the nurse's attention is focused on physiologic stability. Once the patient is stabilized on ECMO, the nurse can shift focus to the prevention of complications, which include bleeding, infection, and skin breakdown.

Allowing time for healing

Since there is no single intervention that results in immediate recovery, the nurse works to create an environment where recovery can occur. In most ECMO cases, the patient's most important ally is time—time to heal damaged lungs, time to allow recovery of heart function after surgery, time to resolve pulmonary hypertension, and time to eliminate excess extracellular fluid. Caring for ECMO patients requires a great deal of patience. Since recovery is a slow process, it does not provide the instant gratification which some ICU staff desire. If the patient is stable and well-supported, the nursing role is not as demanding; however, if there is a dysfunction of the ECMO circuit, the patient can become instantly very unstable, needing the quick and highly skilled response of the ECMO nurse. This exemplifies one challenge inherent to caring for ECMO patients: excelling at both patience with the healing process and crisis management simultaneously.

Time is also important for families. Even if the patient does not recover and survive, ECMO has allowed time to adjust to that reality. While it can be difficult for the nurse to witness, the intense grief displayed by the family prior to a patient's death can be an important step in the grieving process. After all, if the outcome is death, ECMO has afforded the family valuable time to say goodbye to their loved one.[17]

Nursing assessments and interventions

ECMO patients range from newborns with persistent pulmonary hypertension to adults with cardiovascular failure.[18] Many centers organize their ECMO team in a fashion that requires nurses and ECMO specialists to care for patients of all age ranges. Regardless of the patient's age or disease process, the goals of nursing care are essentially the same for all age groups. The means by which these goals are accomplished, however, can be quite different. The following discussion addresses nursing care by system, using an assessment-based approach which allows the nurse to tailor interventions to specific patient needs. The assessments and interventions outlined are not an exhaustive list or the only means to accomplish the stated goals of care. Also, the interventions are not universal. That is, they are assessment-based and individualized to each patient.

Neurologic

The neurologic status of patients on ECMO must be monitored closely due to the potential for brain injury caused by pre-ECMO hypoxia, acidosis, and hypoperfusion. Since most patients are deeply sedated and pharmacologically paralyzed before ECMO, assessment is limited. Allowing the patient to wake from paralysis and deep sedation is the initial step. This situation presents challenges for the nurse and family. The amount of time required to awaken from sedation is unpredictable and can take days. Delay in awakening may be an indication of neurologic injury, placing increased demands on a family already in crisis. Neurologic assessment in newborns is restricted due to the patient's age and development. The pupillary response and fullness of the fontanelle are evaluated for evidence of increased intracranial pressure. The infant is closely observed for signs of seizures. Movement of extremities, tone and visual tracking are also examined as part of the neurologic assessment.[19]

In older children and adults, the neurologic assessment can be more comprehensive. Once again, allowing patients to awaken from sedation is useful as a major complication of ECMO is intracranial hemorrhage (ICH) or infarct. Some patients awaken from deep sedation and are non-responsive to command, may appear visually anxious, and may also thrash around.

This complicates the assessment and generally leads to a decision to return the patient to deep sedation. Some assessment of motor strength is important due to the possibility of unilateral brain injury. The Glasgow Coma Scale is useful for documentation of function, but it is subject to interpretation and can have limited use in small children and patients who are mechanically ventilated.

There are several nursing interventions designed to prevent further neurologic compromise in the ECMO patient. Anticoagulation increases the risk of intracranial hemorrhage and care should be taken to avoid over-heparinization. The presence of a jugular venous cannula can interfere with venous return; elevating the head of the bed and keeping the patient's head in the mid-line position can help to minimize this risk. Other interventions can promote neurologic recovery, including clustering of care, intermittent periods of darkness, and promotion of prolonged rest periods especially at night.

The management of pain and sedation on ECMO can be difficult because the patient is often not sufficiently alert or developmentally able to indicate pain. The degree of sedation varies with institution. Patients are generally maintained at fairly deep levels of sedation, accomplished by a continuous infusion of narcotic as well as an anxiolytic agent.

At the Karolinska Institute, the approach is to manage patients with minimal sedation. Following heavy sedation for cannulation, many patients can be managed with minimal sedation. While tapering sedation doses, the patient may experience a period of excitement and anxiety prior to waking. Early tracheotomy may be performed to eliminate the discomfort caused by the endotracheal tube. Extra staff members may be needed exclusively manage the patient's care and provide psychological support. Constant reassurance is given to the patient, informing the patient about his/her status, repeating this until the patient is lucid enough to understand and remember. Adequate sedation is generally attained with the use of one or two medications, with an additional one at night to promote circadian rhythm. If sedation goals are achieved, the patient is able to read, listen to music, watch television, or use a computer (Table 1).

Respiratory

The respiratory status is assessed continuously by auscultation of breath sounds, determination of respiratory rate and effort, and evaluation for signs of distress such as nasal flaring or retractions. Laboratory measurement of blood gases and bedside measurement of pulse oximetry provide objective indications as to the adequacy of support. Gas exchange is controlled primarily by the membrane oxygenator.

A variety of nursing interventions can improve respiratory status, including maintenance of the airway, mobilization of secretions by positioning and percussion, and clearing secretions from the airway by suctioning. Suctioning is performed with special care due to the risk of pulmonary bleeding with anticoagulation. Deep nasal suctioning is contraindicated for the same reason. Once the patient is placed on ECMO, ventilator settings are adjusted to avoid high peak airway pressure. The same principle must be employed when manually ventilating a patient. Oral care is provided both as a comfort measure and to reduce the risk of ventilator-associated pneumonia. [20]

A common strategy for the management of severe respiratory failure includes prone positioning. While prone positioning can improve gas exchange, there is data to suggest that its use does not impact survival.[21] Prone positioning on ECMO is used routinely in some centers. Two published reports from a single center conclude that there is no additional risk associated with prone positioning in patients on ECMO.[22,23] As with other interventions, an immediate effect may not be seen, but rather slow improvement over time.

Promotion of lung inflation is achieved using a ventilation technique known as "lung conditioning", where 5-10 manual breaths are delivered with a resuscitation bag, utilizing a pressure of 5 cm H_2O above resting peak inspiratory pressure (PIP) and a 5-second hold. This treatment is performed at regular intervals, beginning when the tidal volume shows improvement on "rest settings".

At the Karolinska Institute, the approach to ventilatory support for patients on ECMO takes advantage of the awakened state of the patient. After ECLS is initiated and the ventilator decreased is to rest settings, a total

Table 1. Neurologic assessments and interventions.

Assessment
Pupil checks at regular intervals (more often if using neuromuscular blockade)
Glasgow Coma Scale or similar measure of receptive and motor function
Pain and sedation scoring

Interventions
Administer narcotics and anxiolytics as needed
Elevate the head of the bed, maintaining the patient's head in mid-line position to encourage venous return
Provide periods of stimulation and quiet time
Provide means of distraction (e.g., television, massages, music)
Provide a comforting, restful environment (e.g., pressure relief mattress, dry bedding)
Secure lines and tubes
Utilize additional staff as needed to support the patient's psychological needs

opacification of the lungs often develops. A tracheotomy is often performed to provide good pulmonary toilet. Frequent oral care to prevent nosocomial infection is performed, followed by bacterial and fungal cultures. Hand ventilation with limited pressure helps to mobilize mucous and may provide information about lung compliance. When lung volume increases, aerosol medications such as albuterol, ipratropium bromide, and acetyl cysteine may be added to the treatment regimen. With minimal sedation, the patient can initiate the breath during pressure support ventilation, often resulting in increased tidal volumes. Maintaining normal arterial pH promotes patient-initiated breathing.

Patients placed on ECMO for cardiac support often have normal lung function. The goals are to achieve, then maintain normal pulmonary function. This is extremely important in patients with cyanotic heart disease, as they may not tolerate even minor alterations in lung function. The ventilation strategy is usually based on a goal of normal minute ventilation at low airway pressures. Adults placed on ECMO for cardiac support alone often tolerate extubation. When lung function and blood gases are normal, these patients are generally comfortable without signs of respiratory distress. Removing the endotracheal tube lessens the risk of ventilator-associated pneumonia. As with an intubated patient, pulmonary hygiene is of primary importance (Table 2).

Circulation

Circulatory status is evaluated by assessing the warmth of extremities, urine output, and capillary refill time. Pulses may or may not be palpable if the patient is on VA ECMO and should be normally palpable in patients on VV ECMO.

Inotropic agents such as dopamine, dobutamine, and epinephrine may be used to augment cardiac output. Often the dosages can be weaned after the patient is placed on ECMO either because the systemic perfusion is supported with VA ECMO or the cardiac performance is improved with increased oxygen delivery. Some patients may require vasopressors such as vasopressin, neosynephrine, or norepinephrine due to low systemic vascular resistance.

On VA bypass, the arterial waveform will be dampened, so the quality of pulses will not be a good indicator of systemic perfusion. In patients with an aortopulmonary shunt (i.e., Blalock-Taussig or central shunt), some of the blood will be diverted to the lower resistance pulmonary circuit, affecting the quality of

Table 2. Respiratory assessments and interventions.

Assessment
Respiratory assessment at regular intervals
• Breath sounds
• Presence/absence of effort
• Distress (flaring, retractions)
Assess for air leak if chest tube in place

Interventions
Avoid elevated PIP during manual ventilation with suctioning
Maintain secure airway
Suction airway at regular intervals as needed
Chest physiotherapy with attention to presence of air leak and bleeding risk
Position changes at regular intervals based on comfort, skin integrity, and need for mobilization of secretions; consider prone positioning
"Lung conditioning"
Oral care at regular intervals

pulses in the extremities. Other indicators of adequate perfusion must be used, including warmth of the extremities and renal function.

In all patients, especially those who have had recent surgery, assessment of blood loss and blood volume is of vital importance. This can be extremely challenging in adults and large children. Blood loss >10 cc/kg/hr of blood per hour is common in the immediate post-operative period. At times, it is necessary to assign additional nursing staff to the bleeding patient to keep up with blood loss and transfusion requirements. With large blood losses it is important to replace plasma and platelets, as well as packed red blood cells (PRBCs), to prevent dilutional thrombocytopenia and factor deficiency.

One intervention aimed at providing cardiovascular stability is the maintenance of vasoactive infusions. Ideally, vasoactive medications are infused into a patient line directly, not into the ECMO circuit. The rationale is that in case of a circuit emergency, the patient would continue to receive the vasoactive medications (Table 3).

GI and nutrition

The nursing goals with regard to GI status include prevention of complications and provision of adequate nutrition to assist healing. The most common complications are bleeding, dis-tension, and dysmotility. Pre-ECMO instability can place the patient at risk for bowel ischemia; this is particularly true in newborns. Nursing assessment of GI status includes character and quantity of gastric tube drainage, assessment of bowel sounds, distension, and tenderness. The stomach is decompressed using a nasogastric (NG) or orograstic (OG) tube until it can be determined that the GI tract is functioning. Some centers will begin enteral feedings in older children and adults. Jejunal feeding may be preferred due to the potential for stomach dysmotility, distension, and emesis. There is evidence that feeding directly into the stomach is equally tolerated.[24,25] Once feeding is initiated, ongoing assessment of tolerance is required including evaluation of stooling pattern. A comprehensive assessment of nutrition includes the measurement of daily weight. Although weight is more likely a reflection of fluid balance than nutritional balance, it can be useful for establishing a baseline for convalescence.

NG or OG tubes must be evaluated regularly due to the potential for bleeding from the mucous membranes of the nasopharynx or oropharynx. Management of enteral feeding and bowel elimination is an important part of patient care. Administration of narcotics and sedatives often require the use of stool softeners and laxatives to promote adequate elimination.

Table 3. Circulatory assessments and interventions.

Assessment
Warmth of extremities
Pulses (may be absent on VA support at high blood flows)
Blood volume
Color of extremities (pink, dusky, mottled)
Urine output
Presence/absence of edema

Interventions
Administer vasoactive infusions via a patient line (not via the ECMO circuit)
Maintain adequate blood volume
Position patient to promote optimal perfusion of extremities and minimize dependent edema

If the patient does not have a functional GI tract or is not tolerating enteral feeds, parenteral nutrition is prescribed. Assessment of the tolerance of parenteral nutrition includes the monitoring of blood sugar. Metabolic rate can be measured in patients on ECMO, but it is not highly accurate. It is unclear whether standard tables for calculating caloric requirement are applicable to this unique population. Because ECMO patients frequently require fluid restriction, minimizing non-nutritional fluid administration will help to maximize provision of carbohydrate, fat, and protein (Table 4).

Fluid balance

At the time a patient is placed on ECMO for respiratory support, most patients have some degree of extracellular fluid excess. This cause is multifactorial, including presence of systemic inflammation and capillary leak, and the need for blood volume expansion to maintain adequate cardiac output. Patients may also develop renal failure as a result of pre-ECMO ischemia. Edema is a common finding. Basic nursing care, including patient positioning and prevention of skin breakdown, is very important in the presence of significant edema. Intake and output measurements are useful in assessing progress toward return to a normal fluid balance. In addition, monitoring of electrolytes is important in patients with an altered fluid balance.

Nursing interventions involved in managing fluid balance include maintenance of a urinary catheter and obtaining daily weights, if clinically feasible. A return to the patient's admission or baseline weight is the goal. Patients who are receiving diuretics may develop inadequate intravascular volume, which can affect hemodynamics.

With failure to respond to efforts at correcting fluid balance, a hemofilter may be utilized. The filtration device is placed in-line with the ECMO circuit and can be utilized as a hemofilter or dialysis system depending on patient need. In either case, careful assessment and management of fluid balance and blood volume must be maintained (Table 5).

Skin care

The maintenance of intact skin integrity is essential in preventing complications and improving patient outcomes. A comprehensive skin assessment is best performed with a daily bath and linen change. This should include assessment of IV and cannula sites. ECMO patients with sternal cannulation require particular attention to skin integrity.[26] Also important to the promotion of intact skin integrity is attention to

Table 4. GI and nutrition assessments and interventions.

Assessment

GI assessment at regular intervals including assessment for abdominal distention or tenderness, quality of bowel sounds, tolerance of enteral feeding, character of NG drainage character, and stooling pattern

Nutritional assessment including daily weights, if possible, and calculation of protein and caloric intake

Interventions

Maintain NG/OG tube for feeding and/or decompression

Maintain gastric or jejunal tube for feeding

Administer enteral or parenteral feedings

Promote normal stooling pattern

nutritional status and maintenance of adequate tissue perfusion.

One intervention designed to promote skin integrity is frequent repositioning of the patient to prevent local areas of decreased tissue perfusion. The practice of repositioning varies by institution and on patient stability. An interval of every 3-4 hours is common.[27] Areas prone to breakdown include the back of the head, the sacrum, and heels. Pressure relief surfaces such as airbeds, sheepskin, and gel pads are used to reduce the incidence of pressure ulcers. However, the most important assessment related to the prevention of pressure ulcers is to identify patients at risk, and intervene prior to ulcer development.[28] A protocol for the management of patients with open sternum should be followed including dressing changes and antibiotic use.

Areas of skin breakdown can become a source for infection. In addition, areas of skin entry, including IV and cannulation sites, also increase the risk of infection. Dressings maintained over IV sites and regular treatment of cannulation sites with an antiseptic solution (betadine or clorhexidine) may lessen the likelihood of infection (Table 6).[29]

Bleeding and anticoagulation

Approximately 25% of respiratory support patients and 40% of cardiac support patients experience bleeding complications.[19] Prolonged or severe bleeding may prematurely end the ECMO run. Sites of bleeding or hemorrhage may be intracranial, intrathoracic, or intra-abdominal and can involve cannula, operative, or chest tube sites.

ECMO patients have an increased risk of bleeding because of heparinization as well as circuit platelet and factor consumption. The primary intervention is prevention. To this end, IV lines are left in place and new IV lines are not initiated while on ECMO, un-

Table 5. Fluid balance assessments and interventions.

Assessment
Evaluation at regular intervals for edema, skin turgor, and electrolyte status
Maintain accurate intake and output measurements
Daily weights if clinically feasible

Interventions
Maintain urinary catheter
Calculate intake and output, noting positive or negative fluid balance
Maintenance of hemofiltration or dialysis circuit
Evaluation of electrolyte status
Prevent complications of edema through patient positioning and skin care

Table 6. Skin assessments and interventions.

Assessment
Evaluate for signs of skin breakdown or decreased perfusion
Nutritional assessment
Assessment of skin integrity around IV and cannula sites

Interventions
Frequent repositioning of the patient with close examination of the back of the head, heels, and sacrum
Maintenance of sterile dressings on IV sites
Avoidance of infection of cannula sites with regular inspection and topical antiseptics

less absolutely necessary. Subcutaneous or intramuscular injections are avoided. Blood samples are always obtained from the circuit or patient lines, and never by arterial, venous, or heel stick. Great care is taken with regard to mucus membranes (e.g., suctioning, placement of NG tubes, and oral care). If bleeding begins, it can be difficult or impossible to stop while the patient remains on bypass. Large blood losses are replaced with appropriate blood products. Whole blood activated clotting time (ACT) is lowered. While usually helpful in the control of bleeding, lowering the ACT range places the ECMO circuit at increased risk for thrombosis and increases the likelihood of planned or emergent circuit change. Clotting in the circuit is an unavoidable complication of long-term bypass and fibrinolytic activity in the ECLS circuit is monitored by laboratory assay. Elevated fibrin split products or D-dimers and hypofibrinogenemia are all signs of circuit clotting. The patient can be asymptomatic or present with diffuse bleeding. A change out of the ECLS circuit is the treatment. Often, coagulation parameters normalize 24-48 hours following the circuit change (Table 7).

Caring for the family

In a family-centered care model, the family is included in all aspects of the patient's care. While this can place a strain on the health care team, it allows the family to actively participate in care and decision-making. The term "co-client" has been used to explain the care model in which the nurse cares not only for the patient, but for the family as well.[15]

Each family presents to the health care team a unique set of needs and strengths. Almost certainly they will be in crisis and find their usual coping methods inadequate. The family may have difficulty absorbing information and may need help with basic needs such as housing and meals.

As the patient condition allows, the family can become involved in the care of the patient. They should be apprised of the goals of care, and the indicators of progress, as well as educated about the technology in use. It is important to explain to family members that the patient may appear to be improving and may even be awake and responsive, but may still have no intrinsic lung or heart function. The nurse and ECMO specialist must be clear and thorough when communicating to the family. For example, if a blood gas comes back with an increased PaO_2, the nurse may comment that the blood gas is "better" and this may be interpreted by the family to mean that the patient's condition is improving. In fact, unless active weaning from ECMO is in progress, PaO_2 should not be used as sign of patient improvement.

It is difficult to balance hope for recovery, with emotional preparation for the possibility of death. Hope helps families cope with the

Table 7. Bleeding and anticoagulation assessments and interventions.

Assessment
Assess for signs of active bleeding at IV, incisional, and cannula sites; gastric, chest, or endotracheal tubes; urinary and umbilical catheters; and operative site drains

Interventions
Prevent bleeding by maintaining existing IV lines, avoiding insertion of new IV lines, and careful handling of mucus membranes (suctioning, oral care, NG tube placement)
Monitor platelet count, hematocrit, ACT, and coagulation parameters
Replace blood loss with appropriate blood products as needed

present situation, and allows them to look beyond it to the future.[14] Approaching families with honesty is essential in supporting them during crisis. If a patient develops a devastating complication or is found to have an irrecoverable condition, a family that is well informed will be more prepared to make the decisions surrounding withdrawal of support. At times, the family may even realize the futility of continuing ECLS before it is confirmed by the health care team. Once futility has been determined by the health care team, it important that the physician inform the family about the decision. The family should not be left to decide whether or not to stop ECMO. The physician makes the decision with input from many sources, including medical consultants, family, social workers, and nursing staff.[30] The family's response to the decision to withdraw of support can be quite varied. Although a family may appear to understand the situation and agree to the decision, they may still have hope that the patient will survive and recover.[31]

Supporting a patient and family through end-of-life care is one of the most difficult skills for the ICU nurse to acquire. Every attempt should be made to honor the family's wishes in the process, giving them a sense of control in a situating where they have no control over the outcome. Nurses can be supportive and creative in the grieving process (e.g., create a memory box with photos, take foot imprints of children, provide locks of hair, and other memorabilia). These activities add a personal touch to a painful event.

End-of-life care in the ICU be stressful and in some cases unfamiliar to the ICU nurse. Nurses often suffer along with family members from the death of the patient.[32] Active involvement of the nurse in end-of-life preparation can help to ease this suffering. Collaboration of caregivers helps to meet the unique needs of the patient, family, and staff. The parents can hold the child in their arms, or lay next to their family member while the patient remains on ECMO. These activities require the cooperation of the nurse, ECMO specialist, the respiratory therapist, and physician.

There are a number of staff and workers in the hospital with advanced skills in addressing the issues of death and grief. Pastoral care, social work, palliative care, and bereavement specialists can be valuable resources for the patient, the family, and the staff. Nurses coordinate these interventions (Table 8).

Table 8. Family assessments and interventions.

Assessment
Evaluate the family's coping mechanisms, strengths, and needs on a continual basis
Determine if families have any unique care requests
Inquire about religious practices, beliefs, and customs of the family and patient
Consult pastoral care, palliative care, or bereavement specialists for assistance in meeting family and patient needs

Interventions
Provide frequent and honest feedback about the patient's condition
Promote family involvement in care and decision-making
Encourage families to take breaks from the bedside, as well as to sleep and eat
Provide open visiting
Be consistent in communication with the patient and family members
Encourage family input into decisions regarding withdrawal of support
Allow the family access to the patient to hold or be close to their loved one as appropriate, promote private time with the patient, and religious service or rituals as requested

Conclusion

Nursing care for patients receiving ECMO continues to be an emerging art and science. As health care technologies advance, nurses are obligated to seek education and develop skills to provide safe and therapeutic care. The foundation of the nurse-patient and nurse-family relationship includes provision of comfort and hope. It remains one of the most rewarding tasks of the nurse to pursue the knowledge of how to assist the unique needs of families in crisis.

References

1. Anthony ML, Hardee E. Extracorporeal membrane oxygenation: saving tiny lives. *Crit Care Nurs Clin North Am* 2000; 12:211-217.

2. Estrada EA. ECMO for neonatal and pediatric patients: state-of-the-art and future trends. *Pediatr Nurs* 1992; 18:67-74.

3. Noerr B. ECMO and pharmacotherapy. *Neonatal Netw* 1996; 15:23-31.

4. Suddaby EC, O'Brien AM. ECMO for cardiac support in children. *Heart Lung* 1993; 22:401-407.

5. Tulenko DR. An update on ECMO. *Neonatal Netw* 2004; 23:11-18.

6. Caron EA, Hamblet Berlandi JL. Extracorporeal membrane oxygenation. *Nurs Clin North Am* 1997; 32:125-140.

7. Krause KD, Youngner VJ. Nursing diagnoses as guidelines to care in the neonatal ECMO patient. *J Obstet Gynecol Neonatal Nurs* 1992; 21:169-176.

8. The American Heritage Dictionary of the English Language, 4th ed. Boston, MA: Houghton Mifflin Company; 2000.

9. Ford K, Turner D. Stories seldom told: pediatric nurses' experiences of caring for hospitalized children with special needs and their families. *J Adv Nurs* 2001; 33:288-295.

10. Freire AX, Afessa B, Cawley P, Phelps S, Bridges L. Characteristics associated with analgesia ordering in the intensive care unit and relationships with outcome. *Crit Care Med* 2002; 30:2468-2472.

11. Herr K, Titler MG, Schilling ML. Evidenced-based assessment of acute pain in older adults: current nursing practices and perceived barriers. *Clin J Pain* 2004; 20:331-340.

12. Bird J. Selection of pain measurement tools. *Nurs Stand* 2003; 18:33-39.

13. Chuk PKC. Vital signs and nurses' choices of titrated dosages of intravenous morphine for relieving pain following cardiac surgery. *J Adv Nurs* 1999; 30:858-865.

14. Gelling L. The role of hope for relatives of critically ill patients: a review of the literature. *Nurs Stand* 1999; 14:33-38.

15. Callery P. Caring for parents of hospitalized children: a hidden area of nursing work. *J Adv Nurs* 1997; 26:992-998.

16. Tak YR, McCubbin M. Family stress, perceived social support and coping following the diagnosis of a child's congenital heart disease. *J Adv Nurs* 2002; 39:190-198.

17. Bereavement support following sudden and unexpected death: guidelines for care. *Arch Dis Child Fetal Neonatal Ed* 2002; 87:36-39.

18. ELSO Registry. Ann Arbor, MI: Extracorporeal Life Support Organization; 2004.

19. Voepel-Lewis T, Merkel S, Tait AR, Trzcinka A, Malviya S. The reliability and validity of the face, legs, activity, cry, consolability observational tool as a measure of pain in children with cognitive impairment. *Anesth Analg* 2002; 95:1224-1229.

20. Munro CL, Grap MJ. Oral health in the intensive care unit: state of the science. *Am J Crit Care* 2004; 13:25-33.

21. Guerin C, Gaillard S, Lemasson S. Effects of systematic prone positioning in hypoxemic acute respiratory failure: a randomized

controlled trial. *JAMA* 2004; 292:2379-2387.

22. Haefner SM, Bratton SL, Annich GM, Bartlett RH, Custer JR. Complications of intermittent prone positioning in pediatric patients receiving extracorporeal membrane oxygenation for respiratory failure. *Chest* 2003; 123:1334-1336.

23. Goettler CE, Pryor JP, Hoey BA, Phillips JK, Balas MC, Shapiro MB. Prone positioning does not affect cannula function during extracorporeal membrane oxygenation or continuous renal replacement therapy. *Crit Care* 2002; 6:452-455.

24. Marik PE, Zaloga GP. Gastric versus post-pyloric feeding: a systematic review. *Crit Care* 2003; 7:46-51.

25. Pettignano R, Heard M, Davis R, Labuz M, Hart M. Total enteral nutrition versus total parenteral nutrition during pediatric extracorporeal membrane oxygenation. *Crit Care Med* 1998; 26:358-363.

26. Tabutt S, Duncan BW, McLaughlin D, Wessel DL, Jonas RA, Laussen PC. Delayed sternal closure after cardiac operations in a pediatric population. *J Cardiovasc Surg* 1997; 114:874.

27. Clark M. Repositioning to prevent pressure sores – what is the evidence? *Nurs Stand* 1998; 13:58-64.

28. Phillips L. Pressure ulcers – prevention and treatment guidelines. *Nurs Stand* 1999; 14:56-62.

29. Hadaway L. Skin flora and infection. *J Infus Nurs* 2003; 26:44-48.

30. Thompson BT, Cox PN, Antonelli M. Challenges in end-of-life care in the ICU: statement of the 5th international congress in critical care: Brussels, Belgium, April 2003: executive summary. *Crit Care Med* 2004; 32:1781-1784.

31. Curley MA, Meyer EC. Parental experience of highly technical therapy: survivors and nonsurvivors of extracorporeal membrane oxygenation support. *Pediatr Crit Care Med* 2003; 4:214-219.

32. Jezuit D. Personalization as it relates to nurse suffering: how managers can recognize the phenomenon and assist suffering nurses. *JONAS Healthc Law Ethics Regul* 2003; 5:25-28.

42

New Uses of ECLS

Michael H. Hines, M.D., F.A.C.S.

Introduction

In the years since 1976, when the first patient was successfully supported and removed from ECMO, thousands, particularly infants and children, have benefited from this technology. The ECMO community has taken what it learned from these children and has applied ECMO successfully to adults, particularly those with acute respiratory failure and ARDS. Nevertheless, more recent successes with the use of surfactant, inhaled nitric oxide (iNO), jet ventilation, and high frequency oscillatory ventilation (HFOV) have led to a decline in the need for neonatal ECMO, and some smaller centers have closed their ECMO programs. Several larger institutions have begun to look for other uses for the technology. ECMO professionals and those in even unrelated specialties are attempting to solve a new set of challenges with ECLS technology. Most of the concepts described here are "works in progress" and have not yet been published. These are representative of cutting-edge work going on in extracorporeal support which may, in turn stimulate other new ideas to be investigate and tested.

One excellent example of the benefit of applying one specialty's technology to another specialty's problem is the use of extracorporeal warming in trauma patients with hypothermia-induced coagulopathy. Trauma surgeons have been frustrated with their inability to help hypothermic patients who may bleed to death despite using all conventional therapies. Informal discussions with these surgeons have led to new ideas about how to warm these patients more efficiently. It was believed that ECLS was contraindicated in patients with active bleeding because of the presumed need for anticoagulation. To meet this challenge, new procedures have been developed to warm the blood while not using heparin, leading to the extracorporeal warming protocol described below. Other techniques discussed in this chapter have been developed in similar fashion by applying extracorporeal approaches used for respiratory failure to new problems.

Extracorporeal warming

Over the last decade, much has been learned about the evaluation and treatment of trauma patients, including rapid evaluation with spiral CT scanning, the physiology of resuscitation in the acutely injured patient, and ventilator management of ARDS. The importance of maintaining temperature during the resuscitation phase has also been recognized, and several techniques to prevent and reverse hypothermia have been developed, primarily to avoid its impact on coagulation. However, it remains a challenge to treat patients with severe injuries associated with significant blood loss and hemorrhagic shock. Maintaining adequate blood volume for oxygen delivery in the face of hypothermic coagulopathy. Frequently, the efforts to raise and/or maintain blood temperature in an attempt to correct coagulopathy is offset by continued blood and heat loss from exposure and infusion of cool blood products, despite level I trauma warmers and similar devices. In addition to warming the transfused blood and fluids, techniques such as surface warming and warm intra-peritoneal irrigation have been attempted. However, there remain a small number of patients who seem to have irreversible hypothermia and subsequent coagulopathy despite all efforts. Survival in this group is low.[1] While full cardiopulmonary bypass (CPB) has been used to treat profound hypothermia and exposure, it has generally been avoided in trauma patients with hypothermic coagulopathy because of the requirement for anticoagulation with heparin.

In order to solve this problem, the group at Wake Forest University School of Medicine Winston-Salem, NC, designed a simple circuit that used the very efficient heat exchanger for routine CPB, but without an oxygenator or reservoir, thus removing the need for heparin or other anticoagulation. The circuit contains a small centrifugal pump, is fairly portable, and has been used in the OR, ICU, ER, and for special procedures in radiology. Although only a small number of patients have been treated, the early results are encouraging with several patients surviving to discharge. In principle, resuscitation is altered during the re-warming period as fluid resuscitation is continued, but only crystalloid and packed red blood cells are utilized. It is useless to continue to transfuse other blood products in patients with severe hypothermia. Even the coldest patients can usually be warmed to normothermia (36°C) within ~30 minutes or less. Once raised to this temperature, platelets, cryoprecipitate, and clotting factors in the form of fresh frozen plasma or reconstituted factor complexes are administered. If dramatic improvement in bleeding is not observed, an additional search for surgical bleeding is conducted. Once additional experience is obtained and data collected, the appropriateness and potential applications for this technique can be better determined.

Extracorporeal hyperthermia

In the late 1980s, surgical oncologists began treating patients for peritoneal metastases with intraperitoneal hyperthermia and chemotherapy after debulking of the tumor and reduction of the tumor load. The groups at the University of Texas Medical Branch in Galveston and Louisiana State University at Shreveport investigated the potential uses of systemic hyperthermia in patients with advanced stage lung cancer using a venovenous (VV) ECMO circuit and a modified heat exchanger to achieve temporary blood temperatures in the range of 105°F for several hours. Preliminary results are encouraging and suggest prolonged survival may be achieved with this technique, but much work needs to be done to determine the optimum temperature, length of treatment, impact on survival and morbidity, and safety. The high temperatures cause severe vasodilatation and hypotension and require not only general anesthesia but also intensive monitoring and inotropic support of blood pressure. If preliminary results are a predictor of future results for larger studies, this technique may have a significant impact on a disease with high mortality despite current therapies. Perhaps the technique may be effective on other serious and challenging malignancies such as those seen in gastric, pancreatic, and ovarian cancer.

Elective ECMO support as an alternative to cardiopulmonary bypass

CPB is used in several circumstances in the OR as a method of assisting circulation and oxygenation during a procedure that does not require full cardiopulmonary support. The elective use of VV ECMO techniques has the advantage of simplicity, lower levels of anticoagulation, and the possibility of pre- or post-operative extracorporeal support. Elective support can be used during placement of aortopulmonary shunts in patients with congenital heart disease who cannot tolerate partial occlusion of the great vessels, but who do not require full CPB. Elective extracorporeal support has also been reported during and, temporarily, after complex tracheal reconstructions in newborns with long-segment tracheal stenosis.[2] Planned VV support can also be used for therapeutic bronchoalveolar lavage for complicated pulmonary diseases such as alveolar proteinosis that are currently performed either in a hyperbaric chamber or with associated severe hypoxemia. Patients with morbid obesity present unique challenges to surgeons and anesthesiologists alike, and those with lung disease frequently do not tolerate single lung ventilation for procedures, particularly in the lateral decubitus position relying on the dependent lung for ventilation and gas exchange. Other patients, with and without obesity, that have unstable airways and require intubation for surgical procedures may be supported either urgently when the airway is lost or electively for complex high-risk cases of airway obstruction or compromise from external compression. The disadvantages of using ECMO instead of full CPB are primarily the lack of a reservoir with the ability to continue perfusion during impaired venous return (limiting its effectiveness if there is significant bleeding), the inability to completely empty the heart during support, and the inefficiency of the heating and cooling system when compared to the systems used in CPB. However, the advantages of the ECMO system as described above make it a very valuable addition to the armamentarium.

Extracorporeal interval support for organ retrieval

An examination of the shortcomings of medical science would point to the failure to conquer various forms of cancer, deficient treatments for neurological injury and degenerative disease, and inadequate management of many inherited disorders such as cystic fibrosis. These examples involve shortcomings in understanding and management of the disease processes. The science of transplantation, by contrast, is limited more by the lack of available resources than by incomplete understanding of technique or medical management. There are currently over 89,000 patients on waiting lists for organ transplants, including heart, lung, liver, kidney, pancreas, and intestine.[3] Of these patients, approximately 17-20 die each day not because medical science lacks a treatment, but because of a shortage of resources, namely organs. While research moves ahead on artificial organs such as the Abiocor total artificial heart (Abiomed, Danvers, MA) and in tissue engineering to grow new functioning organs, in the short term, we must try to address the shortage of organs. If every potential organ donor in the U.S. donated his or her organs, the organ shortage and waiting list problem might soon be solved. However, our current systems fall far short of capturing all available donors, due both to poor public education and to inefficiencies in the system itself. The Department of Health and Human Services is currently managing two separate national initiatives to improve the organ donation system. One target is the increased use of non-heart-beating donors (NHBDs) for the recovery of abdominal organs. This approach has been used in several centers around the country; and historically, donation after cardiac death was standard practice prior to changes in the laws that define death. However, the results of the technique were not comparable with traditional heart-beating and living-related donors.

At Wake Forest University and the University of Michigan, a technique has been developed for supporting the abdominal organs after withdrawal of support and the declaration of death, in preparation for harvesting solid organs for transplantation. Unlike traditional methods of infusing large amounts of cold saline solution into the donor after declaration of death, with rapid transport to the OR for harvesting organs, the new technology utilizes extracorporeal support to maintain solid organ perfusion and oxygenation in preparation for harvesting. The technique termed extracorporeal interval support for organ retrieval (EISOR) is also applicable to the brain-dead organ donor who has become unstable before preparations for harvesting are complete. A relatively simple, closed, portable ECMO or CPS circuit is used to support and transport the donors. Femoral cannulas are placed, usually prior to the withdrawal of ventilator support and after the patient is pronounced dead. After five minutes, perfusion of the abdominal organs is initiated. This allows the family to remain with the patient during withdrawal of support and remain until the patient has expired, unlike previous techniques in which care was withdrawn in the OR without family present. Failure of the patient to become asystolic within 1-2 hours of the withdrawal of care is currently a contraindication to harvesting the organs; the procedure is then aborted and the patient moved to a private environment where the family can be present. In order to prevent late resuscitation of the heart, two techniques have been employed. A balloon catheter can be inserted prior to initiation of bypass in the opposite femoral artery, positioned in the mid-thoracic aorta and inflated as the perfusion is initiated. Alternatively, a large dose of lidocaine can be added to the perfusate which will prevent resuscitation of the heart and also vasodilate the abdominal organ vasculature to improve perfusion and cooling of the solid organs. The donor is then transported to the OR and actively cooled to ~25°C. The transplant team then removes the organs just as with a heart-beating donor. The circuit is used to perfuse the abdominal organ block with the preferred solution directly through the femoral cannula, and the venous return is drained outside the circuit as the donor is exsanguinated and the organs harvested. The technique does not preclude harvesting other tissues such as the heart for valves.

Although the numbers remain small and the results unpublished, this procedure has resulted in several successful transplantations of not only kidney, but liver and pancreas as well. There have been very encouraging results that appear to be superior to using cold crystalloid infusions for NHBDs. The ultimate utility of this technique depends on accruing results, and work on designing techniques that will allow the transplantation of intestines and lungs continues.

Artificial placenta

One of the significant challenges in critical care is dealing with the premature lung. The premature infant enters the outside world with insufficient numbers of alveoli as well as surfactant deficiency, and gas exchange is frequently inadequate to support life without the assistance of some form of mechanical support (e.g., conventional mechanical ventilation, high frequency oscillatory ventilation, or jet ventilation). A paradox exists as damage is done to the premature lung parenchyma by the very mechanical ventilatory support designed to treat the lung failure. Many critically ill premature infants sustain long-standing pulmonary problems and a small percentage are afflicted with crippling chronic lung disease (CLD) and pulmonary hypertension. Research is underway to examine the possibility of supporting these newborn patients with some form of extracorporeal support. Significant challenges are size, risk of anticoagulation, and identification of cannulation sites. Conceptually, it would be advantageous to support gas exchange in these infants to allow gentle mechanical ventilation, allowing appropriate development without the iatrogenic injury and subsequent scarring that contributes to CLD.

Total artificial lung

The University of Michigan and The University of Texas at Galveston are continuing research toward development of the total artificial lung.[4] While animal studies demonstrate feasibility, many issues remain, including design of a leak-proof membrane that can sustain long-term exposure to blood. Current models lie external to the chest and have been used in animal models with some success. Much research is required in order to develop a lung capable of long-term function, and which can be totally implanted.

Predicting the future

While futuristic books, television shows, and movies have filled the sky with flying cars for decades, we seem no closer to having them than when we watched George Jetson on television as children. This is less a failure of technologic advancement than a failure of our ability to predict the progress of technology and the many unforeseen discoveries and ideas. In the 1950s and 1960s, the birth of the mainframe computer was marveled at by scientists fascinated with the speed of data manipulation and calculation, even while the device ran with vacuum tubes and magnetic reel-to-reel tapes. Some dreamed that computers would be used in everyday businesses and potentially even in the home, but few imagined that virtually every college student would carry today's laptop computer with them from class to class, with memory capabilities that far exceeded even the highest expectations of the early developers of the computer. Clearly, 50 years ago, the scientists' imaginations focused on the potential new uses of the available technology, yet failed to predict the invention and progress of the microchip and microprocessor. Similarly, here we have described several potential applications of existing technology and extensions of current technology with some modification, but the potential for new ideas and technologies to support is unlimited and just as unpredictable. With minds wide open, we look ahead to the next 50 years of development of new methods of supporting or even replacing various organ functions.

References

1. Jurkovich GJ, Greiser WB, Luterman A, Curreri PW. Hypothermia in trauma victims: an ominous predictor of survival. *J Trauma* 1987; 27:1019-1024.
2. Hines MH, Hansell DR. Elective extracorporeal support for complex tracheal reconstruction in neonates. *Ann Thorac Surg* 2003; 76:175-179.
3. United Network for Organ Sharing. Waiting list candidates for organ transplantation. Available at www.unos.org. Accessed August 2, 2005.
4. Zwischenberger JB. Future of artificial lungs. *ASAIO J* 2004; 50:xlix-xlli.

43

Future of ECLS

Robert H. Bartlett, M.D.

Introduction

In 1990, the National Institutes of Health (NIH) sponsored a workshop on the diffusion of high tech medicine from research to clinical practice using neonatal ECMO as the example.[1] The participants included health care planners, social scientists, biostatisticians, governmental representatives from the NIH and Food and Drug Administration (FDA), and a sizable group of neonatologists and intensivists. At the invitation of the conference coordinator Dr. Linda Wright, the fledgling Extracorporeal Life Support Organization (ELSO) presented the data which formed the basis for the discussion. The conclusion was that neonatal ECMO is a very good example of how complex technology should be developed, recorded, reported, taught, and integrated into clinical practice. Nonetheless, the short history of this technology, which was quite familiar to the researchers, was somewhat overwhelming to the conference participants. One prominent neonatologist was shocked at the pace of development and horrified at the specter of a dozen ECMO cases running simultaneously in a single hospital. Each new group of ECLS providers, currently adult intensivists, will include enthusiasts who are excited by the possibilities, and skeptics who are reluctant to embrace the new technology. If we follow the precedent of research, record-

ing, reporting, and teaching, the result will be steady progress.

In 1990, the future of ECLS was anticipated to include microporous oxygenators; safe, simple automatic pumps; non-thrombogenic surfaces to eliminate bleeding complications; advances in respiratory and cardiac care made possible by ECLS; new approaches to clinical trials; and developing and changing roles of the ECLS specialist and intensive care nurse.[2] Now, 15 years later, we can assess where the technology stands and what lies ahead.

Artificial organs

Membrane lungs

Microporous membrane lungs have the advantages of improved efficiency of gas transfer, lower perfusion pressure, workability of materials, and relatively low manufacturing costs. Almost all membrane lungs used for cardiac surgery are made of microporous materials, usually of hollow fiber configuration. However, they have not replaced the solid silicone rubber Kolobow spiral coil membrane lung for prolonged support. The reason is that, after a few hours, all currently available microporous membrane lungs leak plasma in an unpredictable fashion. When plasma leakage occurs, membrane lung function deteriorates, requiring device replacement. Although a single microporous lung may function well for 5-6 days, the average time to failure is about 2 days, and the problems and expense of frequent and unpredictable membrane lung changes limit their use. Plasma leakage occurs when blood phospholipids are adsorbed onto the surfaces, leading to wetability of the microporous channels and eventually plasma break-through.[3] This problem can be solved in two ways: by coating or including a thin, gas-permeable membrane onto the microporous material, or by making the size of the air spaces on the blood contact surface much smaller. For many reasons, the best design for membrane lungs is blood-outside hollow fiber devices, which is fortunate because it is easier to coat or modify the outside of the small tubes rather than the inside. The development of Mortenson's temporary implantable membrane lung, IVOX (CardioPulmonics, Inc., Salt Lake City, UT) has been a stunning research success.[4] Hundreds of long prosthetic fibers filling the entire vena cava and right atrium are able to remain thrombus-free and functional for weeks. Mortenson's persistence with animal trials and Phase I clinical trials proves not only that non-thrombogenicity is possible, but that the totally implantable prosthetic lung will eventually be a reality. Although the initial trials with the IVOX identified problems with gas exchange capacity and with technical difficulties in placement, these are problems that can be solved. The IVOX clinical investigators had no experience with ECLS, and once given a taste of partial mechanical gas exchange support, were frustrated by the lack of total support capability provided by IVOX. ECLS users, in turn, have been given a taste of the utter simplicity of an implantable device. Everyone has learned more about thrombogenicity. The IVOX and similar devices are still awaiting commercial development. Although there will always be a need for extracorporeal mechanical support, the use of temporary implantable devices for respiratory failure is an attractive possibility.

Extracorporeal circulation can be used to selectively remove all the metabolically produced CO_2, relying on the native lung to supply oxygenation. This concept was originally developed by Gattinoni and Kolobow in the early 1980s and was demonstrated by Gattinoni to be effective in the treatment of severe acute respiratory distress syndrome (ARDS).[5] This technique utilized low flow venovenous (VV) blood flow with an extracorporeal oxygenator and high gas flow to the oxygenator, resulting in total CO_2 removal and a moderate amount of oxygenation. The remainder of the oxygenation was provided by the native lung via static inflation. After Gattinoni's report, this technique was tested by Morris in a small, randomized, controlled trial in which only 40% of patients survived in both the treatment and control groups.[6] Although Morris was assisted by a member of Gattinoni's group, the research team did not have extensive experience with the technique before embarking on the trial. The technique of utilizing CO_2 removal to augment ventilation was emphasized by variations of the Mortenson IVOX by Zwischenberger and others.[7-11] Zwischenberger has also studied the use of a small arterial venous (AV) shunt perfusing a microporous membrane lung. Only 10% of the cardiac output is needed to remove all of the metabolically produced CO_2. Clinical trials of this technique are currently underway in the U.S. and in Europe. The Novalung membrane oxygenator (Novalung GmbH, Hechingen, Germany) is configured with simple connections for AV access to be used for CO_2 removal.

Blood pumps

The servo-regulated roller pump remains the workhorse of prolonged extracorporeal circulation but will be replaced by simpler, safer pumps in the near future. It will be replaced by electronic servo-regulated centrifugal pumps, mechanically servo-regulated peristaltic pumps, or mechanically servo-regulated ventricle pumps. All the new pumps will provide the highest levels of safety without requiring continuous attendance. To achieve this goal, a pump must be able to tolerate sudden inlet occlusion without creating excess suction or hemolysis, sudden outflow occlusion without rupture or hemolysis, and flow regulation based on available venous drainage and/or various physiologic monitors. Even today, half the pumps used for cardiac surgery are centrifugal pumps because the operators favor safe, inadvertent arterial line occlusion without rupture over the expense and the need for an on-line flowmeter. The problem of hemolysis caused by inlet suction is not an issue during cardiac surgery because the pump is attached to a large blood reservoir with centrifugal pumps. The pump can suck air if the reservoir runs dry, but it cannot generate excess suction because the source of venous blood is never occluded. When centrifugal pumps are used for ECLS without a venous reservoir, occasional cessation of venous inflow results in the generation of very high negative pressure, cavitation, and hemolysis. This makes centrifugal pumps unsuitable for ECLS. A Norwegian research team has incorporated a simple negative pressure sensor into a BioMedicus (Medtronic, Eden Prairie, MN) centrifugal pump.[12] The pressure sensor servo-regulates the pump speed to eliminate negative pressure preventing hemolysis. When this system becomes commercially available, it will have major advantages over the roller pump system for ECLS.

Another approach to safe, simple, pumps is the passively-filling peristaltic pump in which a large flaccid pump chamber is stretched over rollers without a back plate to pump against. This concept was developed by the Rhone Poulenc Company 30 years ago and was used for many years as the pump of choice for cardiac surgery and ECLS in France.[13] Rhone Poulenc is no longer in the perfusion business, but now there are at least two other companies with passively-filling peristaltic pumps in development,

and soon will be commercially available.[14,15] The passively-filling peristaltic pump has all of the safety advantages of the centrifugal pump and all the practical advantages (cost, low thrombogenicity, durability) of the roller pump.

Vascular access

As we predicted 10 years ago, VV access for respiratory failure is better than venoarterial (VA) access.[16] The reasons for this are that VV maintains normal pulmonary blood flow, which may enhance lung healing and decrease the risk of microthrombosis; it avoids systemic arterial emboli; it maintains normal cardiac-dependent hemodynamics throughout the course of ECLS; it provides easier vascular access without the risk of arterial access; and it offers relatively greater safety than VA bypass, allowing simplification of management. Improvements to the system should address all of these aspects of VV bypass. Currently, VV bypass is typically carried out with 2 separate large venous access catheters, but in the future, almost all ECLS for respiratory support will be carried out in the VV mode using a single catheter with 2 lumens or single lumen tidal flow systems. In recent years, percutaneous access has become the standard approach in nearly all patients >2 years of age. The use of the Seldinger wire guided technique with sequential dilators and the placement of very large catheters directly has become standard practice worldwide. This has had a remarkable effect on decreasing the incidence of bleeding from cannulation sites.[17] In addition, cannulation can be accomplished quickly and easily under a variety of circumstances, facilitating on-ECMO transport and emergency access. Eventually single catheter VV access will become the standard approach, using either the tidal flow system or double lumen catheter system now widely practiced in neonates. Development of the tidal flow system awaits widespread availability of the French assistance respiratoire extra corporelle (AREC) system, which in turn depends on manufacturers to produce the alternating suction infusion system so successfully used in Paris.[18,19]

Thrombogenicity and anticoagulation

Although our laboratory studies indicated that long-term maintenance of ECLS without bleeding, clotting, and heparin should be possible, the availability of heparin-bonded circuits has not resulted in major changes in the management of ECLS. Systemic heparinization is still required, primarily because if ECLS must be interrupted for any reason stagnant blood in the circuit will clot very quickly. In addition, blood may clot around the outside of vascular access catheters and embolism can result. As expected, the thrombocytopenia and platelet dysfunction which accompanies ECLS has not been eliminated by the availability of heparin-bonded circuits. Nonetheless, the availability of heparin-bonded circuits has allowed the use of ECLS to be instituted in patients with major coagulopathies who are experiencing severe bleeding at the time ECLS is instituted. In the past, this type of coagulopathy and bleeding would have been considered a contraindication to ECLS. Now we have learned that we can go directly on bypass with a heparin-coated circuit in such a patient, control the coagulopathy, and maintain successful extracorporeal support while the bleeding stops. This advance makes it possible to use ECLS for patients who cannot come off conventional cardiopulmonary bypass (CPB) in the OR, patients with major trauma, active bleeding, and patients following major operations, such as thoracotomy for lung transplantation. In this type of patient, we have commonly used heparinized circuits for ECLS with no additional heparin, adding low-dose heparin when the coagulation system has returned to normal and the bleeding has stopped.

Many membrane lungs currently available for cardiac surgery and some of the lungs available in Europe for long-term support are coated with a non-thrombogenic coating. These coatings are preparatory, but all include heparin and some other materials. Heparin coating on the entire extracorporeal circuit has not eliminated the need for systemic heparinization. However, the amount of thrombosis and platelet consumption appears to be considerably improved with both the design of the circuit and the inclusion of non-thrombogenic coatings.

These observations, along with emergent life-threatening hemorrhage in ECLS patients, has led to the practice of decreasing or discontinuing heparin in ECLS patients who have ongoing major bleeding. From the experimental and clinical experience, we have learned that once the extracorporeal circuit has been exposed to blood for a short period of time, even a conventional plastic circuit without heparin bonding can be used for hours or days without clotting as long as high-flow ECLS is maintained. In the future, some combination of surface coating including heparin as well as a modification to minimize platelet adherence, combined with low level anticoagulation in the patient will be used to extend the use of ECLS to intraoperative management and routine management of patients with major coagulopathy and bleeding. This will dramatically change the indications, applications, and complications of extracorporeal support. Various aspects of the technique will have to be altered to allow continuous high flow, eliminating stagnant areas of flow through the elimination of bridges or Luer locks, and maintenance of flow around catheters and access, vessels. Hines and colleagues at Bowman Gray Medical Center have used ECLS for cooling and warming during exsanguinating hemorrhage following trauma. In this circumstance, the patient is allowed to become profoundly anemic through serial dilution and cooled down to a low temperature during repair of the injuries. When major bleeding has been controlled, blood is transfused and the patient is returned to normothermia to facilitate the function of platelets and the fibrin-forming enzymes. This approach is similar to the use of deep hypothermia during cardiac arrest for cardiovascular and neurosurgical operations. It has great promise as a life-saving measure in severe exsanguinating hemorrhage.

The most promising prosthetic surface currently under research is the use of polymers which gradually elute nitric oxide (NO) at the blood surface. NO temporarily inhibits platelet adhesion only for those platelets close to the surface; this mechanism of non-thrombogenicity for normal endothelium can be extended to prosthetic surfaces.[20-22]

Clinical practice of ECLS

It is interesting to see how the clinical supervision of ECLS is developing. Five years ago, it was thought to be likely there would be a dozen patients on ECLS simultaneously in any major medical center, including premature infants, adult ventilator patients, and patients in cardiogenic and hemorrhagic shock. Although ECLS application has not preceded quite that rapidly, in 2005 at the University of Michigan it is common to have 5 patients on ECLS on any given day. Common sense would dictate that one professional team should manage this system in conjunction with intensive care nursing. This team may be composed of a distinct new paramedical profession of ECLS specialists, or the responsibility might ultimately be taken on by subspecialties such as perfusion, respiratory therapy, or nursing. The labor requirements will be similar to the current needs in major ECLS centers, but most of the hour-to-hour management of ECLS will become integrated into specialized ICU nursing. The ECLS specialists will be responsible for cannulation, decannulation, emergency management, circuit priming, general supervision, and preventive maintenance to the patients on extracorporeal support.

ECLS has become routine practice in the last several years because of the standardized system and approach, and because of the development of a new group of health care professionals, the ECLS specialist. The need for ECLS specialists arose because the current systems require continuous attendance for monitoring and management, coagulation control, and management of emergencies. Currently, specialists may be trained in medicine, nursing, respiratory therapy, or perfusion. Extensive didactic, laboratory, and bedside experience are required, because individuals from these various professions do not have the necessary education and training in ECLS management. The ECLS specialist team is essential for making the technique work, and it is also the most expensive component of ECLS. During the next decade, the role of the ECLS specialist will change from continuous bedside supervision to simultaneous supervision of several ECLS patients, generally on an on-call basis. Increased cost efficiency will result when a single nurse/specialist can manage the patient, ventilator, and ECLS simultaneously. However, this will not be possible until the safety features discussed earlier are incorporated into the circuits and intensive care nurses are educated in the details of prolonged extracorporeal circulation.

With improved circuit safety, single vein access, and minimal anticoagulation, indications for ECLS will change from moribund patients to patients with moderately severe respiratory and cardiac failure. ECLS will become an adjunct to conventional ventilation and pharmacologic management rather than something to reserve until standard ventilation and pharmacology has failed. ECLS will be used in patients who are difficult to wean from mechanical ventilation. With improvements in technique and simplification of ECLS, the indications for ECLS will be greatly expanded. Concomitantly, however, other simpler methods of treatment for acute pulmonary and cardiac failure will significantly decrease the need for ECLS. The availability of ECLS has made it possible to study innovative methods of lung management such as inhaled nitric oxide (iNO) and perfluorocarbon liquid ventilation. It is important to remember that our ultimate goal is the safe, successful treatment of patients with severe cardiac and pulmonary failure. When that can be accomplished without the need for complex ECLS, the cycle of laboratory and clinical research on ECLS technology will be complete. We will be ultimately successful when there is no need for this technology, but that time appears to be decades away.

Low flow VV or AV perfusion or intracaval gas exchange may be used to facilitate extubation and allow ambulation, eating, and other activities which are often precluded by intubation and mechanical ventilation. With the improvements in the system outlined above, ECLS will be applied earlier in respiratory and cardiac failure. It will be routinely used for premature infants, trauma patients, older children, and adults with respiratory failure from a variety of causes. ECLS will be used in conjunction with lung transplantation in two ways, to support lung transplantation through acute edema or a rejection crisis, and as a bridge to lung transplantation for children and adults with acute irreversible disease. As currently practiced, ECLS is not appropriate as a bridge to lung transplantation in most circumstances. Good quality donor lungs are rare and are most appropriately used for patients who are not on mechanical ventilators or, in fact, are not hospitalized. To consider lung transplantation in acute lung disease during extracorporeal support will require the development of an implantable or paracorporeal respiratory support system that allows patients to be extubated, discharged from the ICU, stabilized, and kept healthy while awaiting lung transplantation, analogous to patients currently using long-term left ventricular assist devices (LVADs).

ECLS will gain wider application as temporary mechanical support of the circulation in children and adults with cardiac failure. McGovern et al. recently reported that VA ECLS was more effective than balloon pumping or LVADs for support of post-cardiotomy patients with cardiogenic shock.[23] For the reasons outlined above, ECLS will rarely be used as a bridge to cardiac transplantation until the donor supply is increased and the application of mechanical support is simplified.

New applications of ECLS will include ER and cardiac catheterization lab resuscitation in cardiac failure, resuscitation in trauma and hemorrhagic shock, and use as an adjunct to perfusion and temperature control in other types of critical illness. The use of VA extracorporeal support for emergency resuscitation has been reported in a variety of circumstances. More than 300 cases have been collected in a registry of emergency CPB by Hill.[24] Even at this early stage, the results are quite encouraging. Approximately two-thirds of the patients were successfully resuscitated with extracorporeal support, and half of those ultimately recovered. Successful outcome was usually associated with a correctable condition as a cause of the initial cardiac arrest.

The application of ECLS in the management of trauma and resuscitation from hemorrhagic shock will come with the non-thrombogenic system. Exsanguinating hemorrhage from a ruptured liver or duodenal ulcer, for example, may be managed by simultaneous transfusion and volume replacement with quick cannulation for ECLS. Rapid cooling with perfusion will allow total circulatory arrest or continuous cold perfusion at very low flows to permit identification and repair of bleeding vessels or organs, followed by rewarming on bypass.

The success of ECLS for heart and lung failure and the success of intermittent dialysis for acute renal failure have led to the study and early clinical trials of continuous hemofiltration for acute renal failure. Continuous hemofiltration has become standard care for the management of patients with multi-organ failure in the ICU. In this application, continuous hemofiltration has significant advantages over intermittent hemodialysis.[25] Fluid balance is a critical issue in patients with heart and lung failure, and it is common to include a hemofilter in the circuit of patients who are on ECLS for cardiopulmonary support. Blood processing for liver failure requires plasma separation and albumin processing because the toxic molecules in liver failure are all tightly bound to albumin, and hence, is not removed by dialysis or hemofiltration. Early experience with "albumin dialysis" has progressed from laboratory clinical trials and is very promising. Similarly, modules to treat sepsis and modules used for plasmapheresis are under development.

Other uses of ECMO

Many of the lessons learned in ECLS have already been applied to bypass for cardiac surgery such as servo-regulation, mixed venous saturation monitoring, membrane lungs, and standardized descriptors of vascular access catheters. Heparin-bonded, non-thrombogenic circuits will provide a major advance for cardiac operations and other procedures in which extracorporeal circulation with circulatory arrest or control of local blood flow is desirable. The techniques of cardiac surgery without systemic heparin need to be worked out in the laboratory. How to anticoagulate only the blood in the lungs and cardiac chambers and whether thrombosis will occur below an aortic cross clamp are questions that require investigation. With heparin bonded circuits, heparin can be discontinued once the heart is closed, eliminating the dilemma of continued oozing while weaning off bypass versus coming off prematurely to facilitate clotting. Non-thrombogenic surfaces will find major application for other types of artificial organs with blood contact, including dialysis, hemofiltration, and plasmapheresis. The technology of ECLS will be applied to normothermic organ perfusion and preservation.

ECLS has already led to a better understanding of pulmonary pathophysiology. One example is the identification of pulmonary hypertension as the underlying pathophysiology in virtually all cases of respiratory failure in term infants. ECMO studies led to the first identification of progressive irreversible fibrosis as the final common pathway in acute adult parenchymal lung disease.[26] The use of ECLS has drastically changed the management of congenital diaphragmatic hernia (CDH) from a rush to the OR to ICU management until the pulmonary hypertension has been resolved, with elective repair of the hernia days or even weeks after birth. The use of ECLS will permit the evaluation of innovative approaches to lung hypoplasia in the newborn such as chronic static inflation and/or the use of growth factors to stimulate lung growth. Earlier and more extensive use of ECLS will lead to the study of pharmacologic agents to reverse fibrosis and direct delivery of drugs such as antibiotics to treat interstitial disease.

The study of ECLS has brought proper emphasis to the separation of oxygenation from CO_2 removal and the realization that high peak airway pressure during attempted hyperventilation for CO_2 clearance is the major cause of ventilator-induced injury. With this realization, a return to pressure-limited mechanical ventilation has occurred, with ECLS as an adjunct when low pressure mechanical ventilation does not achieve adequate CO_2 clearance. The study of oxygen kinetics and the role of mixed venous saturation monitoring during ECLS has already found its ways into the routine management of intensive care patients. In the ICU, it is common practice to manipulate systemic oxygen delivery (DO_2) to optimize the DO_2 to oxygen consumption (VO_2) ratio. During ECLS it is easy to regulate VO_2 by regulating temperature, and this technique will also find its way into routine ICU management. The use of ECLS facilitates the evaluation of new methods of lung management, particularly nitric oxide inhalation in respiratory failure and perfluorocarbon ventilation in acute lung disease.

Two prospective, randomized trials of ECLS in newborn respiratory failure used adaptive statistical designs, bringing randomized clinical study design to the forefront of discussion.[27,28] This was particularly important because of the evaluation of ECLS as a life support technique. Ethical as well as statistical considerations guided the planning of these studies. Although initially criticized, both the conclusions and the methodology in these studies have stood the test of time, and the use of adaptive designs will simplify prospective, randomized studies in a variety of areas in the future. A third prospective, randomized trial of ECLS in neonatal respiratory failure was conducted in the U.K., supported by the National Health Service.[29] The design of this study, conceived by Field and others, offers a fascinating alternative to adaptive designs. In the U.K. study, all newborn infants with respiratory failure who meet entry criteria in 20 neonatal ICUs were entered into the study. All these patients were being treated with optimal conventional management which varied from center to center. Patients who randomized to ECMO must have parental consent, survive transport to 1 of 4 ECMO centers in the trial, and receive treatment in the ECMO center. Treatment in the 4 ECMO centers was standardized. Therefore, the study was a randomized comparison of neonatal respiratory care as generally practiced throughout the U.K. compared to a standardized approach including ECLS. The endpoint of the study was not only acute survival but 1-year follow-up. A study using this methodology can only be conducted when the management of all the patients can be dictated from a central source, such as the single payor system in the U.K.

The opposite approach was used by Morris et al.[6] in a prospective, randomized evaluation of ECLS for adult respiratory failure. The Morris group evaluated adult patients with acute respiratory failure in a single center over a 3-year period. The patients were randomized to continuing conventional therapy or extra-corporeal CO_2 removal ($ECCO_2R$) following the Gattinoni protocol. The respiratory aspects of both protocols were tightly controlled. They found ~40% survival in both groups, better than expected in conventional treatment and not as good as expected in the $ECCO_2R$ group. This study highlights many of the problems associated with single-center, prospective, randomized studies of a life support technique.

As these studies demonstrate, clinical experiments comparing ECLS to other treatment are difficult because blinding is impossible, therapy is not standardized and changes frequently, an extensive learning period is required before definitive study, and randomization may be refused by families and referring doctors. In the future, the best way to evaluate new methods in life support technology will probably be the approach used by Timmons and Green. A large number of pediatric ICU directors retrospectively collected data on all patients with respiratory failure treated in 1991.[30] Data from 470 patients were pooled into a common database. The database was then evaluated by multi-variate analysis to determine which factors were associated with death or survival. In this study, ECMO was the only treatment variable which was associated with improved survival. Green and others further analyzed the ECMO-treated patients in this database by a matched pairs analysis, which showed that survival was better in ECMO-treated patients compared to matched controls.[31] This approach to evaluation of life support techniques when applied in a prospective fashion has significant advantages over randomized studies and will emerge as the best method of analysis in the future.

Finally, the general success of ECLS in newborn infants has brought the economics and ethics of high tech intensive care to center stage. One author questioned whether the cost of ECMO was justified to save a newborn life.[32] He estimated the cost at $25,000; it is actually about $15,000. The question is certainly valid, although we commonly spend much more than that in the treatment of a single patient with AIDS, cancer, newborn asphyxia, prematurity, and other conditions which have less favorable outcomes. Length of hospitalization and hospital costs were actually found to be lower in neonatal ECLS patients compared to neonates on conventional ventilation.[33] Nonetheless, because ECLS is a highly visible, complex technology, these concerns will arise.

This outline of prospects for the future of ECLS seems at best presumptive and at worst preposterous. However, in 1970 there had been no successful cases, and it was widely held that prolonged extracorporeal support was impossible. By 1980, it had been demonstrated that successful ECLS was possible, but it was widely held that acute lung disease was irreversible in any patient sick enough to need it, and the technique, although possible, was impractical or unnecessary. In 2005 ECLS is standard treatment for some groups of patients. By now, experience has taught us to predict not the limitations but rather the possibilities.

References

1. Bartlett RH, Stolar C. Extracorporeal life support: State of the art. In: NIH Workshop on Neonatal ECMO; January, 1993. NIH Publication No. 93-3399.

2. Bartlett RH. Prospects for the Future. In: Arensman RM, Cornish JD, eds. *Extracorporeal Life Support*. Blackwell; 1993: 337-341.

3. Montoya JP, Shanley CJ, Merz SI, Bartlett RH. Plasma leakage through microporous membranes. Role of phospholipids. *ASAIO J* 1992; 38:M399-405.

4. Mortensen JD. An intravenacaval blood gas exchange (IVCBGE) device. A preliminary report. *ASAIO Trans* 1987; 33:570-573.

5. Gattinoni L, Pesenti A, Kolobow T, Damia G. A new look at therapy of the adult respiratory distress syndrome: motionless lungs. *Int Anesthesiol Clin* 1983; 21(2):97-117.

6. Morris AH, Wallace CJ, Menlove RL, et al. Randomized clinical trial of pressure-controlled inverse ratio ventilation and extracorporeal CO_2 removal for adult respiratory distress syndrome. *Am J Respir Crit Care Med* 1994; 149 (2 Pt 1):295-305.

7. Spears JR, Crilly RJ, Jiang AJ, et al. Stabilization of oxygen-supersaturated water during capillary injection into aqueous media. *Circulation* 1997; 96:4385-4391.

8. Zwischenberger JB, Cox CS, Graves D, Bidani A. Intravascular membrane oxygenation and carbon dioxide removal—a new application for permissive hypercapnia? *Thorac Cardiovasc Surg* 1992; 40:115-120.

9. Cox CS Jr, Zwischenberger JB, Graves DF, Niranjan SC, Bidani A. Intracorporeal CO_2 removal and permissive hypercapnia to reduce airway pressure in acute respiratory failure. The theoretical basis for permissive hypercapnia with IVOX. *ASAIO J* 1993; 39:97-102.

10. Zwischenberger JB, Alpard SK, Conrad SA, Johnigan RH, Bidani A. Arteriovenous carbon dioxide removal: development and impact on ventilator management and survival during severe respiratory failure. *Perfusion* 1999; 14:299-310.

11. Brunston RL Jr, Zwischenberger JB, Tao W, Cardenas VJ Jr, Traber DL, Bidani A. Total arteriovenous CO_2 removal: simplifying extracorporeal support for respiratory failure. *Ann Thorac Surg* 1997; 64:1599-1604.

12. Pedersen TH, Jensen O, Svennevig JL. The construction of a pressure servo-regulator to avoid deleterious negative pressure on the inlet side of the BioMedicus centrifugal pump during ECMO. Presented at: 3rd EESO meeting presentation; 1994; Leicester, U.K.

13. Butrille Y, Chevallet J, Granger A, et al. Rhone-Poulenc oxygenator and associated pumping system. In: Zapol WM, Quint M eds. *Artificial Lungs for Acute Respiratory*

Failure. New York, NY: Academic Press; 1976: 223.

14. Tamari Y, Lee-Sensiba K, Leonard EF, et al. The effects of pressure and flow on hemolysis caused by Bio-Medicus centrifugal pumps and roller pumps. Guidelines for choosing a blood pump. *J Thorac Cardiovasc Surg* 1993; 106:997-1007.

15. Montoya JP, Merz SI, Bartlett RH. Laboratory experience with a novel, non-occlusive, pressure-regulated peristaltic blood pump. *ASAIO J* 1992; 38:M406-411.

16. Delius R, Anderson HL, Schumacher R, et al. Venovenous compares favorably to venoarterial access for extracorporeal membrane oxygenation in neonatal respiratory failure. *J Thorac Cardiovasc Surg* 1993; 106:329-338.

17. Pesenti A, Gattinoni L, Bombino M. Long term extracorporeal respiratory support: 20 years progress. *Intensive and Critical Care Digest* 1993; 12:15-18.

18. Kolobow T, Borell M, Spatola R, Tsumo K, Prato P. Single catheter venovenous membrane lung bypass in the treatment of experimental ARDS. *Trans ASAIO* 1988; 34:35-38.

19. Durandy Y, Chevalier JY, Lecompte Y. Veno-venous extracorporeal lung support: Initial experience in paediatric patients, in neonatal and adult respiratory failure, mechanisms and treatment. In: Gille JP, ed. *Neonatal and Adult Respiratory Failure.* Paris, France: Editions Scientifiques Elsevier; 1989: 159-172.

20. Espadas-Torre C, Oklejas V, Mowery K, Meyerhoff ME. Thromboresistant chemical sensors using combined nitric oxide release/ion sensing polymeric films. *J Am Chem Soc* 1997; 119(9):2321-2322.

21. Annich GM, Meinhardt JP, Mowery KA, et al. Reduced platelet activation and thrombosis in extracorporeal circuits coated with nitric oxide release polymers. *Crit Care Med* 2000; 28(4):915-920.

22. Mellgren K, Friberg LG, Mellgren G, Hedner T, Wennmalm A, Wadenvik H. Nitric oxide in the oxygenator sweep gas reduces platelet activation during experimental perfusion. *Ann Thorac Surg* 1996; 61:1194-1198.

23. Mcgovern GJ. Extracorporeal life support following adult open heart surgery: The allegheny experience. In: Zwischenberger JB, Bartlett RH, eds. *ECMO: Extracorporeal Cardiopulmonary Support in Critical Care.* Ann Arbor, MI: Extracorporeal Life Support Organization; 1995: 473-490.

24. Hill JG. Adult emergency cardiopulmonary support systems. In: Zwischenberger JB, Bartlett RH, eds. *ECMO: Extracorporeal Cardiopulmonary Support in Critical Care.* Ann Arbor, MI: Extracorporeal Life Support Organization; 1995.

25. Bellomo R, Ronco C. Continuous versus intermittent renal replacement therapy in the intensive care unit. *Kidney Int* 1998; 66(suppl):S125-128.

26. Pratt PC, Vollmer RT, Shelburne JD, Crapo JD. Pulmonary morphology in a multihospital collaborative extracorporeal membrane oxygenation project. I. Light micropscopy. *Am J Pathol* 1979; 95:191-214.

27. Bartlett RH, Roloff DW, Cornell RG, Andrews AF, Dillon PW, Zwischenberger JB. Extracorporeal circulation in neonatal respiratory failure: a prospective randomized study. *Pediatrics* 1985; 76:479-487.

28. O'Rourke PP, Krone R, Vacanti J, et al. Extracorporeal membrane oxygenation and conventional medical therapy in neonates with persistent pulmonary hypertension of the newborn: a prospective randomized study. *Pediatrics* 1989; 84:957-963.

29. UK Collaborative ECMO Trial Group. The collaborative UK ECMO (Extracorporeal Membrane Oxygenation) trial: follow-up to 1 year of age. *Pediatrics* 1998; 101:E1.

30. Timmons OD, Havens PL, Fackler JC. Predicting death in pediatric patients with acute

respiratory failure. Pediatric Critical Care Study Group. Extracorporeal Life Support Organization. *Chest* 1995; 108:789-797.

31. Green TP, Moler FW, Goodman DM. Probability of survival after prolonged extracorporeal membrane oxygenation in pediatric patients with acute respiratory failure. Extracorporeal Life Support Organization. *Crit Care Med* 1995; 23:1132-1139.

32. Philips JB. Treatment of PPHN. In: Long WA, ed. *Fetal and Neonatal Cardiology*. Philadelphia, PA: Saunders; 1990: 691-701.

33. Schumacher RE, Roloff DW, Chapman R, Snedecor S, Bartlett RH. Extracorporeal membrane oxygenation in term newborns. A prospective cost-benefit analysis. *ASAIO J* 1993; 39:873-879.

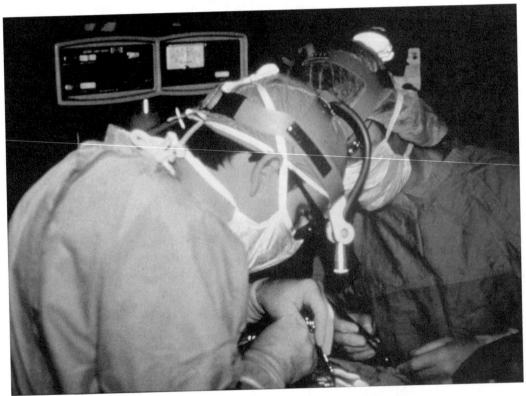
Dr. Bartlett in the operating room.